T0202343

OXFORD MEDICAL PUBLICATIONS

Oxford Handbook of Respiratory Medicine

Published and forthcoming Oxford Handbooks

Oxford Handbook for the Foundation Programme 5e

Oxford Handbook of Acute Medicine 4e

Oxford Handbook of Anaesthesia 4e

Oxford Handbook of Cardiology 2e

Oxford Handbook of Clinical and Healthcare Research

Oxford Handbook of Clinical and Laboratory Investigation 4e

Oxford Handbook of Clinical Dentistry 7e

Oxford Handbook of Clinical Diagnosis 3e

Oxford Handbook of Clinical Examination and Practical Skills 2e

Oxford Handbook of Clinical Haematology 4e

Oxford Handbook of Clinical Immunology and Allergy 4e

Oxford Handbook of Clinical Medicine – Mini Edition 10e

Oxford Handbook of Clinical Medicine 10e

Oxford Handbook of Clinical Pathology

Oxford Handbook of Clinical Pharmacy 3e

Oxford Handbook of Clinical Specialties 11e

Oxford Handbook of Clinical Surgery 4e

Oxford Handbook of Complementary Medicine

Oxford Handbook of Critical Care 3e

Oxford Handbook of Dental Patient Care

Oxford Handbook of Dialysis 4e

Oxford Handbook of Emergency Medicine 5e

Oxford Handbook of Endocrinology and Diabetes 3e

Oxford Handbook of ENT and Head and Neck Surgery 3e

Oxford Handbook of Epidemiology for Clinicians

Oxford Handbook of Expedition and Wilderness Medicine 2e

Oxford Handbook of Forensic Medicine

Oxford Handbook of Gastroenterology & Hepatology 2e

Oxford Handbook of General Practice 5e

Oxford Handbook of Genetics

Oxford Handbook of Genitourinary Medicine, HIV, and Sexual Health 3e

Oxford Handbook of Geriatric Medicine 3e

Oxford Handbook of Infectious Diseases and Microbiology 2e

Oxford Handbook of Integrated Dental Biosciences 2e

Oxford Handbook of Humanitarian Medicine

Oxford Handbook of Key Clinical Evidence 2e

Oxford Handbook of Medical Dermatology 2e

Oxford Handbook of Medical Imaging

Oxford Handbook of Medical Sciences 2e

Oxford Handbook for Medical School

Oxford Handbook of Medical Statistics

Oxford Handbook of Neonatology 2e

Oxford Handbook of Nephrology and Hypertension 2e

Oxford Handbook of Neurology 2e

Oxford Handbook of Nutrition and Dietetics 2e

Oxford Handbook of Obstetrics and Gynaecology 3e

Oxford Handbook of Occupational Health 2e

Oxford Handbook of Oncology 3e

Oxford Handbook of Operative Surgery 3e

Oxford Handbook of Ophthalmology 4e

Oxford Handbook of Oral and Maxillofacial Surgery 2e

Oxford Handbook of Orthopaedics and Trauma

Oxford Handbook of Paediatrics 2e

Oxford Handbook of Pain Management

Oxford Handbook of Palliative Care 3e

Oxford Handbook of Practical Drug Therapy 2e

Oxford Handbook of Pre-Hospital Care

Oxford Handbook of Psychiatry 4e

Oxford Handbook of Public Health Practice 3e

Oxford Handbook of Rehabilitation Medicine 3e

Oxford Handbook of Reproductive Medicine & Family Planning 2e

Oxford Handbook of Respiratory Medicine 3e

Oxford Handbook of Rheumatology 4e

Oxford Handbook of Sport and Exercise Medicine 2e

Handbook of Surgical Consent

Oxford Handbook of Tropical Medicine 4e

Oxford Handbook of Urology 4e

OXFORD HANDBOOK OF
Respiratory Medicine

Fourth edition

Stephen J. Chapman
Consultant in Respiratory Medicine,
Oxford University Hospitals NHS Foundation Trust, Oxford, UK

Grace V. Robinson
Consultant in Respiratory Medicine,
Royal Berkshire NHS Foundation Trust, Reading, UK

Rahul Shrimanker
Consultant in Respiratory Medicine, North Bristol NHS Trust,
Bristol, UK

Chris D. Turnbull
Clinical Lecturer in Respiratory Medicine, University of Oxford,
Oxford, UK

John M. Wrightson
Consultant in Respiratory Medicine,
Oxford University Hospitals NHS Foundation Trust, Oxford, UK

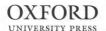

OXFORD
UNIVERSITY PRESS

OXFORD
UNIVERSITY PRESS

Great Clarendon Street, Oxford, OX2 6DP,
United Kingdom

Oxford University Press is a department of the University of Oxford.
It furthers the University's objective of excellence in research, scholarship,
and education by publishing worldwide. Oxford is a registered trade mark of
Oxford University Press in the UK and in certain other countries

© Oxford University Press 2021

The moral rights of the authors have been asserted

First Edition published in 2005
Second Edition published in 2009
Third Edition published in 2014
Fourth Edition published in 2021

Impression: 3

Published in the United States of America by Oxford University Press
198 Madison Avenue, New York, NY 10016, United States of America

British Library Cataloguing in Publication Data
Data available

Library of Congress Control Number: 2020952988

ISBN 978–0–19–883711–4

DOI: 10.1093/med/9780198837114.001.0001

Printed and bound in Italy by
L.E.G.O. S.p.A. Lavis (TN)

Foreword

It is a real privilege to write the forward to this invaluable book. Its continued success as the 'go to bible' for respiratory trainees, and indeed all respiratory practitioners, is a credit to the authors' considerable hard work ensuring the format remains practical and relevant.

The burden of respiratory disease continues to impact significantly on the health of our population. This burden and the needs of respiratory patients, so often under-represented in the past, have now (finally) been appreciated by government: reflected in national policy and the NHS Long Term Plan. A backdrop of exciting clinical trials is advancing treatment options, but also driving increasing sub-specialisation within respiratory medicine. This environment makes it challenging to both keep up to date and meet the aspirations set out to improve outcomes for our patients. The detailed review of all chapters in this new edition keeps the handbook abreast of these advances while ensuring the content is accessible to all respiratory practitioners, not exclusively those studying for the Specialty Certificate Examination.

This fourth edition sees a change in the authorship but, importantly, welcomes on-going input from specialty trainees. It is this balanced approach, alongside the continuity and experience provided from previous editions, which makes this an excellent, comprehensive and user-friendly guide to all aspects of respiratory medicine.

Dr John Park
Consultant Respiratory Physician
Chair, British Thoracic Society Education and Training Committee

Preface

Now in its fourth edition, the overall aim of the *Oxford Handbook of Respiratory Medicine* is to provide a rapid and comprehensive resource for all those involved in respiratory medicine. The layout of the book tries to fulfil the requirement to be able to look up a topic quickly when the clinical need arises, but also to provide further insight into the more difficult areas. We hope that anyone with an interest in respiratory medicine will find this text a rapid and useful reference.

Three of the five authors, Stephen Chapman, Grace Robinson, and John Wrightson, made initial contributions as registrars and now bring a consultant perspective; we welcome new contributions from Rahul Shrimanker and Chris Turnbull, both respiratory registrars at the time of writing.

We acknowledge the enormous contributions of John Stradling and Sophie West as co-authors of previous editions. Their influence, expertise (and idiosyncrasies!) remain evident throughout.

With this fourth edition, we have comprehensively reviewed and updated the entire content and include the latest clinical guidelines and significant research developments.

The handbook is divided into five sections: clinical presentations and approaches to symptoms and problems; the clinical conditions themselves; supportive information; procedures; and useful appendices, containing more technical and reference information.

We hope you find it helpful. Feedback on errors and omissions would be much appreciated. Please post your comments via the OUP website: ✍ http://www.oup.com/uk/medicine/handbooks.

September 2019

Acknowledgements

We offer our grateful thanks to the following friends and colleagues for their reviewing and advice on various sections of this book.

Fourth edition

Dr Rachel Benamore, Dr Stuart Benham, Dr Martin Carby, Mrs Julia De Soyza, Dr Noeleen Foley, Dr Rachel Hoyles, Dr Jeremy Hull, Dr Lennard Lee, Dr James Lordan, Dr Annabel Nickol, Prof Ian Pavord, Mr Mark Unstead, Dr Iara Sequeiros and Dr Diana Slim.

Previous editions

Dr Nicholas Bates, Dr Rachel Benamore, Dr Lesley Bennett, Dr Rachel Bennett, Dr Malcolm Benson, Dr Henry Bettinson, Dr Penny Bradbury, Mrs Debbie Buttar, Dr James Calvert, Mr Peter Close, Dr Jane Collier, Dr Graham Collins, Prof Chris Conlon, Dr Chris Davies, Dr Helen Davies, Prof Rob Davies, Dr Thearina de Beer, Mrs Julia De Soyza, Mrs Joan Douglass, Dr Prosenjit Dutta, Dr Rachael Evans, Dr Julia Fuller, Prof Fergus Gleeson, Dr Helmy Haja-Mydin, Dr Maxine Hardinge, Dr Bernard Higgins, Prof Ling-Pei Ho, Dr Luke Howard, Dr Rachel Hoyles, Ms Elaina Jamieson, Dr Andrew Jeffreys, Dr Clare Jeffries, Prof Nick Maskell, Dr Phil Mason, Dr Kim McAnaulty, Dr Fiona McCann, Dr Sarah Menzies, Dr Alastair Moore, Dr Stuart Mucklow, Dr Annabel Nickol, Dr Jayne Norcliffe, Dr Jeremy Parr, Mrs Lisa Priestley, Dr Ben Prudon, Prof Naj Rahman, Dr Catherine Richardson, Mrs Jo Riley, Dr Peter Sebire, Prof John Simpson Mrs Gerry Slade, Dr Mark Slade, Dr S Rolf Smith, Dr Andrew Stanton, Dr Catherine Swales, Dr Denis Talbot, Dr David Taylor, Dr Catherine Thomas, Dr Estée Török, Mrs Jan Turner-Wilson, Dr David Waine, Dr Ann Ward, Dr Chris Wathen, Dr John Wiggins, and Dr Eleanor Wood.

Contents

Symbols and abbreviations *xv*

Part I Clinical presentations—approaches to problems

1 Breathlessness | 3
2 Chest pain | 7
3 Chronic cough | 11
4 Critically ill patient with respiratory disease | 21
5 Diffuse alveolar haemorrhage | 27
6 Diffuse lung disease | 31
7 Haemoptysis | 43
8 Pleural effusion | 49
9 Post-operative breathlessness | 63
10 Pregnancy and breathlessness | 69
11 Preoperative assessment | 73
12 Pulmonary disease in the immunocompromised—non-HIV | 79
13 Pulmonary disease in the immunocompromised—HIV | 91
14 Sleep and breathing | 99
15 Unexplained respiratory failure | 105

Part II Clinical conditions

16 Acute respiratory distress syndrome | 115
17 Asbestos and the lung | 123
18 Asthma | 141
19 Bronchiectasis | 169
20 Bronchiolitis | 183

189	21	Chronic obstructive pulmonary disease (COPD)
213	22	Connective tissue disease and the lung
231	23	Cor pulmonale
237	24	Cystic fibrosis (CF)
261	25	Drug and toxin-induced lung disease
283	26	Dysfunctional breathing
289	27	Eosinophilic lung disease
297	28	Extreme environments—flying, altitude, diving
305	29	Gastrointestinal disease and the lung
311	30	Hypersensitivity pneumonitis
317	31	Idiopathic interstitial pneumonias
337	32	Lung cancer
381	33	Mediastinal abnormalities
393	34	Paediatric lung disorders
401	35	Pleural effusion
425	36	Pneumoconioses
435	37	Pneumothorax
449	38	Pulmonary hypertension (PHT)
467	39	Pulmonary thromboembolic disease
489	40	Rare lung diseases
517	41	Respiratory infection—bacterial
559	42	Respiratory infection—fungal
585	43	Respiratory infection—mycobacterial
623	44	Respiratory infection—parasitic
629	45	Respiratory infection—viral
655	46	Sarcoidosis
671	47	Sickle cell disease and the lung
677	48	Sleep apnoea and hypoventilation
703	49	Upper airway and tracheal disease
713	50	Vasculitis and the lung

PART III Supportive care

51 Ethical considerations 727
52 Financial entitlements 733
53 Immunosuppressive drugs 739
54 Inhalers and nebulizers 747
55 Intensive care unit (ICU) referral 755
56 Lung transplantation 759
57 Non-invasive ventilation (NIV) 771
58 Oxygen therapy 787
59 Palliative care 799
60 Pulmonary rehabilitation 811
61 Smoking cessation 817

PART IV Practical procedures

62 Airway management 827
63 Bronchoscopy 833
64 Chest drains 851
65 Cricothyroidotomy 861
66 Miscellaneous diagnostic tests 865
67 Pleural biopsy 869
68 Pleurodesis 875
69 Pneumothorax aspiration 881
70 Safe sedation 885
71 Thoracentesis 891
72 Thoracic ultrasound (TUS) 895
73 Thoracoscopy 907
74 Tracheostomy 913

Appendices

921	A1	Blood gases and acid–base balance
935	A2	BMI calculator
937	A3	CT anatomy of the thorax
945	A4	CT patterns of lung disease
957	A5	Drugs used for bronchoscopy and sedation
963	A6	Lung function and cardiopulmonary exercise testing
979	A7	Plain radiograph
983	A8	Radiological investigations and radiation exposure
987	A9	Useful websites

Index   989

Symbols and abbreviations

►►	don't dawdle
↓	decreased
↑	increased
→	leading to
♀	female
♂	male
1°	primary
2°	secondary
~	approximately
≈	approximately equal to
±	plus/minus
>	greater than
<	less than
≥	equal to or more than
°	degree
°C	degree Celsius
α	alpha
β	beta
γ	gamma
+ve	positive
£	pound sterling
®	registered trademark
6MWT	6-minute walk test
α1-AT	α1-antitrypsin
A–a	alveolar to arterial gradient
AAH	atypical adenomatous hyperplasia
A/α1AT	alpha-1 antitrypsin deficiency
Ab	antibody
ABC	airway, breathing, circulation
ABG	arterial blood gas
ABPA	allergic bronchopulmonary aspergillosis
ACCP	American College of Chest Physicians
ACE	angiotensin-converting enzyme
AChR	acetylcholine receptor
ACTH	adrenocorticotropic hormone
AD	autosomal dominant
ADH	antidiuretic hormone
A&E	accident and emergency
AF	atrial fibrillation
AFB	acid-fast bacillus
AFP	alpha-fetoprotein

AHI	apnoea hypopnoea index
AIA	aspirin-induced asthma
AIDS	acquired immune deficiency syndrome
AIP	acute interstitial pneumonia
AIS	adenocarcinoma in situ
AJCC	American Joint Committee on Cancer
ALK	anaplastic lymphoma kinase
ALP	alkaline phosphatase
ALT	alanine aminotransferase
AMS	acute mountain sickness
AMTS	abbreviated mental test score
ANA	antinuclear antibody
ANCA	antinuclear cytoplasmic antibody
ANP	atrial natriuretic peptide
AOT	ambulatory oxygen therapy
APAH	associated pulmonary arterial hypertension
APC	argon plasma coagulation
APDS	activated PI3 kinase delta syndrome
APTT	activated partial thromboplastin time
AR	autosomal recessive
ARDS	acute respiratory distress syndrome
ART	antiretroviral therapy
ASD	atrial septal defect
AST	aspartate aminotransferase
ASV	adaptive servo-ventilation
ATRA	all-trans retinoic acid
ATS	American Thoracic Society
AV	arteriovenous
AVM	arteriovenous malformation
βHCG	beta human chorionic gonadotrophin
BAC	bronchioloalveolar/ bronchoalveolar cell carcinoma
BAL	bronchoalveolar lavage
BCG	bacille Calmette–Guérin
bd	twice a day
BDP	beclomethasone dipropionate
BeLPT	beryllium lymphocyte proliferation test

BHD	Birt–Hogg–Dubé
BHR	bronchial hyperreactivity or hyperresponsiveness
BiPAP	bi-level positive airways pressure
bLVR	bronchoscopic lung volume reduction
BMI	body mass index (kg/m²)
BNF	British National Formulary
BNP	B-type/brain natriuretic peptide
BOOP	bronchiolitis obliterans organizing pneumonia
BOS	bronchiolitis obliterans syndrome
BP	blood pressure
BPD	bronchopulmonary dysplasia
bpm	beats per minute
BSAC	British Sub-Aqua Club
BSI	Bronchiectasis Severity Index
BTS	British Thoracic Society
CABG	coronary artery bypass graft
cAMP	cyclic adenosine monophosphate
CAP	community-acquired pneumonia
CBG	capillary blood gas
CCB	calcium channel blocker
CCF	congestive cardiac failure
CCPA	chronic cavitary pulmonary aspergillosis
CD	Castleman's disease
CEA	carcinoembryonic antigen
CF	cystic fibrosis
CFA	cryptogenic fibrosing alveolitis
CFT	complement fixation test
CFTR	cystic fibrosis transmembrane conductance regulator
cfu	colony-forming unit
Chr	chromosome
CI	contraindication
CK	creatine kinase
Cl⁻	chloride ion
CLD	chronic lung disease
CLL	chronic lymphocytic leukaemia
cm	centimetre
cmH₂O	centimetre of water
CMV	cytomegalovirus
CNS	central nervous system
CO	carbon monoxide
CO₂	carbon dioxide

COHb	carboxyhaemoglobin
COP	cryptogenic organizing pneumonia
COPD	chronic obstructive pulmonary disease
CPAP	continuous positive airway pressure
CPD	continuing professional development
CPET	cardiopulmonary exercise testing
CPK	creatine phosphokinase
CPPE	complicated parapneumonic effusion
CRP	C-reactive protein
CRTH2	prostaglandin-D2 receptor
CSA	central sleep apnoea
CSF	cerebrospinal fluid
CT	computed tomography
CTD	connective tissue disease
ctDNA	circulating tumour DNA
CTEPH	chronic thromboembolic pulmonary hypertension
CTGB	CT guided biopsy
CTPA	computed tomographic pulmonary angiogram
CVA	cerebrovascular accident
CVD	cardiovascular disease
CVID	common variable immune deficiency
CVP	central venous pressure
CXR	chest radiograph
2D	two-dimensional
3D	three-dimensional
d	day
DEXA	dual-energy X-ray absorptiometry
DFA	direct fluorescent antibody
DIC	disseminated intravascular coagulation
DIF	direct immunofluorescence test
DIOS	distal intestinal obstruction syndrome
DIP	desquamative interstitial pneumonitis
DIPNECH	diffuse idiopathic pulmonary neuroendocrine cell hyperplasia
dL	decilitre
DLCO	diffusing capacity for carbon monoxide
DM	dermatomyositis

DNA	deoxyribonucleic acid		EUS	endoscopic ultrasound
DOAC	direct oral anticoagulant		EUS-FNA	endoscopic ultrasound-fine needle aspiration
DOT	directly observed therapy (usually tuberculosis)		EVLP	ex vivo lung perfusion
DPI	dry powder inhaler		FBC	full blood count
DPT	diffuse pleural thickening		FDA	Food and Drug Administration
dsDNA	double-stranded DNA		FDG-PET	18-fluorodeoxyglucose positron emission tomography
DVLA	Driver and Vehicle Licensing Agency		FDS	faster diagnosis standard
DVT	deep vein thrombosis		feNO	fraction of nitric oxide
EBUS	endoscopic bronchial/endobronchial ultrasound		FEV_1	forced expiratory volume in 1s
			$FiCO_2$	fractional inspired carbon dioxide
EBV	Epstein–Barr virus		FiO_2	fractional inspired oxygen
ECG	electrocardiogram		FNA	fine needle aspirate
echo	echocardiogram		FOB	fibre optic bronchoscopy
ECMO	extra corporeal membrane oxygenation		FPAH	familial pulmonary arterial hypertension
ECOG	Eastern Cooperative Oncology Group		FRC	functional residual capacity
ED	emergency department		ft	foot
EDAC	excessive dynamic airways collapse		FVC	forced vital capacity
			γGT	gamma glutamyl transferase
EEG	electroencephalogram		g	gram
eGFR	estimated glomerular filtration rate		GABA	G-aminobutyric acid
EGFR	epidermal growth factor receptor		GBM	glomerular basement membrane
EGPA	eosinophilic granulomatosis with polyangiitis (Churg–Strauss syndrome)		GCS	Glasgow coma scale
			GCT	germ cell tumour
			GI	gastrointestinal
EIA	enzyme immunoassay		GMC	General Medical Council
ELC	emphysema-like change		GM-CSF	granulocyte-macrophage colony-stimulating factor
ELCAP	Early Lung Cancer Action Project		GORD	gastro-oesophageal reflux disease
ELISA	enzyme-linked immunosorbent assay		GP	general practitioner
EMG	electromyogram		GPA	granulomatosis with polyangiitis (Wegener's)
EMU	early morning urine			
ENA	extractable nuclear antigen		GVHD	graft-versus-host disease
ENT	ear, nose, and throat		Gy	gray
EOG	electro-oculogram		h	hour
EPAP	expiratory positive airways pressure		H^+	hydrogen ion
			H2	histamine receptors, type 2
EPD	extended pleurectomy with decortication		HAART	highly active antiretroviral therapy
EPP	extrapleural pneumonectomy		HACE	high altitude cerebral oedema
ERA	endothelin receptor antagonist		HADS	Hospital Anxiety and Depression score
ERS	European Respiratory Society			
ESR	erythrocyte sedimentation rate		HAPE	high altitude pulmonary oedema
ESS	Epworth sleepiness scale/score		Hb	haemoglobin

HCG	human chorionic gonadotrophin		in	inch
HCO_3^-	bicarbonate ion		INR	international normalized ratio
HDU	high dependency unit		IPAH	idiopathic pulmonary arterial hypertension
HFOV	high-frequency oscillatory ventilation		IPAP	inspiratory positive airways pressure
HFNO	high flow nasal oxygen		IPC	indwelling pleural catheter
HGV	heavy goods vehicle		IPF	idiopathic pulmonary fibrosis
HHT	hereditary haemorrhagic telangiectasia		IPPV	intermittent positive-pressure ventilation
HHV	human herpesvirus		IRIS	immune reconstitution inflammatory syndrome
HIV	human immunodeficiency virus			
HLA	human leucocyte antigen		ITMIG	International Thymic Malignancy Interest Group
HOCF	home oxygen consent form		ITU	intensive therapy unit
HOOF	home oxygen order form		IU	international units
HP	hypersensitivity pneumonitis		IV	intravenous
HPLC	high-performance liquid chromatography		IVAD	implantable venous access device
HPOA	hypertrophic pulmonary osteoarthropathy		IVC	inferior vena cava
			IVDU	intravenous drug user
HPS	hepatopulmonary syndrome		JVP	jugular venous pressure
HPV	human papillomavirus		K^+	potassium ion
HR	heart rate		kCO	carbon monoxide transfer factor coefficient
HRCT	high resolution computed tomography		kg	kilogram
HRT	hormone replacement therapy		kHz	kilohertz
HSCT	haematopoietic stem cell transplant		km	kilometre
			kPa	kilopascal
HSV	herpes simplex virus		L	litre
Hz	hertz		LABA	long-acting β_2 agonist
IASLC	International Association for the Study of Lung Cancer		LAM	lymphangioleiomyomatosis
IBD	inflammatory bowel disease		LAMA	long-acting muscarinic antagonist
ICS	inhaled corticosteroids		LCH	Langerhans cell histiocytosis
ICSI	intracytoplasmic sperm injection		LDCT	low-dose CT
ICU	intensive care unit		LDH	lactate dehydrogenase
IFN-γ	interferon gamma		LEMS	Lambert–Eaton myasthenic syndrome
IgE	immunoglobulin E			
IgG	immunoglobulin G		LFT	liver function test
IgM	immunoglobulin M		LIP	lymphoid interstitial pneumonia
IGRA	interferon gamma release assay			
			LMA	laryngeal mask airway
IIDB	industrial injuries disablement benefit		LMWH	low molecular weight heparin
			LOS	lower oesophageal sphincter
IIP	idiopathic interstitial pneumonia		LPA	lasting power of attorney
			LTOT	long-term oxygen therapy
IL	interleukin		LV	left ventricle/ventricular
ILD	interstitial lung disease		LVF	left ventricular failure
ILO	inducible laryngeal obstruction		LVRS	lung volume reduction surgery
IM	intramuscular			

m	metre		N	newton
MAC	*Mycobacterium avium* complex		Na⁺	sodium ion
MART	maintenance and reliever therapy		NaCl	sodium chloride
MC&S	microscopy, culture, and sensitivity		NCEPOD	National Confidential Enquiry into Patient Outcome and Death
MCV	mean corpuscular volume		nd-YAG	neodymium-doped yttrium aluminum garnet
MDI	metered dose inhaler			
MDR-TB	multidrug-resistant TB		NEWS2	revised National Early Warning Score
MDT	multidisciplinary team			
MEN	multiple endocrine neoplasia		ng	nanogram
meq	milliequivalent		NG	nasogastric
MERS	Middle East respiratory syndrome		NHS	National Health Service
			NICE	National Institute for Health and Care Excellence
MERS-CoV	Middle East respiratory syndrome coronavirus		NIMV	non-invasive mechanical ventilation
mg	milligram			
MGIT	mycobacterial growth indicator tube		NIPPV	non-invasive positive pressure ventilation
MGUS	monoclonal gammopathy of uncertain significance		NIV	non-invasive ventilation
			nmol	nanomole
MHRA	Medicines and Healthcare products Regulatory Agency		NNRTI	non-nucleoside reverse transcription inhibitor
MHz	megahertz		NO	nitric oxide
MI	myocardial infarction		NO₂	nitrogen dioxide
MIA	minimally invasive adenocarcinoma		non-REM	non-rapid eye movement sleep
			NOT	nocturnal oxygen therapy
min	minute		NPSA	National Patient Safety Agency
MIP	maximum intensity projection		NRT	nicotine replacement therapy
mL	millilitre		NSAID	non-steroidal anti-inflammatory drug
MMF	mycophenolate mofetil			
mmHg	millimetre of mercury		NSCLC	non-small cell lung cancer
mmol	millimole		NSIP	non-specific interstitial pneumonia
MND	motor neurone disease			
mosmol	milliosmole		NTM	non-tuberculous mycobacteria
MPA	microscopic polyangiitis		NT-proBNP	N-terminal pro-B type natriuretic peptide
MPO	myeloperoxidase			
MRC	Medical Research Council		NYHA	New York Heart Association
MRI	magnetic resonance imaging		O₂	oxygen
mRNA	messenger ribonucleic acid		OCP	oral contraceptive pill
MRSA	methicillin (or multiple) resistant *Staphylococcus aureus*		OCS	oral corticosteroid
			od	once a day
ms	millisecond		ODI	Oxygen desaturation index
MSM	men who have sex with men		OGD	oesophagogastroduodenoscopy
mSv	millisievert			
MTB	*Mycobacterium tuberculosis*		OHS	obesity hypoventilation syndrome
mTOR	mammalian target of rapamycin			
MU	megaunit		OP	organizing pneumonia
MVV	maximum voluntary ventilation		OSA	obstructive sleep apnoea
MwA	microwave ablation		OSAH	obstructive sleep apnoea/hypopnoea

OSAS	obstructive sleep apnoea syndrome
p	probability
PA	posteroanterior
PaCO₂	arterial carbon dioxide tension
PAF	platelet-activating factor
PAH	pulmonary arterial hypertension
PAN	polyarteritis nodosa
PaO₂	arterial oxygen tension
PAP	pulmonary artery pressure
PAS	para-aminosalicylic acid
PAVM	pulmonary arteriovenous malformation
PAWP	pulmonary arterial wedge pressure
PC₂₀	provocative concentration (of histamine or methacholine) causing a 20% fall in FEV₁
PCD	primary ciliary dyskinesia
PCO₂	carbon dioxide tension
PCP	*Pneumocystis carinii* (now *jirovecii*) pneumonia
PCR	polymerase chain reaction
PD	pleurectomy with decortication
PD-1	programmed death protein-1
PDE	phosphodiesterase
PDE-5	phosphodiesterase type-5 inhibitor
PD-L1	programmed death ligand 1
PDT	photodynamic therapy
PE	pulmonary embolus
PEEP	positive end expiratory pressure
PEF	peak expiratory flow
PEFR	peak expiratory flow rate
PEG	percutaneous endoscopic gastrostomy
PERT	pulmonary embolism response team
PESI	pulmonary embolism severity index
PET	positron emission tomography
PFT	pulmonary function test
pGGN	pure ground glass nodule
PHT	pulmonary hypertension
Pi	protease inhibitor
PI3K	phosphoinositide 3-kinase
PM	polymyositis
PMF	progressive massive fibrosis
PO	orally/by mouth

PO₂	oxygen tension
PO₄⁻	phosphate ion
POPH	portopulmonary hypertension
PORT	post-operative radiotherapy
ppb	part per billion
PPH	primary pulmonary hypertension
PPI	proton pump inhibitor
PPO	predicted post-operative
PR	pulmonary rehabilitation
PR3	proteinase 3
PRF	pulse repetition frequency
prn	as required
PRRT	peptide receptor radiotargeted therapy
PS	performance status
PSA	prostate-specific antigen
PSB	protected specimen brush
PSG	polysomnography
PSI	Pneumonia Severity Index
PSN	part solid nodule
PT	prothrombin time
PTH	parathyroid hormone
PTLD	post-transplant lymphoproliferative disorders
PVL-SA	Panton-Valentine leukocidin-producing *Staphylococcus aureus*
PVR	pulmonary vascular resistance
QALY	quality-adjusted life year
qds	four times a day
QoL	quality of life
RA	rheumatoid arthritis
RAD	right axis deviation
RAST	radioallergosorbent test
RBBB	right bundle branch block
RB-ILD	respiratory bronchiolitis-associated interstitial lung disease
RCP	Royal College of Physicians
RCT	randomized controlled trial
REM	rapid eye movement
RER	respiratory exchange ratio
RF	rheumatoid factor
RFA	radiofrequency ablation
RHC	right heart catheterization
RhF	rheumatoid factor
RNA	ribonucleic acid
RNP	ribonuclear protein
ROS1	c-ROS oncogene 1

RQ	respiratory quotient		SVC	superior vena cava
RR	respiratory rate		SVCO	superior vena caval obstruction
RSV	respiratory syncytial virus		SWT	shuttle walk test
RT-PCR	reverse transcriptase polymerase chain reaction		T1RF	type 1 respiratory failure
RV	residual volume; right ventricle/ventricular		T2RF	type 2 respiratory failure
			TB	tuberculosis
RVH	right ventricular hypertrophy		TBB	transbronchial biopsy
s	second		TBM	tracheobronchomalacia
SABA	short-acting β-agonist		TBNA	transbronchial needle aspiration
SABR	stereotactic ablative radiotherapy		tds	three times a day
SACT	systemic anti-cancer therapy		TENS	transcutaneous electrical nerve stimulation
SaO₂	arterial oxygen saturation (usually a percentage)		TFT	thyroid function test
SAP	serum amyloid P		TGC	time gain compensation
SARS	severe acquired respiratory syndrome		TGF	transforming growth factor
			Th2	T helper 2 cell
SARS-CoV	SARS-coronavirus		TIA	transient ischaemic attack
SBE	subacute bacterial endocarditis		TIPS	transjugular intrahepatic portosystemic shunt
SBOT	short-burst oxygen therapy		TKI	tyrosine kinase inhibitor
SBP	systolic blood pressure		TLC	total lung capacity
SBRT	stereotactic body radiation therapy		TLCO	total lung carbon monoxide transfer factor
SC	subcutaneous		TMPT	thiopurine methyltransferase
SCIT	subcutaneous allergen immunotherapy		TNF	tumour necrosis factor
SCL-70	scleroderma antibody (to topoisomerase 1)		TNM	tumour, node, metastasis
			tPA	tissue plasminogen activator
SCLC	small cell lung cancer		TPMT	thiopurine methyltransferase
SCUBA	self-contained underwater breathing apparatus		TR	tricuspid regurgitation
			TRALI	transfusion-related acute lung injury
SD	standard deviation		TSC	tuberous sclerosis complex
SE	side effect		TSH	thyroid-stimulating hormone
SEMAS	self-expanding metal airway stent		TSLP	thymic stromal lymphopoietin
SF-36	Short Form-36		TTF	thyroid transcription factor
SGAD	supraglottic airway device		TTR	transthyretin
SIADH	syndrome of inappropriate secretion of ADH		TU	tuberculin unit
			TUS	thoracic ultrasound
SIGN	Scottish Intercollegiate Guidelines Network		U	unit
			UACS	upper airway cough syndrome
SLE	systemic lupus erythematosus		U&E	urea and electrolytes
SO₂	sulphur dioxide		UICC	Union for International Cancer Control
SO₄⁻	sulphate ion			
SOB	shortness of breath		UIP	usual interstitial pneumonia
spp.	species		UK	United Kingdom
SPPE	simple parapneumonic effusion		URTI	upper respiratory tract infection
SSA	somatostatin analogues			
SSN	sub-solid nodule		US	ultrasound
SUV	standardized uptake value			

USA	United States of America
USS	ultrasound scan
UTI	urinary tract infection
VAP	ventilator-associated pneumonia
VAPSP	volume-assured pressure support ventilation
VATS	video-assisted thoracoscopic surgery
VC	vital capacity
VCD	vocal cord dysfunction
VDT	volume doubling time
VEGF	vascular endothelial growth factor
VGCC	voltage-gated calcium channel

VKA	vitamin K antagonist
V/Q	ventilation-perfusion
vs	versus
VTE	venous thromboembolism
WCC	white cell count
WHO	World Health Organization
wk	week
XDR-TB	extensively drug-resistant tuberculosis
XLA	X-linked agammaglobulinaemia
y	year
ya	years ago
YAG	yttrium–aluminium–garnet
ZN	Ziehl–Neelsen

Part I

Clinical presentations— approaches to problems

1 Breathlessness *3*

2 Chest pain *7*

3 Chronic cough *11*

4 Critically ill patient with respiratory disease *21*

5 Diffuse alveolar haemorrhage *27*

6 Diffuse lung disease *31*

7 Haemoptysis *43*

8 Pleural effusion *49*

9 Post-operative breathlessness *63*

10 Pregnancy and breathlessness *69*

11 Preoperative assessment *73*

12 Pulmonary disease in the immunocompromised— non-HIV *79*

13 Pulmonary disease in the immunocompromised— HIV *91*

14 Sleep and breathing *99*

15 Unexplained respiratory failure *105*

Chapter 1

Breathlessness

Clinical assessment and causes 4
Specific situations 6

Clinical assessment and causes

Physiological mechanisms of breathlessness

Dyspnoea refers to the abnormal and uncomfortable awareness of breathing. Its physiological mechanisms are poorly understood; possible afferent sources for the sensation include receptors in respiratory muscles, juxta-capillary (J) receptors (sense interstitial fluid), and chemoreceptors (sensing $\uparrow CO_2$ and $\downarrow O_2$).

Clinical assessment

All patients need a full history and examination. Key points in the assessment are:

- *Duration and onset* of breathlessness. Box 1.1 groups the causes of breathlessness by speed of onset, although, in practice, some variability and overlap exist. Patients often underestimate the duration of symptoms—enquiring about exercise tolerance over a period of time is a useful way of assessing duration and progression
- *Severity* of breathlessness. Assess the level of handicap and disability by asking about effects on lifestyle, work, and daily activities
- *Exacerbating factors.* Ask about rest and exertion, nocturnal symptoms, and body position. The timing of nocturnal breathlessness may provide clues to the likely cause: left ventricular failure (LVF) causes breathlessness after a few hours of sleep and resolves after about 45min; asthma tends to occur later in the night; laryngeal inspiratory stridor causes noisy breathlessness of very short duration (<1 min); and Cheyne–Stokes apnoeas result in breathlessness that is recurrent and clears each time in <30 s. Orthopnoea is suggestive of LVF or diaphragm paralysis, although it is also common in many chronic lung diseases. Breathlessness during swimming is characteristic of bilateral diaphragm paralysis. Trepopnoea refers to breathlessness when lying on one side as a result of ipsilateral pulmonary disease
- *Associated symptoms*, such as cough, haemoptysis, chest pain, wheeze, stridor, fever, loss of appetite and weight, ankle swelling, and voice change. Wheeze may occur with pulmonary oedema, pulmonary embolism (PE), bronchiolitis, and anaphylaxis, in addition to asthma and chronic obstructive pulmonary disease (COPD)
- *Personal and family history* of chest disease
- *Lifetime employment, hobbies, pets, travel, smoking, illicit drug use, medications*
- *Examination* of the cardiovascular and respiratory systems. Observe the pattern and rate of breathing. Assess for signs of respiratory distress. Look for paradoxical abdominal movement if the history suggests diaphragmatic paralysis. A useful bedside test is to exercise the patient (e.g. by stepping on and off a 15–20 cm block) until their breathlessness occurs, and then measure oximetry immediately on stopping when the finger is still; a fall in O_2 saturation is expected with organic causes of dyspnoea.

Investigations

Initial investigations typically include resting oximetry, peak flow and spirometry, chest radiograph (CXR), and electrocardiogram (ECG). Further tests depend on clinical suspicion; options include full pulmonary function tests (PFTs) with measurement of lung volumes lying and standing, gas transfer and flow–volume loop, bronchial hyperresponsiveness or reversibility testing, maximal mouth or inspiratory sniff pressures, arterial blood gases (ABGs) (with measurement of alveolar to arterial (A–a) gradient), exercise oximetry, ventilation-perfusion (V/Q) scanning and computed tomographic pulmonary angiography (CTPA), high-resolution CT (HRCT), blood tests (full blood count (FBC) and thyroid-stimulating hormone (TSH)), echocardiogram (echo), exercise ECG, and cardiac catheterization.

Box 1.1 Causes of breathlessness grouped by speed of onset

Instantaneous
- Pneumothorax
- PE.

Acute (minutes to hours)
- Airways disease (asthma, exacerbation of COPD, upper airways obstruction)
- Parenchymal disease (pneumonia, pulmonary oedema, pulmonary haemorrhage, acute hypersensitivity pneumonitis)
- Pulmonary vascular disease
- Cardiac disease (e.g. acute myocardial infarction, arrhythmia, valvular disease, tamponade, aortic dissection)
- Metabolic acidosis
- Hyperventilation syndrome.

Subacute (days)
- Many of the above, plus:
  - Pleural effusion
  - Lobar collapse
  - Acute interstitial pneumonia
  - Superior vena cava obstruction
  - Pulmonary vasculitis.

Chronic (months to years)
- Some of the above, plus:
  - Obstructive airways disease (COPD, asthma)
  - Diffuse parenchymal disease (including idiopathic pulmonary fibrosis, sarcoidosis, lymphangitis carcinomatosis)
  - Pulmonary vascular disease (chronic thromboembolic disease, pulmonary hypertension, veno-occlusive disease)
  - Hypoventilation (chest wall deformity, neuromuscular weakness, obesity)
  - Anaemia
  - Thyrotoxicosis.

Specific situations

Causes of breathlessness with a normal CXR

- Airways disease (asthma, upper airways obstruction, bronchiolitis)
- Pulmonary vascular disease (PE, idiopathic pulmonary hypertension, intrapulmonary shunt)
- Early parenchymal disease (e.g. sarcoid, interstitial pneumonias, infection—viral, *Pneumocystis jirovecii* pneumonia)
- Cardiac disease (e.g. angina, arrhythmia, valvular disease, intracardiac shunt)
- Neuromuscular weakness
- Metabolic acidosis
- Anaemia
- Thyrotoxicosis
- Hyperventilation syndrome.

Causes of episodic/intermittent breathlessness

- Asthma
- Pulmonary oedema
- Angina
- Pulmonary embolism
- Hypersensitivity pneumonitis
- Vasculitis
- Hyperventilation syndrome.

Distinguishing cardiac and respiratory causes of breathlessness

- This can be difficult. Many of the clinical features of left heart failure are non-specific and easily confused with respiratory disease (e.g. orthopnoea, wheeze). In chronic cardiac failure, crackles on auscultation and radiological features of pulmonary oedema may be absent, even when the pulmonary capillary wedge pressure is significantly raised (due to adaptive changes from vascular remodelling)
- The presence of emphysema may also render crackles inaudible and lead to atypical CXR appearances of pulmonary oedema
- Chronic left heart failure commonly leads to a restrictive ventilatory defect and reduced gas transfer on PFTs and may also result in pulmonary hypertension
- HRCT features of left heart failure include septal and peribronchovascular interstitial thickening, ground-glass shadowing, pleural effusions, and cardiomegaly
- Resting ECG is useful: in practice, a cardiac cause of breathlessness is unlikely in the setting of a completely normal ECG
- Elevated brain natriuretic peptide (BNP) levels predict the likelihood of left ventricular impairment
- Exercise ECG, echo, and cardiac catheterization may be required
- Cardiac and respiratory diseases can, of course, coexist.

Chapter 2

Chest pain

Introduction to chest pain *8*
Acute pleuritic chest pain *9*
Chronic chest pain *10*

Introduction to chest pain

The majority of patients with chest pain referred for a respiratory opinion have either acute pleuritic pain or persistent, well-localized pain. Cardiac pain rarely presents in this manner, although it should be considered in exertional pain or in the presence of risk factors for ischaemic heart disease.

Within the respiratory system, pain may arise from the parietal pleura, major airways, chest wall, diaphragm, and mediastinum; the lung parenchyma and visceral pleura are insensitive to pain. Processes involving the upper parietal pleura cause a pain localized to that part of the chest. The lower parietal pleura and outer region of the diaphragmatic pleura are innervated by the lower six intercostal nerves, and pain here may be referred to the abdomen. The central region of the diaphragm is supplied by the phrenic nerve (C3, 4, and 5), and pain may be referred to the ipsilateral shoulder tip. Tracheobronchitis tends to be associated with retrosternal pain.

Acute pleuritic chest pain

- Pleuritic pain is sharp, well localized, worse on coughing and inspiration, and the subsequent limitation of inspiration often leads to a degree of breathlessness
- Causes of acute pleuritic chest pain include:
  - Pulmonary infarction (following embolism)
  - Pneumonia
  - Pneumothorax
  - Pericarditis
  - Pleural infection (empyema, tuberculous)
  - Autoimmune disease (e.g. systemic lupus erythematosus (SLE), rheumatoid arthritis (RA))
  - Musculoskeletal
  - Fractured rib
- In addition, consider atypical presentations of serious conditions such as MI, aortic dissection, oesophageal rupture, and pancreatitis. Consider angioinvasive fungi, such as *Aspergillus*, as a cause of pleuritic chest pain in the immunocompromised
- Diagnosis is typically based on 'pattern recognition' of clinical features, followed by selected investigations. Initial investigations typically include chest radiograph (CXR), electrocardiogram (ECG), arterial blood gas (ABGs), serum inflammatory markers, and D-dimers. Further investigations may include V/Q scanning or CTPA, pleural aspiration, and measurement of serum autoantibodies
- PE (see ➔ pulmonary thromboembolic disease p. 472) commonly presents with pleuritic pain, and exclusion of this diagnosis is the usual reason for referral. Assess risk factors for thromboembolic disease. Normal O_2 saturations and PaO_2 in the 'normal' range do not exclude the diagnosis; calculate the A–a gradient (see ➔ p. 924). The presence of a pleural rub is a non-specific sign that occurs with pleural inflammation of any cause
- In young adults, pneumococcal pneumonia may present with acute-onset pleuritic chest pain, although systemic symptoms, such as fever, usually predate the pain by hours
- The pain from pericarditis is pleuritic, but central, and relieved on leaning forward; there may also be a pericardial rub, characteristic ECG features, and a small pericardial effusion on echo
- Musculoskeletal pain may occur as a result of cervical disc disease, arthritis of the shoulder or spine, a fractured rib, or costochondritis (Tietze's syndrome), which often follows a viral infection
- The presence of chest wall tenderness does not invariably indicate a benign musculoskeletal cause; tenderness may be seen in malignant chest wall infiltration and sometimes following pulmonary infarction
- Other features besides pleurisy that may suggest a diagnosis of SLE include rash, photosensitivity, oral ulcers, arthritis, pericarditis, renal or neurological disease, cytopenia, positive antinuclear antibody (ANA) and double-stranded DNA (dsDNA).

Chronic chest pain

- Persistent chest pain that is well localized is typically caused by chest wall or pleural disease. Causes include:
  - Malignant pleural disease or chest wall infiltration
  - Benign musculoskeletal pain
  - Pleural infection (empyema, tuberculous)
  - Benign asbestos-related pleural disease
  - Autoimmune disease (e.g. SLE, RA)
  - Recurrent pulmonary infarction (emboli, vasculitis)
- Pain from malignant chest wall infiltration is often 'boring' in character and may disturb sleep; it is frequently not related to respiration. Causes include 1° lung cancer, 2° pleural malignancy, mesothelioma, and rib or sternal involvement from malignancy (including myeloma and leukaemia)
- Chronic thromboembolic disease tends to present with breathlessness; when chest pain occurs, it is usually episodic, rather than persistent
- As with acute pleuritic pain, investigations are directed by initial clinical suspicion. Consider CT chest, bone scan, serum autoantibodies, FBC and film, serum electrophoresis. CXR may appear normal in malignant chest wall disease.

Chapter 3

Chronic cough

Aetiology and clinical assessment *12*
Treatment *14*
Causes of cough *15*
Chronic cough: asthma, GORD *16*
Chronic cough: rhinitis, post-infectious, ACE inhibitors,
    idiopathic *18*

Aetiology and clinical assessment

Cough is a frequent symptom of many respiratory diseases and is often associated with underlying lung pathology and an abnormal chest radiograph (CXR). Cough can occur in otherwise healthy people and is often a self-limiting symptom. Persistent coughing can be a socially disabling and distressing symptom, for which help is often sought.

- *Acute cough* = cough lasting <3 weeks, usually due to viral upper respiratory tract infection (URTI).
- *Subacute cough* = cough lasting 3–8 weeks
- *Chronic cough* = cough lasting >8 weeks
- Patients with a normal CXR and persistent cough are often grouped under the heading 'chronic cough'
- It can sometimes be difficult to determine the underlying cause
- Susceptible individuals have a heightened cough reflex (therefore coining the term 'cough hypersensitivity syndrome')
- Investigation is warranted, but successful response to therapeutic trials may aid determination of the underlying cause. Centres vary in their approach to this
- Specialist cough clinics suggest they achieve diagnosis and effective treatment in over 80% of patients referred with chronic cough.

Aetiology

In practice, over 90% of cases of chronic cough with a normal CXR are caused by one or more of:

- Cough variant asthma or eosinophilic bronchitis
- Gastro-oesophageal reflux disease (GORD)
- Post-nasal drip (or upper airway cough syndrome), due to perennial or allergic rhinitis, vasomotor rhinitis, or chronic sinusitis.

Cough syncope

Loss of consciousness following violent coughing, a Valsalva-type manoeuvre, which impairs venous return to the heart and provokes bradycardia and vasodilatation (similar to an ordinary faint). Important as car drivers must cease driving until liability to cough syncope has ceased, confirmed by medical opinion; commercial drivers must cease driving and have no cough syncope or pre-syncope for 5 y if they have a chronic respiratory condition, including smoking. If they have asystole due to cough, driving can be considered after pacemaker insertion.

In clinic

Full history can be unhelpful. Although cough is most commonly due to asthma, reflux, or post-nasal drip, there may be no specific symptoms to suggest these diagnoses.

- Duration of cough
- When it tends to occur—night or early morning, after exertion, on exposure to dust, pollen, aerosols, cold air (asthma), after meals or on sitting or bending over (GORD), nocturnal (post-nasal drip and asthma)
- Non-productive or productive and, if so, how much sputum and colour. Significant amounts of sputum usually indicate a 1° lung pathology
- Haemoptysis
- Fever

- Associated symptoms:
  - Shortness of breath (SOB) or wheeze
  - Throat clearing or sensation of post-nasal drip
  - Chest pain
  - Ankle swelling/orthopnoea/paroxysmal nocturnal dyspnoea
  - Dyspepsia
- Previous respiratory disease such as childhood asthma, eczema, or hay fever
- History of sinus disease or perennial rhinitis
- History of previous severe respiratory infections, such as whooping cough, that may have caused bronchiectasis
- Known cardiac disease or valvular heart disease
- Drug history ?ACE inhibitor
- Occupation ?Workplace irritants
- Pets/birds
- Smoker (common cause of persistent cough, dose-related, improves on stopping)
- Use of recreational drugs.

Examination

Usually normal. Look for signs of underlying lung disease or other medical conditions such as heart failure, neurological disease (particularly bulbar involvement). Significant tonsillar enlargement should be excluded, as this is a recognized cause of cough, which can respond to tonsillectomy.

Investigations

Initially

- *Check that CXR is normal*
- *Spirometry* may indicate restrictive or obstructive defect. Performance of spirometry may provoke cough and bronchospasm
- *Methacholine challenge test* (see ➜ p. 868) provides the best positive predictive value for cough due to asthma. Lack of response means cough variant asthma is extremely unlikely. PC_{20} is normal in eosinophilic bronchitis
- *Serial peak flow recordings* twice daily for 2 weeks. >20% diurnal variation suggests asthma. Can be normal in cough variant asthma
- *Induced sputum examination*, if available, for eosinophil count, to suggest either asthma or eosinophilic bronchitis.

Later

- *Consider chest CT* to exclude significant lung disease in patients with refractory cough, even with a normal CXR
- *Consider ENT examination* if predominantly upper respiratory tract disease, resistant to treatment. Consider sinus CT
- *Consider bronchoscopy* if foreign body possible, or history suggestive of malignancy, small carcinoid, endobronchial disease. Perform after CT to help guide bronchoscopist
- *Consider 24h ambulatory oesophageal pH monitoring*
- *Consider oesophageal manometry* for oesophageal dysmotility.

Treatment

The initial treatment of patients with a chronic cough is determined by what the most likely underlying cause is, based on the history and investigations. The key is to give any drug treatment at a high enough dose, and for a long enough time (such as 2–3 months), to be effective.

Symptomatic treatment for cough

Over-the-counter medicines may provide relief, although there is little evidence of a specific pharmacological effect or evidence of clinical benefits. Below is a list of possible treatments:
- *Honey and lemon*—home remedies
- *Dextromethorphan*—a non-sedating non-opiate. Component of many over-the-counter cough remedies. Dose response, with maximum cough reflex suppression at 60 mg (Benylin® preparations, Actifed® preparations, Vicks Vaposyrup® preparations, Sudafed Linctus®, Night Nurse®)
- *Menthol*—short-lived cough suppressant (Benylin® preparations, Vicks Vaposyrup® preparations)
- *Sedative antihistamines*—suppress cough but cause drowsiness. Good for nocturnal cough
- *Codeine or pholcodine*—opiate antitussives—codeine requires prescription. No greater efficacy than dextromethorphan and greater side effect profile
- *Opiates*—prescription. Low-dose morphine sulfate 5–10 mg showed significant improvement in patients with intractable cough in a randomized controlled trial. Side effect profile of opiates, so should be used with caution
- *Gabapentin*—prescription. Neuromodulator used for chronic pain. Not yet licensed for cough, but RCT treatment success in Leicester Cough Questionnaire score, with side effects mostly of nausea and fatigue in 31% on gabapentin, managed with dose reduction (Ryan NM et al. *Lancet* 2012). Starting dose 300 mg/day, with gradual increases until cough suppressed, side effects, or maximum 600 mg tds. Other side effects include diarrhoea, emotional lability, sleepiness, nystagmus, tremor, weakness, peripheral oedema
- *Thalidomide*—can be used in intractable cough due to IPF, with RCT showing significant improvements in cough quality of life (QoL) questionnaires (Horton MR et al. *Ann Intern Med* 2012). Side effects in 74% on thalidomide vs 22% placebo, with constipation, dizziness, and fatigue (for IPF see ➔ p. 320).
- *Afferent nerve receptor (P2X3) antagonists* have shown promise in phase 2 studies and are being further investigated.

Assessing treatment response

Several measures have been developed and validated such as:
- Cough visual analogue scale
- Leicester Cough Questionnaire—cough-specific QoL
- Cough reflex sensitivity measurements—primarily a research tool; subjects inhale increasing doses of either capsaicin or citric acid, with the sensitivity recorded as the dose to cause two or five coughs.

Causes of cough

Respiratory
- Infection: viral upper and lower respiratory tract infection, bacterial pneumonia, tuberculosis (TB), pertussis
- Chronic bronchitis
- Obstructive airways disease: COPD, asthma
- Cough variant asthma
- Eosinophilic bronchitis
- Obstructive sleep apnoea (nocturnal only)
- Lung cancer
- Bronchiectasis, cystic fibrosis
- Interstitial lung disease
- Airway irritants: smoking, dusts and fumes, acute smoke inhalation
- Airway foreign body.

Mediastinal
- External compression of trachea by enlarged lymph nodes (e.g. lymphoma, TB)
- Mediastinal tumours/cysts/masses.

Cardiac
- LVF
- Left atrial enlargement (e.g. severe mitral stenosis).

ENT
- Upper airway cough syndrome, including:
  - Acute or chronic sinusitis
  - Post-nasal drip due to perennial, allergic, or vasomotor rhinitis.

GI
- GORD
- Oesophageal dysmotility, stricture, or pharyngeal pouch causing repeated aspiration
- Oesophago-bronchial fistula.

CNS
Neurological disease affecting swallowing, causing repeated aspiration, such as stroke, multiple sclerosis, motor neurone disease, or Parkinson's disease.

Drugs
- ACE inhibitors
- Some inhaled preparations can cause cough—particularly ipratropium.

Other
- Idiopathic
- Ear wax (vagal nerve stimulation)
- Psychogenic/habitual.

Chronic cough: asthma, GORD

Asthma

Also 'cough variant asthma', 'cough-predominant asthma'. This represents one end of the asthma spectrum, with airway inflammation, but may have minimal bronchoconstriction. There is not always a typical asthma history, but ask about wheeze, atopy, hay fever, or childhood asthma or eczema. Cough may be the only symptom. Cough is typically worse after exercise, in cold air, after exposure to fumes or fragrances, or in the mornings.

- *Spirometry* may be normal, without evidence of airflow obstruction. There may be typical asthmatic diurnal peak flow variability of >20%, or peak flows may be stable
- *Methacholine challenge* should be positive for asthma but does not rule out a steroid-responsive cough. If negative, other causes of cough should be sought
- *Treatment* should be for at least 2 months, with high-dose inhaled steroids. Response may take days or weeks. Bronchodilators may make little difference. If inhaled steroid therapy has been tried unsuccessfully, ensure inhaler technique is optimal and a high dose has been used. Alternatively, prescribe a 2-week course of oral prednisolone 30 mg/day, and assess response. If the cough improves, high-dose inhaled steroids should be continued and slowly reduced after about 2 months. There is a small trial showing leukotriene receptor antagonists decreased cough in people with cough variant asthma; consider using in patients who want to avoid inhaled steroids or in whom they are ineffective
- *Eosinophilic bronchitis* Airway eosinophilia, rarely with peripheral blood eosinophilia, causing heightened cough reflex, but no bronchial hyperresponsiveness/wheeze or peak flow variation. Diagnosis based on negative asthma investigations and induced sputum eosinophilia. Improves with inhaled corticosteroids, usually after 2–3 weeks, or trial of oral prednisolone. Sputum eosinophil count also reduces with treatment. If there is no response, the cough is unlikely to be due to eosinophilic airway inflammation.

GORD

Cough may be related to distal reflux at the lower oesophageal sphincter (LOS) or due to micro-aspiration of acid into the trachea. There may be associated oesophageal dysmotility. LOS reflux is often long-standing and is associated with a productive or non-productive daytime cough, and minimal nocturnal symptoms. It is worse after meals and when sitting down, due to increased intra-abdominal pressure being transmitted to the LOS. Micro-aspiration is associated with more prominent symptoms of reflux or dyspepsia, although these are not always present. Patients may have an intermittent hoarse voice, dysphonia, and sore throat. Cough may be the only symptom of reflux.

Laryngoscopy
May reveal posterior vocal cord inflammation, but this is not a reliable sign.

A trial of treatment
Recommended. This is with a high-dose proton pump inhibitor (PPI) for at least 2, usually 3, months, although longer treatment may be required to control cough. H2 receptor blockers are also effective, and prokinetics like metoclopramide may help as an addition if cough improves but has not gone completely. Other reflux avoidance measures should be carried out: avoiding caffeine, fatty foods, chocolate, excess alcohol, acidic drinks like orange juice, red wine, stop smoking, loose-fitting clothes, sleeping with an empty stomach (avoid eating <4h before bed), sleeping propped up, weight loss if overweight. Surgical fundoplication for reflux-associated cough resistant to drug therapy is not widely used but may be effective in carefully selected cases.

Investigation
If required, due to either treatment failure or because of diagnostic uncertainty, is with 24 h ambulatory pH monitoring, which determines the presence of reflux events, and event markers allow correlation with cough. These may not necessarily be responsible for the cough, so it is not a very specific or sensitive test. Oesophageal manometry can be used to measure the LOS pressure and oesophageal contractions after swallowing to determine the presence of oesophageal dysmotility.

Chronic cough: rhinitis, post-infectious, ACE inhibitors, idiopathic

Rhinitis and post-nasal drip

The term *upper airway cough syndrome (UACS)* is now being used to include all upper airway abnormalities causing cough and is replacing post-nasal drip. *Rhinitis* is defined as sneezing, nasal discharge, or blockage for >1 h on most days for either a limited part of the year (seasonal) or all year (perennial). Rhinitis may be allergic (e.g. hay fever), non-allergic, or infective. The associated nasal inflammation may irritate cough receptors directly or produce a post-nasal drip. These secretions may pool at the back of the throat, giving a sensation of liquid dripping into the back of the throat, which requires frequent throat clearing, or drip directly into the trachea, initiating cough. There may be frequent nasal discharge. A history of facial pain and purulent nasal discharge suggests sinusitis, which can also predispose to post-nasal drip. Symptoms of cough can occur on lying but can be constant, regardless of position. Rhinosinusitis describes inflammation and infection within the nasal passages and paranasal sinuses, with chronic rhinosinusitis defined as symptoms persisting for more than 12 weeks.

ENT examination
May reveal swollen turbinates, 'cobblestone' nasopharyngeal mucosa, nasal discharge, or nasal polyps.

Treatment
Nasal preparations should be taken by kneeling with the top of the head on the floor ('Mecca' position) or lying supine with the head tipped over the end of the bed. Improvements in cough should be found within 2 weeks. Duration of treatment is unclear.
- *Non-allergic rhinitis* Trials suggest the best results are with an initial 3 weeks of nasal decongestants with first-generation antihistamines (which have helpful anticholinergic properties) and pseudoephedrine. Alternatives are nasal ipratropium bromide or xylometazoline. This is then followed by 3 months of high-dose nasal steroids, which are ineffective when used as first-line treatment. Second-generation antihistamines (i.e. non-sedating) are of no use in non-allergic rhinitis
- *Allergic rhinitis* Second-generation oral antihistamine (e.g. cetirizine, loratadine, fexofenadine) and high-dose nasal steroids for 3 months at least
- *Vasomotor rhinitis* Nasal ipratropium bromide for 3 months; nasal steroids may also have a role
- *Chronic rhinosinusitis* Nasal steroids and saline lavage, which should have an effect by 4 weeks, and, if so, treatment should continue, although optimal duration unclear.

Sinusitis

Infection of the paranasal sinuses, which may complicate an URTI and is frequently caused by *H. influenzae* or *S. pneumoniae*. It causes frontal headache and facial pain. Chronic sinusitis may require further investigation with XR or CT, which shows mucosal thickening and air-fluid levels. Surgery may be indicated.

Chronic sinusitis

Treat as for non-allergic rhinitis, but include 2 weeks of antibiotics active against *H. influenzae* such as doxycycline or co-amoxiclav. Medium-term macrolide antibiotics may be helpful.

Post-infectious

Respiratory tract infections, especially if viral in nature, can cause cough. This may take weeks or months to resolve spontaneously, although most settle within 8 weeks. There may be a post-nasal drip contribution. The cough is related to a heightened cough reflex. Associated laryngospasm can occur, which is a sudden hoarseness, with associated stridulous inspiratory efforts and a sensation of being unable to breathe.

Treatment

Antitussives, such as codeine linctus, may ease the symptoms. Inhaled steroids have been tried for the transient bronchial hyperactivity, but there is no trial evidence that these work. Inhaled ipratropium has also been tried, with one report of effectiveness.

ACE inhibitor cough

Occurs with any ACE inhibitor and is related to bradykinin not being broken down by angiotensin-converting enzyme and accumulating in the lung. Occurs in 10–15% of people on ACE inhibitors; more frequent in women. Can occur within weeks of starting the drug, but also up to 6 months; the cough may be initiated by a respiratory tract infection but persists thereafter. Cough usually settles within a week of stopping the drug but may take months. Avoid all ACE inhibitors thereafter and may need to change to an angiotensin receptor antagonist. Stop ACE inhibitor in any patient with a troublesome cough.

Idiopathic chronic cough

Accounts for 20% of referrals to a specialist cough clinic. It is diagnosed after a thorough assessment to exclude an underlying cause. Typically, there is lymphocytic airway inflammation, but there may also be a history of reflux cough. Typically, the patients are middle-aged women with a long-standing dry cough, often starting around the time of the menopause and triggered by an URTI. Organ-specific autoimmune disease is present in up to 30%, particularly hypothyroidism. Treatment is often ineffective.

Recent phase 2 trials of Gefapixant, an oral P2X3 receptor antagonist that works on signals affecting the afferent cough reflex, have shown a 75% decrease in cough frequency compared to placebo in patients with idiopathic chronic cough. Due to the mechanism of action, taste disturbance was a common side effect. Gefapixant and other nerve receptor antagonists are being evaluated in phase 3 studies.

Further information

Irwin et al. Classification of Cough as a Symptom in Adults and Management Algorithms CHEST Guideline and Expert Panel Report. *Chest* 2018;**153**(1): 196–209.

Ryan et al. An update and systematic review on drug therapies for the treatment of refractory chronic cough. *Expert Opin Pharmacother* 2018;**19**: 687–711.

BTS guidelines. Recommendations for the management of cough in adults. *Thorax* 2006;**61**(suppl 1). ℰ http://www.thoraxjnl.com.

Birring SS et al. Development of a symptom specific health status measure for patients with chronic cough: Leicester Cough Questionnaire. *Thorax* 2003;**58**: 339–43.

Chapter 4

Critically ill patient with respiratory disease

Introduction 22
Initial assessment 23
Underlying cause 24
Treatment aims 25

Introduction

Patients often present critically ill to the emergency or the acute medical department with respiratory disease. This may be due to a deterioration or exacerbation of an existing condition, a first presentation of a previously undiagnosed disease, or with respiratory involvement of a systemic disease. As with any critically ill patient, standard management is required initially to stabilize, with the focus then moving to diagnosis and treatment. Often these need to take place in parallel. Depending on the presence of any pre-existing respiratory disease and its nature and severity, it may be important to determine disease-specific treatment and/or treatment limitations ('ceilings of care'), and senior physician input should be sought for this.

Initial assessment

Airway

Is the patient maintaining their airway? Is there snoring or gurgling? Head tilt; chin lift; use suction if good views. Is an airway adjunct necessary? Consider inserting Guedel airway or nasopharyngeal airway if Glasgow Coma Score (GCS) reduced <8. Call intensive care unit (ICU) if intubation and ICU care likely to be necessary, or if the patient is rapidly deteriorating/peri-arrest and full assessment has not yet been possible (see ➲ p. 755).

Breathing

Cyanosis? What is the SaO_2 and associated FiO_2?
- Exclude tension pneumothorax clinically (see ➲ p. 446)
- What is the respiratory rate (RR)?
- Has a blood gas been taken, and what does it show? (see ➲ p. 922)
- Oxygenation adequate? If not, likely to need increased FiO_2 (see ➲ p. 106), or, if this is already maximal, need ventilatory support—involve ICU
- Is the CO_2 low? If hyperventilating and already increased work of breathing to maintain O_2 at current level-may need to increase FiO_2. If FiO_2 already maximal, likely to need ventilatory assistance/nasal high flow oxygen—involve ICU
- Is the CO_2 high (see ➲ p. 106)? Hypoventilating, tiring, or CO_2 narcosis in COPD—consider ventilatory support
- Request an urgent portable chest radiograph (CXR).

Circulation

What is pulse rate, blood pressure (BP), rhythm on cardiac monitor/ECG? What is fluid balance status? Aim to optimize. Ensure IV access secured and blood tests sent. Look at BP, jugular venous pressure (JVP), urine output, peripheral perfusion (capillary refill time). If hypotensive, are they underfilled? Consider fluids. If euvolaemic/overfilled, but hypotensive, with poor urine output, may need inotropic support. Likely to need central venous access to enable central venous pressure (CVP) monitoring, and this will aid drug administration.

Disability

Conscious level: GCS or AVPU (alert, responsive to verbal commands, responsive to pain, unresponsive). Are they confused? Check blood glucose, temperature, pupils, signs of acute neurological disease—neck stiffness, plantar reflexes, tone.

Examination

Temperature, sputum, asterixis, chest signs (pneumothorax, wheeze, silent chest, effusion, consolidation, pulmonary oedema), cardiac murmurs, palpable abdominal organomegaly, skin/nail signs, rash.

Investigations

Immediate tests include full blood count (FBC), clotting screen, C-reactive protein (CRP), urea and electrolytes (U&E), liver function tests (LFTs), and blood cultures before antibiotics.

Underlying cause

If known respiratory disease

This will enable more targeted therapy. Try and obtain recent medical history. Ask patient or their relatives about disease severity, current treatment, plans of clinicians for long-term care (immunosuppression, transplant list, home non-invasive ventilation (NIV), advance directive, lasting power of attorney, etc.). What is the usual current health status—exercise tolerance, activities of daily living? What has caused this deterioration—a potentially reversible process (e.g. infection, drugs, pneumothorax, pulmonary embolus (PE)) or gradual progression of underlying disease? Review CXR, and compare with previous films, if possible.

For more details regarding exacerbations of chronic lung diseases, see ➲ p. 141 (asthma), ➲ p. 189 (COPD), ➲ p. 237 (CF), ➲ p. 169 (bronchiectasis), ➲ p. 317 (IPF), ➲ p. 337 (lung cancer), ➲ p. 671 (sickle cell).

If no known respiratory disease

A full history is required to obtain diagnosis. The patient's cardiorespiratory status and illness severity will determine how brief/full this is. Ask about recent symptoms, travel, contact illness, risk factors for immunocompromise, usual health status, drugs.

For presentation-based differential diagnoses and initial investigation plans, see ➲ p. 3 (breathlessness), ➲ p. 7 (chest pain), ➲ p. 43 (haemoptysis), ➲ p. 79 (immunocompromise), ➲ p. 105 (unexplained respiratory failure), ➲ p. 31 (diffuse lung disease), ➲ p. 27 (diffuse alveolar haemorrhage), ➲ p. 49 (pleural effusion), ➲ p. 69 (pregnancy), ➲ p. 63 (post-operative), ➲ p. 518 (pneumonia), ➲ p. 467 (PE), ➲ p. 435 (pneumothorax), ➲ p. 261 (toxic agents), ➲ p. 703 and ➲ p. 706 (upper airway disease and anaphylaxis), and ➲ p. 360 (SVCO).

Treatment aims

In patients with known severe respiratory disease, with poor pre-morbid state (e.g. very limited exercise capacity, comorbidities, severe dementia), intubation and invasive ventilation may not be appropriate. The patient may have their own views on this or have made a living will/advance directive. Old notes should be reviewed, if possible, and this decision should be discussed with their respiratory consultant or the consultant on call. NIV (see p. 771) may be appropriate.

In patients with known respiratory disease, with an acute exacerbation (infective or non-infective), respiratory and organ support may be indicated to enable them to survive the episode. This should be discussed with their respiratory consultant or the consultant on call and ICU.

In patients with no known respiratory disease, respiratory and organ support may well be indicated to enable them to survive the episode. This should be discussed with the consultant on call and ICU. If they have significant pre-existing comorbidity from a non-respiratory disease (severe cardiac failure, severe dementia), the details of this should be ascertained and discussed with their usual consultant, if possible.

If there is any doubt about a patient's usual health status, or no previous history or notes available, or they are deteriorating before full assessment can be made, full ventilatory and organ support should be considered.

Diffuse alveolar haemorrhage

Causes *28*
Clinical features and investigations *29*
Management *30*

Causes

There are multiple causes (see Box 5.1). One of three underlying histo-pathological abnormalities is seen on lung biopsy samples; pulmonary capillaritis as is seen in systemic vasculitis and anti-glomerular basement membrane (GBM) disease, diffuse alveolar damage in acute respiratory distress syndrome (ARDS) and alveolar haemorrhage in the absence of alveolar damage as is seen in coagulopathies and elevated left sided cardiac pressures.

Bleeding into the alveoli is often a feature of a small-vessel vasculitis of the lungs. Most of this blood tends to remain in the lungs and is not expectorated. Patients with diffuse alveolar haemorrhage may have a background history of vasculitis symptoms over the preceding weeks to months. They can present with slowly progressive dyspnoea with haemoptysis or be acutely unwell with hypoxia. They may require ventilatory support.

Box 5.1 Causes of alveolar haemorrhage

First three are most common:
- **Anti-GBM disease (Goodpasture's)*** see ➔ p. 721
- **Granulomatosis with polyangiitis (GPA/Wegener's)*** see ➔ p. 716
- **Systemic lupus erythematosus*** see ➔ p. 218
- Rheumatoid arthritis see ➔ p. 16
- Microscopic polyangiitis (MPA)* see ➔ p. 720
- Progressive systemic sclerosis see ➔ p. 222
- Polyarteritis nodosa (PAN) see ➔ p. 724
- Mixed connective tissue disease
- Antiphospholipid syndrome
- Behçet's disease
- Essential mixed cryoglobulinaemia
- Endocarditis- or tumour-related vasculitis
- Idiopathic rapidly progressive glomerulonephritis
- Idiopathic pulmonary hemosiderosis
- Leptospirosis
- Isolated pauci-immune pulmonary capillaritis
- Coagulopathy such as disseminated intravascular coagulation (DIC)
- Mitral valve disease
- Bone marrow transplantation (usually within 1 month)
- Drugs: abciximab, all-trans retinoic acid (ATRA), sirolimus, propylthiouracil (PTU), penicillamine, cocaine
- Chemicals: trimellitic anhydride, pyromellitic dianhydrate.

*Indicates conditions commonly considered in the differential diagnosis of *pulmonary-renal syndrome* (diffuse alveolar haemorrhage with glomerulonephritis). Note: conditions causing diffuse chest radiograph (CXR) infiltrate and renal failure may mimic these, e.g. severe cardiac failure, severe pneumonia, leptospirosis.

Clinical features and investigations

Presentation

Abrupt-onset haemoptysis is the most common symptom, although this is not present in one-third of cases. Also cough, dyspnoea, low-grade fever, weight loss, arthralgia, myalgia. There may be a history of chronic sinusitis and other ENT symptoms (granulomatosis with polyangiitis; GPA ≈ Wegener's).

Examination

May be non-specific or may have signs of underlying vasculitis with skin rashes, nail fold infarcts, digital gangrene. Episcleritis, corneal ulceration, epistaxis, nasal crusting, or deafness may be present. Neurological signs, including mononeuritis multiplex, should raise the possibility of vasculitis. Patients may be breathless. Haematuria and proteinuria on urine dip.

Investigations

- May be hypoxic—check SaO_2 ± arterial blood gas
- FBC—?falling Hb/haematocrit
- Clotting profile
- C-reactive protein/erythrocyte sedimentation rate
- Creatine kinase (CK)
- CXR showing bilateral alveolar infiltrates—difficult to distinguish from pulmonary oedema or infection
- Consider chest high resolution computed tomography
- Raised kCO, as increased intra-alveolar Hb is available to combine with carbon monoxide (CO). Abnormal if raised by >30%. If breathless at rest, they will not be able to perform this test, as it requires breath-holding of an air, CO, and helium mixture for 10 s. This test can be used to monitor disease progress
- Bronchoalveolar lavage (BAL) shows bloodstained lavage, which becomes sequentially more so with each washing. Cytology shows hemosiderin-laden macrophages
- Renal involvement: blood and/or protein in the urine, red cell casts, raised urea, and creatinine
- Send blood for urgent complement levels, ANA, ANCA (PR3 and MPO), anti-GBM Ab, anti-dsDNA Ab, antiphospholipid Ab, and rheumatoid factor (RhF)
- Consider biopsy of lung, kidney (if acute glomerulonephritis present), or other affected site if well enough to make a tissue diagnosis. Transbronchial biopsy (TBB) specimens are usually insufficient to make a diagnosis of vasculitis, and a surgical lung biopsy may be required.

Key questions

- Is this isolated lung disease?
- Is there accompanying renal disease?
- Are there other features of an underlying disease?—ENT, joints, etc?

Management

Management of alveolar haemorrhage
- Admit to hospital
- Supportive treatment, with IV fluids, blood transfusion, and O_2, if necessary
- Monitor, paying particular attention to O_2 saturations and keeping them above 92% with O_2 therapy. May need respiratory support with intubation and ventilation or continuous positive airway pressure (CPAP). Monitor Hb, and transfuse, if necessary. Monitor urine output and renal function
- Aim to establish the underlying diagnosis, usually with tissue biopsy
- Treatment with plasma exchange, high-dose steroids and cyclophosphamide, and dialysis, if required.

Chapter 6

Diffuse lung disease

Causes *32*
Clinical assessment and imaging *34*
HRCT diagnosis *36*
Further investigations *38*
Diffuse lung disease presenting with acute respiratory failure *40*

Causes

Diffuse lung disease is common, and its diagnosis is frequently challenging. This chapter describes a diagnostic approach, based on clinical features, imaging, and other investigations; more detailed descriptions of the diseases themselves are presented later in the book. The term 'diffuse lung disease' is used here to describe any widespread pulmonary disease process. Patients typically present with breathlessness and bilateral chest radiograph (CXR) shadowing. The rate of onset and severity of breathlessness are extremely variable, however, and presentations range from an asymptomatic patient with long-standing radiological changes to an acute onset of breathlessness over a period of days, leading rapidly to respiratory failure and death.

Anatomy of diffuse lung disease

An understanding of lung anatomy is helpful when considering the causes of diffuse lung disease and their appearance on high resolution computed tomography (HRCT). Many diffuse lung diseases primarily affect the interstitium ('interstitial lung disease', also described as 'diffuse parenchymal lung disease'), a poorly defined term that refers to the connective tissue fibrous framework of the lung. Centrally, connective tissue surrounds bronchovascular bundles (each consisting of a bronchus and its accompanying pulmonary artery) that originate at the hila. Peripherally, these connective tissue sheaths are in continuity with fibrous interlobular septa, which organize the lung into units called '2° pulmonary lobules', polyhedral structures with approximately 2 cm sides (see Fig. A4.4, ➔ p. 947). Interlobular septa, which define and separate 2° pulmonary lobules, contain lymphatics and venules. A 2° pulmonary lobule contains around 5–12 acini and is supplied at its centre by a bronchiole and pulmonary arteriole.

The term 'interstitial lung disease' is potentially confusing, because many primarily interstitial processes also involve the airways, vasculature, and alveolar airspaces. Disease processes that primarily affect the airways (e.g. bronchiectasis), vessels (e.g. vasculitis), or airspaces (e.g. pneumonia) may also present with diffuse CXR shadowing.

Causes

There are several hundred causes of diffuse lung disease, and it is useful to divide these into groups, based on their rate of onset and aetiology/disease mechanism (see Table 6.1).

Further information

British Thoracic Society. Interstitial lung disease guideline. *Thorax* 2008;**63**(suppl. V): v1–v58.
Rhagu et al. An Official ATS/ERS/JRS/ALAT statement: idiopathic pulmonary fibrosis: evidence-based guidelines for diagnosis and management. *AJRCCM* 2011;**183**(6): 788–824.

Table 6.1 Causes of diffuse lung disease

Disease onset	Cause/mechanism	Examples (common conditions in bold)
Acute (days–weeks)	Infection	**Bacterial** (pneumococcal, staphylococcal, Gram-negative, anaerobic, TB, atypical), viral (influenza, parainfluenza, adeno, respiratory syncytial virus (RSV), cytomegalovirus (CMV), measles, varicella, hanta), fungal (aspergillosis, histoplasmosis, *Pneumocystis jirovecii* pneumonia (PCP))
	Miscellaneous	**Acute respiratory distress syndrome (ARDS)**, acute interstitial pneumonia (AIP), acute hypersensitivity pneumonitis (HP)
Acute or chronic	Drugs	Immunosuppressants (methotrexate, azathioprine, cyclophosphamide); treatment of connective tissue disease (gold, penicillamine, sulfasalazine); cytotoxics (chlorambucil, melphalan, busulfan, lomustine, carmustine, bleomycin, mitomycin); antibiotics (nitrofurantoin, cephalosporins); anti-arrhythmics (amiodarone); illicit (cocaine inhalation, heroin, methadone, talc)
	Toxins	Radiotherapy, high-concentration O_2, paraquat
	Vasculitis/alveolar haemorrhage	Wegener's (GPA), Churg–Strauss (EGPA), Anti-GBM disease, systemic lupus erythematosus (SLE), microscopic polyangiitis (MPA), idiopathic hemosiderosis
	Pulmonary venous hypertension	**Cardiogenic pulmonary oedema**, pulmonary veno-occlusive disease
	Miscellaneous	**Sarcoidosis**, organizing pneumonia (OP), eosinophilic pneumonia, lipoid pneumonia
Chronic (months–years)	Idiopathic interstitial pneumonias (IIPs)	**IPF**, non-specific interstitial pneumonia (NSIP), desquamative interstitial pneumonia (DIP), lymphocytic interstitial pneumonia (LIP), respiratory bronchiolitis-associated interstitial lung disease (RB-ILD)
	Inhalational Inorganic	Asbestosis, coal worker's pneumoconiosis, silicosis, metals, e.g. cobalt, aluminium
	Organic	Hypersensitivity pneumonitis, e.g. bird fancier's lung, farmer's lung
	Connective tissue disease	**Rheumatoid arthritis (RA)**, SLE, scleroderma, poly- and dermatomyositis, ankylosing spondylitis, Sjögren's syndrome, Behçet's disease
	Malignancy	Lymphangitis carcinomatosa, bronchoalveolar cell carcinoma, pulmonary lymphoma
	Miscellaneous	**Bronchiectasis**, Langerhans cell histiocytosis (LCH), amyloidosis, lymphangioleiomyomatosis (LAM), alveolar proteinosis, microlithiasis

Clinical assessment and imaging

History

Clinical features may provide useful clues to the underlying diagnosis. Key points in the history are:

Presenting symptoms

- Breathlessness is the most common symptom, and its rate of onset may be useful diagnostically (see Table 6.1)
- Causes of truly *episodic* breathlessness and CXR shadowing include eosinophilic pneumonia, vasculitis, alveolar haemorrhage, EGPA, HP, cryptogenic organizing pneumonia (COP), allergic bronchopulmonary aspergillosis (ABPA), and pulmonary oedema
- Cough may occur, although its diagnostic value is uncertain; it may be a prominent symptom in IPF, lymphangitis carcinomatosis, HP, OP, sarcoid, and eosinophilic pneumonia. Chronic production of purulent sputum suggests bronchiectasis. Bronchorrhoea (production of large volumes of sputum) may occur with bronchoalveolar cell carcinoma. Haemoptysis suggests alveolar haemorrhage, malignancy, or pulmonary venous hypertension
- Wheeze may occur in asthma associated with eosinophilic pneumonia or EGPA
- Weight loss and fever are non-specific symptoms associated with many diffuse lung diseases.

Other medical conditions, e.g. malignancy, connective tissue disease, HIV infection, other immunosuppression.

Drugs

- Common drug causes of diffuse lung disease are listed in Table 6.1; refer to ℅ http://www.pneumotox.com for a comprehensive database
- Delays of months, or even years, may occur between starting the drug and developing lung involvement
- Illicit drug abuse (crack cocaine or heroin—pulmonary oedema, eosinophilic pneumonitis, diffuse alveolar haemorrhage, interstitial pneumonia; IV drug use—IV talcosis, septic emboli)
- Oily nose drops (lipoid pneumonia).

Occupation, lifestyle, hobbies, and pets

- May involve inhalation of inorganic or organic dusts. Document lifelong employment history, including probable exposure levels, use of protective equipment, and names of employers
- Inorganic dusts associated with development of diffuse lung disease include asbestos, silica, cobalt, beryllium, aluminium, isocyanates, copper sulfate, iron, tin, barium, and antimony
- HP may result from inhalation of organic dusts, such as *Thermoactinomyces* in mouldy hay (farmer's lung), avian proteins or feathers (bird fancier's lung), mushroom compost, mouldy cheese, cork or sugar cane, and isocyanates
- Risk factors for immunocompromise (opportunistic infection, LIP, lymphoma)
- Smoking history (LCH, RB-ILD, DIP, and anti-GBM disease are more common in smokers).

Evidence of extrapulmonary disease
Manifestations of connective tissue disease, vasculitis, sarcoidosis, e.g. arthralgia, skin rash or thickening, ocular symptoms, muscular pain and weakness, Raynaud's, nasal/sinus disease, sicca symptoms, haematuria. Infertility in ♂ (immotile cilia syndrome, cystic fibrosis).

Travel
TB, pulmonary eosinophilia from parasites (tropics), histoplasmosis (north and central USA, parts of South America and Africa), hydatid disease (Middle East, Australasia, Mediterranean).

Family history
α1-antitrypsin (α1-AT) deficiency, rare familial forms of usual interstitial pneumonitis (UIP), and sarcoidosis.

Examination
• Cyanosis and signs of cor pulmonale in severe disease
• Clubbing (IPF, asbestosis, bronchiectasis)
• Basal crackles (IPF, asbestosis, connective tissue disease, pulmonary oedema, lymphangitis, drugs); crackles in bronchiectasis are characteristically coarse
• Absence of crackles, despite a significant CXR abnormality, may be suggestive of sarcoidosis, pneumoconiosis, HP, or LCH
• Squeaks suggest the presence of bronchiolitis and may occur in skin, joint, and eye disease (connective tissue disease, sarcoidosis, vasculitis).

Imaging
CXR
An essential test although rarely diagnostic. Up to 10% of patients with biopsy-proven diffuse lung disease have a normal CXR. Previous CXRs are helpful in assessing disease duration and progression.

Chest HRCT is more sensitive and specific than CXR for diagnosing diffuse lung disease (for HRCT diagnosis, see ➔ Appendix 4). HRCT is often, in itself, diagnostic and should always precede biopsy in the investigation of diffuse lung disease. HRCT also enables assessment of disease extent and optimal biopsy site, if required. HRCT appearance correlates to some extent with disease activity in the interstitial pneumonias: a predominantly 'ground-glass' appearance may signify a steroid-responsive inflammatory state, whereas reticulation and honeycombing are often associated with fibrosis, poor response to treatment, and a worse prognosis.

HRCT diagnosis

HRCT (and, to a limited extent, CXR) appearances can be classified, according to the pattern and distribution of disease and the presence of additional features (see also Appendix 4).

Imaging pattern

Reticular (or linear) pattern

Causes include:
- Interstitial pulmonary oedema
- UIP (reticular shadowing is typically patchy, subpleural, and basal; other features include loss of architecture of 2° pulmonary lobules, honeycombing, traction bronchiectasis)
- Asbestosis (similar features to UIP, often with pleural plaques)
- Connective tissue disease associated fibrosis (similar features to UIP)
- Chronic HP (often associated with regions of ground-glass change, air trapping on expiration, and centrilobular micronodules)
- Drug-induced fibrosis
- Sarcoidosis.

Nodular pattern

Consists of numerous discrete, round opacities 0.1–1 cm in diameter.
- Interstitial processes result in nodularity within interlobular septa, around bronchovascular bundles, and sub-pleurally (e.g. sarcoidosis, which may demonstrate associated perihilar reticular shadowing and lymphadenopathy)
- Airspace diseases may lead to affected acini becoming visible as nodules (e.g. HP, miliary TB, COP, malignancy).

Ground-glass change

An increase in lung density through which pulmonary vasculature is still visible (compare the lung density with that of air within the bronchi). May occur as a result of airspace or interstitial disease and may be patchy or diffuse. Causes include:
- Pulmonary oedema or haemorrhage, ARDS
- HP
- Drugs
- Certain IIPs (NSIP, RB-ILD, DIP, AIP)
- *Pneumocystis jirovecii* pneumonia (PCP)
- Sarcoidosis
- Bronchoalveolar cell carcinoma
- Alveolar proteinosis.

Ground-glass

Appearance may be artefactual, the increased density resulting from breath-holding during expiration. It may also be confused with 'mosaic perfusion' where densities vary in different regions of the lung as a result of either variable perfusion (e.g. in chronic thromboembolic disease) or gas trapping (small airways disease).

Consolidation

Also known as airspace shadowing, it is an increase in attenuation, characterized by air bronchograms (air-filled bronchi superimposed against opacified alveoli) and the loss of visibility of adjacent vessels. It occurs as disease processes infiltrate and fill alveolar airspaces, e.g. with water, blood, pus, malignant cells, or fibrous tissue. Causes include:

- Pneumonia
- Pulmonary oedema or haemorrhage, ARDS
- Drugs
- OP
- Bronchoalveolar cell carcinoma, lymphoma
- Other rare conditions (e.g. eosinophilic pneumonia, alveolar proteinosis).

Cystic change

Refers to well-defined airspaces with a thin wall. Causes include:

- LCH (bizarrely shaped cysts and nodules, apical predominance)
- UIP (subpleural honeycombing)
- PCP
- LIP
- Septic emboli
- LAM (thin-walled cysts, otherwise normal lung)
- Centrilobular emphysema may simulate cystic disease, but there is absence of a well-defined wall.

Interlobular septal thickening

Occurs as a result of processes affecting the lymphatics or venules within interlobular septa such as:

- Pulmonary oedema (smooth thickening)
- Lymphangitis carcinomatosis (irregular, nodular thickening of interlobular septa and bronchovascular bundles, no architectural distortion)
- Sarcoidosis
- UIP.

Imaging distribution

- Upper zone: silicosis, pneumoconiosis, chronic sarcoidosis, HP, ankylosing spondylitis, TB, LCH
- Lower zone: UIP, connective tissue diseases, asbestosis
- Mid-zone: sarcoidosis, pulmonary oedema, PCP
- Peripheral: UIP, eosinophilic pneumonia, drugs (amiodarone), COP
- Sharp borders: radiation pneumonitis.

Additional imaging features

- Lymphadenopathy: sarcoidosis, lymphoma, malignancy, infection, silicosis, berylliosis, LIP
- Pleural effusion/involvement: pulmonary oedema, connective tissue diseases, infection, malignancy, asbestosis, drugs, LAM.

Further investigations

Urine and blood tests

Consider the following investigations:

- Urine dipstick and microscopy for detection of renal disease associated with vasculitis/connective tissue disease
- Erythrocyte sedimentation rate (ESR), C-reactive protein (CRP), full blood count (FBC) (look specifically at the eosinophil count), renal and liver function, CK (?myositis), calcium (increased in >10% of patients with sarcoidosis)
- Autoantibodies (RhF, ANA, ENAs (Ro, La, RNP, Scl-70, Jo-1, Sm))
- ANCA (vasculitis), anti-GBM (Goodpasture's syndrome)
- Serum precipitins (to antigens in HP; poor specificity)
- Serum ACE levels may be increased in sarcoidosis, but this is a non-specific and relatively insensitive test and is unhelpful diagnostically
- HIV testing.

Sputum

- Cytology may be diagnostic in bronchoalveolar cell carcinoma
- Induced sputum may be useful in the diagnosis of PCP and TB.

PFTs

- Useful in assessing progression and severity of disease and response to treatment, but often unhelpful diagnostically
- Typically show restrictive pattern with reduced vital capacity (VC) and transfer factor. Normal values do not exclude mild, early lung disease
- Obstructive pattern rare but may be seen in sarcoidosis, LCH, and LAM; may see mixed picture if coexisting COPD
- Transfer factor may be increased transiently (days) in alveolar haemorrhage. Reduced transfer factor with preserved lung volumes is suggestive of pulmonary vascular disease (pulmonary arterial hypertension or vasculitis) or coexistent emphysema
- Disease progression and response to treatment are best assessed by serial measurements of vital capacity and transfer factor
- Check O_2 saturation and consider ABGs. A fall in O_2 saturation on simple exercise may be tested for in the clinic setting and is a useful clue to underlying lung disease in patients with normal saturation and lung function at rest and an unremarkable CXR.

Cardiac investigations

- *Electrocardiogram (ECG)* Conduction abnormality in sarcoidosis; cardiogenic pulmonary oedema is unusual in the presence of a completely normal ECG
- *Echocardiogram* Assess LV and valvular function if cardiac pulmonary oedema suspected and measure pulmonary arterial pressure (PAP) (e.g. in scleroderma or suspected pulmonary veno-occlusive disease). The presence of a tricuspid regurgitation jet is required in order to assess PAP on echo.

BAL

- Most useful in diagnosis of opportunistic infection (bacterial or fungal pneumonia, TB, PCP), eosinophilic pneumonia, malignancy, alveolar proteinosis, and alveolar haemorrhage
- BAL differential cell counts usually unhelpful diagnostically, although BAL lymphocytosis is typical of HP, sarcoidosis, and LIP, and eosinophilic BAL occurs in eosinophilic pneumonia or drug-induced lung disease.

Lung biopsy

Which patients need a lung biopsy?

In cases of uncertain aetiology, despite clinical assessment and HRCT, lung biopsies often provide a definitive diagnosis. Ideally, they should be taken before treatment is started. The decision to biopsy varies among clinicians and should take into account the individual patient's clinical condition and wishes, and the likely benefit of a definitive diagnosis in terms of predicting treatment response and prognosis. Some take a pragmatic approach when a diagnosis (or group of diagnoses with the same treatment) is likely, but not biopsy-proven, and treat empirically. In some cases, the patient may be too unwell for biopsy and require empirical treatment. Lung biopsy is not usually recommended in patients with typical clinical and HRCT features of IPF, and biopsy of end-stage fibrosis is in general unhelpful in eliciting an underlying aetiology.

Biopsy techniques

TBB provides small samples but relatively high diagnostic yield in diseases with a 'centrilobular' distribution, e.g. sarcoidosis, HP, malignancy, infection (fungi, TB), and OP. Take 4–6 samples. Additional endobronchial biopsies may be diagnostic in sarcoidosis.

Open lung biopsy via thoracotomy or video-assisted thoracoscopic (VATS) biopsy provides larger samples than TBB and have diagnostic yields of at least 90%. Both require general anaesthesia. VATS probably has a lower morbidity and is generally preferred in stable patients; open biopsy is required in ventilator-dependent patients. Open or VATS biopsy is required for histological confirmation of IIPs, vasculitis, lymphoma, LAM, and LCH—the yield of TBB in these conditions is very low.

Percutaneous image-guided biopsy may be useful in the diagnosis of well-localized and dense peripheral infiltrates. A cutting needle biopsy technique is best and, if the lesion(s) abuts the pleural surface, pneumothorax is uncommon.

Diffuse lung disease presenting with acute respiratory failure

The management of patients presenting with diffuse lung disease—particularly ILD—and acute respiratory failure is challenging. These patients are often critically ill with rapidly progressive disease, and a variety of diverse conditions can underlie the typically non-specific presentation with breathlessness, hypoxia, raised inflammatory markers, and diffuse ground-glass infiltrates on HRCT. There is little evidence to guide management, which needs to be on a case-by-case basis. Assessment is largely as outlined earlier in this chapter but with particular emphasis on prompt identification and treatment of reversible causes and early consideration of appropriate ceilings of care/ICU admission.

Causes/differential diagnosis

- Diffuse infection (community-acquired pneumonia (CAP)—including 'atypical', PCP, other fungi, viral, TB)
- LVF
- ARDS
- Drug-induced pneumonitis
- Diffuse alveolar haemorrhage/vasculitis
- Fulminant OP
- AIP
- Acute exacerbation of previously subclinical IPF
- Acute HP
- Acute eosinophilic pneumonia
- Malignancy.

Key points in assessment and treatment

- Have a low threshold for treating *infection*, which, in practice, is difficult to distinguish from many non-infectious causes. Consider PCP. Subacute presentations of infection, such as fungal disease or TB, may rarely mimic ILD
- Look for evidence of *extrapulmonary disease*, particularly involving kidneys (urine dipstick and microscopy), heart, eyes, ENT, skin, muscles, joints. Active disease in these sites may, in some cases, provide a safer biopsy target than the lungs, if histology is required
- Actively consider *drug-induced* lung disease (see ℘ http://www.pneumotox.com): review current and previous medications carefully, and discontinue potentially offending drugs
- *Bloods* FBC (?eosinophilia), renal and liver function, CRP, ESR, CK, urgent immunology (RhF, ANA, ENA profile—including antisynthetase antibodies (anti-Jo-1 (see ➋ p. 220), ANCA (vasculitis), anti-GBM, serum precipitins (to antigens in HP)), HIV testing
- The presence of an antisynthetase antibody, in combination with one or more of interstitial pneumonitis, myositis, and arthritis, is characteristic of *antisynthetase* syndrome. Fever, Raynaud's phenomenon, and mechanic's hands (thick, cracked skin on palms and fingers) may also occur, or pneumonitis may be the sole clinical manifestation. Check anti-Jo-1, which may be positive in myositis-associated acute pneumonitis,

even in the setting of a negative ANA. Other antisynthetase antibodies, such as anti-PL-7 and anti-PL-12, and anti-CADM-140 may underlie rapidly progressive pneumonitis, with or without myositis, but are not yet routinely available
- Consider *echo* to assess LV and valvular function if cardiac pulmonary oedema suspected
- Further *imaging* PE may coexist with ILD, and CTPA with HRCT slices is usually the radiological investigation of choice
- *BAL* is useful in excluding infection but may decompensate seriously ill, hypoxic patients; it is often safer to wait and perform after patients are ventilated. TBBs may increase diagnostic yield, but risk probably outweighs benefit in the majority of patients. *Surgical lung biopsy* may yield a diagnosis that alters management in carefully selected individuals, particularly those with *de novo* lung disease. It can be performed in the ICU on mechanically ventilated patients
- Consider empirical high-dose *steroids* (e.g. IV methylprednisolone 750 mg–1 g on 3 consecutive days, followed by maintenance therapy with 0.5–1 mg/kg/day prednisolone). Fulminant COP is frequently steroid-responsive, and, although robust evidence is lacking, the outcome in AIP may be more favourable following early use of high-dose steroids. Assess the response to steroids over 5–7 days, and then consider further *immunosuppression*, particularly if there is any suggestion of underlying connective tissue disease: IV cyclophosphamide 600–650 mg/m^2 is usually favoured because of relatively rapid onset (often <1 week), with mesna protection against bladder toxicity if total dose exceeds 1 g; a second dose can be given 7–10 days later (depending upon white blood count) or 2-weekly. Empirical 'upfront' treatment with cyclophosphamide, alongside initial IV methylprednisolone, increases the infection risk but may be indicated in severe disease or in suspected severe vasculitis/GPA. Rituximab (a monoclonal antibody that targets peripheral B lymphocytes) or tacrolimus may be of benefit in severely ill patients with connective tissue disease-associated interstitial pneumonitis, particularly antisynthetase syndrome
- Consider *ceiling of care*. High-flow O_2 is almost always needed, and ICU admission and mechanical ventilatory support are usually required. ICU admission is usually appropriate for patients with *de novo* ILD, and it is appropriate to support patients with mechanical ventilation while awaiting a possible response to steroids/immunosuppression. NB: mechanical ventilation is usually considered an absolute contraindication to lung transplantation in the UK. The outcome of mechanical ventilation in patients with IPF is typically very poor, and ICU admission is rarely appropriate in the setting of underlying IPF/extensive fibrotic change.

Further information

British Thoracic Society. Interstitial lung disease guideline. *Thorax* 2008;**63**(suppl. V): v1–v58.

Haemoptysis

Clinical assessment and causes *44*
Investigations *46*

Clinical assessment and causes

Haemoptysis is a common and non-specific symptom and can be a sign of significant underlying lung disease. However, in up to one-third of cases, no cause is found. An early assessment of the likely underlying cause needs to be made and investigations planned accordingly.

Diagnostic approach to haemoptysis

Small-volume haemoptysis is a commonly encountered problem in the outpatient department. It can be safely and efficiently investigated as an outpatient. Massive haemoptysis is usually encountered in the accident and emergency department or in a patient already on the ward with known underlying lung disease. The approaches to small-volume and massive haemoptysis are different.

History

- Past history of lung disease?
- Document volume of blood and whether old (altered) or fresh
- Time course (intermittent, constant)
- Definitely from the airway, and not from the nose or mouth, or haematemesis? (haemoptysis may be swallowed and then vomited)
- Presence of systemic features—associated infection, symptoms consistent with underlying malignancy or vasculitis?

Examination

May be normal or show signs of underlying lung disease, e.g. bronchiectasis, bronchial carcinoma, or symptoms of circulatory collapse.

Causes of haemoptysis

Common

- Bronchial tumour (benign, e.g. carcinoid, or malignant). Haemoptysis is a common presenting feature of bronchogenic malignancy, indicating endobronchial disease, which is usually visible endoscopically
- Bronchiectasis and CF (see ⊃ p. 169). Small-volume haemoptysis is a common feature of bronchiectasis, particularly during exacerbations. It can be a cause of massive haemoptysis from dilated and abnormal bronchial artery branches that form around bronchiectatic cavities
- Active TB. Haemoptysis occurs in cavitating and non-cavitating disease, active disease and inactive disease (e.g. from an old bronchiectatic cavity, which might contain a mycetoma)
- Pneumonia (especially pneumococcal disease)
- Pulmonary thromboembolic disease
- Vasculitides/alveolar haemorrhage syndromes, e.g. GPA (formerly Wegener's), SLE, anti-GBM disease (Goodpasture's syndrome)
- Anticoagulants with any of the above causes.

Rare
- Lung abscess
- Mycetoma
- Fungal/viral/parasitic infections
- Fat embolism
- Foreign body
- Pulmonary endometriosis
- Arteriovenous malformation (AVM), e.g. in hereditary haemorrhagic telangiectasia (HHT) (see ⊃ p. 512)
- Severe pulmonary hypertension (see ⊃ p. 449)
- Mitral stenosis
- Congenital heart disease
- Aortic aneurysm
- *Aspergillus*—invasive fungal disease (intracavity mycetoma) can be a cause of massive haemoptysis
- Coagulopathy, including DIC
- Endometriosis
- Pulmonary hemosiderosis
- Pseudoaneurysm post-aortic surgery
- Iatrogenic, e.g. post-lung biopsy, bronchoscopy.

Investigations

The investigation of small-volume haemoptysis can be carried out as an out-patient, but patients with significant bleeding or a likely serious underlying cause should be admitted if there is clinical concern. Note: beware of the apparently small bleed, which is a sentinel/herald bleed for massive haemoptysis. This is fortunately rare. Massive haemoptysis is more likely to be from a bronchial artery bleed (at systemic pressure) than from a pulmonary artery bleed (low pressure). See Box 7.1.

Outpatient investigations and management

First-line investigations

- *Blood tests* Full blood count, clotting, group and save. If systemic vasculitis is suspected, renal function and a urine dip, with microscopy for casts, are necessary, as well as autoantibodies—start with antinuclear cytoplasmic antibody (ANCA), anti-GBM, and antinuclear antibody (ANA)
- *Sputum* MC&S and acid-fast bacillus (AFB) if infection suspected
- *CXR* may show mass lesion, bronchiectasis, consolidation, or an AVM
- *CT chest* should be done prior to bronchoscopy; prior knowledge of site of abnormality leads to increased pick-up at bronchoscopy. Similarly, a definitive diagnosis, e.g. AVM, may be made from the CT, obviating the need for further investigations. This depends on local resources; CT may miss an upper airway lesion, but bronchoscopy should not. Bronchial artery dilatation may be large enough to be visible on CT with contrast
- *Bronchoscopy* to visualize the airways and localize the site of bleeding. May also be therapeutic, e.g. if a bleeding tumour can be injected with a vasoconstricting agent (adrenaline) or a catheter inserted for tamponade (see Box 7.1)
- *TBB*—if vasculitis suspected.

Second-line investigations

Usually done if first-line investigations fail to demonstrate a cause.
- *Computed tomographic pulmonary angiogram (CTPA)* to exclude PE. Bronchial artery dilatation may be large enough to be visible on a CTPA
- *Bronchial angiogram* Diagnostic and therapeutic. Rare for the actual bleeding site to be identified; more often, the bleeding site is assumed from visualizing a mesh of dilated and tortuous vessels, e.g. around a bronchiectatic cavity. Usually done during an episode of bleeding to maximize the chance of identifying the site of bleeding
- *Bronchial artery embolization* Therapeutic approach to embolize the bleeding artery, usually with coils or glue (specialist centre only). There is a small risk of paraplegia (<1%) if the anterior spinal artery originates from the bronchial arterial circulation and is inadvertently embolized
- *ENT review* The source of the bleeding may be the upper airway
- *Echo* Moderate/severe PHT can cause haemoptysis, especially in a patient on anticoagulants.

Cryptogenic haemoptysis

In about one-third of cases, despite appropriate investigations as described previously, no cause for the haemoptysis can be found. This has a good prognosis. Often the haemoptysis will settle without treatment and will become less worrying to the patient over time, especially as investigations have failed to determine the cause.

▶▶ Box 7.1 Management of massive haemoptysis

Massive haemoptysis (>100 mL blood in 24 h) is a life-threatening emergency, with a mortality of up to 80%. It is extremely distressing for the patient, relatives, and medical staff but is fortunately rare. Investigations will follow treatment, which may be difficult, and is often unsuccessful. In some cases, active treatment may be inappropriate, and palliative treatment with O_2 and opiates may be warranted.

- Airway protection and ventilation:
  - Protection of the non-bleeding lung is vital to maintain adequate gas exchange. This may involve either sitting the patient up or lying on the bleeding side (to prevent blood from flowing into the unaffected lung), or intubation with a double-lumen tube. If intubation is not needed or not appropriate, give high-flow O_2
- Cardiovascular support:
  - Large-bore/central intravenous (IV) access
  - Cross-match blood
  - Fluid resuscitation ± transfusion
  - Correct clotting, e.g. vitamin K 10 mg od; give platelets
  - Inotropes may be required
- Nebulized adrenaline (1 mL of 1:1,000 made up to 5 mL with NaCl 0.9%)
- Oral or IV tranexamic acid (1 g tds, not if in severe renal failure)
- IV terlipressin, 2 mg IV, then 1–2 mg every 4–6 h if continued bleeding
- CXR ± chest CT (depending on stability of patient)
- Early bronchoscopy—diagnostic and therapeutic
- Rigid bronchoscopy (with general anaesthesia) is preferable. May allow localization of the site of bleeding; balloon tamponade with a Fogarty catheter
- Bronchial artery embolization—therapeutic approach to embolize bleeding artery, usually with coils or glue (specialist centre only)
- Surgery—resection of bleeding lobe (if all other measures have failed).

Pleural effusion

Clinical assessment 50
Transudative pleural effusions 54
Exudative pleural effusions 56
Pleural fluid analysis 1 58
Pleural fluid analysis 2 60

Clinical assessment

Pleural effusion is a common presentation of a wide range of different diseases. Commonest causes in the UK and USA (in order): cardiac failure, pneumonia, malignancy, pulmonary embolus (PE).

Priority is to make a diagnosis and relieve symptoms, with minimum number of invasive procedures. The majority of patients do not require a chest drain and can be managed as outpatients. Procedures, such as therapeutic thoracentesis, may be performed readily on a day unit. Consider admission and chest drain insertion for:

- Patients with malignant effusions who are candidates for pleurodesis
- Empyema (pus) or complicated parapneumonic effusion (pleural fluid pH <7.2)—the majority of these effusions are unlikely to resolve without drainage and antibiotics
- Patients who are unwell with an acute massive effusion.

Key steps in the management of the patient with a pleural effusion follow and are also detailed in the diagnostic algorithm in Fig. 8.1.

History, examination, chest radiograph (CXR), and pleural ultrasound (US)

Including a drug history (see ✒ http://pneumotox.com).

Does the patient have an obvious cause for transudative effusions?

For example, heart failure, hypoalbuminaemia, dialysis. If so, this should be treated, with no need for thoracentesis unless atypical features (such as very asymmetrical bilateral effusions, unilateral effusion, echogenicity/septations/nodularity on pleural US, chest pain, or fever) or failure to respond to therapy.

Thoracentesis ('pleural tap'/pleural fluid aspiration)

May be diagnostic and/or therapeutic, depending on the volume of fluid removed. See ➲ p. 892 for procedure details and ➲ p. 58 for pleural fluid analysis. Following diagnostic tap:

- Note pleural fluid *appearance*
- Send sample to biochemistry for measurement of *glucose, protein, and lactate dehydrogenase (LDH)*
- Send a fresh 20–30 mL sample in sterile pot to *cytology* for examination for malignant cells (yield ~60% in malignancy) and differential cell count
- Send samples in sterile pot to *microbiology* for Gram stain and microscopy, culture. For suspected pleural infection, also send pleural fluid in blood culture bottles. Low threshold for acid-fast bacillus (AFB) stain and tuberculosis (TB) culture
- Process non-purulent, heparinized samples in ABG analyser for *pH*
- Consider measurement of cholesterol, triglycerides, chylomicrons, haematocrit, adenosine deaminase, and amylase, depending on the clinical circumstances.

If the patient is breathless, they may benefit from removal of a larger volume of fluid (therapeutic thoracentesis, see ➲ p. 894).

Is the pleural effusion a transudate or an exudate?

Helpful in narrowing the differential diagnosis. In patients with a normal serum protein, pleural fluid protein <30 g/L = transudate, and protein >40 g/L = exudate. In borderline cases (protein 30–40 g/L) or in patients with abnormal serum protein, apply Light's criteria—effusion is exudative if it meets one of following criteria:

- Pleural fluid protein/serum protein ratio >0.5
- Pleural fluid LDH/serum LDH ratio >0.6
- Pleural fluid LDH > two-thirds the upper limit of normal serum LDH.

These criteria are very sensitive in the diagnosis of exudative effusions although may occasionally falsely identify transudates as being exudates, e.g. patients with partially treated heart failure on diuretics may be misidentified as exudates. N-terminal pro-brain natriuretic peptide (NT-proBNP) in pleural fluid or blood may be of use in these cases. Similarly, a total protein gradient (serum-pleural fluid total protein) >31 g/L is suggestive of heart failure.

Further investigations if diagnosis remains unclear

- CT chest with pleural phase contrast (ideally scan prior to complete fluid drainage to improve images of pleural surfaces; useful in distinguishing benign and malignant pleural disease, see ➜ p. 402). Consider CT pulmonary angiography if PE possible, particularly when other tests fail to provide a diagnosis
- Further pleural fluid analysis (see ➜ p. 60), e.g. cholesterol, triglyceride, chylomicrons, haematocrit, adenosine deaminase, amylase, fungal stains. Consider repeat cytology testing
- Pleural tissue biopsy for histology and TB culture using image-guided or thoracoscopic biopsies. These techniques are superior to Abrams' closed pleural biopsy for malignant disease and TB (thoracoscopy has sensitivity of ~100% for TB and >90% for malignancy and allows therapeutic talc pleurodesis at the same time). Use Abrams' biopsy only when TB is strongly suspected and thoracoscopy not available
- Reconsider PE and TB.

Bronchoscopy has no role in investigating undiagnosed effusions, unless the patient has haemoptysis or a CXR/CT pulmonary abnormality. Pleural fluid may compress the airways and limit bronchoscopic views, and so, if bronchoscopy is indicated, it is best performed following drainage of the effusion.

Further information

Light RW. Pleural effusion. *N Engl J Med* 2002;**346**: 1971–7.
Hooper C et al. Investigation of a unilateral pleural effusion in adults: British Thoracic Society pleural disease guideline 2010. *Thorax* 2010;**65**(Suppl. 2): ii4–17.

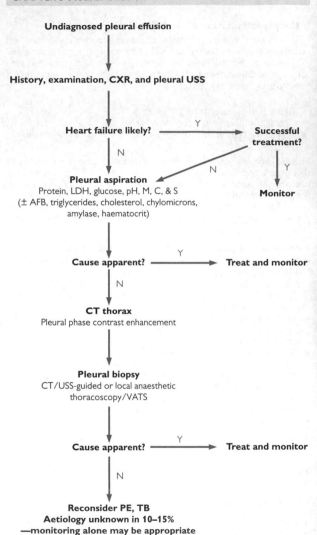

Fig. 8.1 Diagnostic algorithm for the patient with a pleural effusion.

Transudative pleural effusions

Mechanisms

Involve either increased hydrostatic pressure or reduced osmotic pressure (due to hypoalbuminaemia) in the microvascular circulation.

Differential diagnosis

See Table 8.1.

Treatment

Directed at the underlying cause; consider further investigation if failure to respond.

Table 8.1 Causes of transudative pleural effusions

Cause	Notes
Common	
LVF	Investigate further if atypical features (very asymmetrical bilateral effusions, unilateral effusion, chest pain, fever); may be complicated by PE (up to 1/5 of cases at autopsy)
Atelectasis	Common on intensive therapy unit (ITU) or post-operatively (also, hypoalbuminaemia); usually small effusion, may be bilateral; rarely needs investigation
Cirrhotic liver disease ('hepatic hydrothorax')	Ascites often, but not invariably, present; majority right-sided; remove ascites and treat hypoalbuminaemia (see ⊃ p. 306)
Hypoalbuminaemia	
Peritoneal dialysis	Pleural fluid analysis resembles dialysis fluid, with protein <10 g/L and glucose >17 mmol/L
PE	10–20% are transudates (see ⊃ p. 467)
Nephrotic syndrome	Usually bilateral; consider 2° PE if atypical features
Less common	
Constrictive pericarditis	May be unilateral or bilateral
Hypothyroidism	May be transudate or exudate; pleural effusions occur most commonly in association with ascites, pericardial effusion, and cardiac failure, although may be an isolated finding
Malignancy	Up to 5% are transudates
Meigs' syndrome	Unilateral (often right-sided) or bilateral pleural effusions and ascites; occurs in women with ovarian or other pelvic tumours; resolves following removal of tumour
Mitral stenosis	
Urinothorax	Effusion ipsilateral to obstructed kidney with retroperitoneal urine leak, resolves after treatment of obstruction; pleural fluid smells of urine, pH usually low; pleural fluid creatinine > serum creatinine is diagnostic

Exudative pleural effusions

Mechanisms
Involve an increase in capillary permeability and impaired pleural fluid resorption.

Differential diagnosis
See Table 8.2.

Table 8.2 Causes of exudative pleural effusions

Cause	Notes
Common	
Simple parapneumonic effusion (SPPE)	Occurs in 40% of bacterial pneumonias; commonest exudative effusion in young patients (see ➲ p. 518)
Malignancy	Commonest exudative effusion in patients >60y (see ➲ p. 337)
TB	Typically lymphocytic effusion; pleural fluid AFB smear positive in <5% of cases, culture positive in 10–20%, thoracoscopic biopsy histology sensitivity ~100% (see ➲ p. 588). Adenosine deaminase may be a useful 'rule out' test.
Less common	
Complicated parapneumonic effusion (CPPE) and empyema	CPPE defined by pleural fluid pH <7.2 and clinical features of infection, e.g. fever, sweats (see ➲ p. 412); empyema defined by pleural pus
Other infections	Rare; include viral, parasitic, rickettsial, and fungal (e.g. *Aspergillus*, histoplasma, coccidioidomycosis)
PE	80–90% are exudates (see ➲ p. 467)
Rheumatoid arthritis (RA)	Typically low pleural fluid glucose, often <1.6 mmol/L (see ➲ p. 216)
Systemic lupus erythematosus (SLE)	Lupus erythematosus cells in fluid are diagnostic; may respond quickly to prednisolone
Other autoimmune diseases	Eosinophilic granulomatosis with polyangiitis (Churg–Strauss syndrome; intensely eosinophilic fluid), Sjögren's syndrome, scleroderma, dermatomyositis, GPA (Wegener's)
Sarcoidosis	Effusions uncommon
Hepatic, splenic, or subphrenic abscess	
Oesophageal rupture	Initially sterile exudate, followed by empyema; pH <7.2, ↑ salivary amylase, often history of vomiting
Pancreatitis	Pleural fluid pancreatic amylase may be raised
Post-cardiac injury syndrome (Dressler's syndrome) and post-CABG surgery	Pleural effusions common; may be bloodstained (see ➲ p. 423)

(Continued)

Table 8.2 (*Contd.*)

Radiotherapy	May cause small, unilateral effusions up to 6 months after treatment
Uraemia	Effusions frequently resolve after starting dialysis
Chylothorax	Associated with lymphoma, trauma and surgery. Presence of chylomicrons or pleural fluid triglyceride level >1.24 mmol/L (see ⊃ p. 60)
Benign asbestos-related pleural effusion	(See ⊃ p. 126)
Drug-induced	Drugs include amiodarone, β-blockers, bromocriptine, methotrexate, nitrofurantoin, and phenytoin; see ℰ http://www.pneumotox.com for full list; effusions usually resolve following discontinuation of drug
Other, rare causes	Include yellow nail syndrome, cryptogenic organizing pneumonia (COP), amyloidosis, familial Mediterranean fever

Treatment

Involves treatment of the underlying cause, as well as measures to improve breathlessness and remove pleural fluid, e.g. therapeutic thoracentesis (see ⊃ p. 894), intercostal drainage (see ⊃ p. 851), and pleurodesis (see ⊃ p. 875).

Pleural fluid analysis 1

'Routine' pleural fluid analysis comprises assessment of:
- Pleural fluid appearance and other characteristics (see Table 8.3)
- Biochemistry (glucose, protein, and LDH)
- pH measured using a heparinized syringe in a blood gas analyser
- Cytology (for malignant cells and differential cell count (see Table 8.4); ideally fresh 20–30 mL sample)
- Microbiology (Gram stain and culture). Also send blood culture bottles, each inoculated with 5 mL of pleural fluid, if pleural infection likely (increases yield). Low threshold for AFB stain and TB culture

Although considered routine, some of these investigations may be unnecessary, and even misleading, depending on the clinical picture (e.g. microbiological analysis on patients suspected as having transudates).

Additional pleural fluid investigations, such as measurement of cholesterol and triglycerides, haematocrit, glucose, adenosine deaminase, and amylase, may be helpful in certain clinical circumstances.

Table 8.3 Relevance of pleural fluid characteristics

Characteristics	Possible causes
Bloody	Trauma, malignancy, pulmonary infarction, pneumonia, post-cardiac injury syndrome, pneumothorax, benign asbestos-related pleural effusion, aortic dissection/rupture; defined as haemothorax if pleural fluid haematocrit >50% of peripheral blood haematocrit (see ➔ p. 422)
Turbid or milky	Empyema, chylothorax, pseudochylothorax (clear supernatant after centrifuging favours empyema; cloudy after centrifuging suggests chylothorax or pseudochylothorax, see ➔ p. 60)
Viscous	Mesothelioma
Food particles	Oesophageal rupture
Bile-stained	Cholothorax (biliary fistula)
Black	*Aspergillus* infection, metastatic melanoma
Brown, 'anchovy sauce'	Amoebic liver abscess draining into pleural space
Urine odour	Urinothorax
Putrid odour	Anaerobic empyema

Table 8.4 Relevance of pleural fluid differential cell count

Predominant cell type	Possible causes
Neutrophils	Any acute effusion, e.g. parapneumonic, PE
Mononuclear cells	Any chronic effusion, e.g. malignancy, TB
Lymphocytes	TB, especially if >80%; other causes include cardiac failure, malignancy, sarcoidosis, lymphoma, rheumatoid pleurisy, post-CABG, chylothorax
Eosinophils	Often unhelpful; associations include air or blood in pleural space (haemothorax, pulmonary infarct, pneumothorax, previous tap), malignancy, infection (parapneumonic, tuberculous, fungal, parasitic), drug- and asbestos-Induced effusions, EGPA (Churg–Strauss syndrome), or idiopathic
Mesothelial cells	Predominate in transudates; variable numbers in exudates, typically suppressed in inflammatory conditions, e.g. TB. Atypical mesothelial cells may suggest malignancy
Lupus erythematosus cells	Diagnostic of SLE

Pleural fluid analysis 2

Pleural fluid pH and glucose

Pleural fluid pH may be measured using an arterial blood pH analyser. The sample should be appropriately heparinized, e.g. aspirate a few mL of pleural fluid into a pre-heparinized blood gas syringe. Pleural fluid pH is affected by exposure to air (increases pH) or local anaesthetic (decreases pH). Frankly purulent samples should not be analysed—it is unnecessary and might damage the machine.

Normal pleural fluid pH is about 7.6. An abnormally low pH (<7.3) suggests pleural inflammation/infection and is often associated with a low pleural fluid glucose (<3.3 mmol/L or pleural fluid/serum glucose ratio <0.5). The mechanism probably involves increased neutrophil phagocytosis and bacterial or tumour cell breakdown, resulting in the accumulation of lactate and CO_2.

Causes of low pH and low glucose effusions
- CPPE and empyema (pH <7.2 indication for drainage of pleural space, as unlikely to resolve spontaneously; this is not an absolute cut-off—values can vary in each locule of a multiloculated effusion)
- Rheumatoid pleuritis (glucose <1.7 mmol/L in 66% and <2.8 mmol/L in 80% of cases)
- Malignant pleural effusion (associated with advanced disease and poor survival, higher sensitivity of pleural fluid cytological analysis, and failure of pleurodesis)
- Tuberculous pleural effusion
- Oesophageal rupture
- Lupus pleuritis.

Urinothorax is the only transudative effusion that can cause a pH <7.3. An abnormally high (alkaline) pH may rarely occur in the setting of *Proteus* pleural infection.

Pleural fluid triglyceride and cholesterol

Measure in turbid or milky effusions or where chylothorax is suspected.

Chylothorax occurs following disruption of the thoracic duct, and pleural fluid may appear turbid, milky, serous, or bloodstained. The presence of pleural fluid chylomicrons or a pleural fluid triglyceride level >1.24 mmol/L confirms the diagnosis. Causes of chylothorax:
- Trauma or following thoracotomy
- Malignancy (particularly lymphoma)
- Pulmonary lymphangioleiomyomatosis (LAM)
- TB.

Pseudochylothorax

Occurs due to cholesterol crystal deposition in chronic effusions, most commonly due to rheumatoid pleurisy or TB, and may cause a milky effusion; raised pleural fluid cholesterol (>5.17 mmol/L) and cholesterol crystals at polarized light microscopy distinguish it from chylothorax.

Pleural fluid amylase

Abnormal if pleural fluid amylase > upper normal limit for serum amylase, or if amylase pleural fluid/serum ratio >1.0. Causes include:

- Pleural malignancy and oesophageal rupture (both associated with raised *salivary* amylase)
- Pancreatic disease (acute and chronic pancreatitis, pancreatic pseudocyst; associated with raised *pancreatic* amylase).

Note—may be normal early in the course of acute pancreatitis or oesophageal rupture.

Chapter 9

Post-operative breathlessness

Introduction 64
Initial assessment 66
Initial investigations 68

Introduction

The respiratory physician is often asked to see patients who have become dyspnoeic following an operative procedure. The risk of pulmonary complications is greatest with thoracic or upper abdominal surgery, when a degree of respiratory dysfunction and consequent breathlessness due to atelectasis is inevitable. Always rule out upper airway obstruction. See Table 9.1 for possible causes and management.

The four most common causes are:
- Infection/atelectasis
- Pulmonary embolism (PE)
- Pulmonary oedema (due to left ventricular failure (LVF))
- Exacerbation of underlying lung disease such as chronic obstructive pulmonary disease (COPD) or idiopathic pulmonary fibrosis (IPF).

Initial assessment

- Is the patient acutely unwell, needing immediate resuscitation and ventilatory support?
- Comorbid disease and past medical history, especially pulmonary, cardiac, or thromboembolic disease
- Type of surgery:
  - *Thoracic surgery* Consider lobar gangrene (torsion of the remaining lobe causing vascular occlusion) leading to pulmonary infarction with fever and haemoptysis; bronchopleural fistula (often associated with an infected pleural space), leading to sepsis and failure of the underlying lung to re-expand
- Time since surgery:
  - *Early complications (hours)* related to residual anaesthetic effect not adequately reversed, atelectasis, sputum retention, hypovolaemic shock, infection, PE, fat embolism, air embolism, LVF and fluid overload, myocardial ischaemia
  - *Later complications (hours to days)* related to PE, acute respiratory distress syndrome (ARDS), infection, myocardial ischaemia.

Table 9.1 Management of post-operative dyspnoea

Possible cause of dyspnoea	Management options
Basal atelectasis (commoner in smokers and following abdominal or thoracic procedures-mucus in bronchial tree causes small airway obstruction, subsequent alveolar air reabsorption, and collapse of lung segments); collapsed lobe—mucus plugging	Adequate analgesia to encourage expectoration, nebulized saline and bronchodilators, mucolytics, chest physiotherapy, deep breathing. If lung does not re-inflate, consider bronchoscopy to aspirate secretions
Pneumonia—follows atelectasis and lung collapse. Aspiration also possible	If fever and chest signs, give antibiotics for hospital-acquired pneumonia (see ➲ p. 536), adequate analgesia to encourage expectoration, chest physiotherapy
Thromboembolic disease	O_2 as required. Start treatment dose of low molecular weight heparin (LMWH) (if not contraindicated by the operation); Post-operative D-dimer unlikely to be useful. Arrange V/Q scan or CTPA; If in extremis, consider urgent CT or echo and thrombolysis (see ➲ p. 480)
Respiratory failure—opiate overdose or anaesthetic agents causing neuromuscular block not fully reversed Undiagnosed respiratory muscle weakness	Treat the underlying cause. Oxygen, non-invasive ventilation (NIV), or intubation and ventilation may be required. Liaise with ICU as the patient may require transfer for higher monitoring

Metabolic acidosis	Check urea and electrolytes (U&E); look for underlying problem such as renal failure or sepsis
Myocardial ischaemia, myocardial infarction (MI), or acute coronary syndrome	Electrocardiogram (ECG), check troponin. Sublingual or intravenous (IV) glyceryl trinitrate, if required for pain. Start heparin (if not contraindicated by the operation), anti-platelet agents, β-blocker, follow local protocols, in discussion with cardiology team. Urgent referral for 1° angioplasty if MI confirmed
Cardiac failure/fluid overload	O_2, IV furosemide, GTN infusion and inotropes if required. Echo to assess LV
ARDS	Supportive, likely to need mechanical ventilatory support (see ⊃ p. 115)
Phrenic nerve damage causing diaphragmatic paralysis. May occur with thoracic operations such as CABG	Diagnose on lung function tests, chest radiograph (CXR), and clinically decreased diaphragm movement. Advise to tilt whole bed (head up) when sleeping. Nerves may recover but can take 2+ years. Nocturnal continuous positive airway pressure (CPAP) or NIV may improve symptoms
Fat embolism following long bone fracture, especially with reaming and manipulation	O_2, IV fluids, supportive care
Laryngeal spasm	Reassurance, O_2 if required
Anaemia	Cross-match and transfuse. Identify if ongoing bleeding source
Myasthenia gravis crisis precipitated by anaesthetic agents	May need intubation and ventilation. Stop all anticholinesterases. Consider plasma exchange and IV immunoglobulin. Urgent neurology input

Initial investigations

- O_2 saturations and ABG on O_2 (if required)
- ECG
- CXR—compare with preoperative CXR, if available
- Full blood count and clotting screen
- U&E & venous lactate
- See if preoperative oximetry and spirometry were performed. There should be a record of the O_2 saturation on the anaesthetic chart.

A D-dimer level is unhelpful, as it will be raised by many different intra- and post-operative mechanisms. CRP and WCC are also largely unhelpful, as these are frequently raised post-operatively.

Pregnancy and breathlessness

Causes 70
Investigations 72

Causes

Normal physiological changes of pregnancy

- Elevated serum progesterone levels stimulate respiratory drive and lead to an increased tidal volume and raised minute ventilation, with only a modest increase in O_2 consumption. The subsequent fall in maternal pCO_2 facilitates foetal CO_2 transfer across the placenta; any cause of maternal hypercapnia leads quickly to foetal respiratory acidosis. Respiratory rate is unaffected by pregnancy. Elevation of the diaphragm occurs due to the enlarging uterus, leading to a reduced functional residual capacity (FRC), although diaphragm function is normal and VC is unaffected. Peak flow and FEV_1 are unaffected by pregnancy
- Increased cardiac output occurs due to an increase in heart rate (HR) (by about 15 beats/min) and stroke volume; peripheral resistance falls. Blood pressure (BP) is reduced in the first and second trimesters by 10–20 mmHg but is normal at term. Peripheral pulses tend to be increased in volume. Dependent oedema is common. Third heart sound and ejection systolic murmurs are commonly heard. May hear venous hums in the neck
- Raised levels of coagulation factors and impaired fibrinolysis, combined with venous stasis, result in a significantly increased risk of venous thromboembolism (VTE)
- Upper airway oedema, particularly in the setting of pre-eclampsia, may predispose to upper airways obstruction during sleep, but rarely frank obstructive sleep apnoea (OSA). OSA tends to occur in obese women and may be associated with impaired foetal growth and pre-eclampsia. Snoring in pregnancy is a poor predictor of OSA.

Causes of breathlessness in pregnancy

Causes are listed in Box 10.1. In general, breathlessness may be due to:
- Normal physiological changes of pregnancy. Up to 70% of pregnant women experience a degree of breathlessness, perhaps as a result of the increase in ventilation. Tachypnoea is a useful sign, as it is abnormal in pregnancy and suggests an underlying disease process
- New disease process. Pulmonary embolism (PE) is the commonest and is a major cause of maternal death. Other rare, but serious, causes include amniotic fluid embolism and acute respiratory distress syndrome (ARDS)
- Exacerbation of chronic respiratory or cardiac disease. Asthma is the commonest. Unsuspected underlying disease may present for the first time in pregnancy, e.g. structural heart disease such as mitral stenosis, or lymphangioleiomyomatosis (LAM). Pulmonary hypertension (PHT) is associated with a particularly poor prognosis during pregnancy. Patients with interstitial lung disease (ILD) and vital capacity (VC) <1 L should also consider avoiding pregnancy. In patients with cystic fibrosis (CF), the presence of PHT, or FEV_1 <60% predicted are associated with a worse outcome.

Box 10.1 Causes of breathlessness in pregnancy

Pulmonary
- Exacerbation of pre-existing lung disease, e.g. asthma, CF, LAM
- Pneumonia
  - Bacterial, including TB, aspiration
  - Viral, particularly varicella, influenza
  - Fungal, particularly coccidioidomycosis
- Aspiration pneumonitis
- Pulmonary metastases from choriocarcinoma (very rare).

Pleural
- Pneumothorax, particularly during labour
- Small asymptomatic effusions post-partum
- Ovarian hyperstimulation syndrome (very rare).

Vascular
- Venous thromboembolism
- Amniotic fluid embolism
- Air embolism
- Aortic dissection
- PHT.

Cardiogenic pulmonary oedema
- Exacerbation of pre-existing cardiac disease, e.g. valvular or congenital disease
- Peripartum cardiomyopathy.

Non-cardiogenic pulmonary oedema
- Iatrogenic fluid overload
- Tocolytic therapy (used to inhibit uterine contractions in preterm labour)
- ARDS due to pre-eclampsia, sepsis, massive haemorrhage, amniotic fluid embolism.

Other
- Anaemia
- Oesophageal rupture
- Hemidiaphragm rupture.

Investigations

Liaise with your obstetrics team, as well as with paediatricians and anaesthetists, if delivery is approaching. Management of specific conditions is discussed in the individual disease chapters in Part 2.

The following investigations may be affected by the pregnancy itself:

- *ABGs* Normal maternal pO_2 >13.3 kPa and pCO_2 3.7–4.3 kPa. A compensatory fall in serum bicarbonate (to 18–22 mmol/L) occurs, resulting in an average pH of 7.44. During the third trimester, perform ABGs in an upright position, as pO_2 may be 2.0 kPa lower when supine. A–a gradient is unaffected during pregnancy, except when supine near term

- *Blood tests* In normal pregnancy, white cell count (WCC), platelets, ESR, D-dimers, and fibrinogen are usually raised, and serum creatinine levels reduced. D-dimer is increased from about 6 weeks' gestation to 3 months post-partum. C-reactive protein (CRP) is not significantly affected. BNP levels are not affected by pregnancy itself and so elevated BNP may be a useful pointer towards a cardiac cause

- *Chest radiograph (CXR)* may show increased pulmonary vasculature due to normal increase in cardiac output. Required for diagnosis of pneumonia and pneumothorax. With abdominal shielding, the radiation doses to mother and baby are very small, and CXR should be performed if clinically indicated. Lateral CXR carries a greater radiation exposure and should be avoided

- Further investigation to exclude PE should be guided by local policy (see ➋ p. 484). *Leg vein ultrasound (US)* should be performed first if there are symptoms and signs of a deep vein thrombosis (DVT). If DVT is confirmed in the setting of clinical features suggestive of PE, then treatment can continue without the need for radiation exposure from further imaging. *Ventilation-perfusion (V/Q) scans* are associated with a higher radiation dose to the foetus and, as such, a slightly higher risk of childhood cancer, whereas *computed tomographic pulmonary angiogram (CTPA)* carries a greater maternal radiation dose and, in the setting of the hormonal changes within the breast during pregnancy, leads to an increased lifetime risk of breast cancer in the mother. The ventilation component of a V/Q scan can often be omitted during pregnancy, reducing the radiation dose. CTPA should be performed if CXR is abnormal and PE suspected. CTPA can also identify other pathology such as aortic dissection in haemodynamically unstable patients.

Preoperative assessment

Introduction 74
History and investigations 75
Management options 76

Introduction

The respiratory physician may be asked to assess a patient prior to elective or emergency surgery. These patients are usually those with pre-existing respiratory disease such as chronic obstructive pulmonary disease (COPD). Patients are now often also referred to respiratory units following positive screening for obstructive sleep apnoea (OSA).

- The usual functional status of the patient should be determined
- Their respiratory function should be optimized, if possible, with medication changes where appropriate
- Consider preoperative continuous positive airway pressure (CPAP) in those with confirmed OSA

These patients may require ventilatory support post-operatively. Ultimately, the decisions regarding fitness for surgery rest with the surgeon and the anaesthetist.

Box 11.1 Risk factors for perioperative complications
- Thoracic or upper abdominal surgery
- Anaesthetic length >3.5 h
- Smoker
- Chronic lung disease
- Raised $PaCO_2$
- Moderate or severe OSA
- Raised serum bicarbonate
- Current respiratory symptoms
- Poor performance status
- Concurrent cardiac disease
- Obesity
- Older age

History and investigations

- Risk factors for perioperative complications are shown in Box 11.1
- Usual functional state and exercise tolerance (those with an exercise tolerance of <5 m will struggle to wean off a ventilator)
- Assess day-to-day symptoms: preoperative infections/symptoms increase the risk of post-operative complications
- O_2 saturations on air and after exertion such as walking or climbing up and down a step for 2 min. Cardiopulmonary exercise test (CPET) may be necessary (see ⊃ p. 976)
- Arterial blood gas (ABG) on air, if saturations <94%. *Risk of surgery increases as the $PaCO_2$ increases*
- Spirometry, with bronchodilator reversibility testing. *Risk of surgery increased if FEV_1 <0.8L*
- Chest radiograph -CXR—if 65 y+ and no CXR in last year, or if acute respiratory symptoms
- History of snoring or apnoea
- Consider screening tool for OSA such as STOP-BANG (see Box 11.2)
- ECG
- Echo, if cardiac function compromised.

Management options

- Smoking cessation reduces post-operative complications. The optimal time to stop preoperatively is not known but the longer the better
- If airflow obstruction offer optimal bronchodilator therapy: long-acting β2 agonist (LABA), long-acting muscarinic antagonist (LAMA), or LABA/LAMA
- Consider regular nebulized bronchodilators in inpatients
- Regular inhaled steroid, if evidence of steroid reversibility/eosinophilia
- Preoperative course of oral steroids, if evidence of steroid reversibility/ eosinophilia
- Preoperative course of antibiotics, if evidence of infection
- Consider pulmonary rehabilitation: reduced length of stay and complication rates with preoperative exercise
- Inspiratory muscle training as part of organized preoperative exercise reduces length of stay and atelectasis/ pneumonia risk
- High-intensity interval training of unproven significance in terms of post-operative complication rates
- Consider chest physiotherapy with deep breathing exercises
- Consider CPAP if moderate or severe OSA present
- Alert anaesthetist to OSA diagnosis if present, anaesthetic and recovery can be modified
- Consider measuring bicarbonate levels: an elevated serum bicarbonate identifies a particularly high-risk group
- Optimize nutrition
- Lose weight if overweight/obese.

Further information

Lumb. Preoperative respiratory optimization: an expert review. *Anaesthesia*. 2019;**74:Supp 1**: 43–48.

Chiu et al. Diagnostic accuracy of the Berlin questionnaire, STOP-BANG, STOP, and Epworth sleepiness scale in detecting obstructive sleep apnea: a bivariate meta-analysis. *Sleep Med Rev.* 2017;**36**: 57–70.

Box 11.2 STOP-BANG: screening tool for OSA

Patients complete each of the following:

- **S**noring: Do you **Snore** loudly (loud enough to be heard through closed doors or your bed-partner elbows you for snoring at night)?
- **T**ired: Do you often feel **Tired, Fatigued, or Sleepy** during the daytime (such as falling asleep during driving or talking to someone)?
- **O**bserved: Has anyone **Observed** you **Stop Breathing** or **Choking/Gasping** during your sleep?
- **P**ressure: Do you have or are you being treated for **High Blood Pressure?**
- **Body Mass Index** more than 35 kg/m²
- **Age** older than 50 y?
- **Neck** size large (measured around Adam's apple)
  - Men >17 in/43 cm
  - Women >16 in/41 cm
- **Gender**: Male?

1 point for each positive criterion:

- 0–2 Low risk of OSA
- 3–4 Intermediate risk of OSA
- 5–8 High risk of OSA

In preoperative populations the STOP-BANG score (using a cut-off of ≥3) has a sensitivity of 90% and 36% specificity for identifying OSA.

In those with intermediate or high scores consider performing overnight pulse-oximetry or sleep study to confirm diagnosis before surgery, if surgery can be delayed. If not inform the anaesthetist so that intra-/peri-operative management can be optimized.

Chapter 12

Pulmonary disease in the immunocompromised—non-HIV

Clinical assessment 80
Further investigations 82
Causes 84
Differential diagnosis of pulmonary complications based on time course after transplantation 86
Treatment 88

Clinical assessment

- Pulmonary disease is a significant cause of morbidity and mortality in the immunocompromised, and its diagnosis and management are challenging. In the UK, this is encountered most commonly in the setting of immunocompromise secondary to cytotoxic chemotherapy, haematological malignancy, immunosuppression post-transplant (particularly renal and haematopoietic stem cell transplant (HSCT, including bone marrow, cord blood, and growth factor-stimulated peripheral blood transplantation)), prolonged corticosteroid use, and HIV (see ➔ p. 92)
- Most pulmonary diseases present in a similar manner in the setting of immunocompromise, with fever, dyspnoea, dry cough, chest pain, and often hypoxia. This non-specific clinical presentation, combined with the large number of possible causes, makes reaching a precise diagnosis difficult; the diagnosis remains unclear in up to 10% of cases, even at autopsy
- For causes of pulmonary infiltrates in the non-HIV-infected immunocompromised see ➔ p. 84, and treatment see ➔ p. 88; pleural effusion in this patient group is outlined in Box 12.1. Specific conditions are described separately (e.g. invasive aspergillosis, see ➔ p. 564; *Pneumocystis jirovecii* pneumonia (PCP), see ➔ p. 570).

> **Box 12.1 Pleural effusion in non-HIV immunocompromise**
> Causes of pleural effusion in non-HIV immunocompromised patients include cardiac failure and fluid overload, PE, drug-related, parapneumonic (bacterial, including *Nocardia*; fungal, e.g. PCP), or related to underlying disease (e.g. leukaemic infiltrates, lymphoma, chylothorax, myeloma). Pleural effusions are common after liver transplant: usually right-sided or bilateral transudates and resolve by third week; may require drainage if symptomatic.

Clinical assessment

In the *history*, the underlying cause of immunocompromise and the timing of respiratory disease onset may provide clues to the diagnosis. The rate of disease onset may also suggest possible causes:

- *Acute onset* (<24 h) bacterial pneumonia, viral pneumonitis (e.g. CMV), pulmonary oedema or haemorrhage, PE, ARDS
- *Subacute onset* (days) fungi (e.g. *Pneumocystis*, *Aspergillus*), bacteria (e.g. *Nocardia*, *Legionella*), viral (e.g. CMV), drug-induced pneumonitis
- *Chronic onset* (weeks) malignancy, mycobacteria, fungi.

Chest *examination* may suggest the extent of pulmonary involvement, although this can be misleading and there are often no abnormal signs (e.g. in PCP, or bacterial pneumonia in the setting of neutropenia). Assess fluid status; pulmonary oedema is common following transplantation. Extrapulmonary involvement may be helpful in suggesting a pathogen, e.g. cutaneous lesions (herpes simplex and varicella-zoster; necrotic lesions from *Pseudomonas* and other Gram-negative bacteria, mycobacteria, and fungi; subcutaneous abscesses in *Staphylococcus aureus* and *Nocardia*), CNS involvement (*Pseudomonas*, *Aspergillus*, *Cryptococcus*, *Nocardia*, mycobacteria, *Streptococcus pneumoniae*, *Haemophilus influenzae*, varicella-zoster).

Initial investigations

- *CXR* appearance is very variable: may be normal or show consolidation, nodular infiltrate, or diffuse shadowing. CXR is of limited diagnostic value, as appearances are non-specific and atypical presentations are common; the 'first-choice' diagnosis based on CXR is correct in only one-third of cases. CXR may, however, be helpful in monitoring disease progression and response to treatment
- *Blood and pleural fluid* (if available) sampling for microscopy and culture. Consider blood CMV viral load PCR, galactomannan (component of *Aspergillus* cell wall), beta-D glucan (component of *Candida*, *Aspergillus*, and *Pneumocystis* cell walls), urinary *Legionella* antigen
- *Sputum examination* is often of little diagnostic value in immunocompromised patients, with the exception of TB. Send sputum for acid-fast stain and mycobacterial culture, fungal stain, and culture. Induced sputum has a low yield for PCP in non-HIV patients
- *The degree of hypoxia* is often not appreciated; measure O_2 saturations, and consider ABGs. Severe hypoxia tends to be more commonly associated with infection due to bacteria, viruses, or *Pneumocystis* than with mycobacteria or fungi.

Is immediate antibiotic treatment required?

Immediate empirical treatment with broad-spectrum antibiotics prior to further investigation should be considered, depending on the nature of immunological defect and local hospital policy. In general, neutropenic patients with fever are at significant risk of developing overwhelming sepsis and should receive prompt antibiotic cover, irrespective of the CXR appearance and presence or absence of respiratory symptoms/signs. More invasive diagnostic procedures can then be reserved for patients who deteriorate or fail to improve within a period of observation (e.g. 2–3 days). In non-neutropenic patients, depending on the clinical circumstances, it is often possible to withhold treatment until definitive investigations have taken place.

Further investigations

More invasive diagnostic techniques are usually required for a definitive diagnosis.

CT chest

- Specific indications not yet defined. May not be needed in typical cases of bacterial pneumonia or PCP
- Useful in identifying the location and extent of pulmonary disease, and aiding invasive sampling procedures
- Often detects pulmonary disease in the presence of a normal CXR— consider if respiratory symptoms or unexplained fever, but normal CXR
- May be diagnostic, e.g. PE (CTPA), lymphangitis carcinomatosis, invasive aspergillosis ('halo' and 'air crescent' signs).

Bronchoscopy with BAL

- First-line investigation; consider early in management. Diagnostic in about 60% of patients overall; up to 70% of patients with infection. Results in change to treatment in ~50% of cases overall. Complications are rare
- Useful in the diagnosis of bacterial pneumonia, PCP (sensitivity 80–90%), CMV (sensitivity 85–90%), aspergillosis (sensitivity 50%), TB, malignant disease, diffuse alveolar haemorrhage, and alveolar proteinosis
- BAL fluid analysis: routine microscopy and culture for bacteria; additional stains and culture for fungi, mycobacteria, *Nocardia*; silver or immunofluorescence stain for *Pneumocystis*; respiratory viral screen; panfungal PCR; galactomannan
- Consider additional tests on BAL fluid: cytology (including flow cytometry) for malignant cells; inspection of sequential BAL returns and cytology for hemosiderin-laden macrophages if alveolar haemorrhage suspected; *Cryptococcus* antigen detection; CMV PCR; *Toxoplasma gondii* PCR
- TBB has a slightly higher sensitivity than BAL for the diagnosis of infection but carries a risk of bleeding and pneumothorax, which can be serious complications in this patient group; it is not usually performed at initial bronchoscopy, although may be considered, e.g. if lymphangitis is suspected.

Lung biopsy

Consider as a second-line investigation if BAL is non-diagnostic. Options include:

- *Repeat bronchoscopy with transbronchial lung biopsy* is useful in the diagnosis of malignancy, mycobacteria, fungi, OP, and drug-induced lung disease
- *VATS or open lung biopsy* has a greater diagnostic yield than TBB, although it is unclear if this can be directly translated into an improved survival. Results in change to treatment in <50% of patients, and complications may be serious
- *Percutaneous image-guided fine-needle aspiration (FNA) or biopsy* for investigation of peripheral nodules.

Causes

Causes of pulmonary disease in the immunocompromised can be broadly divided into infectious and non-infectious; multiple disease processes are common. The nature and timing of immunosuppression may provide clues to the cause(s) of pulmonary disease—for solid organ (kidney and liver) transplantation see p. 86, HSCT see p. 86, HIV see p. 96, and lung transplantation see p. 766.

Infectious causes (>75% of cases)

Infection is the commonest cause of respiratory disease in the immunocompromised. The nature of immunological defect may suggest the likely infectious agent:

• *Neutropenia or impaired neutrophil function* (e.g. 2° to leukaemia or cytotoxic treatment): Bacteria (*P. aeruginosa*, *S. aureus*, *S. pneumoniae*, *E. coli*, *Klebsiella*, *H. influenzae*, *Nocardia*), fungi (*Aspergillus*, *Candida*, mucormycosis)
• *Impaired T-lymphocyte function* (e.g. 2° to transplantation, cytotoxic treatment, high-dose steroids, lymphoma, HIV): Fungi (PCP, *Cryptococcus neoformans*, *Candida*, endemic mycoses), viruses (CMV, herpes simplex, varicella-zoster), bacteria (mycobacteria, *Listeria*, *Legionella*, *Nocardia*), parasites (*Toxoplasma gondii*)
• *Hypogammaglobulinaemia or impaired B-lymphocyte function* (e.g. 2° to myeloma, acute and chronic lymphocytic leukaemia, lymphoma): Encapsulated bacteria (*S. pneumoniae*, *H. influenzae*).

Considerable overlap exists between immune deficiencies however, and the pattern of infection will be further modified by prophylactic treatment, e.g. CMV and PCP prophylaxis.

Non-infectious causes (<25% of cases)

Often present with similar, if not identical, clinical and radiological features to infection, and signs (e.g. fever) do not reliably differentiate between them. Causes include:

• *Pulmonary oedema*, e.g. following renal transplant or HSCT
• *ARDS*, e.g. 2° to sepsis, drugs, transfusion-related acute lung injury, aspiration, 'engraftment syndrome' following HSCT
• *Drug-induced disease* Causes include ATRA (all-trans retinoic acid), antithymocyte globulin, azathioprine, bleomycin, busulfan, carmustine, chlorambucil, cyclophosphamide, cytosine arabinoside, hydroxycarbamide, liposomal amphotericin B, melphalan, mitomycin, methotrexate, sirolimus
• *Respiratory involvement from the underlying disease*, e.g. lymphoma, leukaemic infiltration, lymphangitis, connective tissue disease, leukostasis with very high leucocyte counts in leukaemia
• *Pulmonary embolism* May be complicated by secondary infection; clinical/radiological features may be confused with invasive aspergillosis; may be more common after renal transplant
• *Radiation-induced pulmonary disease* Pneumonitis (dyspnoea; clear margins on CT; typically follows lung radiotherapy; may be delayed and triggered by later chemotherapy treatment, so-called radiation recall pneumonitis) or OP (cough; extends beyond radiation field on CT; typically follows breast radiotherapy).

- *Diffuse alveolar haemorrhage* may complicate leukaemia and HSCT; similar clinical presentation to that of pneumonia; haemoptysis is rare; multilobar CXR/CT infiltrates; diagnostic criteria include exclusion of infection, progressively bloodier returns from BAL of three different subsegmental bronchi, and ≥20% of alveolar macrophages hemosiderin-filled (may require several days to appear); reported mortality ranges 30–100%
- *'Idiopathic pneumonia syndrome'* following HSCT; breathlessness with hypoxia and multilobar CXR/CT infiltrates; infection excluded with BAL and ideally a second later investigation (e.g. repeat BAL or lung biopsy); diffuse alveolar damage or interstitial pneumonitis on biopsy; mortality >70%
- *Engraftment syndrome* comprises fever, ARDS, and erythematous rash during marrow recovery post-HSCT
- *Bronchiolitis obliterans syndrome (BOS)* following allogeneic HSCT (from sibling or unrelated individual; occurs only extremely rarely following autologous procedure); typically associated with other forms of chronic graft-versus-host disease, e.g. cutaneous; gradual onset of dry cough, dyspnoea; CXR often normal; fixed obstructive spirometry with FEV_1 <75% predicted and ≥10% decline over <2 y, FEV_1/FVC ratio <0.7, and RV >120% predicted; air trapping and bronchial dilatation on HRCT (request expiratory images); exclude/treat airways infection
- *Cryptogenic organizing pneumonia*
- *Post-transplant lymphoproliferative disease* may complicate allogeneic HSCT or solid organ transplant, most commonly lung (see ⊃ p. 769)
- *Pulmonary alveolar proteinosis*
- *Pulmonary veno-occlusive disease*
- *Pulmonary cytolytic thrombi*
- *Pulmonary metastatic calcification* may complicate chronic renal failure and rarely progress after transplantation; CXR shows single or multiple nodules or patches of consolidation, may not appear calcified; CT typically diagnostic
- *Right hemidiaphragm dysfunction* is common after liver transplant and usually not relevant clinically.

Multiple disease processes

About 30% of patients have two or more disease processes accounting for their respiratory involvement. Secondary infection with a different infectious agent (commonly *Aspergillus* or Gram-negative bacteria such as *P. aeruginosa*) may complicate either a primary respiratory infection or a non-infectious process such as PE. Secondary infection is associated with a poor prognosis; consider particularly in patients who deteriorate after an initial response to treatment and in patients who are neutropenic.

Differential diagnosis of pulmonary complications based on time course after transplantation

Haematopoietic stem cell transplant

First month post-transplant (prolonged neutropenia pre-engraftment)
- Infection (*Pseudomonas aeruginosa, E. coli, Klebsiella pneumoniae, H. influenzae, S. aureus, Legionella* species, *Aspergillus*, influenza, RSV, parainfluenza 3, human metapneumovirus)
- Pulmonary oedema
- ARDS
- Transfusion-related acute lung injury
- Drug-induced lung disease
- Diffuse alveolar haemorrhage
- Idiopathic pneumonia syndrome.

Months 1–3 (impaired cellular immunity post-engraftment, related in part to immunosuppressive drugs and GVHD)
- Infection (Gram-negative bacteria, *Nocardia*, CMV, RSV, parainfluenza 3, herpes simplex, PCP, strongyloides, toxoplasmosis)
- Drug-induced lung disease
- Diffuse alveolar haemorrhage
- Idiopathic pneumonia syndrome
- Engraftment syndrome (timing coincides with neutrophil engraftment)
- Post-transplant lymphoproliferative disease
- Pulmonary veno-occlusive disease.

Months >3 (poor lymphocyte function, particularly following allogeneic HSCT)
- Infection (Gram-positive bacteria, CMV, RSV, parainfluenza 3, herpes simplex, varicella-zoster, *Nocardia*, TB, non-tuberculous mycobacteria, PCP, *Aspergillus*, endemic mycoses e.g. *Histoplasma*)
- Bronchiolitis obliterans syndrome (pulmonary GVHD; may occur up to 5 y post-allogeneic HSCT, typically within first 2y)
- Organizing pneumonia and other interstitial lung disease (LIP, NSIP)
- Pleuroparenchymal fibroelastosis
- Post-transplant lymphoproliferative disease
- Pulmonary veno-occlusive disease.

Solid organ transplantation

First month post-transplant (recent surgery ± ICU)
- Nosocomial bacterial infection (Gram-negative, *S. aureus* including MRSA, *Legionella*)
- ARDS
- Pulmonary oedema
- Drug-induced lung disease
- Pulmonary embolism
- Pleural effusion (especially after liver transplant)
- Right hemidiaphragm dysfunction (after liver transplant).

Months 1–6 (maximal immunosuppression)
- Opportunistic infection (CMV, PCP, *Nocardia*, *Aspergillus*, *Scedosporium apiospermum*)
- Drug-induced lung disease
- Post-transplant lymphoproliferative disease.

Months >6 (reduction in immunosuppression, unless rejection)
- Common community-acquired pathogens (*H. influenzae*, *S. pneumoniae*, *Legionella*, TB, non-tuberculous mycobacteria, PCP, endemic mycoses e.g. *Histoplasma*, viruses e.g. influenza, parainfluenza, adenovirus, RSV)
- Opportunistic infection (see under Months 1–6)
- Post-transplant lymphoproliferative disease
- Pulmonary metastatic calcification.

Treatment

Antimicrobials

Depending on the clinical circumstances, antimicrobials may need to be started prior to definitive investigations (see ➲ p. 81), although blood cultures should always precede antibiotic treatment. Choice of antimicrobial depends on the underlying condition and local hospital policy.

- In general, most neutropenic patients are treated with broad-spectrum antibiotics providing both Gram-positive and Gram-negative cover, e.g. piperacillin/tazobactam; antifungals are considered if slow response to treatment or subsequent deterioration. Consider adding vancomycin if MRSA is a possibility
- Treatment for CMV and PCP is associated with significant side effects and ideally should be based on a definitive diagnosis. In unwell patients who are strongly suspected to have PCP, treatment (see ➲ p. 572) can be started immediately, as BAL *Pneumocystis jirovecii* stains remain positive for up to 2 weeks
- Antituberculous treatment should only rarely be administered in the absence of a microbiological diagnosis.

Diuretics

Fluid overload and pulmonary oedema are common following renal transplantation and HSCT, and typical clinical and radiological signs may be disguised; consider a trial of diuretics.

Steroids

- Despite a lack of RCT-evidence, prednisolone (1 mg/kg/day PO or methylprednisolone 1 g IV daily for 3 days) is often considered in the treatment of drug- or radiation-induced lung disease, engraftment syndrome, diffuse alveolar haemorrhage, and idiopathic pneumonia syndrome following HSCT. Ideally, exclude underlying infection prior to starting steroids
- Prednisolone (40–80 mg daily PO) is also recommended for the treatment of PCP in patients with respiratory failure (see ➲ p. 572)
- Bronchiolitis obliterans syndrome (BOS), following allogeneic HSCT, is usually treated with increased immunosuppression (typically oral prednisolone 1 mg/kg/day with rapid taper) together with '**FAM**' therapy: inhaled **F**luticasone (most clinicians use high dose ICS/LABA combination), **A**zithromycin (typically 250 mg three times weekly), and **M**ontelukast. Superadded airways infection is common and should be treated aggressively. Consider treatment of gastro-oesophageal reflux, pulmonary rehabilitation, inhaled LAMA, extracorporeal photopheresis, and lung transplantation in severe or progressive BOS.

Supportive treatment

Administer supplementary O_2 (or high-flow nasal oxygen) to maintain saturations 94–98%. Respiratory failure in immunocompromised patients is associated with a poor outcome; mortality following intubation and mechanical ventilation ranges 60–100%. Carefully consider appropriate ceilings of care, including suitability for intubation and mechanical ventilation.

Surgery

Surgical wedge resection or lobectomy may be considered in the treatment of invasive aspergillosis, either acutely for lesions adjacent to pulmonary vessels that are judged to have a significant risk of massive haemoptysis, or at a later date for residual lesions at risk of reactivation with further chemotherapy.

Pulmonary disease in the immunocompromised—HIV

Clinical assessment 92
Causes of respiratory disease in HIV infection 96
Further investigations and treatment 97

Clinical assessment

HIV is associated with a reduction in cell mediated immunity, reflected in low CD4 counts. Widespread use of antiretroviral therapy (ART) and antimicrobial prophylaxis means life expectancy is now near normal. Respiratory disease remains common in the setting of HIV, and patients should be managed in consultation with an HIV specialist.

Major causes of respiratory disease in the HIV-infected patient are listed on p. 96. Specific conditions are described separately (e.g. *pneumocystis jirovecii* pneumonia (PCP), see ⊃ p.570; tuberculosis (TB), see ⊃ p. 585). Key management steps are as follows:

Clinical assessment

- As with other causes of immunocompromise, clinical features of respiratory disease in HIV-infected patients are non-specific: breathlessness, cough, fever, weight loss, and fatigue are common. Respiratory symptoms are not always present
- Ask about treatment and compliance with ART and PCP prophylaxis
- Source of HIV infection may be relevant: human herpesvirus-8 (HHV-8) related Kaposi's sarcoma occurs almost exclusively in HIV infected men who have sex with men (MSM); TB and bacterial pneumonia are more common in IV drug users (IVDUs)
- Travel history may be useful: infection with 'endemic mycoses' (histoplasmosis, blastomycosis, coccidioidomycosis) is well recognized in the USA but rare in the UK
- Careful examination may provide clues to the diagnosis. Pulmonary Kaposi's sarcoma is unusual in the absence of disease elsewhere; palatal Kaposi's sarcoma, in particular, is predictive of pulmonary involvement. Extrapulmonary mycobacterial disease is common and may involve the liver, lymph nodes, pericardium, and meninges.

Investigations

Chest radiograph (CXR)

- CXR changes are relatively non-specific. Appearances of bacterial pneumonia may be atypical, e.g. diffuse bilateral infiltrates mimicking PCP. TB may present with focal or diffuse CXR consolidation
- PCP classically appears as bilateral perihilar infiltrates that progress to alveolar shadowing; more unusual patterns include small nodular infiltrates or focal consolidation; CXR is normal in 10% of cases. Pneumothorax is suggestive of PCP although may also occur with TB
- Pleural effusion or hilar/mediastinal lymphadenopathy are unusual in PCP and are more suggestive of mycobacterial infection or Kaposi's sarcoma. Lung cancer is also a common cause
- Common causes of CXR cavitation are PCP, TB (with high CD4 count), *P. aeruginosa*, fungi, *R. equi*, Nocardia. Cavitation is relatively unusual in TB, occurring late in the course of HIV
- Common causes of pleural effusion in HIV infection are Kaposi's sarcoma, parapneumonic effusion, TB, cardiac failure, lymphoma, and lung cancer.

CD4 count

May be useful in narrowing the differential diagnosis: bacterial infection, including TB, occurs at any stage of disease, although infection is more severe at lower CD4 counts; PCP and atypical presentations of TB occur most commonly at CD4 <200 × 10⁶/L; NTM, Kaposi's sarcoma, *P. aeruginosa* pneumonia, and lymphoma occur late in the disease (CD4 <50 × 10⁶/L). A recent increase in CD4 count (following the introduction of ART) may suggest an immune reconstitution inflammatory syndrome (IRIS, see Box 13.1).

Blood cultures

Should be taken prior to antimicrobial treatment. Bacteraemia is relatively common with bacterial pneumonia in HIV, particularly with *S. pneumoniae* infection. Bacteraemic TB may occur in advanced disease.

Other blood tests

Raised inflammatory markers are a non-specific finding. Antigen testing may be useful for some fungal diseases. Raised beta D glucan levels may be useful in the diagnosis of PCP or invasive aspergillosis.

Sputum

Induced sputum may assist the diagnosis of PCP and mycobacterial disease. Induced sputum has a sensitivity of about 60% for the diagnosis of PCP. TB is more likely to be smear-negative in the setting of HIV, as cavitation is less common. Induced sputum should be obtained in a negative-pressure room.

Other cultures

Consider sampling urine, stool, lymph node, or bone marrow in suspected mycobacterial disease, as extrapulmonary disease is common.

Computed tomography (CT) chest

Useful in looking for evidence of respiratory disease in patients with symptoms but a normal CXR, and may be helpful in directing invasive diagnostic procedures. CT is also of benefit in the diagnosis and staging of Kaposi's sarcoma and lymphoma.

Box 13.1 IRIS

IRIS (immune restoration disease or paradoxical reaction) is a clinical syndrome resulting from restored immunity to infectious or non-infectious antigens, following the introduction of ART. The mechanism is uncertain but probably includes partial recovery of the immune system or an exuberant host-antigen response with host genetic susceptibility. It is more likely in the context of current infection due to mycobacteria, herpes, varicella, and cytomegalovirus (CMV). The clinical features can be diverse and depend on the underlying infectious or non-infectious agent. A clinically silent infection may be 'unmasked' as the CD4 count rises, and may be associated with an excessive inflammatory response. The commonest clinical features are fever, lymphadenopathy, and worsening respiratory symptoms. New pulmonary infiltrates and pleural effusions are common. TB-IRIS tends to develop within 2 months of the start of ART, and central nervous system (CNS) TB-IRIS is reported up to 10 months after ART initiation. Treatment with corticosteroids appears to be effective, although no randomized controlled trial (RCT) data exist. Various regimes are suggested, including methylprednisolone 40 mg bd and prednisolone 20–70 mg od for up to 7 weeks. Infectious agents must also be treated, and, in the very unwell, this may mean empirical treatment for PCP and TB and high-dose steroids while awaiting confirmatory microbiology.

Causes of respiratory disease in HIV infection

Infectious

Bacteria
- *Streptococcus pneumoniae*
- *Haemophilus influenzae*
- *Staphylococcus aureus*
- Gram-negative bacteria, especially *Pseudomonas aeruginosa*
- *Nocardia asteroides*
- *Rhodococcus equi.*

Mycobacteria
- *Mycobacterium tuberculosis*
- *Mycobacterium avium complex* (MAC)
- *Mycobacterium kansasii.*

Viruses
- Influenza
- Parainfluenza
- Respiratory syncytial virus (RSV)
- Herpes simplex
- Adenovirus
- CMV.

Fungi
- *Pneumocystis jirovecii* (PCP)
- *Aspergillus* spp.
- *Cryptococcus neoformans*
- Endemic mycoses.

Parasites
- *Strongyloides stercoralis* (hyperinfection syndrome).

Non-infectious
- Malignancy
  - Kaposi's sarcoma
  - Lung cancer
  - Non-Hodgkin's lymphoma
  - Chronic obstructive pulmonary disease COPD
- IRIS
- Drug-induced lung disease
- Cardiogenic pulmonary oedema (e.g. 2° to cardiomyopathy)
- HIV-associated pulmonary arterial hypertension (PAH)
- Interstitial pneumonitis
  - Non-specific interstitial pneumonitis
  - Lymphocytic interstitial pneumonitis.

Further investigations and treatment

Bronchoscopy and bronchoalveolar lavage (BAL)

- Bronchoscopy and BAL are safe and frequently diagnostic in this patient group and should be considered early in management, particularly in the presence of a diffuse CXR abnormality or following non-diagnostic induced sputum analysis. BAL should also be considered in patients with a localized CXR abnormality that has not responded to a trial of broad-spectrum antibiotics
- BAL fluid analysis: routine microscopy and culture for bacteria; additional stains and culture for fungi, mycobacteria, *Nocardia*; silver or immunofluorescence stain for *Pneumocystis*; cytology, including flow cytometry for malignant cells; respiratory viral polymerase chain reaction (PCR). Consider additional tests such as *Cryptococcal* antigen detection; CMV PCR; panfungal PCR; galactomannan
- Both *Nocardia* and *Rhodococcus equi* stain weakly acid-fast and so may be confused with mycobacteria
- Kaposi's sarcoma appears as 'raised bruises' in the trachea or bronchial tree on bronchoscopy; routine biopsy is not usually recommended, as diagnostic yield is low and significant haemorrhage may occur
- Lung cancer is more common in the setting of HIV, typically affecting relatively young patients with mild to moderate immunocompromise.

Lung biopsy

If bronchoscopy and BAL are non-diagnostic, consider repeat bronchoscopy with transbronchial biopsy (TBB) or surgical lung biopsy. TBB has a greater sensitivity than BAL, but potentially serious complications (such as pneumothorax or haemorrhage) are significantly more common.

Treatment

- Consider broad-spectrum antibiotics and empirical treatment for PCP (high-dose co-trimoxazole, and steroids if the patient is in respiratory failure; see ⊃ p. 572). BAL *Pneumocystis* stains remain positive for up to 2 weeks despite treatment, and so empirical treatment for PCP should not be delayed pending bronchoscopic confirmation if the patient is unwell and this diagnosis is suspected
- In the absence of another identifiable cause, consider empirical treatment directed at TB, pending sputum and BAL culture results
- Further antimicrobial treatment can be directed at specific pathogens isolated from BAL or biopsy
- Although isolation of *Aspergillus* spp. from respiratory samples may reflect contamination or colonization, consider treatment with voriconazole if isolated from BAL in setting of severe immunocompromise (CD4 $<30 \times 10^6$/L)
- Supportive therapy with O_2; consider nasal high flow oxygen/ respiratory support. PCP is the commonest cause of respiratory failure requiring intensive care unit (ICU) admission in HIV-positive patients. It was historically considered to carry a very high mortality rate, although recent studies have reported more favourable outcomes and ICU admission for invasive ventilation should be considered.

Sleep and breathing

History *100*
Examination and investigations *102*

History

The problem

Sleep apnoea and related problems are now a common reason for referral to many respiratory units. This is due to much better recognition of the syndromes and the increasing prevalence of obesity. Respiratory units with sleep services are seeing increasing numbers of patients, primarily for possible obstructive sleep apnoea (OSA), and, therefore, most patients tend to be sleepy. Referrals for insomnia are not usually encouraged.

Patients arrive at a respiratory sleep unit for several different reasons. They are commonly:
- Concerns that the patient may have sleep apnoea
- Concerns that an obese individual may have obesity hypoventilation
- Loud snoring, with the patient or spouse seeking advice
- Referrals from the ENT department who may be considering offering surgery for snoring and wish to exclude OSA first
- Excessive daytime sleepiness, diagnosis unclear
- Pre-operative assessment, particularly pre-bariatric surgery, as prevalence of OSA very high
- Other nocturnal symptoms such as sleepwalking, panic arousals, etc.

Thus, in sleep outpatients, the issues revolve around making the correct diagnosis of the excessive daytime sleepiness or nocturnal symptoms (and referring on, if appropriate), offering simple advice for snoring, or putting the patient through the continuous positive airway pressure (CPAP) induction programme.

Some units perform a sleep study first, on the basis of an appropriate referral letter, as it is more efficient; others see the patient first and then book a sleep study if indicated (usually >95% are studied). For the purposes of this account, it is assumed that the patient is seen first.

History

A clear history of the exact presenting complaint is obviously necessary, concentrating on the following points when OSA is suspected (a full discussion is available in the section on OSA; see ➔ pp. 678–692).
- Sleepiness: how severe, what does it interfere with, over how long has it been coming on, and does it impair quality of life. The Epworth sleepiness scale (ESS) is useful as part of the assessment of this (see Fig. 14.1); scored out of 24: 0–9 is considered normal, and >9 excessively sleepy. It is only a guide and should be interpreted with the overall history
- Important to differentiate sleepiness (tendency to nod off, due to inadequate sleep) from tiredness (feelings of exhaustion due to many causes, often without a tendency to nod off). OSA usually causes sleepiness more than tiredness, although this is not always so clear-cut, especially in women
- Snoring and apnoeas. Best assessed from a witness: how loud, continuous, intermittent, and are there recognized 'stopping breathing' or choking episodes during sleep?
- Other OSA symptoms such as nocturia and restless sleep

- History of weight and neck size increases over the last 5–10 y (recent weight gains common)
- History of nasal or other ENT surgery (previous palate surgery increases discomfort of CPAP)
- Previous medical history (certain risk factors such as mandibular surgery, hypothyroidism, acromegaly, Down's, Prader–Willi, etc.)
- Previous cardiovascular/cerebrovascular history especially AF and hypertension history (may influence decision to treat)
- Alcohol and smoking history (both worsen OSA)
- Occupation (is it vigilance-critical?)
- Shift working (may exacerbate the sleepiness from OSA)
- Driving issues: such as sleepiness while driving and 'near misses' or actual sleep-related accidents (sensitive issue requiring careful discussion)
- Does the patient drive for a living and what kind of vehicle or licence?

If OSA seems unlikely, then other causes of sleepiness need to be considered more carefully, concentrating on the commonest (see Box 14.1).

Box 14.1 Alternative diagnoses for excessive daytime sleepiness

- Depression, often missed
- Lifestyle issues—alcohol, late night working, shift work, caffeine excess, family circumstances, etc.
- Drugs—β-blockers and psychoactive drugs (e.g. antidepressants, sedatives, opiates, and anxiolytics)
- Narcolepsy—e.g. associated with cataplexy (loss of muscle tone in response to emotion, which can be subtle), sleep paralysis (paralysis on wakening for seconds to minutes), and prolific vivid dreaming (sleep onset or during naps)
- Periodic limb movements during sleep—associated with restless legs during the day. Association with renal failure, iron deficiency, and diabetes mellitus
- Post-severe head injury or cranial irradiation (hypothalamic damage)
- Post-infectious (e.g. Epstein–Barr virus)
- Idiopathic (sometimes hereditary)
- Certain neurological disorders such as myotonic dystrophy, Parkinson's disease, and previous stroke
- Simply being at the sleepier end of the normal spectrum
- The symptom may really be tiredness such as in 'ME' or insomnia, when the ESS is usually low
- Circadian rhythm disorders—tendency to sleep/awaken early or late reducing sleep opportunities. Can be variant of normal or insomnia/sleepiness due to blindness.

Examination and investigations

Examination of these patients is often relatively unhelpful.

In OSA, the main features to look for are

- Neck circumference (best measure of the obesity contribution to the cause of OSA, >17in) and body mass index (BMI)
- Oropharynx, often crowded with boggy mucosa, enlarged tonsils (Mallampati score can be used; see ➲ Fig 48.9 p. 702)
- Teeth, crowding suggests retrognathia/micrognathia (and mandibular advancement devices require sound teeth)
- Nasal patency (how easy will nasal CPAP be?)

Further assessment may be required

See Box 14.2

- Assessment of respiratory function, signs of cor pulmonale, FEV_1/VC ratio, and SaO_2 (associated COPD increases likelihood of being in type II ventilatory failure, so-called overlap syndrome)
- Standing to lying VC: >20% fall suggests diaphragm weakness
- BP (may influence decision to treat OSA)
- Endocrinology: hypothyroidism, acromegaly, Cushing's, diabetes
- Evidence of a neuromuscular disorder including a previous stroke
- Paradoxical abdominal movements during inspiration in a supine position suggesting diaphragmatic weakness
- Evidence of heart failure (central sleep apnoea (CSA), or Cheyne–Stokes respiration, which can produce overnight oximetry tracings similar to those of OSA).

Box 14.2 Clinic tests to perform

- Blood gas estimation if respiratory failure suspected (these OSA patients will require more urgent treatment)
- Thyroid function (hypothyroidism not always clinically obvious) plus other hormone tests, if indicated
- Routine haematology and biochemistry (prevalence of type 2 diabetes will be high in this overweight population)
- Some would recommend a fuller cardiovascular risk assessment, including cholesterol, fasting triglycerides, glucose, and folate, since these patients are often in a high-risk group (untreated 10 y cardiovascular event risk typically predicted to be about 35%).

Other scenarios

If it is known already that the patient has OSA, then a joint decision between the doctor and the patient needs to be made as to whether to undergo a trial of treatment (usually CPAP). This will depend mainly on the symptom severity vs. the perceived inconvenience of the treatment. Recent evidence suggests that even relatively asymptomatic patients with OSA, presenting to a sleep clinic, may benefit from a trial of CPAP, thus to quote, 'if in doubt, blow up the snout'. However, an abnormal sleep study is rarely a reason in its own right for CPAP. Weight loss works but is rarely achievable. Other causes must not be missed (e.g. hypothyroidism, tonsillar hypertrophy) simply because CPAP is available.

EPWORTH SLEEPINESS SCALE

Name:.......................Hospital number...................Date:....................

Your age (Y)...........Your sex (Male= M/Female=F)..................
- How likely are you to doze off or fall asleep in the situations described in the box below, in contrast to feeling just tired?
- This refers to your usual way of life in recent times.
- Even if you haven't done some of these things recently try to work out how they would have affected you.
- Use the following scale to choose the *most appropriate number* for each situation:-

0 = Would *never* doze   2 = *Moderate* chance of dozing
1 = *Slight* chance of dozing   3 = *High* chance of dozing

Situation	Chance of dozing
Sitting and reading	❏
Watching TV	❏
Sitting, inactive in a public place (e.g. a theatre or a meeting)	❏
As a passenger in a car for an hour without a break	❏
Lying down to rest in the afternoon when circumstances permit	❏
Sitting and talking to someone	❏
Sitting quietly after a lunch without alcohol	❏
In a car, while stopped for a few minutes in the traffic	❏
Thank you for your cooperation	Total score = ❏

Fig. 14.1 Epworth Sleepiness Scale questionnaire.

Reproduced from Murray W. Johns—A New Method For Measuring Daytime Sleepiness: The Epworth Sleepiness Scale. *Sleep* 1991;**14**: 540–545, with permission from Associated Professional Sleep Societies, LLC.

If the patient has come via ENT and is being considered for pharyngeal surgery, then the respiratory physician's role is to dissuade the patient from this route, as the objective success rate is poor and the hazards significant. The presence of significant untreated OSA is a contraindication to surgery. All other approaches to snoring, such as the use of mandibular advancement devices, should be considered first and pharyngeal surgery regarded as the last resort of the totally desperate.

For further information on OSA management see ➔ pp. 684–689.

Unexplained respiratory failure

Causes *106*
Clinical assessment and management *110*

Causes

Definition

Respiratory failure is conventionally divided into type I (hypoxia only, PaO_2 <8 kPa) and type II (hypoxia and hypercapnia, $PaCO_2$ >6 kPa): they are conceptually quite different. Type I is an increased A–a O_2 gradient (implying increased V/Q mismatch), with adequately increased alveolar ventilation maintaining a normal $PaCO_2$. The causes are numerous, including most of respiratory medicine, and requires the usual 'history, examination, and investigations'.

A more difficult, less common clinical scenario is an unexplained rise in $PaCO_2$ (>6 kPa, type II), with no obvious cause following a standard assessment. This may occur in the outpatient, ward, A&E, or ICU setting.

Pathophysiology

A rise in $PaCO_2$ can be due to V/Q mismatch with inadequate compensatory hyperventilation, e.g. overwhelming asthma, when there will also be a large A–a gradient indicating this increased V/Q mismatch. However, it can also be due to inadequate ventilatory drive or primary ventilatory pump failure where the A–a gradient will usually be normal. The following list contains mainly the causes that might not have been suspected from the initial assessment but, for completeness, also includes some more obvious causes. The conditions with asterisks are the ones most commonly discovered when the cause is not immediately obvious.

Failure of drive

Brainstem abnormality

- Polio and post-polio syndrome* (exact mechanism unclear)
- Brainstem stroke (involvement of respiratory centres bilaterally)
- Arnold–Chiari malformation—herniation of cerebellum into foramen magnum, compressing the brainstem
- Syringobulbia—expansion of a fluid compartment in the middle of the spinal cord extending up into the medulla (can be associated with Arnold–Chiari malformation)
- Surgical damage during operations for Arnold–Chiari and syringobulbia
- Encephalitis
- Brainstem tumour
- Congenital hypoventilation syndrome—usually presents soon after birth, can be later; abnormalities of neural crest development due to increased number of 'alanine repeats' in one of the homeobox genes (*PHOX2B*).

Suppression

- Sedative drugs, including alcohol, opiates, etc.*
- Compensatory hypoventilation following metabolic alkalosis (hypokalaemic alkalosis, diuretic-induced, prolonged vomiting).

Pump failure

Neurological (particularly if diaphragm involved)

- Myopathies
  - Acid maltase deficiency (Pompe's), diaphragm paralysis commonly occurs early*
  - Duchenne muscular dystrophy
  - Myotonic dystrophy
  - Several other very rare primary or secondary myopathies, e.g. limb girdle, hypothyroid, drugs (hydroxychloroquine)
- Neuropathy
  - MND* can affect diaphragm early on
  - Bilateral diaphragm paralysis*, e.g. trauma, bilateral neuralgic amyotrophy (also known as 'brachial neuritis', inflammatory damage to nerves of lower brachial plexus—cause unknown)
  - Guillain–Barré
  - Spinal muscular atrophy (autosomal recessive affecting spinal cord motor neurons)
  - High cord transection
  - Lyme disease (neuralgic amyotrophy/phrenic nerve palsy)
- Neuromuscular junction abnormalities
  - Myasthenia gravis*
  - Lambert–Eaton myasthenic syndrome (LEMS)
  - Botulism
- Anti-acetylcholine esterase inhibition
  - Organophosphates (see ➔ pp. 270–271)
  - Botulism
- Mixed
  - Post-ITU ('critical care neuropathy'), post-muscle relaxants*.

Chest wall

- Obesity, especially abdominal (obesity hypoventilation syndrome)*
- Raised abdominal pressure, 'abdominal compartment (or hypertension) syndrome', e.g. ascites, or gut and mesentery oedema
- Scoliosis*
- Post-thoracoplasty (usually 'three stage', many ribs caved in, starting from the top down—done for TB prior to effective chemotherapy)
- Flail chest
- Pneumothorax/large pleural effusion
- Severe ankylosing spondylitis.

Airways obstruction/mixed

- Unrecognized COPD/severe asthma*
- OSA and additional COPD/obesity/muscle weakness,[1] sometimes called 'overlap syndrome'.

---

* The conditions most commonly discovered when the cause is not immediately obvious.

The ventilatory loading effects of obesity, COPD, and OSA commonly summate to produce ventilatory failure when each on their own would not be regarded as of sufficient severity. Estimating the contribution each is making to an individual's ventilatory failure can influence therapy and expectations of success, e.g. if OSA dominant (severe OSA), the ventilatory failure is likely to respond to CPAP; dominant COPD (FEV1 <25% predicted) will need maximal lower airways bronchodilator therapy (thresholds only for general guidance), but the likely poor response of the lower airways obstruction will mean that even limited additional weight reduction and/or treatment of milder OSA may be useful in this situation.

Clinical presentation

Slow onset

In several of the conditions listed previously, e.g. acid maltase deficiency, MND, and scoliosis, the onset of ventilatory failure can be insidious and include:

- General fatigue and/or hypersomnolence
- Awakenings from sleep, characteristically every ~2 hours, corresponding to periods of REM sleep
- Headaches on awakening
- Morning confusion
- Morning cyanosis
- Ankle oedema (fluid retention, cor pulmonale, from the hypoxia)
- Orthopnoea, particularly if diaphragmatic weakness
- Dyspnoea standing in a swimming pool (this usually indicates diaphragm paralysis, as the pressure of water, even at 1m depth, pushes the unopposed diaphragm further up into the chest)
- Swallowing difficulties (often MND) or other evidence of a more generalized proximal neuromuscular problem.

Apparent rapid onset

Sometimes, the significance of these symptoms is missed for a while, and a relatively trivial respiratory tract infection, a general anaesthetic, or the prescription of a ventilatory depressant tips the balance and the patient goes into severe ventilatory failure, with impaired conscious level or coma. These individuals will end up ventilated on ICU and may be difficult to wean, or present again with ventilatory failure a few weeks after discharge.

Clinical assessment and management

History, examination, and investigations

History

Carefully taken history, e.g. symptoms of subtle weakness prior to presentation, episode of shoulder pain (neuralgic amyotrophy), past history of polio, orthopnoea (diaphragm weakness), drug history. Often this is not available, as the patient may present unconscious.

Examination

Thorough examination, particularly neurological, e.g. fasciculation, diaphragm weakness 'abdominal paradox' (when supine, inward drawing of abdomen on inspiration or sniffing—masked if on positive pressure ventilation), myotonia, as well as rarer signs seen in some of the conditions listed previously.

Blood gases taken breathing air (following >20min off extra O_2)
- Degree of CO_2 retention
- Presence of a base excess indicating chronicity of CO_2 retention
- Calculate A–a gradient to detect any V/Q mismatch (see ◑ p. 921)
- In pure hypoventilation, there should be no significant A–a gradient (<2 kPa), unless there is 2° basal atelectasis from poor lung expansion and/ or obesity.

Pulmonary function tests (PFTs)

(See ◑ p. 963)
- Presence of unexpected severe airways obstruction
- Reduced VC (neurological or chest wall)
- Further fall of VC on lying down (>20% change, definitely abnormal)— indicative of diaphragm paralysis. If supine VC is <25% predicted, very likely to be the main cause of the raised $PaCO_2$
- Mouth pressures, sniff pressures, or transdiaphragmatic pressures; not much more helpful than the % fall in VC on lying down.

Specific tests—for some of the conditions listed previously such as:
- EMG studies—MND, myotonia
- MRI (gadolinium-enhanced)—Arnold–Chiari, brainstem lesion, syrinx
- CPK—some myopathies
- Sleep study—e.g. (i) REM desaturation (early marker of ventilatory failure, when supine VC has usually dropped below 60% predicted normal), (ii) continuous nocturnal hypoventilation (when supine VC has dropped below 40% predicted), and (iii) additional OSA
- Cough peak flow—when less than 270 L/min in a stable patient introduce strategies to aid an effective cough (or earlier depending on symptoms)
- Blood film for abnormal lymphocyte cytoplasmic vacuolation (mainly acid maltase deficiency)
- Muscle biopsy—acid maltase deficiency (glycogen-containing vacuoles and low enzyme levels).

Management

Management of the underlying condition, if possible, is paramount. Weak expiratory muscles and weak laryngeal adduction prevent effective coughing, with an increased incidence of serious chest infections. Clearing retained secretions can be a major problem. Physiotherapists can help teach patients and their carers sputum clearance techniques (cough peak flow <270 L/min is a useful indicator of the need for the need of cough assist techniques/devices). Increasing the lung volume, prior to coughing, with positive pressure devices (e.g. using the patient's own ventilator, intermittent positive pressure device 'The Bird', or simple bag and face mask) and 'breath stacking' techniques generate a higher expiratory flow with improved sputum clearance. Mechanical insufflator/exsufflator 'cough assist' devices are available that both increase inspiratory volume and speed expiratory flows. Their acute and prophylactic role is still being evaluated.

Lying down and sleeping with the *whole bed tipped head up* by about 15–20° greatly improves ventilation in the presence of bilateral diaphragm paralysis or major abdominal obesity. Just elevating the top half of the bed and bending the patient in the middle, leaving the abdomen and legs horizontal, does not work. The abdominal contents have to descend into the pelvis to effectively 'offload' the diaphragm. This posture will also improve the ability to wean from assisted ventilation.

When the underlying condition is irreversible, the decision will need to be taken as to whether long-term NIV is appropriate (see ⊃ pp. 782–783).

Further information

Bott et al. Guidelines for the physiotherapy management of the adult, medical, spontaneously breathing patient. *Thorax* 2009:**64(S1)**: i1–51.

Part II

Clinical conditions

16 Acute respiratory distress syndrome *115*

17 Asbestos and the lung *123*

18 Asthma *141*

19 Bronchiectasis *169*

20 Bronchiolitis *183*

21 Chronic obstructive pulmonary disease (COPD) *189*

22 Connective tissue disease and the lung *213*

23 Cor pulmonale *231*

24 Cystic fibrosis (CF) *237*

25 Drug and toxin-induced lung disease *261*

26 Dysfunctional breathing *283*

27 Eosinophilic lung disease *289*

28 Extreme environments—flying, altitude, diving *297*

29 Gastrointestinal disease and the lung *305*

30 Hypersensitivity pneumonitis *311*

31 Idiopathic interstitial pneumonias *317*

32 Lung cancer *337*

33 Mediastinal abnormalities *381*

34 Paediatric lung disorders *393*

35 Pleural effusion *401*

36 Pneumoconioses *425*

37 Pneumothorax *435*

38 Pulmonary hypertension (PHT) *449*

39 Pulmonary thromboembolic disease *467*

40 Rare lung diseases *489*

41 Respiratory infection—bacterial *517*

42 Respiratory infection—fungal *559*

43 Respiratory infection—mycobacterial *585*

44 Respiratory infection—parasitic *623*

45 Respiratory infection—viral *629*

46 Sarcoidosis *655*

47 Sickle cell disease and the lung *671*

48 Sleep apnoea and hypoventilation *677*

49 Upper airway and tracheal disease *703*

50 Vasculitis and the lung *713*

Acute respiratory distress syndrome

Pathophysiology and diagnosis *116*
Management and complications *120*

Pathophysiology and diagnosis

Definition and epidemiology

Acute respiratory distress syndrome (ARDS) is not a single entity but represents the severe end of a spectrum of acute lung injury due to many different insults. Manifests as acute and persistent lung inflammation with increased vascular permeability. Most commonly seen on the ITU where about 10–20% of such patients will have ARDS depending on the definition. The 2012 'Berlin Definition' of ARDS requires:

- Respiratory symptoms within 1 week of known clinical insult
- Bilateral opacities consistent with pulmonary oedema on chest radiograph (CXR) or computed tomography (CT)
- Respiratory failure must not be fully explained by cardiac failure or fluid overload. Echo may be required to exclude hydrostatic pulmonary oedema
- Oxygenation impairment, defined by PaO_2/FiO_2 ratio at least ≤300 mmHg (40 kPa) despite positive end-expiratory pressure (PEEP) ≥5 cmH$_2$O:
  - Mild ARDS—PaO_2/FiO_2 >200 mmHg (27 kPa)
  - Moderate ARDS—PaO_2/FiO_2 >100 mmHg (13 kPa)
  - Severe ARDS—PaO_2/FiO_2 ≤100 mmHg (13 kPa).

Other ARDS grading scores exist, e.g. Murray lung injury score (based on plain CXR findings, oxygenation, PEEP level, and respiratory system compliance).

Pathophysiology

Inflammatory damage to the alveoli, either by locally produced pro-inflammatory mediators or remotely produced and arriving via the pulmonary artery. These mediators recruit neutrophils, which release proteases and reactive oxygen species causing capillary and alveolar damage. Changes in pulmonary capillary permeability allow fluid and protein leakage into the alveolar spaces with pulmonary infiltrates. The alveolar surfactant is diluted with loss of its stabilizing effect, resulting in diffuse alveolar collapse and stiff lungs. This leads to:

- Gross impairment of ventilation-perfusion (V/Q) matching with shunting, causing arterial hypoxia and very large A–a gradients. There are usually enough remaining functioning alveoli such that hyperventilation maintains CO_2 clearance; thus, hypercapnia is infrequently a problem
- Pulmonary hypertension (PHT) will develop 2° to the hypoxia, but this may be helpful (aids V/Q matching), rather than deleterious
- Reduced compliance (stiff lungs) due to loss of functioning alveoli (alveolar collapse, filled with fluid and protein) and hyperinflation of remaining alveoli to their limits of distension.

Common causes

There are many causes of pro-inflammatory mediator release sufficient to cause ARDS, and there may be more than one present. Common causes, in order of prevalence:

- Sepsis/pneumonia (risk increased with alcoholism and cigarette smoking)
- Gastric aspiration (even if on a proton pump inhibitor (PPI), indicating that a low pH is not the only damaging component)
- Trauma/burns (via sepsis, lung trauma, smoke inhalation, fat emboli, and possibly direct effects of large amounts of necrotic tissue).

Less common causes

- Acute pancreatitis
- Transfusion-related acute lung injury (TRALI), caused by any blood product (possibly due to human leucocyte antigen (HLA)/white blood cell antibodies, commoner with older blood products, >6U); usually occurs within a few hours of transfusion. No specific therapy or evidence of steroid response
- Transplanted lung—worse if lung was poorly preserved
- Post-bone marrow transplant as bone marrow recovers
- Drug overdose, e.g. tricyclic antidepressants, opiates, cocaine, aspirin
- Near drowning
- Following upper airway obstruction; mechanism unclear.

The course of ARDS is fairly characteristic. *Phase 1* is the early period of diffuse alveolar damage and hypoxaemia with pulmonary infiltration. *Phase 2* (fibroproliferative) develops after a week or so as the pulmonary infiltrates resolve and, on histology, seems to be associated with an increase in type II pneumocytes (surfactant producers), myofibroblasts, and early collagen formation. *Phase 3* (fibrotic) occurs in some. This is a fibrotic stage that leaves the lung with cysts, deranged micro-architecture, and much fibrosis on histology.

Clinical features

ARDS should be considered in any patient with a predisposing risk factor who develops severe hypoxaemia and a widespread diffuse pulmonary infiltrate. Approximately 1–2 days following the clinical presentation of the precipitating cause (sepsis, aspiration, etc.), there is rapidly worsening dyspnoea (± a dry cough) and hypoxaemia, requiring rapidly escalating amounts of supplemental O_2 up to 100% via a non-rebreathe system (see p. 788). Coarse crackles in the chest. Intubation and ventilation are nearly always required, although initiating HFNO or continuous positive airway pressure (CPAP) via a face mask at 5–10 cmH$_2$O with 100% O_2 can improve oxygenation temporarily.

Diagnosis

There are no specific tests that allow a confident diagnosis, and exclusion of other more specifically treatable diagnoses is required. The cause for the ARDS needs to be established and prevented from continuing or re-curring, if possible. The CXR or CT shows diffuse alveolar infiltrates and air bronchograms, similar in appearance to cardiogenic pulmonary oedema or diffuse pulmonary haemorrhage. Changes are worst in dependent areas.

Differential diagnoses include:

• *Left ventricular failure (LVF)* (may be excluded on clinical grounds, echo, or, less commonly, checking pulmonary capillary wedge pressure <18 mmHg)
• *Diffuse alveolar haemorrhage* (e.g. Goodpasture's, GPA/Wegener's, and systemic lupus erythematosus (SLE); clues will include a drop in Hb, blood in the airways and pulmonary secretions, and other clinical features of one of these disorders; see ➲ p. 28)
• *ILD* (e.g. AIP or fulminant OP; see ➲ p. 332 and ➲ p. 330)
• *(Idiopathic) acute eosinophilic pneumonia*
• *Cancer and lymphangitis carcinomatosis.*

Some centres advocate lung biopsy to exclude alternatives, although most reserve biopsy for cases when the differential diagnosis includes conditions for which management would be changed (e.g. fungal infection, vasculitis, cryptogenic organizing pneumonia (COP)).

Management and complications

Management

The essential aspects of management are to treat the precipitating cause, provide best supportive care with adequate oxygenation, and avoid further damage from barotrauma, hyperoxia, and nosocomial infections. Mechanical ventilation with positive end expiratory pressure (PEEP) and higher inflation pressures are almost always required to maintain oxygenation (SaO_2 values in the low 90s are entirely adequate). There is evidence that high inflation pressures may worsen ARDS directly (micro-barotrauma); therefore, try to maintain plateau pressures <30 cmH_2O.

Many ventilation strategies have been tried to reduce the high inflation pressures that result from the stiff lungs (low compliance). For example, using low tidal volume ventilation to reduce inflation pressures (6 mL/kg ideal body weight, compared with 12 mL/kg) reduces mortality by 9% and increases ventilator-free days. Use of higher PEEP (attempt to open collapsed alveoli) has been shown in a meta-analysis to improve oxygenation and is associated with a lower intensive care unit (ICU) mortality for patients with PaO_2/FiO_2 ≤200 mmHg (27 kPa). Reducing the minute ventilation and allowing the $PaCO_2$ to rise (permissive hypercapnia) also reduces the inflation pressures.

Prone ventilation has been tried in an attempt to improve V/Q matching, and initial increases in PaO_2 are observed. A meta-analysis suggested a possible survival advantage for those with severe hypoxia, and a 2013 randomized controlled trial (RCT) (PROSEVA) has shown a significant reduction in both 28- and 90-day mortality for patients with severe ARDS, although trial limitations prevent generalization to all patients.

Several different artificial surfactants have been tried to attempt improving lung compliance, although good delivery to the abnormal areas is unlikely. Although effective in animal models, the RCTs have been negative in humans.

Haemodynamic monitoring, guided by central venous catheters, has a similar efficacy to pulmonary artery catheters, but is associated with a halving in catheter-related complications (mostly, arrhythmias).

Different degrees of hydration have been compared, with reduced fluid balances improving gas exchange and shortening duration of mechanical ventilation. Secondary analysis of a cohort study suggested that a negative day 4 fluid balance is associated with decreased mortality, although this was not confirmed in a randomized study.

High-dose steroids have been used, but there is evidence of harm as well as benefit, and minimal evidence of overall improved survival. Some ARDS-related diseases, such as acute eosinophilic pneumonia, usually show good response to steroid therapy. A 2019 Cochrane Review suggested that steroids may reduce early mortality, but low certainty; no consistent evidence of difference to duration of ventilation or late mortality. Certain subgroups may do slightly better and others worse, e.g. steroids are possibly beneficial during the first 14 days, but detrimental thereafter.

Extracorporeal membrane oxygenation/CO_2 removal will buy time and allow the lung to 'rest', but these techniques are very expensive and it is difficult to demonstrate any long-term benefit.

Table 16.1 summarizes the latest UK ARDS recommendations

Table 16.1 Latest UK ARDS recommendations

Strongly in favour	
Tidal volume	≤6 mL/kg ideal body weight
	Plateau pressure ≤30 cmH₂O
Prone position	For moderate/severe ARDS
	≥12 hours/day
Weakly in favour	
Conservative fluid management	
Higher PEEP	For moderate/severe ARDS
Neuromuscular blockers	For moderate/severe ARDS
	Using 48 hr cisatracurium infusion
Extra corporeal membrane oxygenation (ECMO)	Severe ARDS, high lung injury score or hypercapnic pH <7.2
Weakly against	
Inhaled vasodilators	
Strongly against	
High-frequency oscillatory ventilation (HFOV)	

Complications

- The high ventilation pressures lead to barotrauma: pneumothorax, surgical emphysema, pneumomediastinum. Pneumothorax may be lethal but difficult to detect on a CXR in the supine patient
- Nosocomial infections occur in about half the patients, making surveillance mini-bronchoalveolar lavages (BALs) important
- Myopathy associated with long-term neuromuscular blockade, high steroid doses, and poor glycaemic control
- Non-specific problems of venous thromboembolism (VTE), gastro-intestinal (GI) haemorrhage, inadequate nutrition.

Prognosis

Improved over the last 20 y, probably due to improvements in supportive care and ventilator strategies, rather than an ability to modify the inflammatory process and its subsequent repair. Prognosis is worse with intra-pulmonary causes. Early deaths are usually due to the precipitating condition, and later deaths to complications. Over half of the patients will survive with varying residual lung damage, although the pulmonary function tests (PFTs) often show only minor restrictive abnormalities (and reduced kCO), indicating the considerable capacity of the lung to recover. A prospective cohort study showed that 6-minute walking test (6MWT) distance remained decreased (at 76% predicted), even at 5 y.

Future developments

The optimal level of PEEP in a particular patient is difficult to predict. Inadequate PEEP allows more atelectasis, but too high PEEP contributes to overdistension of remaining alveoli and further barotrauma when there are no more 'recruitable' alveoli. Ways to estimate the best PEEP are under investigation. HFOV has been around a long while, but the OSCILLATE and OSCAR randomized trials suggested a lack of benefit, with possible harm associated with its use. Recently, liquid ventilation with perfluorochemicals has been tried. These dense O_2-carrying liquids reduce the heterogeneity of ventilation by nullifying the requirement for surfactant, thus recruiting the collapsed alveoli. There are improvements in oxygenation but no evidence yet of clinically meaningful outcomes.

Nitric oxide (NO) has been tried, with clear improvements in oxygenation but very little effect on survival and is associated with renal impairment. The mode of action is not clear and may be more than just vasodilatation. Inhaled prostacyclin is similarly unconvincing. Anti-inflammatory and anti-oxidant therapies are still very much in the experimental phase.

Further information

Griffiths MJD et al. Guidelines on the management of acute respiratory distress syndrome. *BMJ Open Respir Res.* 2019;**6**(1): e000420.

Asbestos and the lung

Asbestos *124*
Benign asbestos-related pleural disease *126*
Asbestosis *128*
Mesothelioma: diagnosis *130*
Mesothelioma: treatment and outcome *134*
Compensation for asbestos-related diseases *138*

Asbestos

Asbestos consists of a family of naturally occurring hydrated silicate fibres that may be subdivided into two groups:

- Curly *serpentine* fibres, of which chrysotile (white) is the only fibre currently in commercial use
- Straight needle-like *amphiboles*, which comprise crocidolite (blue), amosite (brown), anthophyllite, tremolite, and actinolite.

Fibres have a predisposition to localize to the pleura. They differ in their lung clearance kinetics and pathogenic potential; amphibole fibres clear more slowly from the lung and are more carcinogenic than chrysotile. While asbestos usage in developed countries is restricted, the use of chrysotile asbestos in developing economies continues to rise.

Mechanisms of exposure

Occupational exposure

Accounts for the majority of cases of asbestos-related disease and includes:

- Mining, milling, and transport of asbestos
- Use of asbestos products, e.g. in construction and demolition, floor tiling, insulation, fireproofing, textiles, friction materials (brake linings), ship building, pipefitting, electrical repair, boiler fitting and lagging, carpentry, plumbing, and welding.

Domestic exposure

May include:

- Relatives of asbestos workers exposed to 'carry home' asbestos in hair or clothes
- Following remodelling or renovation in contaminated buildings
- Local geological exposure from natural deposits, e.g. areas of central and south-east Turkey, north-west Greece, and Corsica
- Urban environment (although undisturbed and non-friable asbestos building insulation is not considered hazardous).

A complete occupational history is essential if asbestos-related disease is suspected and should include the method of exposure, with dates and names of employers. This information may be of medicolegal importance and ideally should be elicited during the first consultation.

Asbestos-related lung disease

Comprises:

- Benign asbestos-related pleural disease
  - Pleural plaques
  - Benign asbestos-related pleural effusion
  - Diffuse pleural thickening
  - Rounded atelectasis
- Asbestosis
- Mesothelioma
- Lung cancer (multiplicative risk from smoking).

Other diseases linked to asbestos exposure include pericarditis and perhaps head and neck and GI cancers. Whether asbestos exposure truly leads to an increased risk of lung cancer in the absence of asbestosis remains controversial.

Asbestos-related disease typically exhibits a long latency period of 20–40 y from exposure. Peak industrial asbestos use in the UK occurred in the early 1970s, and asbestos-related disease is likely to remain common for at least the next 20 y. The incidence of mesothelioma is forecast to peak in 2015–2020 in Europe.

All deaths should be notified to the coroner if asbestos-related disease is suspected or proven.

Benign asbestos-related pleural disease

Pleural plaques

- Most common manifestation of asbestos exposure
- Discrete areas of white or yellow thickening on the parietal pleura; may calcify. Histologically, these are acellular, avascular areas of hyaline collagen fibrosis
- Bilateral and occur particularly on the posterolateral chest wall (particularly adjacent to ribs), over the mediastinal pleura, and on the dome of the diaphragm but are absent in the costophrenic angles
- Develop 20–30 y after exposure; incidence (but not the extent of plaques) increases with longer duration of exposure; found in up to 50% of asbestos-exposed workers and may also occur after low-dose exposures
- Usually asymptomatic although, if extensive, may be associated with mild breathlessness due to pleural restriction
- Effect on pulmonary function is uncertain: most studies have failed to demonstrate abnormal lung function, although otherwise unexplained mild airways obstruction or restriction has been described in some populations of asbestos workers with pleural plaques—the mechanism of this is unclear, although it may reflect asbestos-induced small airway disease or early interstitial fibrosis, respectively
- High resolution computed tomography (HRCT) is more sensitive than chest radiograph (CXR) in detecting pleural plaques
- There is no evidence that plaques are pre-malignant
- Asymptomatic plaques are no longer eligible for compensation in England and Wales but are in Scotland and Northern Ireland (see ⮕ p. 138)
- Tuberculosis (TB), trauma, and haemothorax may each cause single pleural plaques; multiple plaques are highly suggestive of asbestos exposure.

Benign asbestos-related pleural effusions

- Relatively early manifestation of asbestos pleural disease; usually occurs within 10 y of exposure
- Development is considered to be dose-dependent although can occur after minimal exposure
- Typically small and unilateral and may be asymptomatic or occasionally associated with pleuritic pain, fever, and dyspnoea
- Usually resolve spontaneously over a few months, although some recur
- The pleural effusion is an exudate, often bloodstained, with no characteristic findings on pleural fluid analysis
- Diagnosis depends on a history of asbestos exposure and the exclusion of other causes, including mesothelioma
- Benign asbestos pleurisy may precede the development of diffuse pleural thickening; there is no clear association with mesothelioma
- Treat symptomatically, with pleural aspiration for breathlessness and non-steroidal anti-inflammatory drugs (NSAIDs) for pain.

Diffuse pleural thickening (DPT)

- Consists of extensive fibrosis of the visceral pleura, with areas of adhesion with the parietal pleura and consequent obliteration of the pleural space
- Unlike pleural plaques, its margins are ill-defined, and it may involve the costophrenic angles, apices, and interlobar fissures
- Development appears to be dose-related and may follow recurrent asbestos pleurisy
- On CXR, it may be defined as a smooth, uninterrupted pleural opacity, extending over at least a quarter of the chest wall, with or without obliteration of the costophrenic angles; on CT, the pleural density extends >8 cm craniocaudally, 5 cm laterally, and is >3 mm thick
- Symptoms are relatively common and comprise exertional breathlessness and chest pain, which can be chronic and severe
- May lead to significant restrictive pulmonary function impairment (with normal lung carbon monoxide transfer factor (TLCO)), especially if the costophrenic angle is obliterated; hypercapnic respiratory failure has been described
- Pleural biopsy may be required to distinguish it from mesothelioma
- Treatment is difficult; decortication often fails to result in clinical or functional improvement
- Patient may be eligible for compensation (see ➲ p. 138).

Rounded atelectasis

(Also known as folded lung, Blesovsky syndrome, or shrinking pleuritis with atelectasis.)

- Develops as contracting visceral pleural fibrosis; ensnares and then twists the underlying lung, resulting in the distinctive radiological appearance of a rounded or oval pleural-based mass of 2.5–5 cm in diameter
- Asbestos exposure is the most common cause, although any cause of pleural inflammation may result in rounded atelectasis
- CT is often diagnostic, demonstrating a 'comet tail' of vessels and bronchi converging toward the lesion, adjacent thickened pleura, and volume loss in the affected lobe
- An atypical appearance may require positron emission tomography (PET)/CT ± biopsy to exclude malignant disease
- Typically asymptomatic, although breathlessness or dry cough may occur
- Usually stable or slowly progressive, and no specific treatment is required
- Surgical decortication may improve symptoms but frequently results in reduced lung volumes and is not generally recommended.

Further information

American Thoracic Society Statement. Diagnosis and initial management of non-malignant diseases related to asbestos. *Am J Respir Crit Care Med* 2004;**170**: 691–715.

Asbestosis

Definition

Chronic interstitial fibrosis resulting from asbestos inhalation.

Causes

Factors affecting disease development include:
- *Degree and length of asbestos exposure* A clear dose-response relationship exists; usually seen in workers with many years of high exposure although may follow a very high exposure of short duration, resulting in a shorter latency period
- *Fibre type* Amphibole fibres are probably more fibrogenic than chrysotile, although most exposures are mixed fibre types
- *Cigarette smoking* increases the severity and rate of progression of asbestosis.

Latency period from first exposure to clinical disease is usually at least 15–20 y and may be >40 y.

Clinical features

Insidious onset of breathlessness, dry cough. Bibasal late-inspiratory crackles, clubbing in 40% of cases. May progress to respiratory failure, cor pulmonale.

Differential diagnosis

Includes other causes of interstitial fibrosis, particularly usual interstitial pneumonia (UIP).

Investigations

- *CXR* Bilateral symmetrical reticulonodular pattern, primarily affecting the lower lobes peripherally, which may extend upwards to involve the mid- and upper zones; may progress to honeycomb lung. Massive bilateral upper lobe fibrosis (without lower lobe involvement) is rare but well described. Associated pleural thickening or plaques may be seen and suggest a diagnosis of asbestosis, rather than UIP. Classification is based on size, thickness, and profusion of opacities. CXR insensitive to early disease; may be normal in 15–20% of symptomatic biopsy-proven asbestosis
- *HRCT* is more sensitive than CXR and is abnormal in 10–30% of cases with a normal CXR. Features include basal 'ground-glass' opacities (seen early in the disease), parenchymal bands, subpleural curvilinear lines and opacities, interlobular septal thickening, signs of fibrosis (traction bronchiectasis, loss of lobular architecture, honeycombing in advanced disease) and pleural plaques
- *PFTs* are classically restrictive with reduced lung volumes and transfer factor, although obstructive or mixed patterns may also occur (perhaps reflecting asbestos-induced small airway disease)
- Analysis of *sputum* or *BAL* may demonstrate asbestos bodies, although sensitivity is limited. The finding of interstitial fibrosis, in the absence of asbestos bodies, on *lung biopsy* makes asbestosis unlikely. Asbestosis demonstrates fewer fibroblastic foci than with UIP pattern fibrosis although visceral pleura is frequently mildly fibrotic. Analysis of material for asbestos bodies is only very rarely indicated, usually for research or litigation purposes.

In general, CXR and HRCT show only limited correlation with physiological disease severity.

Diagnosis

Gold standard is pathological demonstration of fibrosis with mineralogical quantification of asbestos bodies. The College of American Pathologists and Pulmonary Pathology Society have defined a 5-point scheme for grading asbestosis:

- Grade 0—fibrosis confined to bronchiolar walls
- Grade 1—fibrosis extends only to first-tier alveoli
- Grade 2—fibrosis involves alveolar ducts and second-tier alveoli
- Grade 3—fibrosis of all alveoli between respiratory bronchioles
- Grade 4—honeycombing.

In practice, histology is rarely required, and a diagnosis can be made on the basis of a history of significant asbestos exposure, with appropriate delay between exposure and disease, and radiographic evidence of fibrosis (particularly when seen with pleural plaques).

Treatment

- No pharmacological treatment is of proven benefit
- Supportive management, including supplementary O_2, as required, influenza and pneumococcal immunization, smoking cessation, compensation if exposure was occupational (see ⮑ p. 138).

Prognosis

Varies widely. After removal from exposure, progression occurs in 5–40% of patients over 10 y; progression is faster following greater exposure, although rapid progression over 1–2 y is unusual and more in keeping with UIP. Fewer CXR opacities after exposure are associated with better prognosis. Increased risk of developing lung cancer.

Mesothelioma: diagnosis

Definition

Malignant tumour of mesothelial surfaces (most commonly the pleura), usually resulting from asbestos exposure.

Causes

Asbestos is the major single cause, and there is a history of occupational asbestos exposure in up to 90% of cases. All types of asbestos can cause mesothelioma—amphibole is the most potent, but also evidence for chrysotile. Mean latent interval between first exposure and death is around 40 y; cases are rare with latency <15 y. Not dose-related (unlike asbestosis or bronchogenic cancers) and no evidence for a threshold asbestos dose below which there is no risk, although the risk at low exposure levels is small. No significant association with smoking. The mechanism through which asbestos fibres result in mesothelioma is unclear; possibilities include direct irritation of the parietal pleura, disruption of mitosis, generation of toxic O_2 radicals, and stimulation of mitogen-activated kinases leading to proto-oncogene activation.

Other causes of mesothelioma include non-asbestos fibres, e.g. erionite, which is found in rocks in Cappadocia, Turkey—mesothelioma accounts for up to a quarter of all adult deaths in local villages. Evidence for Simian Virus 40 (contaminated polio vaccine in 1950s/60s) is limited. Rare cases of mesothelioma caused by ionizing radiation or chest injury are described. 'Spontaneous' mesothelioma in children is also documented.

Clinical features of pleural mesothelioma

- Chest pain (typically dull ache, 'boring', diffuse, occasionally pleuritic), breathlessness; a small proportion are asymptomatic. Profuse sweating may occur
- Consider in any patient with a pleural effusion or pleural thickening, particularly if chest pain is present
- Rarely may present with persistent chest pain and a normal CXR
- Weight loss and fatigue uncommon at presentation (<30% of cases), but are prominent as disease progresses
- Clubbing is very rare (<1%)
- Chest wall invasion may be seen (especially at thoracentesis sites)
- Bilateral pleural involvement is unusual at presentation
- Paraneoplastic syndromes are described, e.g. disseminated intravascular coagulation (DIC).

Differential diagnosis

Includes benign asbestos pleural effusion, DPT, and adenocarcinoma involving the pleura.

Investigations

Pleural fluid

Aspiration typically reveals an exudative straw-coloured or bloody effusion. Cytological analysis may provide the diagnosis (sensitivity range 32–84%) and is often useful in excluding other pathology, e.g. adenocarcinoma. Poor at diagnosing sarcomatoid mesothelioma. Pleural fluid glucose and pH may be low in extensive tumours. Mesothelioma may track through the chest wall along thoracentesis sites; avoid repeated pleural aspiration if the diagnosis is suspected.

Imaging

CXR and CT features include:

- Moderate to large unilateral pleural effusion, usually with pleural nodularity and enhancement following pleural contrast, and involvement of mediastinal pleura
- Localized pleural mass or thickening without free fluid
- Uniform encasement of lung, resulting in small hemithorax
- Local invasion of chest wall, ribs, heart, mediastinum, hilar nodes, and diaphragm; transdiaphragmatic spread and invasion of contralateral pleura
- Associated pleural plaques or interstitial fibrosis in a minority of cases.

The role of magnetic resonance imaging (MRI) is unclear—it may provide additional information in some cases, e.g. chest wall invasion, although is rarely required. PET/CT may have a role in distinguishing benign and malignant pleural disease (although TB pleuritis, talc, and chronic pleural inflammation cause 18-fluorodeoxyglucose (FDG) avidity), as well as identifying lymph node spread for staging, and can help to select sites for image-guided biopsy.

Biopsy

Diagnosis usually requires histological confirmation, except when the patient is too unwell or too frail for biopsy. Ultrasound (US)- or CT-guided cutting needle biopsy and thoracoscopic biopsy of pleural masses have a high diagnostic yield and should be used in preference to blind (Abrams') biopsy techniques. Early use of thoracoscopy may both provide a diagnosis and enable treatment of large effusions with talc pleurodesis, thereby avoiding repeated non-diagnostic procedures with attendant problems of needle-track spread.

Histological subtypes

- Epithelioid (50% of cases; may be confused with adenocarcinoma; better prognosis)
- Sarcomatoid (or fibrous; includes lymphohistiocytoid and desmoplastic patterns; worse prognosis)
- Mixed (biphasic; contains both subtypes).

Immunohistochemistry is key to making the diagnosis. British Thoracic Society (BTS) guidelines suggest used of two positive mesothelial stains (e.g. calretinin, cytokeratin 5/6, Wilms tumour 1, and podoplanin-D240) and two negative (adeno)carcinoma stains (e.g. thyroid transcription factor (TTF) 1, carcinoembryonic antigen (CEA), and Ber-EP4). Difficulty with sarcomatoid mesothelioma which frequently does not display mesothelial markers. Electron microscopy of histopathological specimens may also help to distinguish mesothelioma from adenocarcinoma.

Staging

Guidelines recommend using 8th edition of tumour, node, metastasis (TNM) staging (see Box 17.1) and stage groupings (see Table 17.1), which predict survival.

Table 17.1 Mesothelioma staging and survival

Stage	TNM classification	Median survival (months)	5y survival (%)
IA	T1 N0 M0	23	16
IB	T2–3 N0 M0	20	13
II	T1–2 N1 M0	19	10
IIIA	T3 N1 M0	14	8
IIIB	T4 N0–1M0	14	5
	T1–4 N2 M0		
IV	Any T, any N, M1	10	0

Imaging may underestimate extent of disease, and accurate staging would require surgical exploration. Poor prognostic features include transdiaphragmatic muscle invasion and involvement of mediastinal lymph nodes, ♂ gender, age >75, chest pain, poor performance status, high WCC, thrombocytosis, and non-epithelioid histology. A low standardized uptake value on PET may also be prognostically beneficial.

Various prognostication scores are available, including LENT (see → p. 406) and Brims' decision tree analysis (places patients into four groups with differing survival according to weight loss, performance status, Hb, albumin and histology (medians: group 1–34 months; group 2–18 months; group 3–12 months; group 4–7 months)).

Box 17.1 8th edition of the TNM staging system for mesothelioma (IASLC/UICC/AJCC)

Extent of 1° tumour (T)

Tx 1° tumour cannot be assessed

T0 No evidence of 1° tumour

T1 Tumour limited to ipsilateral pleura

T2 Tumour involving ipsilateral pleura with either:
   (a) diaphragm muscle involvement
   (b) extension into lung

T3 Locally advanced resectable tumour. Involving ipsilateral pleura with:
   (a) endothoracic fascia involvement
   (b) mediastinal fat involvement
   (c) resectable chest wall tumour
   (d) involvement of outer part pericardium

T4 Locally advanced unresectable tumour. Involving ipsilateral pleura with:
   (a) diffuse or multifocal chest wall disease
   (b) extension to peritoneum
   (c) extension to contralateral pleura
   (d) extension to mediastinal organs
   (e) extension into spine
   (f) extension through pericardium ± pericardial effusion ± myocardial tumour.

Regional lymph nodes (N)

Nx Cannot be assessed

N0 No regional lymph node metastasis

N1 Ipsilateral bronchopulmonary, hilar, or mediastinal nodes

N2 Contralateral mediastinal, ipsilateral, or contralateral supraclavicular nodes.

Distant metastasis (M)

Mx Cannot be assessed

M0 No distant metastasis

M1 Distant metastasis present.

Mesothelioma: treatment and outcome

Treatment

Management of pleural effusions

Early definitive treatment is key; repeated pleural aspirations should be avoided. Talc pleurodesis can be achieved either using a chest drain or at thoracoscopy, depending on local resources. Pleurodesis is not possible if the lung does not re-expand following drainage of pleural fluid ('trapped lung') and the resulting recurrent pleural effusions are difficult to manage; indwelling pleural catheters (IPCs) allow fluid drainage without needle aspiration and are useful in this situation. 1° use of IPCs is reasonable, dependent on patient preference (see ⟴ p. 858).

Radiotherapy

Routine prophylactic radiotherapy to procedure tracts is no longer recommended after two RCTs (SMART and PIT) demonstrated no differences in rate of procedure tract metastases. Pre- and post-surgical radiotherapy is also not recommended unless in the context of clinical trials. Palliative radiotherapy provides pain relief in a proportion of patients with chest wall pain (including related to tract metastases) but is less useful in the treatment of breathlessness or superior vena caval obstruction (SVCO).

Surgery

Five types of surgery have been used—extrapleural pneumonectomy (EPP), extended pleurectomy with decortication (EPD; lung-sparing with complete macroscopic resection including diaphragm/pericardium if required), pleurectomy with decortication (similar to EPD but no resection of diaphragm/pericardium), partial pleurectomy, and thoracoscopy with pleurodesis, but their roles require further investigation. Trimodal therapy (chemotherapy, followed by EPP and radiotherapy) was evaluated in the MARS randomized feasibility study for 'resectable disease', finding the EPP group to have a shortened survival without any gain in QoL, although the study has been controversial. Operative mortality is ~7–16% for EPP and ~4% for PD. The MesoVATS RCT comparing talc pleurodesis vs video-assisted thoracoscopic surgery (VATS) partial pleurectomy showed similar overall survival at one year (57% talc; 52% VATS) but a significantly higher complication rate and length of hospital stay for surgery. Latest 2018 BTS guidelines recommends *not* using partial pleurectomy over talc pleurodesis, *not* using EPP, and *not* using EPD (unless in the context of a clinical trial). Studies are ongoing, including comparison of pleurectomy+decortication with IPC.

Systemic anti-cancer therapy

Patients with good performance status should be considered for chemotherapy. Pemetrexed (an inhibitor of DNA synthesis proteins, e.g. thymidylate synthase) plus cisplatin has an objective response rate (tumour shrinkage of >50%) of 41% and conveys a survival advantage of just under 3 months when compared with cisplatin alone. Cisplatin/pemetrexed combination is a frequently used combination, although carboplatin may be substituted for cisplatin in those at increased risk of toxicity. Addition of bevacizumab (vascular endothelial growth factor (VEGF) inhibitor) to cisplatin/pemetrexed improves survival from median 16.1 to 18.8 months in one study (with increased hypertensive and thrombotic complications) but this is not presently licensed in UK for this purpose. Ongoing treatment of an individual may be guided by objective metabolic responses based on PET/CT. Other studies have shown that addition of raltitrexed (also an inhibitor of thymidylate synthase) to cisplatin improves survival by 2.5 months.

General management

Early involvement of a pain relief and palliative care service is required. Ensure adequate analgesia: opiates and NSAIDs for chest wall pain; consider amitriptyline, pregabalin, or gabapentin for neuropathic pain (from intercostal nerve or vertebral involvement); nerve blocks or cordotomy may be required. Breathlessness may be multifactorial, e.g. pleural effusion, lung compression, wall restriction, pericardial involvement, anaemia, pain, anxiety, and fear. Discuss compensation issues (see ⊃ p. 138). Liaise with general practitioner (GP), specialist nurse, palliative care teams. Remind GP that all deaths have to be reported to the coroner. The Coroners' Society of England and Wales and BTS have encouraged coroners to avoid postmortems where biopsy has already confirmed mesothelioma. A coronial inquest is opened and adjourned soon after death but may take ~3 months for the full inquest to complete.

Clinical course

Median survival is 4–12 months from diagnosis. Typically progresses by local extension, sometimes leading to involvement of the contralateral lung or peritoneum, SVCO, cardiac tamponade, or spinal cord compression. Distant metastases are common (50% at autopsy), although occur late and are rarely clinically apparent.

Peritoneal mesothelioma

Rarer than pleural mesothelioma, it may be associated with more prolonged asbestos exposure. Remains intra-abdominal in most cases. Clinical features include abdominal discomfort, weight loss, ascites, and, in some cases, organ involvement (e.g. intestinal obstruction). Fine needle aspirate (FNA) of omental masses may provide a diagnosis, although laparoscopy is often required. Prognosis is worse than for pleural mesothelioma, with median survival 7.4 months. No treatment is of proven benefit.

Mesothelioma has also been described affecting *other serosal surfaces* such as pericardium and tunica vaginalis.

Future developments

- Several biomarkers have shown promise in mesothelioma diagnosis, but none are recommended as sole diagnostic tests. Mesothelin (expressed on the surface of mesothelial cells) is an FDA-approved diagnostic and prognostic marker for mesothelioma, with serum sensitivity 60% and specificity 81% and PF sensitivity 75% and specificity 76% in meta-analysis. Other malignancies can raise levels (including ovarian, pancreatic, and lung carcinomas, lymphoma). Other potential markers include megakaryocyte-potentiating factor, osteopontin, and fibulin-3. They may also have a role in disease monitoring and outcome prediction but further studies required.

- Studies of gene expression in tumour samples may prove to be useful in both distinguishing mesothelioma from adenocarcinoma and in predicting prognosis
- Likely therapeutic role of immunotherapy using checkpoint inhibitors (e.g. anti-PD-1 antibody (pembrolizumab, nivolumab±ipilimumab)/ anti-PD-L1 antibody (durvalumab)). Randomized trials currently recruiting. Novel therapeutic strategies using antimesothelin monoclonal antibodies, gene therapy, anti-angiogenic agents, and photodynamic therapy are in development.

Further information

Woolhouse I et al. British Thoracic Society Guideline for the investigation and management of malignant pleural mesothelioma. *Thorax* 2018;**73**(Suppl 1): i1-i30.
http://www.iaslc.org/Research-Education/IASLC-Staging-Project/Staging-Educational-Materials

Compensation for asbestos-related diseases

Identification of asbestos exposure is essential for the patient to be able to claim compensation. Patients are not eligible for compensation if their exposure occurred while they were self-employed. There are two principal sources of support and compensation.

From the government

Apply to the Department for Work and Pensions for Industrial Injuries Disablement Benefit, using form BI100PD (health care team fill in form BI100PN(A)). Available for the following diseases:
- DPT
- Asbestosis
- Lung cancer associated with DPT or asbestosis or some asbestos exposure (disablement automatically assessed as 100%)
- Mesothelioma (disablement 100%).

There must be a clear history of asbestos exposure at work. Compensation is not available for pleural plaques alone. If successful and employer is no longer in business, may apply for a single payment from the government under the Pneumoconiosis, etc. (Workers' Compensation) Act 1979. The value of compensation reflects the degree of disability from which the patient is considered to suffer and their age at diagnosis (in 2019, lump sums were between £14K and £92K dependent on age). Next of kin may also claim within 12 months posthumously but receive less. Since 2014, the Diffuse Mesothelioma Payment Scheme, funded by insurers and administered by a claims management company (mesoscheme.org.uk) (for those whose employer/insurer is not contactable, lump sum is £87K–£271K, age dependent. Other governmental payments will reduce amount.

For patients who have had secondary asbestos exposure from their partner, and the self-employed, other benefits may be available, including the 2008 Diffuse Mesothelioma payment (lump sum (between £14K and £92K, age dependent, less for dependents)).

Further possible benefits—Constant Attendance Allowance, Exceptionally Severe Disablement Allowance, Employment and Support Allowance, Disability Living Allowance, Personal Independence Payments and Reduced Earnings Allowance. The War Disablement Pension scheme may provide compensation for disease resulting from asbestos exposure with HM forces.

From the courts: Civil law

Compensation directly from a previous employer. Can be claimed from the employer's insurer, even if the employer is now out of existence. Advise patient to seek advice as soon as possible from a solicitor with relevant experience. Claims must be initiated within 3 y of the individual's first awareness that they have an asbestos-related disease; attempts to initiate claims after 3 y may be statute-barred. Inform the patient of this, and document the conversation in the medical notes. In England and Wales, a Court of Appeal ruling in 2006 concluded that pleural plaques alone should now no longer be considered an indication for compensation, and a subsequent 2007 appeal failed to overturn this ruling in the House of Lords. Subsequent 2011 legislation in Scotland and Northern Ireland has made plaques compensable in these countries. Awards for asbestosis range from £15,000 to £50,000, depending on symptoms and the degree of disability; such patients may accept an interim settlement, allowing further claims to be made, or may wish to take a greater 'once and for all' award and forego their right to further claims in the event of mesothelioma developing. Typical awards for mesothelioma are £45,000–£50,000, with additional amounts awarded for care and future loss of wages and pension; total compensation may be ± £100,000 (or significantly more for younger patients). Successful claims have also been made for mesothelioma occurring in relatives who had 2° exposure to asbestos while washing work clothes.

Further information

Guide to Industrial Injuries Disablement Benefits (DB1) gives guidance on IIDB, Pneumoconiosis, etc. (Workers' Compensation) Act 1979 and other benefits: ℛ http://www.gov.uk/ government/publications/industrial-injuries-disablement-benefits-technical-guidance/ industrial-injuries-disablement-benefits-technical-guidance

ℛ http://www.gov.uk/industrial-injuries-disablement-benefit

ℛ http://www.mesothelioma.uk.com

Asthma

Definition, epidemiology, pathophysiology, aetiology *142*
Clinical features *144*
Investigations *146*
Acute severe asthma *148*
Chronic asthma: management *152*
Chronic asthma: additional treatment options *156*
Non-pharmacological management *158*
Difficult/refractory asthma *160*
Asthma in pregnancy *162*
Occupational asthma *164*
Management of occupational asthma *166*
Vocal cord dysfunction *167*
Allergic rhinitis (hay fever) *168*

Definition, epidemiology, pathophysiology, aetiology

Asthma is a chronic inflammatory disorder of the airway characterized by bronchial hyperreactivity to a variety of stimuli, leading to a variable degree of airway obstruction, some of which may become irreversible over many years.

It is a clinical diagnosis based on:
- A history of recurrent episodes of wheeze, chest tightness, breathlessness, and/or cough, particularly at night
- Evidence of generalized and variable airflow obstruction, which may be detected as intermittent wheeze on examination or via tests such as peak expiratory flow (PEF) measurement.

Epidemiology

It is the commonest chronic respiratory disease in the UK, with a prevalence of 10–15%. There is a wide variation in disease prevalence worldwide, with highest levels seen in English-speaking countries (where there is also a high prevalence of sensitization to common aeroallergens). The reason for the increasing worldwide prevalence over the last few decades is unclear.

Pathophysiology

Asthma is increasingly recognized as a heterogeneous condition. The most common underlying pathology is that of chronic eosinophilic bronchitis/bronchiolitis. Airway inflammation is seen, with cellular infiltration by T helper 2 (Th2) cells, lymphocytes, eosinophils, and mast cells. There is large and small airway involvement, and cytokine production (e.g. IL-13, IL-4, IL-5, and cysteinyl-leukotrienes).

Up to 25% of asthma is thought to be non-eosinophilic. Neutrophilic airway inflammation makes up the largest proportion of this group and this may be driven by persistent airway infection. A minority of asthma has little airway inflammation, with smooth muscle dysfunction the predominant pathology. These non-eosinophilic groups are associated with a poorer short-term response to inhaled corticosteroids and oral corticosteroids and may turn out to need a different treatment strategy.

Airway obstruction occurs due to a combination of:
- Inflammatory cell infiltration
- Mucus hypersecretion with mucus plug formation
- Airway smooth muscle contraction.

Airway obstruction due to the first two factors is typically not bronchodilator responsive and is particularly likely to be the present in patients with an asthma attack. Non-specific (corticosteroids) and specific (monoclonal antibodies) anti-inflammatory treatments are effective for the treatment and prevention of these episodes.

This may become irreversible over time due to:
- Basement membrane thickening, collagen deposition, and epithelial desquamation
- Airway remodelling occurs in chronic disease, with smooth muscle hypertrophy and hyperplasia. This is now recognized as increasingly important in the pathophysiology of the most difficult to treat chronic asthma.

Aetiology

This is due to a combination of genetic and environmental factors, with many different genes identified.

Immunological mechanisms

A subgroup of asthma is atopic and therefore react to antigen challenge by producing specific IgE from B-lymphocytes. This leads to the formation of IgE-antigen complexes that bind to mast cells, basophils, and macrophages, leading to the release of preformed mediators, e.g. histamine, IL-5, and other eosinophil chemotactic factors resulting in type 2, eosinophilic inflammation. Allergy is not demonstrated in up to 50% of asthma. Non-allergic mechanisms involving the irritation and insult to the airway epithelium, such as environmental triggers, are also thought to provoke a type 2 response. These factors cause bronchoconstriction and airway oedema.

Prostaglandins, leukotrienes, kinins, and histamine are all important 2° messengers involved in the inflammatory response.

The innate immune response to infection can cause persistent neutrophilic airway inflammation.

Genetic factors

A hereditary component to asthma and atopy is well established, and a number of chromosomes and linkages are implicated. The multiple mechanisms and 2° messengers involved in asthma make the contribution of the effects of specific genes difficult to determine. Established susceptibility loci include the genes ADAM33, GPRA (G protein related receptor for asthma), and ORMDL3, a member of a gene family that encodes transmembrane endoplasmic reticulum proteins. The latter was identified by a genome-wide screen, and its function and role in the pathogenesis of asthma is not yet clear.

Hygiene hypothesis

This suggests that asthma may be a by-product of modern 'first world' cleanliness. Early life exposure to bacterial endotoxin switches off the allergic response (by reducing Th2-mediated pathways), and when this exposure is lost, the likelihood of developing allergic diseases, such as asthma, increases considerably. Large epidemiological studies support this hypothesis.

Environmental factors

The increasing prevalence of asthma appears to be associated with a rising standard of living worldwide, and not just in westernized societies. This has implicated a number of environmental factors. A number of explanations are speculated (but not proven), including dietary changes, a reduction in childhood infections, increased immunization, or a combination of all three.

Phenotypic differences

It is increasingly recognized that 'asthma' is likely to represent a number of different 'diseases' or sub-phenotypes, rather than one disease with a unifying pathological mechanism. Sub-phenotypes may differ in underlying pathophysiology, clinical features, and disease course, and research aimed at clearly identifying such disease subgroups (e.g. through the use of biomarkers, such as blood eosinophilia, or the host genetic profile) is ongoing.

Further information

Haldar P et al. Cluster analysis and clinical asthma phenotypes. AJRCCM 2008;**178**(3): 218–224.
Brusselle G et al. Eosinophils in the Spotlight: Eosinophilic airway inflammation in nonallergic asthma. Nature Medicine 2013;**19**: 977–979.

Clinical features

- Cough
- Shortness of breath (SOB)
- Wheeze
- Chest tightness.

Classically, these are variable, intermittent, worse at night, associated with specific triggers, e.g. pollens, cat and dog dander, and non-specific triggers, e.g. cold air, perfumes, and bleaches, due to airway hypersensitivity. Asthma may be labelled 'cough variant' or 'cough predominant' when cough is the major symptom (see Box 18.1).

Examination

- May be entirely normal
- Classically, expiratory wheeze is heard
- Chest deformity/hyperinflation—long-standing/poorly controlled asthma
- Severe life-threatening asthma may have no wheeze and a silent chest.

Diagnosis

Asthma is a clinical diagnosis but should be supported by objective measurements. Important to:

- Identify provoking factors, e.g. cold air, bleach, perfume, and environmental aeroallergens (grasses, pollen, hay), and any occupational exposures
- Assess disease severity. Longitudinal studies show greater decline in lung function in asthmatics than non-asthmatics—greater still in asthmatics who smoke.

Don't forget to look for/ask about:

- Nasal symptoms–obstruction, rhinorrhoea, hyposmia
- Atopic dermatitis/eczema/hay fever
- Allergies, including food allergy (see Box 18.2)
- Reflux/gastro-oesophageal reflux disease (GORD) disease (treating reflux may improve symptoms that have been wrongly attributed to asthma, particularly cough)
- Laryngo/pharyngeal reflux (hoarse voice, throat clearing, acid in throat)
- Triggers, including exercise, menstruation
- Social situation/stresses
- Aspirin sensitivity (associated with later-onset asthma and nasal polyps; see Box 18.3)
- Family history.

Box 18.1 The diagnosis is based on the presence of:
- Symptoms (cough, wheeze, breathlessness)
- Day-to-day peak flow variability (>15% variability or reversibility to inhaled β_2 agonist)
- Airway hyperresponsiveness.

Consider the diagnosis of asthma in:
- Recurrent cough, episodic breathlessness, and wheeze
- Chest tightness
- Isolated or nocturnal cough
- Exercised-induced cough or breathlessness
- Hyperventilation syndrome (see ➲ p. 284).

Box 18.2 Oral allergy syndrome
A subset of patients sensitized to aeroallergens, such as tree and grass pollens, develop localized lip angio-oedema after ingestion of specific fruits that share cross-reactive epitopes with pollen allergens. The reaction occurs immediately after ingesting the fruit. Cooked fruit is usually tolerated, presumably because the culpable proteins are denatured with cooking. Birch pollens cross-react with apples, hazelnuts, and potato. Ragwort shares epitopes with melon and bananas.

Box 18.3 Aspirin-induced asthma (AIA) (Samter's triad)
- Defined as asthma, nasal polyps, and aspirin sensitivity.
- Asthma is precipitated by ingestion of aspirin or other NSAIDs
- Occurs in up to 20% of asthmatics and is commoner in women
- The mechanism is thought to be via aspirin inhibition of the cyclo-oxygenase pathway, with excess leukotriene production via the lipo-oxygenase pathway
- BAL and urine in AIA patients show excess leukotrienes post-aspirin exposure
- Loss of anti-inflammatory prostaglandin E2 may also be important.

Investigations

The number of investigations required depends on the probability of the diagnosis from the history, simple spirometry, and peak flow recordings. Most patients referred for a respiratory opinion will already have completed home peak flow recordings and have had a chest radiograph (CXR). Repeating PEFs may still be of benefit. Objective evidence of asthma is important before starting long-term therapy with potentially harmful drugs, e.g. high-dose inhaled steroids. For differential diagnoses, see Box 18.4.

Baseline investigations

- *Peak flow recording/simple spirometry* looking for variability and response to treatment. Airway obstruction leads to decreased PEF and forced expiratory volume in 1s (FEV_1); often normal between episodes of bronchospasm. If persistently normal, the diagnosis must be in doubt. Comparing reading over time and between episodes of normality and high symptoms is of use. The diagnosis is highly likely if:
  - 20% diurnal PEF variation on >3 days/week, in a week of peak flow diary measures
  - FEV_1 ≥15% decrease after 6 min exercise
  - FEV_1 ≥15% (and 200 mL) increase after 2-week trial of oral steroid (30 mg prednisolone od)
- *Bronchodilator reversibility testing* FEV_1 ≥15% (and 200 mL) increase after a single dose of a short-acting β_2 agonist therapy (e.g. salbutamol 4 puffs (400 micrograms) by metred dose inhaler (MDI) with spacer or 2.5 mg by nebulizer) or 200 micrograms bd of inhaled beclomethasone or equivalent for 6–8 weeks. A 400 mL improvement is strongly suggestive of asthma; smaller improvements are less sensitive and need careful interpretation.

Further investigations (if required)

- *Blood tests*
  - Full blood count (FBC; eosinophilia is common in asthma, but, if the total eosinophil count is unusually high, consider eosinophilic granulomatosis with polyangiitis (EGPA; Churg–Strauss syndrome))
  - IgE (associated atopy, i.e. positive skin prick tests to common allergens, often with associated allergic rhinitis and eczema)
  - Specific IgEs if other environmental triggers suspected
- Fractional exhaled nitric oxide concentration (FeNO) has been shown to be useful in monitoring asthma to determine optimum inhaled corticosteroid dose. FeNO may also be useful in diagnosis (but is not a very specific measure). Normal values are 5–25 ppb, values ≥50 ppb are highly suggestive of eosinophilic airway inflammation. FeNO levels are lowered by inhaled corticosteroids and in current smokers. FeNO testing may be used as an aid to assess compliance, e.g. with a FeNO suppression test with monitored inhaled corticosteroids
- There is increasing evidence that elevated FeNO and blood eosinophils are independent and additive prognostic biomarkers of the risk of asthma attacks and are predictive of the likelihood of response to anti-inflammatory treatment including biological drugs. Assessment of these biomarkers is essential in patients with severe asthma. It is likely that risk assessment using these biomarkers will become part of standard clinical practice in the next few years

- *CXR* if atypical symptoms. May show hyperinflation or evidence of localized abnormality simulating wheeze, e.g. adenoma (rare)
- *Skin prick tests* to define atopic constitution or identify potential triggers
- *Methacholine/histamine challenge* measures bronchial hyperresponsiveness (BHR) as a PC_{20}, the dose (provocative concentration) of agent (histamine or methacholine) causing a 20% fall in FEV_1. Asthma is suggested by a PC_{20} <8 mg/mL (the lower the PC_{20}, the more likely the diagnosis is asthma). Normal subjects have a PC_{20} >16 mg/mL. The absence of BHR virtually excludes the diagnosis of asthma; however, the presence of BHR does not prove asthma
- *Bronchial provocation tests* aim to demonstrate bronchospasm to an inhaled agent, usually occupational. The response to an aerosolized sample of a suspected agent may be useful if the diagnosis of occupational asthma is suspected, but PEF recordings at home, work, and on holiday may be more useful. Should only be carried out in a tertiary referral centre, under expert supervision
- *Induced sputum analysis* Sputum eosinophilia may help confirm the diagnosis. Rarely available in routine clinical practice
- *Aspergillus* Specific IgE to *Aspergillus* or skin tests may be useful if *Aspergillus* sensitivity is a concern. See → p. 562 IgG to *Aspergillus* if ABPA is a possibility
- *Laryngoscopy/ENT examination* Useful if concerns about nasal symptoms or obstruction, e.g. from polyps, or to exclude upper airway obstruction, or a vocal cord abnormality
- *Bronchoscopy* Rarely needed. Its main use is to exclude an obstructing airway tumour, e.g. carcinoid. Eosinophilic airway inflammation may be seen on bronchial biopsy
- *Lung biopsy* is very occasionally needed in those in whom no adequate explanation for persistent and minimally reversible airflow obstruction is seen, to exclude another cause, e.g. bronchiolitis obliterans.

Box 18.4 Important differential diagnoses in asthma

Consider especially if unusual features in the history, or poor correlation between objective measures and symptoms, or poor treatment response:

- Upper airway obstruction (breathlessness, noisy, stridulous breathing, low peak flows out of proportion to FEV_1)
- Foreign body aspiration
- Tumour, especially tracheal (but can respond to steroids)
- Congestive cardiac failure (CCF) (young patient with a murmur)
- Vocal cord dysfunction (VCD)
- Hyperventilation syndrome
- Chronic thromboembolic disease or primary pulmonary hypertension (PPH)
- Interstitial lung disease
- EGPA (Churg–Strauss syndrome) and other eosinophilic lung diseases
- Bronchiolitis (see → p. 183)
- Gastro-oesophageal reflux disease (GORD).

Acute severe asthma

As of 2017, asthma still accounts for over 1,400 deaths per year in the UK.

Most asthma deaths occur outside hospital

- Often in patients with a label of mild or moderate asthma (60% of deaths)
- In those receiving inadequate medical treatment and/or supervision
- In those who have been symptomatically deteriorating and may have already sought medical help
- Associated with adverse behavioural and psychosocial factors
- See Box 18.5 for hospital management of acute asthma.

Fatality in asthma is due to cardiac arrest 2° to hypoxia and acidosis—reversal of hypoxia is paramount.
  Give high-flow O_2.

Risk factors for fatal or near-fatal asthma

- Previous near-fatal asthma, e.g. previous ventilation or respiratory acidosis
- Three or more classes of asthma medication
- Repeated A&E attendances (especially within the last 12 months)
- Previous admission for asthma (especially within the last 12 months)
- High β_2 agonist use
- Adverse behavioural or psychosocial features such as:
  - Non-adherence with asthma medications or follow-up
  - Self discharge from hospital
  - Alcohol or drug abuse
  - History of psychiatric illness

Initial assessment of acute asthma

See Box 18.5

- Clinical features e.g. tachypnoea, tachycardia, silent chest
- PEF expressed as a percentage predicted or, more usefully, percentage of the patient's best PEF (within 2 years)
- Pulse oximetry
- Arterial blood gases are required in patients with a SpO_2 <92%. In acute asthma the pCO_2 is initially low due to hyperventilation. A normal CO_2 may indicate fatigue
- CXR is not routinely recommended in the absence of suspected pneumothorax or consolidation, life-threatening asthma, or failure to respond to initial treatment
- Life-threatening or near-fatal asthma attacks require hospital admission.

Severity of acute asthma

Moderate acute asthma
- Increasing symptoms
- PEF ≥50–75% predicted or best
- No features of acute severe asthma
- 1 h following treatment in A&E, patients with PEF ≥75% predicted or best may be discharged home with appropriate changes to their asthma medication in the absence of concerns, e.g.:
  - Significant ongoing symptoms
  - Compliance concerns
  - Living alone
  - Psychological problems or learning difficulties
  - Previous near-fatal asthma
  - Nocturnal presentation
  - Pregnant
  - Exacerbation despite adequate oral steroid pre-presentation.

Acute severe asthma
Defined as any of:
- PEF 33–50% predicted or best
- Respiratory rate (RR) ≥25
- Heart rate (HR) ≥110
- Inability to complete sentence in one breath
- May be able to be discharged if respond well to initial treatment as above.

Life-threatening asthma
Any one of:
- PEF ≤33% predicted or best
- SaO_2 ≤92% (needs arterial blood gases (ABG))
- PaO_2 ≤8 kPa
- Normal CO_2 (4.6–6 kPa)
- Silent chest
- Cyanosis
- Poor respiratory effort
- Bradycardia/arrhythmia/hypotension
- Exhaustion
- Altered conscious level.

Near-fatal asthma
- Raised $PaCO_2$, and/or
- Needing mechanical ventilation with raised inflation pressures.

▶▶Box 18.5 Hospital treatment of acute asthma

- Airway—ensure no upper airway obstruction
- Breathing—give high-flow O_2
- Circulation—gain intravenous (IV) access.

Monitoring
- Record PEF on arrival in A&E, 15–30 min after starting treatment, and regularly thereafter, according to response
- Record O_2 saturation, and maintain 94–98%
- ABG for pH and $PaCO_2$ (if saturation <92% or other severe features)
- Record and document HR and RR
- Measure glucose and potassium
- O_2—high concentration (40–60%) and high-flow mask, e.g. Hudson
- CXR to exclude infection/pneumothorax.

NB CO_2 retention, following administration of high-flow O_2, is not a problem in acute asthma. A high CO_2 indicates a near-fatal attack and should precipitate urgent intensive care unit (ICU) review for invasive ventilatory support, **not** controlled O_2 therapy. CO_2 is often low (due to hyperventilation), thus a normal CO_2 may indicate a tiring patient.

Treatment
- β2 *agonist*—inhaled or nebulized, e.g. nebulized salbutamol 2.5–5 mg, driven by O_2
  - Give repeated doses or continuous, e.g. 5–10 mg/h
  - Use IV only if inhaled therapy cannot be used reliably (rarely the case)
  - Note: risk of hypokalaemia with $β_2$ agonist and steroids. Repeated use of $β_2$ agonists may lead to lactic acidosis
- *Anticholinergic*—nebulized ipratropium bromide (500 micrograms 4–6 hourly) added to $β_2$ agonist therapy may improve bronchodilatation in acute severe asthma
- *Steroids*—the earlier given in an attack, the better the outcome
  - Oral is as effective as IV
  - Dose 40–50 mg PO prednisolone, continuing for at least 5 days or until recovery. There is no agreed definition of recovery, but sensible to continue oral steroids until peak flow is maintained for 5–7 days. The dose can be stopped abruptly (assuming the patient continues on inhaled steroid). This does not apply to patients on repeated doses or long-term steroids where a longer and weaning course may be appropriate
  - Inhaled corticosteroids should be continued (or started as soon as possible) as part of the chronic disease management plan
- *IV magnesium sulfate*—immediately if acute severe and if poor response to above therapies, 1.2–2 g IV infusion over 20 min. The safety and efficacy of repeated doses have not been assessed. Nebulized magnesium sulfate is not recommended in adults.
- *IV aminophylline*—some patients may respond; give if poor response to initial therapy in acute severe or life-threatening disease
  - Dose—5 mg/kg loading dose over 20 min, followed by continuous infusion of 0.5–0.7 mg/kg (500 mg in 500 mL normal saline or 0.5% glucose at 0.5 × body weight in kg/mL/h). If on maintenance therapy, do not give loading dose, but start continuous infusion

- Note: needs therapeutic drug monitoring. Side effects: nausea, arrhythmias, palpitations. Cardiac monitoring is required
- *Antibiotics*—only give if definite infective element to the exacerbation. Most exacerbations are due to viruses, especially the common cold. *C. pneumoniae* and *M. pneumoniae* are also implicated
- *IV fluids*—patients are often dehydrated. Hypokalaemia (due to β_2 agonists) must be corrected
- *Intramuscular (IM) adrenaline*—may be useful if near arrest, while awaiting ICU support.

ICU referral

Liaise with ICU early! Better to discuss early a patient who does not subsequently need ICU input, than to find you and your patient in difficulty with no ICU bed. See Box 18.6.

There is very little evidence to support the use of NIV in the management of asthma in the ICU setting. There is no evidence to support its use outside of ICU. Hypercapnic respiratory failure in acute severe asthma is an urgent indication for endotracheal intubation.

Box 18.6 When to discuss with ITU
- Worsening PEF despite treatment
- Worsening hypoxia
- Hypercapnia (or rising CO_2 even if not yet >6 kPa)
- Falling pH
- Exhaustion/poor respiratory effort
- Drowsiness/confusion
- Respiratory arrest.

Discharge

Consider discharge when:
- Reduced β_2 agonist dose
- Off nebulized drugs and on inhalers ≥24 h
- PEF ≥75% predicted or best
- Minimal PEF diurnal variation
- Appropriate education has been given.

Prior to discharge, consider:
- Reason for the exacerbation. Could it have been avoided?
- Check patient's self-management plan/asthma action plan
- Check inhaler technique (see ➔ p. 752)
- Discharge on an inhaled steroid containing inhaler
- Book an appointment with GP or practice nurse for within 2 days
- Book chest clinic appointment with respiratory physician or specialist nurse within 1 month

Further reading

Royal College of Physicians. Why asthma still kills, The National Review of Asthma Deaths (NRAD). 2014.
BTS/SIGN British guideline on the management of asthma. 2019 ♪ https://www.brit-thoracic.org.uk/quality-improvement/guidelines/asthma/

Chronic asthma: management

Aim to minimize symptoms and prevent exacerbations, prevent the potential consequences of long-standing airway inflammation leading to airway remodelling and chronic unresponsive airway obstruction, and improve quality of living (QoL) (see Box 18.7).

The emphasis should be on education, self-management, and personal asthma action plans. Aim for:

- Minimal day and night symptoms
- No exacerbations
- Normal lung function and prevention of lung function decline with the development of fixed airflow obstruction
- No limit to physical activity
- Minimum steroid dose.

Treatment guidelines use a step-up/step-down approach, starting treatment at the level appropriate to disease control, based on the history, spirometry, and medication usage.

> **Box 18.7 The main aims during outpatient review**
> - Ensure the diagnosis is correct and that symptoms are due to asthma and not coexistent/alternative pathology (e.g. reflux, dysfunctional breathing, etc.)
> - Aim for no symptoms/normal lung function on minimal treatment
> - Ensure an action plan is in place for exacerbations
> - Identify patients at risk of an adverse outcome.

Pharmacological management

Incorporating 2019 British Thoracic Society (BTS)/Scottish Intercollegiate Guidelines Network (SIGN) guidelines for the management of asthma. Therapy should be escalated and reduced through these steps to find the lowest dose of medications that adequately controls symptoms. Inhaler technique (including a spacer if used) and treatment adherence should be assessed at each stage.

Intermittent reliever therapy

Patients with a diagnosis of asthma should be prescribed a short-acting bronchodilator to relieve symptoms. Intermittent reliever therapy alone is not recommended for the treatment of established asthma.

- Inhaled short-acting β_2 agonist or ipratropium bromide
- Ten puffs/day (two or more canisters/month) is a marker of poorly controlled disease.

Regular preventer therapy

- Inhaled steroids are the most effective preventer drugs in achieving asthma control
- Start at 200 micrograms/day beclomethasone dipropionate (BDP) or equivalent in a twice-daily dose
- Titrate steroid dose to symptoms, aiming for lowest effective dose
- Local steroid side effects only (oral *Candida*, dysphonia) from BDP ≤800 micrograms/day

- Possible dose-related bone density effects at this dose or above
- Fluticasone provides equal clinical activity to budesonide at half dosage. Mometasone is an alternative inhaled steroid; the current limited evidence suggests it is equivalent to twice the dose of BDP. Ciclesonide is a pro-drug, and the available evidence suggests it may have fewer local oropharyngeal side effects and less systemic activity than conventional inhaled steroids. Qvar® (BDP) has a smaller particle size and may be of benefit in some.

Initial add-on therapy
- If asthma remains uncontrolled despite taking 200–800 micrograms/day inhaled steroid, add a long-acting β_2 agonist (LABA). A combination inhaled corticosteroid (ICS)/LABA preparation is generally preferred to ensure continued ICS usage with LABA and improve adherence
- If there is no response to a LABA, consider stopping it and increase the inhaled steroid dose
- The combination of an inhaled corticosteroid and LABA is licensed as maintenance *and* reliever therapy (MART therapy), if a rapid-onset LABA, e.g. formoterol, is used in the context of a personal asthma action plan.

Additional add-on therapies
- Ensure definite benefit is obtained from any of these subsequent drugs before continuing—stop and consider an alternative drug if no benefit
- Increase inhaled steroid dose to 800 micrograms BDP/day or equivalent
- Leukotriene receptor antagonist—limited evidence as add-on therapy in adults but produces a benefit in some. Trial for 4 weeks and stop if no benefit

Specialist therapies
- If asthma remains uncontrolled despite the above steps, refer for specialist care
- Tiotropium bromide—some evidence of reduced exacerbation frequency when added to ICS/LABA. Further studies ongoing
- Theophylline may be trialled but *needs therapeutic drug monitoring* as has side effects, for example, nausea
- If control is inadequate on 800 micrograms BDP equivalent with a LABA, can increase inhaled steroid dose to 2,000 micrograms BDP equivalent in a combination inhaler
- Continuous or frequent use of oral steroids. Asthma that is not controlled on the above treatments may require long-term oral steroids. Aim is to control asthma using the lowest possible doses.

  These patients should be under the care of a specialist asthma service
- Risk of side effects if on oral steroids for >3 months or 3–4 courses/year
- Warn patient of potential side effects (hypertension, diabetes, cataracts, gastric erosions), and ask GP to monitor. Start osteoporosis prophylaxis with calcium and vitamin D, or a bisphosphonate. Document baseline bone densitometry in those receiving prednisolone for >3 months (see € p. 742).

Monoclonal antibody therapy

Recent advances in severe asthma have yielded new monoclonal antibody therapies. These are for the treatment of severe, eosinophilic asthma.

Omalizumab

Monoclonal antibody against IgE, has been shown to reduce asthma exacerbations, improve asthma symptom and QoL scores and is licensed for atopic individuals with difficult-to-control asthma. Omalizumab is given as a subcutaneous injection 2–4 weekly. The dose depends on the patient's weight and serum IgE concentration; around two-thirds of patients respond. The serum IgE should be 30–700 IU/mL, with higher IgE levels acceptable at higher body weights. 2013 National Institute for Health and Care Excellence (NICE) approved for severe persistent allergic asthma, which is unstable despite optimized standard therapy (continuous oral steroid or >4 courses/year). Response is assessed at 16 weeks. No evidence for oral steroid-sparing effect. Can now be self-administered at home.

Mepolizumab

Monoclonal antibody against IL-5. NICE approved for use in severe, eosinophilic (blood eosinophil count ≥ $0.3*10^9$ cells/L) with continuous or frequent (≥4) oral corticosteroid use in the last 12 months despite optimized standard therapy. Given as a subcutaneous injection of 100 mg 4 weekly. Shown to reduce asthma exacerbations by around 50% and to reduce maintenance oral corticosteroid dose by 50% compared to placebo. Treatment response assessed at 12 months. Can be self-administered at home.

Benralizumab

Monoclonal antibody against the IL-5 receptor-alpha. NICE approved for severe eosinophilic asthma, either blood eosinophil count ≥ $0.3*10^9$ cells/L with continuous or frequent (≥4) oral corticosteroid use in the last 12 months or blood eosinophil count ≥$0.4*10^9$ cells/L with continuous or frequent (≥3) oral corticosteroid use in the last 12 months. Given as a subcutaneous injection of 30 mg 8 weekly after the initial 3 doses are given 4 weekly. Similar exacerbation and oral corticosteroid reduction to mepolizumab.

Reslizumab

Monoclonal antibody against IL-5. NICE approved for severe eosinophilic asthma (blood eosinophil count ≥ $0.4*10^9$ cells/L) with continuous or frequent (≥3) oral corticosteroid use in the last 12 months. Given as an intravenous infusion 4 weekly. Similar exacerbation reduction as mepolizumab and benralizumab. Oral steroid sparing effects are being investigated.

Dupilumab

Monoclonal antibody against the IL-4 receptor-alpha. Dupilumab blocks the action of IL-4 and IL-13. Proven efficacy in moderate-severe type 2 asthma (as evidenced by the blood eosinophil count and/or FeNO) in reducing exacerbations and in oral steroid reduction. Licensed for use in asthma and also has a license for atopic dermatitis and nasal polyps, both conditions that often coexist with asthma. Currently undergoing evaluation by NICE.

Additional points

- *Regular review* To ensure patients are on appropriate treatment for their disease severity and are maintained on the lowest possible inhaled steroid dose. This may include adherence/prescription reviews. Step down treatment if patient stable for 3 months or more. Step down inhaled steroid by reducing dose by 25% at 3-monthly intervals. The Royal College of Physicians (RCP) has suggested three routine questions for monitoring (see Box 18.8)
- *Asthma action plan* All patients with severe asthma should have an agreed written asthma action plan (self-management plan), their own peak flow meter, and regular checks on compliance and inhaler technique. A self-management plan should include specific advice about recognizing loss of asthma control and action to take if asthma deteriorates. Patients may be advised to increase their ICS dose fourfold at the start of an exacerbation to try and avoid a course of OCS. This may be achieved by adding an additional ICS inhaler to ICS/LABA combinations. The previous recommendation of doubling the dose of inhaled steroid at the start of an exacerbation is unproven.

Box 18.8 Monitoring morbidity—the three RCP questions

In the last week or month:
- Have you had difficulty sleeping because of your asthma symptoms (including cough)?
- Have you had your usual asthma symptoms during the day (cough, wheeze, chest tightness, or breathlessness)?
- Has your asthma interfered with your usual activities (e.g. work, housework)?

Chronic asthma: additional treatment options

Steroid-sparing drugs

For example, methotrexate, oral gold, and ciclosporin—may be useful if other treatments are unsuccessful. They may reduce long-term steroid requirements, but all have side effects and need haematological surveillance. There are very few data to support their use, and significant variability in response. Guidelines suggest a 3-month trial, once other drugs have proven unsuccessful, with treatment in a centre with experience of their use. The use of these agents has become superfluous in the biological era as biological treatments targeting IL-5 and IL-4/13 have emerged as highly effective oral corticosteroid (OCS) sparing agents

Continuous subcutaneous terbutaline

Has no RCT evidence to show efficacy or safety in asthma.

Macrolides

Increasing evidence suggests azithromycin may reduce the rate of severe exacerbations across phenotypes of asthma (AMAZES study). They should be considered in patients who continue to exacerbate despite treatment optimisation. Their effect is being further studied, as are concerns regarding antibiotic resistance and non-tuberculous mycobacteria (NTM) infection with long-term macrolide use.

Bronchial thermoplasty

This is the application of controlled radiofrequency energy to the airway wall, using a specialized catheter at bronchoscopy. It heats the tissue to about 65°C, reducing muscle mass in the small and medium-sized airways, with several airways treated under direct vision at each session. Three separate sessions are required to treat all accessible airways. There is limited evidence to suggest that it can reduce exacerbations of asthma. Adverse events are common in the period immediately after the procedure. The optimum target group for this treatment has not yet been identified. Bronchial thermoplasty can be considered at a specialist centre in patients who have poorly controlled asthma despite optimum medical therapy.

Future developments

New steroids

Research for 'dissociated steroids' is ongoing. These are steroids in which the useful anti-inflammatory effects (mediated by transcription factor inhibition) are dissociated from the side effects (mediated via glucocorticoid DNA binding). Safer steroids, e.g. ciclesonide, a once-a-day inhaled steroid, appear to have an improved side effect profile. Ciclesonide is a pro-drug, activated by airway esterases, with fewer side effects due to high degrees of protein binding.

Cytokine targets

The cytokines IL-33, IL-25, and thymic stromal lymphopoietin (TSLP) are epithelial alarmins thought to be involved in the pathogenesis of type-1, neutrophilic inflammation and type 2, eosinophilic inflammation. Studies evaluating monoclonal antibodies targeting these are currently underway.

Oral anti-inflammatory drugs

Oral antagonists of the prostaglandin-D2 receptor, CRTH2, have been shown to reduce eosinophilic airway inflammation. These are being further evaluated in phase 3 studies.

Inhaled steroid strategy

Recent evidence suggests that prn ICS/LABA is more effective than short-acting β-agonist (SABA) alone and just as effective as regular ICS preventer in preventing asthma exacerbations despite a lower daily ICS dose. This is being further investigated as a treatment strategy.

Further information

Normansell et al. Omalizumab for chronic asthma in adults and children. *Cochrane Database Syst Rev* 2014;(1).

Pavord ID et al. Mepolizumab for severe eosinophilic asthma (DREAM): a multicenter, double-blind, placebo-controlled trial. *Lancet* 2012;**380**: 651–659.

Gibson et al. Effect of azithromycin on asthma exacerbations and quality of life in adults with persistent uncontrolled asthma (AMAZES): a randomised, double-blind, placebo-controlled trial. *Lancet* 2017;**390**(10095): P659–P668.

Non-pharmacological management

Allergen avoidance

May reduce severity of disease in sensitized the individual; however, despite theoretical benefits, it is generally hard to demonstrate the benefit of allergen avoidance in clinical trials. House dust mite control measures need to be comprehensive—there is no current evidence to support it, although trials are ongoing. Pet removal may be useful, if the history is suggestive and sensitivity has been demonstrated by skin prick testing or raised specific IgE levels.

Smoking cessation

May reduce asthma severity. Current and previous smoking reduces the effect of inhaled steroid; these individuals may need higher steroid doses.

Complementary therapies

No consistent evidence of benefit.

Dietary manipulation

No consistent evidence and none supported by interventional trials.

Weight reduction

In obese asthmatics weight reduction leads to improved control.

Immunotherapy

No clear benefit of subcutaneous or sublingual immunotherapy. Not recommended for the treatment of asthma.

Breathing techniques

A Cochrane review of breathing exercises concluded that there was no evidence of improvement in lung function, but showed improved QoL scores.

Further information

NICE guidelines Bronchial thermoplasty for severe asthma. 2018 ℘ https://www.nice.org.uk/guidance/ipg635
BTS/SIGN British guideline on the management of asthma. 2019 ℘ https://www.brit-thoracic.org.uk/quality-improvement/guidelines/asthma/
℘ http://www.ginasthma.com.

Difficult/refractory asthma

Patients with difficult asthma are a small subgroup of asthma patients (5–10%). There is no universally accepted definition of difficult asthma, but it refers to a clinical situation where a prior diagnosis of asthma exists, and asthma-like symptoms and asthma attacks persist despite prescription of high-dose asthma therapy. These individuals have disease that is difficult to treat, evidenced by high-maintenance medication requirements or persistent symptoms and airflow obstruction, with multiple exacerbations, despite high medication use. They have high numbers of admissions and cause significant anxiety to their families and medical staff. There is a wide range of disease severity, including those with highly labile disease and those with severe, more chronic airflow obstruction. It is important to try and identify 'difficult to treat' asthma due to factors such as treatment adherence, smoking, and psychological comorbidity from treatment refractory asthma. Treatment non-adherence is over-represented in patients with difficult asthma.

Difficult asthma should be systematically assessed by a multidisciplinary difficult asthma service.

Diagnosis of refractory asthma

- Confirm the asthma diagnosis is correct—this will mean going back through the notes and retaking a thorough history
- Confirm reversible airflow limitation now or in the past (as for non-refractory asthma; see ➋ p. 146)
- Consider other diagnoses for cough, breathlessness, and wheeze, and investigate for potential exacerbating diseases:
  - COPD/smoking/α1-AT deficiency
  - Bronchiectasis/cystic fibrosis (CF)
  - Sinus disease—consider ENT review
  - EGPA (Churg–Strauss syndrome)/eosinophilic syndromes—consider antinuclear cytoplasmic antibody (ANCA)
  - Systemic disease—thyroid disease or vasculitis
  - Allergic bronchopulmonary aspergillosis (ABPA)—consider *Aspergillus* IgE and IgG/skin tests/total IgE
  - VCD—consider laryngoscopy
  - Hyperventilation syndrome/dysfunctional breathing
  - Gastro-oesophageal reflux—consider oesophagogastroduodenoscopy (OGD)/24 h pH study
  - Upper airway obstruction—consider CT or bronchoscopy
  - Obstructive sleep apnoea (OSA)—consider sleep study
  - Obesity
  - Cardiac dysfunction—consider echo and/or cardiological opinion
  - Psychiatric/emotional issues/depression/2° gain—consider psychiatry or psychology review
  - Functional wheeze by breathing near residual volume.

Refractory asthma

Before labelling a patient as 'refractory', compliance must be confirmed. This is usually done by checking pharmacy prescription records, using inhaler devices monitoring medication usage, i.e. 'chipped inhalers', FeNO suppression testing, or by measurement of plasma prednisolone or early morning cortisol levels.

Treatment
Is that of non-refractory asthma, with inhaled LABA and high-dose inhaled corticosteroids (see ➲ p. 152). Ensure treatment trials are adequate and adhered to.
- In patients unable to tolerate a prednisolone dose <20 mg/day, corticosteroid pharmacokinetic studies may be useful. However, <25% of patients with severe asthma show clinically significantly increased prednisolone clearance (usually a specific reason can be identified such as concomitant use of enzyme-inducing medication). IM steroid, e.g. triamcinolone 100 mg, may be useful if compliance is a major problem, should give an adequate steroid level for 1 month
- Inflammatory biomarkers markers, e.g. sputum or plasma eosinophil counts or FeNO, may be useful to assess medication response
- Anti-inflammatory and immunomodulating drugs (specialized centre only). Include methotrexate, ciclosporin, oral gold, and IV gamma-globulin. None of these have been studied in an RCT in this group of patients, and none have demonstrated improvement in airway hyperresponsiveness
- Macrolide antibiotics have anti-inflammatory and immune modulatory effects, reducing airway reactivity and inflammation, and have been shown to reduce oral steroid requirements and reduce exacerbation rate in non-eosinophilic asthma. Persistence of airway infection by *H. influenzae*, *C. pneumoniae*, and *Mycoplasma* is increasingly recognized as a contributory factor in persistent airflow obstruction and recurrent exacerbations, and macrolide antibiotics may act in this situation to clear persistent infection. Use, e.g. azithromycin 250 mg, on alternate days or 3 times a week, or 500 mg twice weekly. Risk of hearing loss, see ➲ p. 250 for guidance.

'Steroid-resistant' asthma
This subgroup of patients represents a very small proportion of refractory asthma patients. They are likely to be the non-eosinophilic end of the spectrum. Middle-aged obese women, often with other additional diagnoses, are over-represented in this group. They require supportive treatment, without high doses of corticosteroids. Diagnoses other than asthma are likely, and investigation should be directed towards these. Whether they represent a further 'asthma phenotype' is unclear.

Further information
BTS/SIGN British guideline on the management of asthma. 2019 ℘ https://www.brit-thoracic.org.uk/quality-improvement/guidelines/asthma/
Robinson DS et al. Systematic assessment of difficult-to-treat asthma. *Eur Respir J* 2003;**22**: 478–483.

Asthma in pregnancy

Pregnancy can affect asthma.

- Asthma can affect the outcome of pregnancy
- Prognosis—1/3 worsen, 1/3 improve, 1/3 no change
- Asthma course is likely to be similar in successive pregnancies
- Severe asthma is more likely to deteriorate than mild asthma
- Most exacerbations occur late, in the second and third trimester, and are due to viral infections and non-adherence to inhaled corticosteroid.

Pre-pregnancy counselling

- Asthmatics must continue normal asthma medication
- Give smoking cessation advice
- Monitor the pregnant asthmatic closely
- Severe exacerbations in pregnancy are associated with low birthweight infants, an effect similar to maternal smoking in pregnancy.

Acute asthma in pregnancy

- Risk to foetus of uncontrolled asthma outweighs any small risk of drugs
- Asthma medications are generally safe in pregnancy—treat acute asthma as you would for non-pregnant patients
- Inhaled steroids should be continued.
- Drug therapy as for non-asthmatics, including inhaled and oral corticosteroids
- Maintain O_2 saturation >94–98%
- Continuous foetal monitoring during acute severe asthma
- Liaise with obstetrician if acute severe asthma

Leukotriene receptor antagonists

Limited safety data available for use in pregnancy. Should not be withheld if required for achieving asthma control.

Monoclonal antibody therapy

Omalizumab is not approved for use in pregnancy but registry data suggests that it is safe. Often continued during pregnancy due to the risk of poor asthma control on pregnancy. Data for the newer, anti-IL-5 drugs are awaited but animal models do not suggest any risk of harm.

Management during labour

- Acute asthma is rare in labour (probably due to high sympathetic drive)
- Close liaison between the respiratory and obstetric teams is paramount, with close foetal monitoring
- Management should be as for non-pregnant individuals (see ➲ p. 148), maintaining the O_2 saturation >94–98%. There is no RCT data for magnesium sulfate, although it is used in eclampsia
- Regional anaesthetic blockade is preferable to general anaesthesia
- Prostaglandin E_2 may be safely used for induction of labour
- Prostaglandin $F_2\alpha$ (for post-partum bleeding) should be used with extreme caution due to the risk of inducing bronchospasm
- Give parenteral hydrocortisone, 100 mg 6–8-hourly, during labour if on oral prednisolone at >7.5 mg daily for >2 weeks prior to delivery.

Breastfeeding
- An asthmatic mother may reduce the chance of atopy in her child by breastfeeding; current opinion is divided
- Prednisolone is secreted in breast milk, but the infant is exposed to only tiny, and clinically irrelevant, doses.
- Use asthma medications as normal during lactation.

Occupational asthma

- This is asthma due to specific workplace sensitizers and may account for 10% of adult-onset asthma
- The diagnosis is often difficult to make
- Early diagnosis is important, as earlier removal from the workplace in affected individuals leads to a better outcome
- It is different to asthma exacerbated by irritants in the workplace and can occur in individuals with or without prior asthma.

- Agents induce asthma through immunological and non-immunological mechanisms. Immunological disease appears after a latency period of exposure; thus, it is necessary for the worker to be sensitized to the causal agent. Non-immunological disease is characterized by the absence of a latent period and occurs after accidental exposure to high concentrations of a workplace irritant. This is irritant-induced asthma (previously named reactive airways dysfunction syndrome), usually caused by exposure to, e.g. smoke, vapours, or fumes, with a strong temporal relationship between irritant exposure and the development of asthma-type symptoms
- The latency between first exposure and symptom onset can be long and depends on the sensitizing agent—an accurate history therefore includes current and past exposures
- Once sensitized, re-exposure to very low concentrations can provoke symptoms
- May be associated with rhinitis and urticaria
- Improves away from work but can take several days to settle.

Risk factors
- Atopy
- HLA type (e.g. *HLA-DQB1*0503* associated with isocyanate allergy)
- Smoking (especially for high molecular weight agents).

Diagnosis
- Confirm the diagnosis of asthma
- Confirm the relationship between asthma and work exposures
- Find the specific cause
- There are two useful screening questions:
  - Is your asthma worse when at work?
  - Does your asthma improve when away from work or on holiday?

Document lung function deterioration in the workplace, usually by serial peak flow recording at work, at home, and on holiday.

Bronchial provocation/challenge testing using suspected agent—*only* in specialized centres, but difficulties with testing and producing a valid test substance mean that a negative specific bronchial challenge in a worker with otherwise good evidence of occupational asthma is not sufficient to exclude the diagnosis.

Skin prick testing/specific IgE for certain sensitizers (although a positive test only indicates sensitization which can occur with or without disease).

Document
- The range of chemicals used, and look up the literature on their propensity to cause asthma (see Table 18.1)
- Working practices
- Use of personal protective equipment.

Serial PEF recording in occupational asthma
- Record every 2 h from waking to sleep
- For 4 weeks, while no changes to treatment
- Document home/work periods and any holidays
- Analysis is best made by experts, usually using a criterion-based analysis system, e.g. OASYS (a computer program that plots and interprets serial peak flow recordings; see ॐ http://www.occupationalasthma.com)
- Patients may be sensitized to >1 agent, and >300 agents have been identified.

Table 18.1 Causes of occupational asthma

Sensitizing agent	Occupational exposure
Low molecular weight agents (act as haptens)	
Isocyanates	Paint spraying, adhesives, polyurethane foams
Acid anhydrides	Epoxy paint, varnish, resins, baking
Metals	Welding, plating, metal refining
Glutaraldehyde and other disinfectants	Health care workers
Drugs	Pharmaceutical industry
High molecular weight agents	
Amine dyes	Cosmetics, hair dyes, rubber workers
Wood dusts, bark	Textile workers, joiners, carpenters
Animal-derived antigens	Vets, laboratory workers (20% affected)
Biological enzymes	Detergent industry, pharmaceuticals
Plant products	Bakers, hairdressers
Fluxes, colophony	Solderers, electronics industry

Management of occupational asthma

- Identify the cause
- Remove the worker from exposure
- Support continued employment away from the cause, if at all possible
- Early diagnosis and removal from exposure are important factors for a good outcome
- Improvement in FEV_1 may be maintained for 1 y following last exposure, and for up to 2 y for non-specific responsiveness
- The decision to remove the patient from the workplace should not be taken lightly and should be made by a consultant with experience of occupational lung disease
- The employee may be eligible for *industrial injuries disablement benefit* (no proof of negligence is required) see p. 737.

Vocal cord dysfunction

A proportion of patients labelled as having severe asthma will have symptoms originating from the upper airway. This can be due to VCD and/or so-called 'upper airway hyperresponsiveness'; these are different but overlap. VCD is likely to arise from interrelationships between laryngeal hyperresponsiveness and autonomic imbalance, with inputs from potential aetiological/aggravating factors, e.g. reflux, psychological stress, hypocapnia (hyperventilation). Increased laryngeal hyperresponsiveness can occur following respiratory tract infections and possibly asthma itself. Upper airway hyperresponsiveness may include more than just the larynx, but this is not clear.

Patients will typically present with asthma symptoms, with associated triggers, e.g. odours, cold air. They typically have no reduction in peak flow or response to asthma medications (though this is possible).

A careful history will reveal shortness of breath that is of short duration, worse on inspiration, and extremely sudden in onset, with symptom-free periods.

Pathogenesis
- Recent upper respiratory tract infection (URTI), may take months to settle
- Post-nasal drip/chronic sinusitis
- GORD with micro-aspiration
- Chronic laryngitis
- Hyperventilation in association with anxiety/panic
- It is postulated that the origin of the vocal cord closure may stem from a reflex airway protective mechanism.

Diagnosis
Based on excluding other causes of cough and breathlessness. It may be suggested by hearing a more stridulous noise and lack of basal wheeze. The gold standard is visualization of abnormal vocal cord movement at laryngoscopy, where there is excessive adduction of the anterior two-thirds of cords with the creation of a posterior 'glottic chink', although this finding may not always be present at the time of study. Inducible laryngeal obstruction (ILO) can occur on exercise and can be evaluated using dynamic, exercise laryngoscopy. The flow–volume loop should show inspiratory flow limitation, with 'stuttering' of the flow.

Treatments
(for which there are no RCTs)
- Speech therapy
- Psychology input
- Coughing and cough suppression techniques
- Local botulinum injections

Further information
Hull et al. Laryngeal dysfunction: assessment and management for the clinician. *AJRCCM* 2016;**194**(9): 1062–1072.
Stanton AE, Bucknall CE. Vocal cord dysfunction. A review. *Breathe* 2005;**2**: 31–37 (℞ http://www.ers-education.org/publications/breathe/archive/september-2005.aspx).

Allergic rhinitis (hay fever)

This is the syndrome of nasal discharge or blockage, with nasal and/or eye itching and sneezing. It is often associated with post-nasal drip, cough, fatigue, and with significant morbidity. Allergic rhinitis is defined as perennial if the symptoms occur all year round, and seasonal if occurring at a particular time of year. The prevalence is increasing and affects up to 15% of the UK population. Up to 30% of patients with persistent allergic rhinitis have asthma.

Aetiology

The lining of the nose is in continuum with the lower respiratory tract, and inflammation of the upper and lower airways often coexists. Common aeroallergens provoking seasonal allergic rhinitis are tree pollen in the spring and grass pollen in the summer months. Perennial rhinitis usually reflects allergy to indoor allergens such as house dust mite (the provoking allergen is a digestive enzyme that is shed in the faeces), cat salivary protein, cockroaches, or animal dander.

Pathophysiology

Symptoms occur following the inhalation of allergen to which the subject is sensitized and against which they have IgE antibodies. These antibodies bind to mast cell IgE receptors, with the release of mediators, including tryptase and histamine, causing symptoms immediately after exposure.

Diagnosis

Usually made from the history, which should identify the triggers to the disease. The main differential diagnosis is with sinusitis due to bacterial infection and upper airway involvement due to vasculitis. Asthma is common in association with rhinitis, and treatment of rhino-sinusitis in association with asthma leads to improved asthma control. Up to 50% of asthma patients will have allergic rhinitis.

Treatment

- Allergen avoidance—this may be easier said than done. It can take up to 20 weeks to remove cat allergen from a house. Keeping car and house windows shut may help avoid pollen. Pollen counts are highest in the afternoon and early evening. Wearing sunglasses may reduce the ill-understood 'photic-sneeze' reflex, commoner in allergic rhinitis sufferers.
- Desensitization with increasing doses of the subcutaneous allergen is of debatable value, and includes a small risk of anaphylaxis during therapy
- Non-sedating antihistamines improve sneezing and itching but have less effect on nasal blockage
- Topical intranasal steroid, e.g. budesonide, triamcinolone
- Topical anticholinergics, e.g. ipratropium, may be useful for rhinorrhoea, if uncontrolled with topical nasal steroids
- Topical sodium cromoglicate may be beneficial, particularly for allergic conjunctivitis
- Decongestants, e.g. oxymetazoline, may help, but rebound nasal blockage and tachyphylaxis are a potential problem if used regularly
- Leukotriene receptor antagonists (e.g. montelukast) may be beneficial.

Chapter 19

Bronchiectasis

Epidemiology, pathophysiology, and causes *170*
Clinical features and diagnosis *174*
General management *176*
Further management *180*

Epidemiology, pathophysiology, and causes

Definition

Irreversible abnormal dilatation of one or more bronchi, with chronic airway inflammation. Associated chronic sputum production, recurrent chest infections, and airflow obstruction.

Epidemiology

UK 2013 data suggests a prevalence of around 500/100,000 (female>male). The exact prevalence is unknown but recent epidemiological studies suggest it is increasing. The advent of high resolution computed tomography (HRCT) scanning may now lead to the diagnosis of more subtle (and possibly subclinical) disease.

Pathophysiology

An initial (usually infectious) insult is needed to damage the airways. Disordered anatomy leads to 2° bacterial colonization, perpetuating inflammatory change and damaging the mucociliary escalator. This prevents bacterial clearance and leads to further airway damage. Major airways and bronchioles are involved, with mucosal oedema, inflammation, and ulceration. Terminal bronchioles become obstructed with secretions, leading to volume loss. A chronic host inflammatory response ensues, with free radical formation and production of neutrophil elastase, further contributing to inflammation. Bronchial neovascularization, with hypertrophy and tortuosity of the bronchial arteries (which are at systemic pressure), may lead to intermittent haemoptysis.

Aetiology

The causes of bronchiectasis are many and varied (see Table 19.1). Determining the aetiology of the condition may lead to different management if, for example, the underlying cause is found to be cystic fibrosis (CF), rather than an immune deficiency. The cause is idiopathic in around 50% of cases, and these are likely to be due to an (as yet unidentified) impairment in host defence.

The most important cause to exclude is CF (see ➔ p. 237). Even relatively mild bronchiectasis diagnosed in middle age can be due to CF; this diagnosis will alter management, with:

- Involvement of the multidisciplinary CF team
- Attention to other potential problems, e.g. GI disease, diabetes
- Family screening
- Fertility issues.

Consider investigations for CF (cystic fibrosis transmembrane conductance regulator (CFTR) mutation screen and sweat test; see ➔ p. 239) if:

- Predominantly upper lobe disease
- Persistent *S. aureus* infection
- Malnutrition ± malabsorption, diabetes
- Family history of bronchiectasis (consider CF, primary ciliary dyskinesia (PCD), activated PI3 kinase delta syndrome (APDS))
- Associated subfertility or infertility
- Age <40 at presentation and no other cause for bronchiectasis identified.

Table 19.1 Causes of bronchiectasis

Congenital	Pulmonary sequestration
Post-infective	Tuberculosis
	Whooping cough (if infection in a localized area)
	Severe pneumonia
	Non-tuberculous mycobacteria (NTM) (see ➲ p. 618)—there is some debate as to whether the bronchiectasis seen in association with NTM (classically in elderly ♀) is caused or secondarily infected by NTM
Immunodeficiency	1°—common variable immune deficiency (CVID), X-linked agammaglobulinaemia (XLA, usually diagnosed in childhood), activated PI3 kinase delta syndrome (APDS, due to rare activating PI3Kd mutations; causes bronchiectasis which is often familial, with *H. influenza* and *S. pneumoniae* infection; other features may include herpes virus infection, cytopenias, elevated IgM, and lymphoma), Good syndrome (immunodeficiency with current or prior thymoma)
	2°—HIV, chronic lymphocytic leukaemia, nephrotic syndrome
Mucociliary clearance abnormalities	
Airway diseases	Cystic fibrosis
	Primary ciliary dyskinesia (see ➲ p. 506) chronic obstructive pulmonary disease (COPD)
	Asthma
	A1AT Deficiency
	Allergic bronchopulmonary aspergillosis (ABPA)
Toxic insults	Aspiration
	Inhalation (toxic gases, chemicals)
Mechanical insults	Foreign body aspiration
	Extrinsic lymph node compression
	Intrinsic (intraluminal) obstructing tumour

Associated diseases	Bronchiectasis is associated with a number of systemic diseases, so cough and sputum production in these conditions should trigger referral to determine the cause:
	Rheumatoid arthritis (RA) (up to 35% of RA patients have bronchiectasis) (see ➔ p. 216)
	Connective tissue diseases, e.g. Sjögren's syndrome, systemic lupus erythematosus (see ➔ p. 218)
	Ulcerative colitis and Crohn's disease (see ➔ p. 310)
	Chronic sinusitis
	Yellow nail syndrome
	Marfan's syndrome

Clinical features and diagnosis

Suspect bronchiectasis in a patient with recurrent episodes of 'bronchitis' over several years prior to presentation, including those with COPD with frequent exacerbations and/or positive sputum for *P. aeruginosa*.

Diagnosis

Usually made clinically, with HRCT chest for confirmation.

Investigations are aimed at:

- Confirming the diagnosis
- Identifying a treatable underlying cause for the bronchiectasis (possible in about 50%)
- Optimizing management to prevent exacerbations and lung damage.

Essential investigations

- *Chest radiograph (CXR)* sensitivity is only 50%, classically shows 'ring shadows' and 'tramlines'—indicating thickened airways, and the 'gloved finger' appearance. Consolidation around thickened and dilated airways
- *HRCT* chest (slices ≤1mm, with high spatial frequency reconstruction) is 97% sensitive in detecting disease. Typically shows airway dilatation to within 1cm of the lung periphery, bronchial wall thickening, and the airway appearing larger than its accompanying vessel (signet ring sign). Expiratory scans may be useful to demonstrate post-obstructive air trapping/mosaic perfusion, indicative of small airways disease. If the bronchiectasis is localized to a single lobe, CT is useful to determine whether a central obstructing lesion is present. Contiguous 3mm slices are needed to exclude a central airway lesion if there is associated haemoptysis. Symptoms correlate with wall thickening and mucous plugging on CT scan. The radiological term 'traction bronchiectasis' refers to airway dilatation 2° to airway distortion, seen with chronic severe interstitial fibrosis. These patients rarely have clinical features of bronchiectasis
- *Lung function* FEV_1/FVC and flow-volume loop
- *Sputum microbiology* Standard microscopy, culture, and sensitivity (MC&S), acid-fast bacillus (AFB), and fungal cultures
- *PFTs* with reversibility testing
- *Immunoglobulins* A, M, G
- *Aspergillus* precipitins, *Aspergillus*-specific radioallergosorbent test (RAST), total IgE (see p. 562).

Additional investigations

- *CFTR mutation screen and sweat test* (see ➲ p. 239)
- *Autoantibodies* (ANA, RhF, dsDNA) if associated arthritis/connective tissue disease
- *Vaccination response* to tetanus, *H. influenza B*, and pneumococcal antibodies. If pneumococcal antibodies are low, arrange vaccination with 23 valent polysaccharide pneumococcal vaccine and repeat antibody testing 6 weeks later; failure to generate adequate pneumococcal antibody levels is suggestive of an immunodeficiency (e.g. IgG subclass deficiency), and referral to an immunologist may be required
- *Detailed immunological investigation* (including neutrophil and lymphocyte function studies, genetic analysis)
- *Skin tests/RAST* to identify specific sensitizers (usually *Aspergillus*)
- *Bronchoscopy* to exclude a foreign body if suggested by CT; obtain microbiological samples if unusual clinical presentation or failure to respond to standard antibiotics
- *Nasal nitric oxide +/- brushings/biopsy* (in tertiary centre) to assess ciliary beat frequency with video microscopy to exclude PCD in those with risk factors
- *A1AT levels* if deficiency suspected
- *Barium swallow/oesophageal imaging* if recurrent aspiration suspected
- *Vasculitis screen (RF, ANCA, ANA, ENA, and anti-CCP antibodies)* if connective disease/arthritis/vasculitis associated bronchiectasis suspected
- *HIV serology.*

General management

The main aims of management of non-CF bronchiectasis are:
- Treatment of any underlying medical condition
- Prevention of exacerbations and progression of underlying disease by daily physiotherapy. The options for airway clearance include:
  - Active cycle of breathing technique—this involves breathing control with forced expiration (huffing) using variable thoracic expansion
  - Postural or autogenic drainage
  - Cough augmentation—using flutter valves/cough insufflator/high-frequency oscillation/positive pressure devices
  - Exercise regimes—important to prevent general deconditioning
  - The physiotherapist is also vital during admission for exacerbations to help clear tenacious sputum
  - Nebulized saline or hypertonic saline may improve airway clearance, although there is no RCT data to support its use in non-CF disease
- Reduction of bacterial load and prevention of 2° airway inflammation and damage with antimicrobial chemotherapy
- Supportive treatment—treatment of associated airflow obstruction
- Optimize nutrition
- Refer for pulmonary rehabilitation if breathlessness limits activities of daily living
- Refer for surgery in rare cases, for localized resection of affected area
- Refer for lung transplantation if indicated (see ᗡ p. 759).

Antimicrobial chemotherapy

- This may be intermittent for exacerbations only (for mild disease) or long term for more severe disease. Antibiotics may be oral, nebulized, or IV
- Regular sputum surveillance will ensure the likely colonizing organism is known
- *In vivo* sensitivity may be different to *in vitro* sensitivity
- Patients need a higher antibiotic dose and for a longer time period (usually 10–14 d) than people without bronchiectasis
- Antibiotic treatment choice depends on the severity of the underlying disease
- Treatment response is usually assessed by a fall in sputum volume and change to mucoid from purulent or mucopurulent sputum, with an improvement in systemic symptoms, spirometry, and C-reactive protein (CRP)
- *Pseudomonas*-colonized patients have more frequent exacerbations, worse CT scan appearances, and a faster decline in lung function.

Exacerbation treatment

An exacerbation is usually a clinical diagnosis, with an increase in sputum volume and tenacity and with discoloration. It may be associated with chest pain, haemoptysis and wheeze, and systemic upset—fevers, lethargy, and anorexia. The CRP is not always elevated. Treatment depends on the potential pathogens and resident flora. Nebulized bronchodilators and regular physiotherapy (as an inpatient or outpatient) may also be needed.

Exacerbation of mild bronchiectasis
- Antibiotics for exacerbations only (tailored to the colonizing organism—review previous sputum microbiology)
- Sputum samples should be sent for MC&S prior to starting antibiotics, but empirical treatment can be started while awaiting culture results
- In the absence of prior positive microbiology, amoxicillin 500 mg–1 g tds or doxycycline 100 mg bd for 10–14 days
- Use a higher-dose oral regime, e.g. amoxicillin 1 g tds for 2 weeks or augmentin 625 mg tds, especially if colonized with *H. influenzae*
- A 2-week course of oral ciprofloxacin at 500–750mg bd if *Pseudomonas aeruginosa* colonized. Counsel re: photosensitivity and tendinitis risk; stop if ankle pain; avoid in patients with long QT interval or known vascular aneurysm
- If early relapse, with a return to purulent sputum within 6–8 weeks, consider a longer course of oral antibiotics, e.g. amoxicillin 500 mg bd or doxycycline 100 mg od for 6 weeks. If treatment failure, change to appropriate IV antibiotics until clinical improvement.
- For those requiring long term prophylactic antibiotics, continuation of a stable antibiotic regime is preferable to rotating antibiotics
- A new growth of methicillin-resistant *S. aureus* (MRSA) (1st isolation or regrowth in the context of intermittently positive cultures) should be treated aiming for eradication

Exacerbation of more severe bronchiectasis
Chronic suppressive antibiotics aim to prevent progression of disease by reducing bacterial load and preventing ongoing inflammation, thereby reducing morbidity and improving quality of living.
- Antibiotics are usually given for at least 2 days after the sputum has cleared—often for 2 weeks
- If oral antibiotics fail, IV treatment is required. This may mean inpatient admission or could involve long-line insertion, patient education in self-administration of IV antibiotics, and involvement of a home care team.
- Regular, planned cyclical IV antibiotics may be required in those with more frequent exacerbations

First isolate of Pseudomonas aeruginosa
- Initial treatment is a 2-week course of oral ciprofloxacin 500–750 mg bd (see caution notes above)
- If this fails and the patient still has *Pseudomonas* on sputum culture, guidelines recommend consideration of IV antibiotics, usually an anti-pseudomonal penicillin (minimum 2 weeks) with nebulized colistin, gentamicin or tobramycin for 3 months
- Combination IV antibiotics (anti-pseudomonal penicillin and aminoglycoside) are only needed if there is a lack of clinical response and /or resistance to one or more anti-pseudomonal antibiotics. Aminoglycoside antibiotic drug levels need careful monitoring as risk of toxicity is high in this patient group
- Consider long-term therapy with daily nebulized colistin or gentamicin to reduce levels of *Pseudomonas* in colonized patients with frequent exacerbations. This may need to be in combination with a macrolide antibiotic if the exacerbation frequency is high. Challenge testing is required prior to starting regular nebulized antibiotics to ensure no significant bronchoconstriction.

Macrolide antibiotics

These have both antibacterial and immunomodulatory properties and decrease mucous production, alter inflammatory mediator release, and inhibit *Pseudomonas* virulence factors and biofilm formation. Five trials have reported beneficial effects of macrolides in bronchiectasis, with reduced exacerbation rates and improved lung function and symptoms. The drugs are well tolerated, though concerns have been raised about antimicrobial resistance with long-term use.

Prior to starting a long-term macrolide:

- Counsel re: risk of hearing loss, caution in those with impaired hearing and poor balance
- Check liver function at 1 month and then 8 weekly
- Avoid if creatinine clearance <30 ml/min
- Avoid concomitant nephrotoxic drugs
- Baseline electrocardiogram (ECG) to assess QTc interval
- Exclude active NTM infection with at least one sputum sample negative for NTM
- Azithromycin 250–500 mg 3 times weekly or 500 mg twice weekly are possible regimes
- An 'antibiotic holiday' may be recommended e.g. over the warmer, summer months

The Bronchiectasis Severity Index (BSI) includes clinical, microbiological, and radiological features, and has been validated in predicting mortality, exacerbations, and hospital admissions and thus may be useful in defining disease severity. ◌ http://www.bronchiectasisseverity.com

Further management

- *Self-management plan* Patients need an individual plan for exacerbations, which usually involves having a supply of home antibiotics; for an example see ℘ https://www.brit-thoracic. org.uk/standards-of-care/quality-standards/bts-bronchiectasisquality-standards
- Treatment of associated *airflow obstruction*/*wheeze* with inhaled steroids and/or bronchodilators if there is an additional disease process causing this e.g. the bronchiectasis is in the context of asthma or COPD. There is no indication for inhaled steroids in isolated bronchiectasis. This also applies to oral steroids, leukotriene receptor antagonists, phosphodiesterase type 4 (PDE4) inhibitors and methylxanthines
- There is no specific treatment for abnormalities of *mucociliary function*, although β_2 agonists may enhance airway clearance
- *Nebulized hypertonic saline* (7%) may aid sputum clearance, although bronchospasm may limit its use
- *Acetylcysteine* may reduce sputum viscosity. If required a 6-month trial is recommended
- *Annual influenza and pneumococcal vaccinations*
- *Osteoporosis prophylaxis* (if on long-term steroids)
- *Reflux* treatment if aspiration
- Associated *rhinosinusitis* is seen in up to 70% (see ➔ p. 709). Treat with nasal steroid; consider antibiotics if infection likely
- *Nutrition* Treat weight loss or low body mass index (BMI) aggressively as this is associated with a poorer prognosis
- *Immunoglobulin replacement therapy* Patients found to have immunoglobulin deficiency should be referred to an immunologist for further assessment. IV immunoglobulin replacement therapy is usually given once or twice monthly, as a day case or weekly subcutaneous at home
- *Oxygen* For those with ventilatory failure, use the same criteria long-term oxygen therapy criteria as for COPD (see ➔ p. 792)
- *Non-invasive ventilation (NIV)* Hypercapnic ventilatory failure due to end-stage disease may need long-term nocturnal NIV. This can also be used as a bridge to transplantation
- *Surgery* This is the only potential curative treatment, with resection of a single chronically infected lobe occasionally being of benefit. It is much less commonly needed now, as the incidence of single lobe disease related to previous severe childhood pneumonia is falling. In some cases, bronchiectasis can recur at a later date in other lobes
- *Transplant* Most commonly performed for CF bronchiectasis, but referral may be warranted for severe non-CF-related disease (see ➔ p. 759)
- *Nebulized DNase (dornase alfa)* Evidence indicates this may be harmful in non-CF bronchiectasis; not recommended.

Complications of bronchiectasis

- Infective exacerbation
- Haemoptysis—small-volume haemoptysis (increasing during exacerbations) is common. Massive haemoptysis (usually from tortuous bronchial arteries around damaged lung) is a life-threatening emergency (see ➲ p. 47)
- Pneumothorax
- Respiratory failure
- NTM infection
- ABPA
- Cardiovascular disease—the incidence of cardiovascular events is higher in those with bronchiectasis, the rate correlates with severity of disease and frequency of exacerbations

Bronchiectasis and *Aspergillus*

- ABPA—excessive immune response to environmental fungus *Aspergillus* (most commonly *fumigatus* species); may be the cause of bronchiectasis (suspect particularly if upper lobe disease), as mucus plugs become impacted in distal airways, causing airway damage and subsequent dilatation (see ➲ p. 562)
- Aspergilloma—*Aspergillus* may colonize a previously formed cavity. This is extremely difficult to treat. Most commonly, it causes systemic upset and haemoptysis (see ➲ p. 566).

Further information

Hill AT, et al. Guideline for non-CF bronchiectasis. *Thorax* 2019;74(Suppl 1): 1–69.
O'Donnell AE. Bronchiectasis Update. Curr Opin Infect Dis. 2018;31(2): 194–198.
NICE bronchiectasis guideline 2018 (NG117). ꝏ http://www.nice.org.uk

Bronchiolitis

Pathophysiology and causes *184*
Management *186*

Pathophysiology and causes

Definition and epidemiology

Bronchioles are small airways of <2 mm diameter, lined by bronchial epithelium and with no cartilage in their walls. Terminal bronchioles lead to alveoli. Many bronchioles need to be affected by disease before a patient becomes symptomatic, when there will be increased airway resistance unresponsive to β$_2$ stimulants. Bronchiolitis is poorly understood and is a mixture of conditions.

Disease seems to affect bronchioles in two main ways:
- Affecting the bronchioles in isolation, with non-specific injury causing subsequent epithelial damage and inflammation, e.g. viral bronchiolitis
- As a bronchiolitis associated with other airway disease where the bronchiolitis may be more of an incidental finding, along with other pathologies, e.g. cryptogenic organizing pneumonia (COP), hypersensitivity pneumonitis (HP), respiratory bronchiolitis-associated interstitial lung disease (RB-ILD), Langerhans cell histiocytosis (LCH).

Pathophysiology

This is unclear. There is probably an initial injury to the epithelium of the bronchioles with subsequent inflammation. Adjacent alveoli are often also involved. There are two main pathological patterns of bronchiolitis. Both can exist in the same patient.
- *Proliferative bronchiolitis* More common of the two patterns. Non-specific reaction to bronchiolar injury, with organizing exudate within the bronchiolar lumen. Proliferation of intraluminal fibrotic buds, called Masson bodies, seen in bronchioles, alveoli, and alveolar ducts. Associated alveolar wall inflammation and foamy macrophages in alveolar spaces. May completely or partially resolve. Tends to be more responsive to steroids. The pathology merges with that of COP (see ⊃ p. 330)
- *Constrictive bronchiolitis* Less common. Concentric narrowing of the bronchiolar wall due to cellular infiltrates ± smooth muscle hyperplasia, which may cause extrinsic compression, obliteration, distortion, mucus collection, peribronchiolar fibrosis, and scarring. Patchy in distribution. Typically, progressive and unresponsive to steroid therapy. Usually leads to respiratory failure and death.

In practice, these are the commonest situations in which a diagnosis of bronchiolitis is useful:
- Viral bronchiolitis (e.g. respiratory syncytial virus (RSV))
- Post-lung transplant (bronchiolitis obliterans syndrome (BOS), see ⊃ p. 768)
- Post-bone marrow transplant
- Connective tissue disease (usually rheumatoid arthritis (RA))
- In association with ILD and airways disease
- Diffuse pan-bronchiolitis (including Japanese pan-bronchiolitis)
- Causes of bronchiolitis are listed in Box 20.1

Clinical features

Insidious onset of cough and dyspnoea over weeks to months. There may be an associated medical history, such as recent viral illness, transplant, connective tissue disease, or vasculitis, or a history of mineral dust or drug exposure.

Box 20.1 Causes of bronchiolitis

Proliferative bronchiolitis (associated with OP)
Commoner causes
- COP (see ➜ p. 330)
- HP (see ➜ p. 311)
- Chronic eosinophilic pneumonia (see ➜ p. 294)
- Connective tissue disease—RA, polymyositis, dermatomyositis (see ➜ p. 213)
- Post-bone marrow, heart, and lung transplant
- Organizing acute infection—mycoplasma, *Legionella*, influenza, cytomegalovirus (CMV), HIV, *pneumocystis jirovecii* pneumonia (PCP).

Rarer causes
- Acute respiratory distress syndrome (ARDS) (see ➜ p. 115)
- Vasculitides, including GPA (formerly Wegener's) (see ➜ p. 713)
- Drug-induced reactions such as L-tryptophan, busulfan, cocaine
- Chronic thyroiditis
- Ulcerative colitis
- Radiation or aspiration pneumonitis
- Distal to bronchial obstruction
- Common variable immunodeficiency syndrome.

Constrictive bronchiolitis
Commoner causes
- Connective tissue disease, particularly RA, especially women in their 50s and 60s, with long-standing RA. May be related to penicillamine or gold therapy. May improve with TNF-α inhibitor therapy
- Infection—viral (adenovirus, RSV, influenza, parainfluenza), mycoplasma.

Rarer causes
- 'Chronic rejection phenomenon' in heart, lung, bone marrow transplants—affects up to 65% of lung transplant patients after 5 y post-transplant and is the 1° cause of late death, BOS (see ➜ p. 768). Patients taking statins post-transplant have a lower incidence of this; reasons unclear
- Diffuse pan-bronchiolitis (including Japanese pan-bronchiolitis)
- Following inhalation injury: mineral dusts, such as asbestos, silica, iron oxide, aluminium oxide, talc, mica, coal, sulphur dioxide, nitrogen oxide, ammonia, chlorine, phosgene—may develop cough days to weeks after exposure
- Drug reaction
- Hypersensitivity reactions
- Ulcerative colitis
- Cryptogenic. Rare, mostly women >40. Cough and dyspnoea. PFT: progressive airflow obstruction and air trapping. total lung carbon monoxide transfer factor (TLCO) decreased, no bronchodilator response.

Management

Investigations
- *PFTs* Obstructive defect may be found, with air trapping and no bronchodilator reversibility in constrictive bronchiolitis. Proliferative bronchiolitis can cause a restrictive or mixed defect. Impaired TLCO in both
- *CXR* can be normal or may show hyperinflation, especially with constrictive bronchiolitis. Also diffuse infiltrates with proliferative bronchiolitis, which may be migratory
- *HRCT* is helpful and may be performed prone in full expiration. (Prone CT is used to minimize any gravity-dependent changes). Normal bronchioles are too small to be seen; indirect signs of disease may be hyperinflation, air trapping, causing a mosaic pattern and subsegmental atelectasis. Bronchioles with thickened walls due to inflammation and dilatation may be seen. CT is also useful to assess for signs of associated ILD
- *Open or thoracoscopic lung biopsy* may be required to make the diagnosis, as TBBs are usually inadequate. The small airways need particularly careful examination.

Management
- Treat any underlying disorder
- Cough suppressants
- Long-term macrolide antibiotics, such as erythromycin 200–600 mg/ day, may improve symptoms, lung function, and mortality, especially in those with *diffuse pan-bronchiolitis* and *cryptogenic bronchiolitis*. Erythromycin lowers the neutrophil count by an unknown mechanism and reduces the number of lymphocytes
- Steroids are effective in cases of proliferative bronchiolitis and can treat the associated OP, e.g. 0.5–1 mg/kg prednisolone/day, maximum 60 mg/day. They may also be beneficial in bronchiolitis due to inhalation injury, both in early and later stages. Relapse of the bronchiolitis may occur on stopping steroids.

Bronchiolitis: specific conditions

Diffuse pan-bronchiolitis
This is a distinct condition and used to be thought of as rare outside Japan. Described 30 ya in Japan as a condition involving both the upper and lower respiratory tracts, with bronchiolar inflammation and chronic sinusitis. An infectious aetiology was postulated as the cause, but no particular organism has been consistently found. It can be familial and is associated with HLA-B54 (specific to East Asians) and A11 (Korea). Rarely seen in people of Asian descent living abroad. More prevalent in men, mean age at presentation 45, occurs particularly in non-smokers. Chronic sinusitis can precede the chest symptoms often by years. Most patients have a productive cough with copious purulent sputum, exertional dyspnoea, wheeze, and weight loss. There may be progressive respiratory failure with signs of cor pulmonale and crackles and wheezes on auscultation.

More recently, a very similar clinical condition has been described outside Japan, with sinusitis as a less common feature. This diffuse version is also an idiopathic inflammatory and suppurative disorder of the respiratory bronchioles, causing progressive and severe airways obstruction. It is presumably very similar to the Japanese variety and probably under-recognized.

- *PFTs* are obstructive although may show a mixed pattern, with minimal airway hyperresponsiveness. TLCO is reduced
- *CXR and CT* may show diffuse ill-defined nodules (sometimes 'tree-in-bud'), bronchiectasis, and air trapping
- *Sputum cultures* may repeatedly show growths of *Haemophilus influenzae*, *Pseudomonas aeruginosa*, and less commonly *Streptococcus pneumoniae*, *Klebsiella pneumoniae*, or *Staphylococcus aureus*. These should be treated but can be difficult to eradicate
- *Cold agglutinins* may be positive; mycoplasma tests are negative
- *BAL* shows marked neutrophilia, along with mild blood neutrophilia
- *Open or thoracoscopic lung biopsy*, although this may not be considered necessary in areas where pan-bronchiolitis is prevalent. Bronchiolar histology is characteristic, although not pathognomonic, with a transmural infiltrate of lymphocytes, plasma cells, and foamy macrophages. The intraluminal exudates may be organized to form a polypoid plug.

Treatment

Low-dose erythromycin 400–600 mg/day for 6 months to 2 y confers a significant survival benefit. Most likely related to its anti-inflammatory and immunomodulatory effects (inhibits many cytokines), as well as reducing mucin secretion, rather than through its antibacterial effects. Untreated, 50% 5 y mortality. With treatment, >90% 10 y survival. Azithromycin 250–500 mg three times a week may be a suitable alternative but less experience. Relapses occur but usually respond to macrolides again.

Acute bronchiolitis

This is a seasonal epidemic viral infective illness, common in infants <2 y, who present with coryza, low-grade fever, cough, wheezing, tachypnoea, respiratory distress, hyperinflation, and tachycardia. It is most commonly caused by RSV, but also adenovirus, influenza, parainfluenza, rhinovirus, human metapneumovirus, coronavirus, and human bocavirus. *Mycoplasma* and *Chlamydophila* cause a similar picture of wheeze and lower respiratory tract infection. In adults, acute bronchiolitis is caused by the same organisms but is less severe.

- *CXR* may be normal or show hyperinflation, occasionally with patchy opacities, consolidation, and collapse
- *Histologically*, there is acute and chronic inflammation of bronchioles, with necrosis, sloughing, oedema, and inflammatory exudates in the bronchiolar lumen.

Treatment

Supportive, with O_2 and fluids. Steroids and bronchodilators may be given if severe, but systematic reviews in children show no significant outcome benefit.

Further information

Ryu JH et al. Bronchiolar disorders. *Am J Respir Crit Care Med* 2003;**168**: 1277–1292.
Smyth RL, Openshaw PJ. Bronchiolitis. *Lancet* 2006;**368**: 312–322.
Poletti V et al. Diffuse panbronchiolitis. *Eur Respir J* 2006;**28**: 862–871.
Koyama H, Geddes DM. Erythromycin and diffuse panbronchiolitis. *Thorax* 1997;**52**: 915–918.

Chronic obstructive pulmonary disease (COPD)

Definition, aetiology, pathology, and clinical features *190*
Investigations *192*
Non-pharmacological management of stable COPD *196*
Pharmacological management of stable COPD *198*
COPD exacerbations *202*
Management of exacerbations *206*
Surgical/bronchoscopic treatment *208*
α1-antitrypsin (α1-AT) deficiency *210*

Definition, aetiology, pathology, and clinical features

Chronic obstructive pulmonary disease (COPD) is common and is mostly caused by smoking. Patients with COPD represent a large proportion of inpatient (~12% of all general medical admissions) and outpatient work for the chest physician. COPD encompasses a number of underlying pathologies including chronic bronchitis and emphysema.

Definition
- Fixed airflow obstruction – post bronchodilator FEV_1/FVC ratio <0.7
- Persistent respiratory symptoms.

Aetiology
95% of cases are smoking-related, typically >20 pack years. COPD occurs in 10–20% of smokers, indicating that there is probable genetic susceptibility. COPD is increasing in frequency worldwide, particularly in some developing countries, due to high levels of smoking, but also because of biomass fuel exposure. Smoking tobacco with marijuana increases COPD risk. It can also be caused by environmental and occupational factors, e.g. dusts, chemicals, air pollution. Reduced maximal attained lung function due to events during gestation, birth, or childhood may also be a risk factor for developing COPD.

Pathology
- Airflow limitation and gas trapping—chronic inflammation and fibrosis of small airways, characterized by CD8 lymphocyte, macrophage, and neutrophil infiltration, with release of pro-inflammatory cytokines. Airflow limitation in the small airways leads to gas trapping and static hyperinflation. Recurrent infections may perpetuate airway inflammation
- Emphysema and gas exchange abnormalities due to alveolar wall destruction, causing irreversible enlargement of airspaces distal to the terminal bronchiole (the acinus), with subsequent loss of elastic recoil and hyperinflated lungs
  - Panacinar emphysema can occur with dilated airspaces evenly distributed across acini
  - Centriacinar or proximal emphysema can occur with dilated air spaces found in association with the respiratory bronchioles
  - Periacinar or paraseptal emphysema can occur with dilated air spaces at the edge of the acinar unit and abutting a fixed structure such as the pleura or a vessel
- Mucous gland hyperplasia, particularly in the large airways, with mucus hypersecretion and therefore a chronic productive cough. Other mucosal damage from smoke:
  - Squamous metaplasia: replacement of the normal ciliated columnar epithelium by a squamous epithelium
  - Loss of cilial function: this leads to impairment of the normal functioning of the mucociliary escalator—another reason for the chronic productive cough
- Thickened pulmonary arteriolar wall and remodelling occur with hypoxia. Leads to increased pulmonary vascular resistance, pulmonary hypertension (PHT), and impaired gas exchange.

The cause of the increase in airways resistance, and hence expiratory flow limitation, is multifactorial. Small airway inflammation reduces the airway lumen. Emphysema destroys the radial attachments to the small airways, which normally hold them open and resist dynamic compression.

COPD is increasingly being recognized as having features not only of pulmonary, but also systemic, inflammation, and this may be the cause of the comorbidities found in patients with COPD. Daily activities are often modified to avoid dyspnoea, which can lead to deconditioning, muscle weakness, and wasting, meaning standing and walking become even harder. This leads to a vicious cycle of inactivity. An approach to assessing COPD in the outpatient clinic is listed in Box 21.2.

Clinical features
- Dyspnoea
- Chronic cough, may be productive
- Wheeze
- In advanced disease systemic features such as fatigue, weight loss, and anorexia may be seen.

Significant airflow obstruction may be present before the patient is aware of it. COPD is rare below 35 y and should prompt consideration of alternate diagnoses.

History
- Smoking history. Pack years. Are they still smoking?
- Occupational and industrial exposures
- History of exacerbations
- Presence of comorbidities
- Impact on patient's life

Signs
Depend on the severity of the underlying disease. Physical examination may well be normal. Signs present may include:
- Raised respiratory rate
- Hyperexpanded/barrel chest
- Prolonged expiratory time >5s, with pursed lip breathing
- Use of accessory muscles of respiration
- Quiet breath sounds (especially in the lung apices) ± wheeze
- Quiet heart sounds (due to overlying hyperinflated lung)
- Possible basal crepitations
- Signs of cor pulmonale and CO_2 retention (ankle oedema, raised jugular venous pressure (JVP), warm peripheries, plethoric conjunctivae, bounding pulse, polycythaemia. Flapping tremor if CO_2 acutely raised).

Further information
NICE Chronic obstructive pulmonary disease in over 16s: diagnosis and management. 2018. ℰ www.nice.org.uk/guidance/ng115

GOLD Global strategy for the diagnosis, management, and prevention of chronic obstructive pulmonary disease. 2019. ℰ www.goldcopd.org

Investigations

Pulmonary function tests

Spirometry is the key diagnostic test for COPD.

- Obstructive spirometry and flow–volume loops; $FEV_1/FVC < 0.7$ (post-bronchodilation)
- Reduced FEV_1 to <80% predicted or FEV_1 >80% with other respiratory symptoms, e.g. cough or breathlessness. COPD airflow limitation severity scale is shown in Table 21.1 and Medical Research Council (MRC) dyspnoea scale in Box 21.1.
- FEV_1 is the measurement of choice to assess progression of COPD, but it correlates weakly with the degree of dyspnoea. Changes in FEV_1 do not reflect the decline in a patient's health
- Minimal bronchodilator reversibility (<15%, usually <10%) and minimal steroid reversibility (how to perform these, see ➔ p. 968). It is not necessary to test these in most patients but is useful if there is diagnostic uncertainty or if the patient is thought to have both COPD and asthma
- Raised total lung volume, FRC, and RV because of emphysema, air trapping, and loss of elastic recoil
- Decreased total lung carbon monoxide transfer factor (TLCO) and kCO because presence of emphysema decreases surface area available for gas diffusion.

Chest radiograph (CXR)

Not required for diagnosis, and repeated CXR is unnecessary, unless other diagnoses are being considered (most importantly, lung cancer or bronchiectasis).

- Hyperinflated lung fields, with attenuation of peripheral vasculature 'black lung sign'; >7 posterior ribs seen
- Flattened diaphragms (best CXR correlate of post-mortem degree of emphysema)
- More horizontal ribs
- May see bullae, especially in lung apices, which, if large, can be mistaken for a pneumothorax due to loss of lung markings (CT can differentiate).

Consider checking α1-AT levels (see ➔ p. 210), full blood count (FBC) to ensure not anaemic or polycythaemic (suggesting persistent hypoxia), thyroid function test (TFT) if unduly breathless. C-reactive protein (CRP) is slightly increased in COPD but decreases after steroid treatment. It may be related to the presence of comorbidities and may aid the assessment of the systemic effects of COPD, particularly in the research setting. Electrocardiogram (ECG) and echo to assess cardiac status if features of cor pulmonale.

Diagnosis

Based on the history of smoking and progressive dyspnoea, with evidence of irreversible airflow obstruction on spirometry. Asthma is the most important differential diagnosis. Asthma is steroid- and bronchodilator-responsive. Nearly all patients with COPD will have a smoking history; this is not universal in asthma. Symptoms are common under the age of 35 in asthma; rare in COPD. Chronic productive cough is common is COPD and uncommon in asthma. Breathlessness is progressive and persistent in COPD but variable in asthma. In asthma, there is significant diurnal or day-to-day variability of symptoms, and night-time waking with shortness of breath (SOB) or wheeze is common; these symptoms are uncommon in COPD. Some patients have both.

Table 21.1 Airflow limitation severity according to GOLD guidelines 2019 for patients with $FEV_1/FVC < 0.7$. Based on post-bronchodilator FEV_1

Mild	$FEV_1 \geq 80\%$ predicted
Moderate	$50\% \leq FEV_1 < 80\%$ predicted
Severe	$30\% \leq FEV_1 < 50\%$ predicted
Very severe	$FEV_1 < 30\%$ predicted

Box 21.1 Modified MRC dyspnoea scale

- Grade 0: Not troubled by breathlessness except on strenuous exercise
- Grade 1: Short of breath when hurrying or walking up a slight hill
- Grade 2: Walks slower than contemporaries on level ground because of breathlessness or has to stop for breath when walking at own pace
- Grade 3: Stops for breath after walking about 100 m or after a few minutes on level ground
- Grade 4: Too breathless to leave the house, or breathless when dressing or undressing.

Table 21.2 BODE index

Variable	Points on BODE index			
	0	1	2	3
FEV$_1$ (% predicted)	≥65	50–64	36–49	≤35
Distance walked in 6min (m)	≥350	250–349	150–249	≤149
MRC dyspnoea scale	0–1	2	3	4
BMI	>21	≤21		

BODE index (see Table 21.2) is a simple grading system for COPD, using *B*ody mass index (BMI), airflow *O*bstruction, *D*yspnoea, and *E*xercise capacity as its scoring variables. It has been shown to be better than FEV$_1$ at predicting risk of hospitalization and death in patients with COPD, as it is multidimensional. Patients are scored as having a BODE index of 0–10, with higher scores indicating a higher risk of death. It is being increasingly used, with recommendations to calculate it in the clinical setting to give prognostic information (Celli BR et al. *New Engl J Med* 2004; 350: 1005–1012).

Non-pharmacological management of stable COPD

Aims of COPD management should include:
- Ensuring the diagnosis is correct
- Stopping smoking
- Optimizing treatment by minimizing symptoms where possible
- Helping the patient maintain their quality of life (QoL)
- Minimizing exacerbations.

Management should be delivered by a multidisciplinary team (MDT).

No treatment has yet been shown to modify disease progression in the long term, except for stopping smoking.

Smoking cessation

The only intervention proven to decrease the smoking-related decline in lung function is complete smoking cessation. All patients with COPD who smoke should be encouraged to stop at every opportunity. Fig. 21.1 shows the accelerated decline in FEV_1 in susceptible smokers and the delay in this acceleration from stopping smoking; susceptible smokers, however, never regain the original curve. Nicotine replacement therapy (NRT) should be used to aid smoking cessation (see ➔ p. 817).

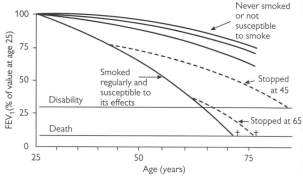

Fig. 21.1 Modification of the Fletcher–Peto diagram of FEV_1 decline in susceptible smokers.

Education

Can improve ability to manage illness and stop smoking.

Pulmonary rehabilitation

A multidisciplinary programme, with RCT evidence that it improves exercise tolerance, QoL, and reduces hospital admissions. Muscle mass, particularly in the lower limbs, is reduced in people with COPD, compared with age-matched healthy controls. This is an independent predictor of mortality and disability, independent of the severity of the underlying lung disease, and may reflect the systemic nature of COPD. The mainstay of rehabilitation is graded exercise to improve muscle function but also includes breathing techniques and education.

Programmes vary but are usually run on an outpatient basis over several weeks, with multidisciplinary involvement (see ⮕ p. 811). Should be made available to all appropriate patients with COPD, including after hospitalization for acute exacerbation.

Diet

Weight loss is recommended if the patient is obese to minimize respiratory effort. OSA/OHS may coexist as part of an overlap syndrome (see ⮕ p. 677). If the patient is very breathless, calorific intake may be low and a catabolic state may exist. Compared with people with a normal BMI, low BMI is associated with impaired pulmonary status, decreased diaphragm mass, lower exercise capacity, and increased mortality rate. Nutritional supplementation may therefore be necessary. Maintaining body weight and muscle mass correlates well with survival.

Self-management plan

Important for patients on how to respond promptly to symptoms of an exacerbation

Psychosocial support

Practical support at home, day centres; car disability badge; assess for signs of anxiety and depression.

Box 21.2 An approach to COPD in the outpatient clinic

- Establish diagnosis and severity—PFTs, CXR
- Ensure there are no other causes for symptoms, e.g. anaemia, pulmonary embolism (PE), heart failure, interstitial lung disease (ILD), thyroid dysfunction, pneumothorax, large bulla, arrhythmia, depression
- Consider chest CT only if CXR abnormalities require clarification or symptoms disproportionate to spirometry or if surgery being considered
- Encourage the patient to stop smoking
- Review current treatment—optimize bronchodilatation and inhaled steroids
- Assess whether there is any need for a nebulizer
- Check O_2 saturation and perform blood gas if ≤92%. Consider long-term oxygen therapy (LTOT)
- Refer for pulmonary rehabilitation if appropriate
- Consider sputum culture if persistent purulent sputum
- Check vaccinations are up to date
- Involve respiratory nurse specialist for input in the community, if appropriate
- Follow up in clinic if ongoing medical issues, including whether patient may be a lung transplant candidate (see ⮕ p. 759). Otherwise, discharge back to general practitioner (GP)
- Inform GP of all the above decisions.

Pharmacological management of stable COPD

Pharmacological management aims to relieve symptoms and reduce exacerbations but will not modify disease. Increase treatment in a stepwise fashion. Exacerbations require additional therapeutic support (see ● p. 203).

GOLD and National Institute for Health and Care Excellence (NICE) guidelines differ on the indications and starting medications for inhaled therapy in COPD. GOLD suggests using a combination of the severity of airflow limitation and the exacerbation risk to decide on inhaled treatments (Table 21.1) whereas NICE use the presence or absence of asthmatic features.

Inhaled therapy

Inhaled therapy is the mainstay of COPD treatment and achieves maximal disease control in the majority of patients.

Simple pulmonary function testing may not show significant bronchodilator reversibility of FEV_1, but bronchodilators provide therapeutic benefit in the long term by reducing dyspnoea, perhaps by decreasing chest hyperinflation, and reducing exacerbations. Clinical trials of inhaled steroids have shown a reduction in exacerbation frequency and severity in COPD, but no slowing in lung function decline. There is evidence of increased risk of pneumonia with inhaled steroids.

- All patients should have short-acting β_2 agonists, as required, for symptom relief
- For symptoms of airflow limitation/obstruction start a long-acting bronchodilator, either a long-acting β2 agonist (LABA), a long-acting muscarinic antagonist (LAMA), or a LABA/LAMA combination. If a single agent is used and there are persistent symptoms, escalate to dual bronchodilator therapy. Studies have shown that LABA/LAMA combinations are superior to monotherapy
- If exacerbations are the main problem (2 or more/year, or one requiring hospital admission), start an inhaled corticosteroid (ICS)/ LABA combination. ICS alone should not be used in the treatment of COPD.
- If persistent symptoms and/or exacerbations then escalate to triple therapy with ICS, LABA, and LAMA combination. New combination inhalers offer all 3 classes of drug in one inhaler
- Nebulizer therapy is indicated if the patient is unable to use inhalers or if they are disabled or distressed with breathlessness despite maximal inhaler therapy. Only those with a clear response, i.e. reduction in symptoms or improvement in activities of daily living, should continue with long-term domiciliary nebulized treatment (usually with salbutamol and ipratropium), as there is a significant placebo effect.

Other medications for COPD

Oral methylxanthines

Theophyllines, for example, can be used as maintenance therapy and may improve symptoms. Add after inhaled bronchodilators and trial of inhaled steroids; continue only if symptoms improve. Method of action is unclear, but they may have an anti-inflammatory effect. Care regarding therapeutic/ toxic levels, especially in elderly patients.

Oral steroids

Not recommended as a maintenance therapy in COPD. It may, however, be difficult to withdraw them in patients with severe COPD following an exacerbation. If so, keep the dose as low as possible, and prescribe osteoporosis prophylaxis if indicated. Warn regarding steroid side effects, and document.

Phosphodiesterase-4 inhibitors

Roflumilast is approved by NICE for patients with COPD with an FEV_1 < 50% predicted and ≥2 exacerbations in the past 12 months despite triple inhaled therapy. This should be started under specialist care.

Mucolytics

Carbocisteine, mecysteine hydrochloride, for example, may benefit some patients with chronic productive cough to facilitate expectoration by reducing sputum viscosity. Prescribe for a 4-week trial period, and only continue if there is evidence of improvement. Meta-analyses show mucolytics cause a significant decrease in the number of COPD exacerbations and decrease the number of days of disability, although the benefit may only apply if the patient is not taking inhaled steroids. Worth trying in those with moderate to severe COPD, with frequent or prolonged exacerbations, or those repeatedly in hospital with COPD exacerbations. Caution if known peptic ulcer disease.

Prophylactic antibiotics

Azithromycin has been shown to reduce exacerbations in COPD in non- and ex-smokers. There is no evidence of benefit in current smokers. A dose of 250 mg 3x/week may be used in patients with frequent (4 or more per year) exacerbations despite optimal inhaled therapy. Prior to starting treatment check baseline ECG (QT interval), liver function tests, and sputum culture (including acid-fast bacillus (AFB) culture—NTM infection is a contraindication to long-term macrolide use). Repeat LFTs after 4 weeks of treatment. Assess response at 3–6 months. Counsel patients to contact healthcare if they develop hearing loss/tinnitus.

Oxygen

Can be used as LTOT as described; see ➲ p. 787.

Vaccination

Influenza vaccine annually and pneumococcal vaccine. Meta-analysis showed a decrease in exacerbations occurs 3 weeks after receiving influenza vaccine, and there is no evidence of an earlier increase in exacerbations due directly to vaccination.

Non-invasive ventilation

There is some evidence to suggest that patients with hypercapnia, 2–3 weeks following hospital admission with a COPD exacerbation associated with decompensated hypercapnic respiratory failure, may benefit from long-term nocturnal non-invasive ventilation (NIV) to reduce further exacerbations/hospital admission. Refer these patients to a NIV service for review (see ➲ p. 771).

Palliative care/respiratory sedation

Use of low-dose sedatives, such as morphine sulfate solution 2.5–10 mg prn or diazepam 2 mg bd, can be used as a palliative measure (see ➋ p. 799) aiming to relieve the sensation of dyspnoea and associated anxiety in those with severe COPD. Dose may need to be titrated against any rise in CO_2 (surprisingly uncommon). Patients with a high symptom burden/end-stage disease may benefit from referral to a palliative care service and MDT assessment.

Further information

P. Murphy et al. Effect of home noninvasive ventilation with oxygen therapy vs oxygen therapy alone on hospital readmission or death after an acute COPD exacerbation. A randomized clinical trial. *JAMA* 2017;**317**(21).

KA Albert et al. Azithromycin for prevention of exacerbations of COPD. *NEJM* 2011; **365**: 689–698.

Kopsaftis et al. Influenza vaccine for chronic obstructive pulmonary disease (COPD). *Cochrane Database Syst Rev* 2018; 6.

COPD exacerbations

Exacerbations are defined as an acute worsening of symptoms that result in additional therapy. They can cause considerable morbidity in those with limited respiratory reserve. Exacerbations may range from mild, requiring only an increase in short-acting β-agonist (SABA) use, to severe requiring urgent hospital assessment +/- ventilatory support.

It has been recognized that significant numbers of patients do not regain their premorbid lung function or QoL following an exacerbation, and those with frequent exacerbations experience a more rapid FEV_1 decline than those with fewer exacerbations. Exacerbation frequency increases with COPD severity. Exacerbations are 50% more likely in winter. The assessment and management of COPD exacerbations is outlined in Box 21.3.

Causes

The main cause of exacerbations is thought to be viral infection, although other causes include bacterial infection and environmental factors. Common bacterial pathogens are *Haemophilus influenzae*, *Streptococcus pneumoniae*, and *Moraxella catarrhalis*, and the commonest viral pathogens are rhinovirus, RSV, influenza, parainfluenza, coronavirus, human metapneumovirus, and adenovirus. Consider the possibility of PE or pneumothorax as differential/coexisting diagnoses.

Symptoms

Include increased cough, increased sputum volume and/or purulence, increasing dyspnoea or wheeze, chest tightness, increasing ankle oedema (due to cor pulmonale).

Pathophysiology

There is increased airway resistance due to bronchospasm, mucosal oedema, and increased sputum. This worsens expiratory flow limitation, and expiration takes longer. Shallow rapid breathing further limits the time for expiration. This promotes dynamic hyperinflation, and this itself causes mechanical compromise within the lung and the airway. Maximal recruitment of the accessory muscles is required, and thoraco-abdominal dyssynchrony is often present.

Box 21.3 Management summary: acute exacerbation of COPD

- Assess the severity of the exacerbation by measuring respiratory rate (RR), O_2 saturations, degree of air entry, tachycardia, BP, peripheral perfusion, conscious level, mental state
- Exclude a tension pneumothorax clinically
- If hypoxic, give controlled 24–35% O_2 via Venturi face mask to aim for SaO_2 88–92%, O_2 should be prescribed.
- Salbutamol nebulizer; establish venous access.
- Check blood gas—arterial is the gold standard
- Request a CXR
- Perform ECG
- Check bloods for white cell count (WCC), CRP, potassium, etc.
- Optimize volume status
- Take a brief history, if possible. Important to assess normal functional status such as exercise tolerance and requirement for help with activities of daily living. Medical records may be helpful regarding severity of disease and previous decisions regarding ventilation or resuscitation
- Nebulized bronchodilators—salbutamol 2.5–5 mg and ipratropium 500 micrograms on arrival and 4–6 hourly. Run nebulizer with air, not O_2
- Continued O_2 therapy, aiming to maintain saturations between 88% and 92%. Repeat blood gases after 60 min to ensure improvement if hypoxic or acidotic. Repeat if clinical deterioration
- Consider antibiotics
- Oral steroids
- Consider IV aminophylline if not improving with nebulizers
- Consider intensive care—ideally, consultant-led decision with the patient, their family, and ICU regarding invasive mechanical ventilation. Document in the medical notes. Consider resuscitation status
- Consider NIV if pH <7.35 and PCO_2 >6.5 kPa following initial medical management and optimization of O_2 therapy, see p. 771. Decide if this is the ceiling of therapy
- Deep vein thrombosis (DVT) prophylaxis
- Early mobilization and nutrition.

Prognostic scores

Can be used to predict mortality from COPD exacerbations. A commonly used score (see Table 21.3) is the DECAF (Dyspnoea, Eosinopenia, Consolidation, Acidaemia, and atrial Fibrillation). A score of 0 conveys an inpatient mortality of <1% compared to score of 5, which had an inpatient mortality of 70%. A score of ≤1 can be used to help decide which patients are suitable for outpatient treatment.

Table 21.3 The DECAF Score

Variable	Score
Dyspnoea	
eMRCD 5a	1
eMRCD 5b	2
Eosinopenia (<0.05 ×10⁹/l)	1
Consolidation	1
Acidaemia (pH <7.3)	1
Atrial fibrillation	1
Total DECAF Score	**6**

Further information

J Steer et al. The DECAF Score: predicting hospital mortality in exacerbations of chronic obstructive pulmonary disease *Thorax* 2012;**67**.

Intermediate care hospital-at-home in COPD: BTS guideline. *Thorax* 2007;**62**: 200–210.

Management of exacerbations

- Assess the severity of the exacerbation: increase in dyspnoea, tachypnoea, use of accessory muscles, new cyanosis, pedal oedema, confusion
- Exclude alternative diagnoses such as pneumothorax, PE, pulmonary oedema
- Can the patient self-care and self-medicate? In the presence of severe symptoms, with possible comorbid disease and decreased functional activities, the patient is likely to need hospital management
- Investigate with CXR, arterial blood gas (ABGs), ECG, FBC, and urea and electrolytes (U&Es). Admission arterial pH is the best predictor of survival. A respiratory acidosis should prompt close monitoring and repeat assessment after an hour of optimal medical treatment. A pH <7.25 is associated with a rapidly rising mortality. A raised pH may imply an alternative diagnosis, not associated with worsening airways obstruction. Check theophylline level if patient is taking regularly; consider sending sputum for culture if it is purulent.

Treatment

Antibiotics

If sputum purulent, fever/pyrexia, high CRP, new changes on CXR.

Systemic steroids

For all patients with exacerbations of COPD who are admitted to hospital or are significantly more breathless than usual. Give prednisolone 30 mg/day for 5 days, unless there are specific contraindications. Optimum dose and length of steroids not established. This improves FEV_1 and symptoms, and shortens recovery time. Avoid long-term steroid treatment due to side effects. If the patient has a longer course of steroids, or repeated courses due to repeated exacerbations, the dose will need to be tailed off slowly. Frequent short courses of steroids may merit long-term bone protection.

Inhaled or nebulized bronchodilators

Breathless, unwell patients may benefit from nebulizer therapy in the acute period to reduce symptoms and improve airflow obstruction.

Controlled O_2 therapy

Start with 24–35% via Venturi face mask, with oximetry, ABGs, or capillary gas monitoring. Aim saturations between 88% and 92%, balancing hypoxia, hypercapnia, and pH (see ➲ p. 921). Too little O_2 causes anaerobic metabolism and metabolic acidosis (probably SaO_2 >80% would prevent this); too much O_2 (SaO_2 >92%) can cause hypercapnia and a respiratory acidosis. A deteriorating pH to below 7.25 has a much poorer prognosis. Make sure your instructions to the ward staff are clear as to the need to keep the SaO_2 within this window by changing the % O_2 delivered as necessary. Falling conscious level is the best clinical marker of significant CO_2 retention and acidosis.

IV aminophylline

Evidence is lacking, but it may be beneficial, particularly if the patient is wheezy and has not improved with nebulizers alone. Give a loading dose, unless the patient is on regular oral aminophylline, followed by a maintenance infusion. Monitor aminophylline levels daily. Main side effects are tachycardia and nausea. *Cardiac monitoring required.*

Non-invasive ventilation

The treatment of choice for respiratory acidosis in COPD which has not responded to initial medical treatment. Has been shown to markedly reduce mortality. Appropriate for conscious patients with ongoing respiratory acidosis (pH <7.35 or less), hypoxia, and hypercapnia (PCO_2 >6.5 kPa). May avoid intubation. Ceiling of treatment should be determined before its use (see ➲ p. 771).

Intubation/intensive care

If the patient is not responding to medical therapy, or NIV is contraindicated (e.g. low Glasgow Coma Scale (GCS), vomiting), a decision regarding invasive mechanical ventilation needs to be made. This may be considered to be appropriate if the patient usually has a good functional status, with minimal comorbidity. These decisions should ideally be discussed with the patient, their family, their consultant, and the ICU consultant and documented in the medical notes. Resuscitation decisions should also be made.

Early rehabilitation and nutrition

To prevent muscle wasting and deconditioning.

Acute respiratory assessment service/'hospital at home'

Respiratory nurse-led service supporting early discharge of COPD patients after hospital assessment and providing ongoing respiratory care at home. CXR, SaO_2, and baseline spirometry (if this is first presentation) should be performed prior to discharge. Reduces length of inpatient stay and hence is an economic alternative. Unsuitable patients are those with impaired GCS, acute confusion, pH <7.35, acute changes on CXR, concomitant medical problems requiring inpatient stay, insufficient social support (including living far from the hospital and not having a telephone), new hypoxia with SaO_2 <90%, and unable to provide O_2 at home.

Future directions

A preliminary study by Bafadhel et al. (*AJRCCM* 2012;**186**: 48–55) has suggested that a biomarker directed approach to giving oral steroids during exacerbations, based on the blood eosinophil count, may be superior to current practice. Further studies are investigating this. Monoclonal antibody therapies targeting various inflammatory pathways in COPD are being investigated.

Surgical/bronchoscopic treatment

Lung transplant

In young patients (below 60–65 y) with severe disease, often due to α1-AT deficiency, lung transplant may be an option. Local transplant teams will advise regarding local criteria (see ➔ p. 759).

Bullectomy

Suitable for selected patients who are breathless, have FEV_1 <50% predicted, and isolated large bulla seen on CT. Improves chest hyperinflation.

Lung volume reduction techniques

Resection or collapse of areas of emphysema to reduce chest hyperinflation and improve diaphragmatic function, elastic recoil, physiology of the lungs, and hence functional status of the patient.

Patients who may be considered are those with FEV_1 20–30% predicted, with symptomatic dyspnoea despite maximal medical therapy, and with heterogeneously distributed emphysema on CT, giving areas to target. $PaCO_2$ should be <7.3 kPa and TLCO >20% predicted. Patients should have completed pulmonary rehabilitation and have stopped smoking. Preoperative assessment: PFTs, 6-minute walking test (6MWT), QoL, and dyspnoea indicators.

Current options for lung volume reduction include surgical resection and bronchoscopic lung volume reduction through the placement of endobronchial valves or coils.

Endobronchial valves—Bronchoscopic lung volume reduction surgery (bLVR)

Refers to techniques to reduce emphysematous hyperinflation via a flexible bronchoscope and thus avoid potential mortality and morbidity associated with surgery. The evidence supports one-way valves, placed bronchoscopically within the segmental and subsegmental bronchi that supply the hyperinflated lobes. They allow mucus to leave the bronchus but no air to enter. It is a minimally invasive variation on lung volume reduction surgery (LVRS), with the aim of improving lung function and QoL. A multicentre RCT (VENT) has been completed of best medical care (including pulmonary rehabilitation) vs best medical care plus unilateral endoscopic bronchial valve, with CT determination of lobe to target. There were 321 patients randomized, FEV_1 15–45% predicted. There were small, but significant, improvements in FEV_1 and 6MWT in the valve group, with those with intact interlobar fissures on CT having a much greater improvement than those with incomplete fissures (which allow collateral ventilation, and thus occluding the segmental bronchi with valves does not isolate the lobe). Therefore, endobronchial valves are only suitable for patients with intact, or largely intact fissures which can be measured using CT and functionally at bronchoscopy (CHARTIS technique). LVRS may be an option for those with non-intact fissures as below.

Other endobronchial treatments

Endobronchial coils, biological sealants, and thermal airway (steam to cause inflammation, and subsequent fibrosis and contraction) have also been used in small studies. These procedures are only undertaken as part of clinical studies currently.

Lung volume reduction surgery (LVRS)

Surgery is performed in specialist centres via median sternotomy or by thoracoscopy. Improvements are seen in FEV_1 and RV, dyspnoea, and QoL scores. These effects are maximal 2–6 months post-surgery. Symptomatic improvement is sustained for about 2–4 y. Post-operative complications: persistent air leak >7 days in 30–40%, pneumonia in up to 22%, respiratory failure in up to 13%. Reported post-operative mortality 2.5–15%.

The National Emphysema Treatment Trial (NETT, Michigan, USA)

randomized 1,218 patients to receive medical treatment or LVRS. Mean FEV_1 of the subjects was 27% predicted. LVRS was found to only be beneficial in those with upper lobe predominant emphysema and a poor exercise tolerance. There was an excess mortality for patients with FEV_1 < 20% predicted, TLCo < 20% predicted or homogenous emphysema and so LVRS is not recommended for these groups.

Further information

Herth FJF et al. Efficacy predictors of lung volume reduction with Zephyr valves in a European cohort. *Eur Respir J* 2012;**39**: 1334–1342.

Sciurba FC et al. A randomized study of endobronchial valves for advanced emphysema. *N Engl J Med* 2010;**363**: 1233–1244.

Naunheim KS et al. Long-term follow-up of patients receiving LVRS vs. medical therapy for severe emphysema by the NETT research group. *Ann Thoracic Surg* 2006;**82**: 431–443.

Fishman A et al. A randomized trial comparing lung-volume-reduction surgery with medical therapy for severe emphysema. *N Engl J Med* 2003;**22**: 2059–2073.

α1-antitrypsin (α1-AT) deficiency

This is an inherited condition that is associated with the early development of emphysema. It is relatively common (estimated 1 in 2,000–5,000 individuals) and is probably under-diagnosed, as it is often asymptomatic in non-smokers.

Pathophysiology

α1-AT is a glycoprotein protease inhibitor produced by the liver. It is secreted via the bloodstream into the lungs and opposes neutrophil elastase, which destroys alveolar wall connective tissue. Elastase is produced in increased levels by pulmonary neutrophils and macrophages in response to smoking and lung infections. If α1-AT is deficient, the elastase cannot be opposed, and subsequently basal emphysema develops. The disease is worse in smokers and can cause COPD at a young age (40s and 50s). There may also be associated liver dysfunction, chronic hepatitis, cirrhosis, and hepatoma, as abnormal protein secretion accumulates in the liver. Predisposition also to skin disease (panniculitis) and vasculitis (especially ANCA +ve).

Genetics

α1-AT deficiency is inherited as an autosomal co-dominant disorder. So far, >100 different alleles have been identified for this gene (*SERPINA 1*) on the long arm of chromosome 14. The commonest alleles are the M allele (normal), the partially defective S allele, and the almost fully defective Z allele (lysine is substituted for glutamic acid at position 342, leading to abnormal folding, preventing post-translational processing with retention within cells), commonest in Scandinavia.

- MM, the normal phenotype. Background population risk of emphysema
- MS, MZ have 50–70% of normal α1-protease inhibitor (Pi) levels. Background risk of emphysema
- SZ, SS have 35–50% of normal levels; 20–50% risk of emphysema
- Homozygous ZZ has only 10–20% of normal levels. 80–100% risk of emphysema.

Screening

Should be carried out, especially in patients <40 with COPD or minimal smoking history or family history. Also patients with unexplained liver disease should be screened. Send blood for α1-AT concentrations and genotyping if levels are low. Siblings should be screened and the particular importance of not smoking and avoiding passive smoking emphasized. Non-smokers are usually asymptomatic.

Treatment

Includes usual therapy for COPD. Smoking cessation is essential. Specialist centre involvement recommended. Specific treatment is known as augmentation therapy, with ideally weekly, but also 2-weekly or monthly infusions, of purified α1-AT from pooled human plasma. This raises concentrations in serum and epithelial lining fluid above the protective threshold. A number of RCTs have shown a small reduction of disease progression as measured by CT. It has been suggested as a treatment by the European Respiratory Society. It should not be used in current smokers or those with PiSZ or PiMZ genotypes as there is no evidence of efficacy in these groups. It is expensive, and its cost effectiveness in terms of cost per year of life saved is high. It is, however, the only specific therapy available at present. Lung volume reduction therapies (see p. 208) may be considered. Lung transplantation is an option if patient meets referral criteria (see p. 759).

Future developments

Inhaled α1-AT may provide a way of delivering the enzyme to the lower respiratory tract to have its action locally and potentially reduce inflammation. Gene therapy is under development, finding ways of delivering the α1-AT gene into the cell. Other strategies include inhibition of hepatic polymerization of α1-AT, promotion of hepatic secretion, inhibition of neutrophil elastase by synthetic inhibitors to avoid the use of human plasma, and pegylation of α1-AT to prolong its serum half-life.

Further information

M. Miravitlles et al. European Respiratory Society statement: diagnosis and treatment of pulmonary disease in α1-antitrypsin deficiency. *ERJ* 2017;**50**.

α1-antitrypsin deficiency UK support group. ℛ http://www.alpha1.uk.

Connective tissue disease and the lung

Differential diagnosis and standard tests *214*
Rheumatoid arthritis (RA) *216*
Systemic lupus erythematosus (SLE) *218*
Idiopathic inflammatory myopathies *220*
Systemic sclerosis *222*
Sjögren's syndrome *224*
Ankylosing spondylitis *225*
Behçet's syndrome *226*
Autoantibodies: disease associations *228*

Differential diagnosis and standard tests

Patients with connective tissue diseases often develop pulmonary complications, for which they should be referred to a chest physician. Patients typically present with symptoms of dyspnoea, cough, fever, or chest pain. They may often already be on immunosuppressive drugs.

Differential diagnosis

In practice, a few tests (see Box 22.1) will help distinguish the main differential diagnoses.

Opportunistic pulmonary infection
- May be in those on immunosuppressive drugs or functionally immunosuppressed from underlying disease
- Any usual organism, but also tuberculosis (TB), non-tuberculous mycobacteria (NTM), *Pneumocystis jirovecii*, fungi, cytomegalovirus (CMV)
- Often acute onset, with non-specific features of low-grade fever, productive cough, raised inflammatory markers
- Can be very unwell and need full supportive treatment with intensive care unit (ICU)
  - For further information, see ⊃ p. 755.

Often inflammation or fibrosis
- Usually more indolent presentation, with dry cough and dyspnoea, but can become acutely unwell on background of chronic lung disease
- Fine inspiratory crackles on auscultation
- Consider development of pulmonary hypertension (PHT) in patients with systemic sclerosis.

New pathology
- Unrelated to the original condition, including pulmonary thromboembolic disease, heart failure.

Drug side effects
- Methotrexate—pneumonitis occurs in 5% of patients receiving methotrexate. Potentially life-threatening. Mortality 15–20%. Cough, fever, dyspnoea, widespread crackles, restrictive defect, and pulmonary infiltrates on chest radiograph (CXR) and computed tomography (CT). Peripheral eosinophilia in 50%. Bronchoalveolar lavage (BAL) lymphocytosis. Usually subacute onset but may be sudden. Usually within 4 months of starting methotrexate. Non-specific histological findings. No more common in those with pre-existing lung disease. Treatment: stop the drug; commence steroids (usually oral prednisolone, rarely high-dose methylprednisolone), and avoid methotrexate in the future. Can be reversible. Can get mild intractable cough with methotrexate
- Leflunomide—pneumonitis may occur although appears to be rare; consider this diagnosis, and discontinue the drug if new or worsening respiratory symptoms. Avoid leflunomide in patients with pre-existing interstitial lung disease (ILD)

- Anti-TNF-α therapy—includes infliximab (a monoclonal antibody), etanercept (a receptor fusion protein), and adalimumab (a humanized IgG1 antibody). All may predispose to severe infection (viral, bacterial, fungal), particularly when used in association with other immunosuppressants. Opportunistic infection is common, including *Pneumocystis jirovecii* pneumonia (PCP) and mycobacterial disease (both TB, see ⊃ pp. 586–597, and NTM, see ⊃ pp. 618–621). The risk of mycobacterial disease appears to be less with etanercept than with infliximab and adalimumab. All patients should be screened for latent TB prior to starting anti-TNF-α drugs (see ⊃ pp. 610–611). Concern has also been raised that these drugs may lead to increased rates of malignancy, and there is a dose-dependent increase in cancer diagnoses in RA patients treated with infliximab. ILD may worsen on these drugs; consider stopping anti-TNF-α if pre-existing ILD worsens
- Penicillamine—causes obliterative bronchiolitis in RA. Can also cause HP and a pulmonary-renal syndrome causing alveolar haemorrhage. May respond to stopping the drug
- Gold—alveolar opacities seen on high-resolution CT (HRCT), with associated fever and skin rash. BAL lymphocytosis. Treatment: stop the drug, and commence steroids. Usually reversible.

Box 22.1 Standard tests to consider for the investigation of these patients

- SaO₂ and blood gas
- CXR mainly to exclude consolidation/pneumothorax
- HRCT
- Routine sputum culture ± mycobacterial and fungal
- Pulmonary function tests (PFTs), including kCO
- Autoantibody (see ⊃ pp. 228–229) and inflammatory marker levels
- Bronchoscopy and BAL (with differential cell count)
- Transbronchial or very rarely video-assisted thoracoscopic surgery (VATS) lung biopsy.

For an approach to:
- Diffuse lung disease, see ⊃ p. 31
- Diffuse alveolar haemorrhage, see ⊃ p. 27
- Pulmonary disease in the immunocompromised host (non-HIV), see ⊃ p. 79.

Further information

British Society for Rheumatology. Rheumatoid arthritis guidelines on safety of anti-TNF therapies. *Rheumatology* 2010;49: 2217–2219.

Rheumatoid arthritis (RA)

- Persistent deforming symmetrical peripheral arthropathy with non-articular manifestations, including vasculitis
- Pulmonary/pleural disease is commoner in men and occasionally occurs before the development of joint problems
- Pneumonia is common, causing 15–20% of RA deaths.

Pleuritis

Frequent, occurring in >30% of patients and usually mild. Pleuritic pain, with no obvious other cause.

Pleural effusion

Usually asymptomatic. Typically exudative, with a low glucose, a low pH, a lymphocytosis, may be pseudochylous (see ➔ p. 60). Often associated with other lung manifestations. Need to exclude other causes for effusion. If problematic, may require drainage and steroids (see ➔ p. 422).

Pulmonary fibrosis

Similar to the idiopathic interstitial pneumonias (IIPs) (see ➔ p. 317), minor pulmonary fibrosis found in up to 60% of patients in lung biopsy studies, but significant/symptomatic disease only in 5%. Symptomatic disease is unusual. Tends to occur in patients with multisystem disease, including vasculitis, and those with nodules, seropositive disease, and high antinuclear antibody (ANA) titres. More common in men and smoking is a risk factor for fibrosis development.

- *Presents* with progressive dyspnoea and cough
- *Examination* Clubbing and bilateral basal crepitations
- *PFTs* Low kCO, restrictive pattern
- Radiologically and histologically usual interstitial pneumonia (UIP) pattern, with subpleural basal reticular pattern, but can be like non-specific interstitial pneumonia (NSIP)
- *Treatment* Prognosis is much worse than other connective tissue disease-ILD, some studies suggest nearly as progressive as idiopathic pulmonary fibrosis (IPF). Steroids or immunosuppressants do little to change the course but should be tried. Studies in anti-fibrotics are ongoing.

Acute pneumonitis also recognized, which presents with rapidly deteriorating dyspnoea and development of respiratory failure, or acute deterioration on a background of chronic fibrosis. Acute pneumonitis tends to be more steroid-responsive.

Pulmonary nodules

Fewer than 5% of patients with RA. Usually found incidentally on imaging. Occur in seropositive disease, and are associated with nodules elsewhere (elbows and fingers). Single or multiple; may measure up to 7 cm, mainly subpleural or along interlobular septa. May cavitate and rarely cause haemoptysis or pneumothorax. Main differentials are lung cancer or vasculitis. Usually followed on CT to ensure stability. They typically show mild uptake on positron emission tomography (PET). May need biopsy to exclude malignancy.

Organizing pneumonia (OP)

Multifocal consolidation, with fever, dyspnoea, cough and weight loss, not responding to antibiotics. Can be disease- or drug-induced (gold) or have no obvious cause (for further information, see ➲ pp. 330–331). Confirmed by transbronchial, CT guided biopsy (CTGB), or VATS (if high level suspicion for cancer) showing acini filled with loose connective tissue and a variable inflammatory infiltrate. Often a dramatic response to steroids. May need long-term immunosuppression.

Small airways disease and obliterative bronchiolitis

Mild small airways disease found in about a third when looked for on HRCT, but often asymptomatic with variable histology. Obliterative bronchiolitis is a rarer problem, with lymphocytic infiltration of terminal bronchioles progressively obliterated by inflammatory connective tissue.

- May present with dyspnoea, dry cough, and hyperinflated chest, with basal crepitations and mid-inspiratory 'squeak or squawk'
- *PFTs* Irreversible obstructive pattern, hypoxia
- *CXR* Hyperinflation, no infiltrates
- *HRCT* Mosaic pattern
- *Biopsy* shows destruction of terminal bronchiolar wall by granulation tissue, effacement of the lumen, and replacement of the bronchiole by fibrous tissue
- Irreversible pathology, unresponsive to treatment. May rapidly progress
- Can give trial of oral steroids, continuing with high dose inhaled steroids if response. Penicillamine was thought to be a causative factor, but the evidence for this weak. Consider transplant.

Vasculitis

Rarely involves the lung and very rarely causes pulmonary haemorrhage. Rare cause of PHT.

Cricoarytenoid arthritis

Present in 75% of patients with RA by fibreoptic laryngoscopy and HRCT, but rarely symptomatic. Commoner in women. Unrelated to lung fibrosis. Causes sore throat, hoarse voice, upper airways obstruction with stridor, or obstructive sleep apnoea (OSA). Flow–volume loop may be abnormal. May need continuous positive airway pressure (CPAP)/tracheostomy and steroids—oral and joint injection.

Bronchiectasis

Often subtle with minimal clinical features but may be found in 30%. Diagnosis made on HRCT.

Sjögren's syndrome

Causing mucosal drying, often in association with ILD, produces dry cough and increased airway infections (see ➲ p. 224)

Caplan's syndrome

RA, single or multiple chest nodules, and coal-worker's pneumoconiosis, see ➲ pp. 428–429 (now rare).

Further information

Amital A et al. The lung in rheumatoid arthritis. *Press Med* 2011;**40**: e31–48.

Systemic lupus erythematosus (SLE)

- Multi-organ autoimmune disease, mainly affecting women
- dsDNA antibodies present in high titres, and these may pathogenic
- Can also get a drug-induced lupus syndrome (see Box 22.2), improves on stopping drug
- Pulmonary disease (lung, vasculature, pleura, diaphragm) often seen and may be a presenting feature of the disease
- American College of Rheumatology classification—see Box 22.3.

Pleural disease

Common, found in up to 50% of patients. Often asymptomatic but may have dyspnoea or pleuritic pain due to pleuritis with a pleural rub. ('Pleuritic' pain may also be musculoskeletal.) Often bilateral and exudative, with a neutrophilia, or a lymphocytosis in chronic effusion. Can be haemorrhagic. Rarely develop fibrothorax. Pleural biopsy findings non-specific. Need to exclude other causes for effusion. If symptomatic, may need treatment with NSAIDs or steroids.

Atelectasis

Associated with pleurisy or effusion.

Diffuse ILD

Occurs in up to 70% of patients in CT/autopsy series, but usually mild and asymptomatic. Radiologically usually NSIP. Only 5% develop clinical disease similar to UIP, with dyspnoea, cough, and basal crackles. May be associated with pleuritic pain. PFTs show restrictive defect with reduced kCO. Rarely, progressive and severe.

Acute lupus pneumonitis

In <2%, severe illness with mortality rate >50%. Cough, dyspnoea, fever, pleuritic pain, hypoxia. Widespread crackles. CXR shows infiltrates, which may be widespread. Histologically, non-specific acute alveolar injury. Need to exclude infection, pulmonary oedema. Treatment: steroids and cytotoxic drugs may be necessary, may have good response. Can progress to chronic interstitial pneumonitis.

PHT

Due to pulmonary vasoconstriction, rather than pulmonary vasculitis. Commoner in those with Raynaud's phenomenon. Associated with poorer prognosis: 50% 2 y mortality. Diagnosed on echo. Need to exclude PE as a cause, especially in those with antiphospholipid antibodies. Treatment as for idiopathic PHT (see ᗐ pp. 460–465).

PE

Commoner in the 20–30% with antiphospholipid antibodies.

'Shrinking lung syndrome'

Dyspnoea (± episodic pleurisy) caused by reduced lung volumes and poor respiratory reserve, probably due to diaphragmatic muscle weakness. Small lungs on CXR. Normal lung parenchyma on CT. Restrictive lung function tests, with normal/high kCO. May improve with steroids.

Alveolar haemorrhage

Rare. May be life threatening. Can have associated glomerulonephritis. Acute dyspnoea, with infiltrates on CXR. Raised kCO. Treat with high-dose steroids + cyclophosphamide.

Organizing pneumonia (OP or bronchiolitis obliterans)

See ➔ pp. 330–331

Box 22.2 Drug-induced lupus—causative drugs

These include:

- Isoniazid
- Procainamide
- Hydralazine
- Quinidine
- Minocycline
- Penicillamine
- Anticonvulsants.

Box 22.3 Criteria of the American College of Rheumatology for the classification of SLE

SLE if four or more criteria present, serially or simultaneously, during any interval:

- Malar rash
- Discoid rash
- Photosensitivity
- Oral ulcers
- Non-erosive arthritis: ≥2 peripheral joints
- Pleuritis or pericarditis
- Renal disorder: proteinuria >0.5 g/24 h or 3+ persistently, or cellular casts
- Neurological disorder: seizures or psychosis (having excluded drugs or other causes)
- Haematological disorder: haemolytic anaemia or leukopenia (<4.0 × 10^9/L on two or more occasions), lymphopenia (1.5 × 10^9/L on two or more occasions), thrombocytopenia (<100 × 10^9/L)
- Immunological disorder: raised anti-dsDNA antibody, anti-Sm antibody, positive finding of antiphospholipid antibodies
- ANA in raised titre (in the absence of drugs known to be associated with drug-induced lupus).

Further information

Keane M, Lynch J. Pleuropulmonary manifestations of SLE. Rare diseases 7. *Thorax* 2000;**55**: 159–166.

Idiopathic inflammatory myopathies

Idiopathic inflammatory myopathy associated interstitial lung disease can be the prominent feature (anti-synthetase syndrome) or as part of:
- Dermatomyositis (DM), which has a characteristic rash
- Amyopathic dermatomyositis, which has the typical skin changes of DM but no clinical signs of muscle weakness
- Polymyositis (PM), which causes symmetrical proximal muscle weakness
- For diagnostic criteria see Box 22.4.

Raised serum muscle enzymes. Myositis-specific antibodies and myositis associated antibodies are positive. DM is frequently associated with underlying malignancy (particularly if anti-TIF1 or anti-NXP2 positive), including lung, oesophagus, breast, colon, and ovary, so therefore needs thorough investigation. Pulmonary complications are a common and frequent cause of death. As with other connective tissue diseases, differentiation of the pulmonary problems from those due to drugs and infection is important.

ILD

In 20–30%. Commoner in anti-synthetase syndrome if anti-MDA5 positive, or if associated with anti-PM-Scl antibodies. Less common when DM is associated with malignancy. Patients present with dyspnoea, cough, arthralgia, and fevers, with fine bibasal crackles.
- *HRCT* shows patchy consolidation and peripheral reticular pattern
- *Histology* Wide variation, with UIP, NSIP, COP, and diffuse alveolar haemorrhage all reported, related to steroid response
- May require treatment with steroids, cyclophosphamide, or rituximab (after consultation with rheumatology as national commissioning policy for rituximab allows funding only if certain criteria are fulfilled).

Anti-synthetase syndrome
A subset, often with ILD as the dominant feature. Other features include polyarthritis, fever, Raynaud's, mechanics hands, dysphagia, and pericarditis (particularly PL7 positive), with or without myositis. They have serum antibodies to one or more of the aminoacyl-transfer RNA synthetases, a family of intracytoplasmic enzymes involved in protein synthesis. Antibodies to Jo-1 (20–30%), PL-7 (5–10%), PL-12 (5–15%), OJ, EJ, and KS are recognized and should be specifically tested for (myositis blot). ANA is often negative and specific request for these tests may be required. Anti-Ro antibodies in addition to anti-Jo increase the risk of rapidly progressive ILD.

Anti-MDA5 antibodies
Patients with anti-MDA5 antibodies often present with skin rash, with no or mild muscle weakness. While this only accounts for ~7% of idiopathic inflammatory myopathies, anti-MDA5 antibodies are often associated with a rapidly progressive ILD.

Organizing pneumonia

Poorer prognosis if associated with features of fibrosis.

PHT

Commoner with Jo, PL12, and PL7 antibodies.

Pulmonary vasculitis

Causing haemoptysis (rarely alveolar haemorrhage).

Aspiration pneumonia

In 20%, associated with marked increase in mortality. Caused by dysphagia and pharyngeal muscle weakness and regurgitation.

Ventilatory failure

Due to intercostal and diaphragm muscle weakness. Restrictive defect on PFTs with preserved gas transfer if isolated muscle weakness.

Spontaneous pneumomediastinum

Occurs rarely (acute retrosternal pain, neck, and face subcutaneous emphysema), usually in association with ILD, in DM more often than PM.

Box 22.4 Diagnostic criteria for idiopathic inflammatory myopathy

- Muscle weakness
- Objective symmetrical proximal muscle weakness, either upper or lower limbs (or both)
- Neck flexion weakness relative to neck extension
- Proximal leg weakness relative to distal leg strength
- Skin changes
- Heliotrope rash (purple discolouration of the eyelids)
- Gottron's papules (erythematous to violaceous papules over extensor surfaces of joints involving fingers, elbows, knees, malleoli and toes)
- Gottron's sign (erythematous to violaceous macules over extensor surfaces, that are not palpable)
- Dysphagia or oesophageal dysmotility
- Elevated serum muscle enzymes: CK, LDH, AST, or ALT
- Typical auto-antibody findings
- Typical muscle biopsy findings
- *MRI is also commonly used to identify myositis*

Adapted from the 2017 European League Against Rheumatism/American College of Rheumatology Classification Criteria for Adult and Juvenile Idiopathic Inflammatory Myopathies and Their Major Subgroups.

Further information

Lundberg et al. 2017 European League Against Rheumatism/American College of Rheumatology Classification Criteria for Adult and Juvenile Idiopathic Inflammatory Myopathies and Their Major Subgroups. *Arthritis & Rheum* 2017;**69**: 2271–2282.

Barsotti and Lundberg. Myositis an evolving spectrum of disease. *Imm Medicine* 2018;**41**: 46–54.

Systemic sclerosis

This disease affects women more than men (4:1), has HLA associations, and often presents in the fifth decade. It is largely a clinical diagnosis, and there are several types:

- *Limited cutaneous* (many have CREST syndrome). 60% of systemic sclerosis cases. Patients often have long-standing Raynaud's, developing non-pitting oedema of the fingers, which become 'sausage-shaped'. Develop thick, shiny skin after a few weeks to months. Later, they can develop skin changes on the hands, face, and neck, microstomia, digital and facial telangiectasia, intra- and subcutaneous calcification, and oesophageal dysmotility (74%). Patients can also develop pulmonary fibrosis (26%), PHT (21%), and cardiac (9%), oesophageal (90%), and renal disease (8%), but less common than in diffuse cutaneous disease
- *Diffuse cutaneous* Abrupt-onset disease, with widespread symmetrical itchy, painful swelling of fingers, arms, feet, legs, and face, and associated constitutional symptoms. There is oedema, which is replaced by tight, shiny skin, bound to underlying structures extending proximal to the wrists, within a few months. There is cutaneous thickening, as well as hypo- or hyperpigmentation. Raynaud's phenomenon is present, as well as skin sclerosis on the trunk and upper arms, arthropathy, renal disease (18%), pulmonary fibrosis (41%), PHT (17%), cardiac disease (12%), and GI disease (90%)
- *Overlap syndromes*, or mixed connective tissue diseases, have features of systemic sclerosis, together with those of at least one other autoimmune rheumatic disease such as SLE, RA, PM. Over time, other organ involvement may develop and evolve into a more defined disease
- *Systemic sclerosis sine scleroderma* Vascular or fibrotic visceral features without skin scleroderma. May or may not have Raynaud's phenomenon. May develop ILD, oesophagitis, arrhythmias, malabsorption, pseudo-obstruction, renal failure (>2% of cases)
- *Environmentally induced* Contentious but may result from exposure to vinyl chloride, pesticides, or epoxy resins.

  Pulmonary complications are the most common cause of death.

Pulmonary fibrosis

Seen at post-mortem in up to 80% of patients. ANA is positive in 60% and of speckled or nucleolar type. Pulmonary involvement is seen, particularly if Scl-70 antibody is present. All antibody groups may develop ILD, often more severe with anti-topoisomerase I antibodies. Micro-aspiration from oesophageal dysmotility may be contributory.

- *Present* with dyspnoea and a history of Raynaud's
- *Examination* Signs of systemic sclerosis, fine bibasal crackles
- *PFTs* show restrictive defect and reduced kCO. Rapidly falling kCO is a poor prognostic sign. HRCT shows mostly NSIP pattern but can be UIP pattern. VATS lung biopsy is rarely required unless concerned about other pathologies (such as malignancy/vasculitis)

- *Treatment* with steroids, cyclophosphamide, or mycophenolate mofetil (MMF). An RCT of oral cyclophosphamide vs placebo in patients with active alveolitis and scleroderma-related ILD showed a modest, but significant, effect on forced vital capacity (FVC), dyspnoea, and quality of life. An RCT showed comparable effects of MMF to cyclophosphamide on FVC over two years, and MMF might be better tolerated. In those with fibrosis nintedanib slows the reduction in FVC compared to placebo and has recently been granted FDA approval in the US
- *Prognosis* Systemic sclerosis-associated ILD has a better prognosis than IPF. This may be related to slower disease progression, immune-modulatory therapy slows progression. Associated increased risk of lung cancer. Studies of antifibrotics are ongoing.

PHT

May be isolated or 2° to ILD. Isolated PHT is characteristic of limited cutaneous disease, especially in those with cutaneous telangiectasias and anti-centromere antibodies. Pathologically similar to primary pulmonary hypertension (PPH). Subintimal cell proliferation, endothelial hyperplasia, and the obliteration of small intrapulmonary vessels.
- *Presents* with dyspnoea, right ventricle (RV) hypertrophy, and right heart failure
- *Diagnosis* by echo or right-heart catheter
- *Treatment* as for PPH (see ◑ pp. 460–465). May respond to prostacyclin infusions or may need transplant
- *Prognosis* Better than for those with PPH.

Chest wall limitation

Via skin scleroderma over chest ('hide-bound chest'); very rare.

Organizing pneumonia

See ◑ pp. 330–331.

Aspiration pneumonia

Uncommon and due to oesophageal dysmotility.

Bronchiectasis

Often seen on HRCT, but much less commonly of clinical significance.

Further information

McMahan ZH, Hummers LK. Systemic sclerosis—challenges for clinical practice. *Nat Rev Rheumatol* 2013;9: 90–100.

Tashkin DP et al. Scleroderma Lung Study Research Group. Cyclophosphamide versus placebo in scleroderma lung disease. *NEJM* 2006;**354**: 2655–66.

Tashkin et al. mycophenolate mofetil versus oral cyclophosphamide in scleroderma-related interstitial lung disease: Scleroderma Lung Study II (SLS-II), a double-blind, parallel group, randomised controlled trial *Lancet Respir Med* 2016;**4**: 708–719.

Distler et al. Nintedanib for systemic sclerosis-associated interstitial lung disease. *NEJM* 2019; **380**: 2518–2528.

Sjögren's syndrome

- Inflammation, lymphocytic infiltration, and destruction of primarily the salivary and lachrymal glands
- Keratoconjunctivitis sicca or xerostomia (dry eyes and dry mouth) is usually evidence of 1° disease but, when associated with connective tissue disease, especially RA, is 2° Sjögren's
- Classical sicca syndrome includes dry eyes and mouth, with parotid or salivary gland enlargement
- Pulmonary involvement occurs in about 25%, commoner in women and in their 60s.

Pleuritic

Can cause pleuritic chest pain.

Airways disease

Bronchial hyperresponsiveness, chronic bronchitis, bronchiectasis, and small airways disease. Mild abnormalities on PFTs, rarely significant.

Dry cough

Atrophy of mucus gland in trachea and bronchi and lymphoplasmocytic infiltrate (xerotrachea). Possibly a higher incidence of chest infections. Treatment: nebulized saline, physiotherapy, inhaled steroids.

Diffuse lung disease

Develops later, often asymptomatic, but may have cough, dyspnoea, and crackles on examination. PFTs show a restrictive defect and NSIP, LIP, or UIP pattern on CT.

Lymphoma

Unusual but is 40 times more common in Sjögren's syndrome, especially in patients with high levels of immunoglobulins, autoantibodies, and cryoglobulins. Usually non-Hodgkin's B-cell lymphoma. Can mimic OP.

OP

Can cause organising pneumonia (OP).

Pleural thickening/effusion

Rare.

PHT, thromboembolism

Rare.

Ankylosing spondylitis

- Chronic inflammatory disease causing spinal ankylosis with sacroiliac joint involvement
- 90% of Caucasian patients are HLA-B27 +ve.

Pulmonary fibrosis

Occurs in 5–15%, especially those with advanced disease. Typically bilateral in the upper lobes. May develop cysts/cavities and become colonized with *Aspergillus*.

Pleural involvement

Pleuritis and apical pleural thickening.

Restrictive defect

Due to costovertebral rigidity causing fixed restrictive deformity of the thorax, rarely leading to respiratory failure with nocturnal hypoventilation. Nocturnal NIV may be indicated.

Behçet's syndrome

- Systemic vessel vasculitis involving arteries and veins of all sizes, with recurrent painful oral ± genital ulceration, skin lesions, arthritis, and chronic relapsing uveitis, which can cause blindness
- Marked geographical distribution, with greatest prevalence in Turkey, Iran, and Japan. Mainly young adults
- Musculoskeletal, skin, neurological, GI, and major artery and vein involvement.

Pulmonary vascular disease

Aneurysms, arterial and venous thrombosis, and pulmonary infarcts in <5%. Recurrent haemoptysis is the main manifestation. This can be massive and fatal. Pulmonary aneurysms are seen as non-cavitating shadows on CXR and confirmed by CT. These are associated with DVT, therefore making anticoagulation difficult due to possible haemoptysis from the aneurysm.

Pleural effusion, eosinophilic pneumonia

Both rare.

Autoantibodies: disease associations

Antinuclear antibody (ANA)	+ve in
SLE	99%
RA	32%
Juvenile RA	76%
Chronic active hepatitis	75%
Sjögren's syndrome	68%
Behçet's disease	64%
Polyarteritis nodosa	
Myasthenia gravis	
Autoimmune thyroid disease	
Extensive burns	
Normal controls *ANA often negative in anti-synthetase syndrome*	0–2%
Extractable nuclear antigen (ENA)	**(done by lab if ANA +ve)**
Anti-dsDNA—SLE	
Anti-Sm—SLE	
Anti-centromere—limited scleroderma	
Anti-Scl-70—lung fibrosis in scleroderma	
Anti-Jo-1 and other synthetases—myositis	
Anti-Ro—Sjögren's, SLE, foetal heart block	
Anti-RNP—SLE, scleroderma, myositis, mixed connective tissue disease, and RA	
PR3(c)-ANCA (proteinase 3)—GPA (Wegener's)	
MPO(p)-ANCA (myeloperoxidase)—microscopic polyangiitis	
RhF	**+ve in**
RA*	70–80%
Sjögren's syndrome	<100%
Felty's syndrome	<100%
Systemic sclerosis	30%
Still's disease	Rarely +ve

Infective endocarditis	<50%
SLE	<40%
Normal controls	5–10%

Also: Neoplasms, after radio-or
chemotherapy
   Hyperglobulinaemic states
   Dermatomyositis

*Anti-CCP (cyclic citrullinated peptide) is much more specific to RA than RF and positive in
60–70% of RA.

Chapter 23

Cor pulmonale

Definition, causes, and pathophysiology 232
Clinical features and investigations 234
Management 235

Definition, causes, and pathophysiology

Cor pulmonale is the traditional term for changes in the cardiovascular system resulting from the chronic hypoxia (and usually hypercapnia) of chronic lung disease leading to pulmonary hypertension (PHT). PHT is precapillary due to raised pulmonary vascular resistance, is usually mild-moderate and does not tend to progress; a subgroup of patients may develop severe PHT, disproportionate to their lung disease (see ⊃ p. 449). Presents with peripheral oedema.

Cor pulmonale can occur in most situations where there is chronic hypoxia (see Box 23.1):

- Most often in the setting of hypoxic and hypercapnic chronic obstructive pulmonary disease (COPD)
- Hypoventilation syndromes (scoliosis, neuromuscular diseases, obesity)
- Much less common when there is no associated rise in $PaCO_2$ (e.g. with interstitial lung diseases (ILDs), altitude, right-to-left shunts).

It is often also referred to as 'right heart failure', which is misleading as the cardiac output in cor pulmonale is usually *normal or high* with *increased* peripheral perfusion (hence, the 'bounding pulse' and warm peripheries of type II ventilatory failure). If allowed time to adapt, the right ventricle (RV) can generate much higher pressures (e.g. in idiopathic pulmonary arterial hypertension (IPAH)) than are usually seen in cor pulmonale in response to the hypoxia. In true right heart failure, the RV fails to develop an adequate cardiac output, e.g. following right-sided myocardial infarction (MI) or pulmonary emboli (PEs) that occlude a large proportion of the pulmonary vascular bed, this rarely occurs in cor pulmonale. This also produces a raised jugular venous pressure (JVP), as occurs in the fluid overload of cor pulmonale, but, in contrast, there will of course be a low cardiac output and poor peripheral perfusion.

> **Box 23.1 Cor pulmonale results from the following sequence of events**
> - Lung disease causes hypoxia, cyanosis, and sometimes polycythaemia
> - Hypoxia acutely causes pulmonary vasoconstriction and chronically causes pulmonary vascular remodelling
> - This leads to pulmonary hypertension
> - In addition, hypoxia is sensed both within the kidney and via the carotid body, generating increases in sympathetic activity and renal vasoconstriction
> - Increased sympathetic activity (and other mechanisms) leads to renal retention of salt and water
> - This extra salt and water are mainly held in the capacitance vessels (the large veins), often with a raised JVP
> - If vascular permeability rises (particularly when the $PaCO_2$ rises, producing peripheral vasodilatation and an increase in capillary pressure), extra fluid accumulates in dependent tissues.

Patients often present with their first episode of ankle swelling during an exacerbation of their COPD when, for the first time, the $PaCO_2$ rises and the PaO_2 falls, far enough to provoke the above events. Body weight may not actually rise very much with the onset of ankle oedema; however, the extra salt and water, retained in the capacitance vessels leading up to the exacerbation, move into the subcutaneous tissues, probably due to the CO_2-induced vasodilatation, raising mean capillary hydrostatic pressure.

Loss of pulmonary vascular bed from emphysema also contributes to the raised pulmonary artery pressure (PAP), and the ECG often shows RV hypertrophy, although this is not sensitive. Echocardiography is the best non-invasive test, but it is often not possible to obtain good images (hyper-inflation of COPD or obesity). Right heart catheter is the gold-standard test but is rarely necessary unless estimated PAP is disproportionately high on echo (>40 mmHg). During an exacerbation, extra hypoxia will produce further rises in PAP, with which the hypertrophied RV usually copes, helped by the raised JVP providing a larger pre-load to increase RV filling. Excessive diuresis can lead to a true fall in right-sided output due to inadequate filling of the RV.

Clinical features and investigations

- Features of the underlying disease causing the hypoxia, e.g. COPD/bronchiectasis
- Easily visible veins and a raised JVP
- Cyanosis and a suffused conjunctiva (polycythaemia and vessel dilatation from the raised CO_2)
- Sometimes marked polycythaemia, very rare consequences due to hyperviscosity
- Peripheral vasodilatation, with a 'bounding' pulse and warm peripheries
- Ankle swelling and pitting oedema
- RV hypertrophy (sternal heave uncommon, masked by hyperinflated lung between heart and chest wall; more often seen with the higher pressures of IPAH
- Tricuspid incompetence (not usually severe)
- CXR—enlarged pulmonary arteries/underlying lung disease
- FBC—may have associated polycythaemia
- Oximetry—cor pulmonale is unlikely if awake SaO_2 >92%
- Blood gases—cor pulmonale progressively more likely as PaO_2 drops below 8 kPa (equivalent $SaO_2 \approx 91\%$) and $PaCO_2$ rises above 6 kPa
- ECG—may indicate right axis deviation (RAD), p pulmonale (right atrial hypertrophy), and right bundle branch block (RBBB)
- Echo—dilated or hypertrophied RV, tricuspid regurgitation (TR), providing estimate of PAP, and exclude other diagnoses such as a patent atrial septal defect (ASD)
- Overnight oximetry—to reveal unexpected degrees of hypoxia, e.g. from obstructive sleep apnoea (OSA), obesity, neuromuscular disease
- Consider referral for right heart catheter where PHT disproportionate (>40 mmHg).

Management

Cor pulmonale is a marker of poor prognosis in COPD, with a five-year survival rate of ~50%. It is not clear if this relates to PHT or the severity of the COPD. Long-term oxygen therapy is the main treatment in patients with cor pulmonale and hypoxia (PaO$_2$ <8.0 kPa) and improves survival.

Minimal ankle oedema needs no treatment. 'Trimming' the ankles to normal is unnecessary and may reduce RV output by reducing RV filling. If the oedema is more substantial, then the following may help:

• Treat underlying condition to raise PaO$_2$ and lower PaCO$_2$
• Raise PaO$_2$ through added O$_2$; provide long-term O$_2$ at home
• In hypoventilation syndromes, home overnight non-invasive ventilation is likely to be the correct management
• Promote a limited diuresis with judicious use of diuretics
• Always elevate legs when sitting
• Some will venesect if haematocrit exceeds 0.6, but no RCT evidence of physiological benefit or a reduction in hyperviscosity complications.

Treating the blood gas disturbance and improving burdensome peripheral oedema are the main therapeutic aims. The long-term O$_2$ trials showed that improving the PaO$_2$ was useful, not that lowering the PAP was important. Specific agents used to lower pulmonary artery pressures used in PAH have not been shown to help in cor pulmonale.

Further information

Weitzenblum E and Chaouat A. Cor pulmonale. *Chron Respir Dis* 2009; 6: 177–185.

Cystic fibrosis (CF)

General principles *238*
CF microbiology: overview *240*
CF antibiotics 1 *242*
CF antibiotics 2 *244*
Management of exacerbations *246*
Intravenous antibiotic administration *248*
Pulmonary interventions *250*
Pulmonary complications *252*
Nutrition and gastrointestinal disease *254*
Other extrapulmonary disease *256*
Supportive care and future developments *258*

General principles

Definition and pathophysiology

- Cystic fibrosis (CF) is a multi-system disease due to mutations in the gene encoding the CF transmembrane conductance regulator (CFTR), a complex chloride channel
- CFTR is essential for regulating chloride permeability across epithelial tissues and, in addition, has other complex cellular roles (e.g. CFTR downregulates the epithelial sodium channel and influences expression of other genes including those involved in inflammatory responses, ion transport, and cell signalling)
- Loss of CFTR function or quantity causes inadequate hydration of mucous secretions. In the lungs this results in defective mucociliary clearance, mucus obstruction of the luminal space, and colonization with pathogenic bacteria. Recurrent cycles of infection and inflammation contribute to lung damage and subsequent development of bronchiectasis
- In the pancreas, the exocrine ducts become blocked by secretions, leading to pancreatic destruction, pancreatic enzyme insufficiency, and CF-related diabetes.

Multidisciplinary care

- A multidisciplinary team (MDT) approach is essential, comprising respiratory physician, specialist nurse, physiotherapist, pharmacist, dietician, social worker, and psychologist, with regular additional input from gastro-enterology and endocrine teams
- Ongoing care of CF patients moves to the adult CF centre at the age of 16–18 y, although a period of transitional care should begin between ages 14–16 y
- Improved treatment of CF has led to an increase in survival, and the majority of UK CF patients are adults. The median predicted survival for a baby born with CF now is 47 y.

Genetics

- Autosomal recessive disease, with a carrier frequency of 1 in 25 in Caucasians; 1 in 2,500 UK live births have CF. CF is rare in Afro-Caribbeans but is seen in patients of Asian origin in the UK
- Heterozygote advantage through resistance to diarrhoeal disease may have led to persistence of *CFTR* mutations at relatively high population frequencies, despite the previously lethal homozygous form
- Over 2,000 different mutations in the *CFTR* gene are recognized and can be classified on the basis of the mechanism by which they cause disease (Table 24.1)
- The most common mutation in the UK is F508del (previously termed DeltaF508; a deletion of three nucleotides, causing the loss of a phenylalanine at residue 508), with a decreasing prevalence from north-west to south-east Europe. Half of patients with CF in England are F508del homozygous; 90% carry at least one F508del allele
- Thirteen other mutations have a frequency >1% (e.g. G542X (3.4%), G551D (2.4%), W1282X (2.1%), 3905insT (2.1%))

- CF is characterized by wide variation between patients in disease severity, rate of progression, and, to an extent, organ involvement. This phenotypic variation reflects: (i) class of *CFTR* mutation (correlates with pancreatic status but not with severity of lung disease); (ii) polymorphism in non-*CFTR* 'modifier' genes (e.g. *IFRD1*, which regulates neutrophil function); (iii) environmental factors (e.g. treatment adherence, socio-economic factors, access to care, pathogen-specific factors).

Screening

In the UK, neonatal heel-prick for immunoreactive trypsinogen measurement is offered routinely as part of a national screening programme. Positive samples are tested for common *CFTR* mutations and, if needed, a second trypsinogen screen, followed by sweat testing.

Diagnosis

Patients are usually diagnosed with CF as neonates or children (genetic screening, family history, failure to thrive, meconium ileus, rectal prolapse, cough, recurrent chest infections). Diagnosis is based on the presence of two disease-causing *CFTR* mutations, along with a positive sweat test (sweat chloride concentration >60 mmol/L, usually 90–110 mmol/L) and compatible clinical features. Sweat chloride levels are usually lower in CF that presents in adulthood (borderline is 40–60 mmol/L; <40 is considered normal although can occur in CF).

CFTR-related disease

CFTR-related disease refers to patients with mild manifestations of CFTR dysfunction such as single organ involvement (e.g. late-onset bronchiectasis, congenital bilateral absence of the vas deferens, or idiopathic pancreatitis). These typically occur with 'milder' *CFTR* mutations (classes IV or V) that result in residual CFTR function, and patients tend to be pancreatic-sufficient. A grey area exists between CF and CFTR-related disease, and, in some cases, a firm diagnosis is not possible on initial investigation but becomes apparent during follow-up; note that CF remains a clinical diagnosis.

Table 24.1 Classes of *CFTR* mutation

Class I	Defective protein synthesis, e.g. G542X
Class II	Defective protein maturation and trafficking, e.g. F508del
Class III	Impaired chloride channel opening (gating), e.g. G551D
Class IV	Defective channel ion transport (conductance), e.g. R117H
Class V	Defective splicing
Class VI	Accelerated turnover at cell surface

CF microbiology: overview

Chronic pulmonary sepsis and its complications account for much of the morbidity and mortality in CF. The airways of a CF patient are chronically colonized by pathogenic bacteria from an early age. Bronchiectasis is usually established by a young age.

- Patients commonly expectorate variable volumes of purulent sputum, even when well
- When organism levels are high, patients may feel generally unwell or more tired, or have anorexia, weight loss, temperature >38°C
- They may have symptoms of dyspnoea, increased volume of more purulent sputum, haemoptysis, wheeze, and chest ache
- Examination and chest radiograph (CXR) can be unchanged from normal during exacerbations
- With effective antibiotic treatment, FEV_1 levels should rise to the pre-infection normal. If they do not, further antibiotics may be necessary, and other diagnoses or unusual organisms should be considered
- In practice, the FEV_1 is the most reliable marker of disease progression and can be used to assess overall decline, as well as to determine an exacerbation and response to treatment (as peak expiratory flow rate (PEFR) would be used in asthma).

Organisms

Airway colonization changes over time, with increasing age, and organisms become more resistant to antibiotics. Typical progression of organism colonization with time is *Staphylococcus aureus*, followed by *Haemophilus influenzae*, and then *Pseudomonas aeruginosa* (see Fig. 24.1). Goals of management should be initially to prevent infection, then to eradicate it, and finally to control the infection. Material for culture should be collected; most commonly sputum, but bronchoalveolar lavage (BAL) if necessary. Polymicrobial infection is common.

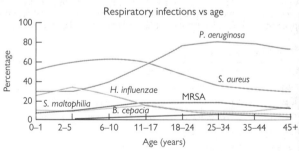

Fig. 24.1 Prevalence of selected respiratory pathogens in patients with CF over time.

Reproduced from Goss C, *Thorax* 2007; **62**: 360–367 with the kind permission of *BMJ*.

CF antibiotics 1

Antibiotic courses in patients with CF need to be longer and at higher doses than in non-CF patients. Indications for treatment in adults include any new isolate from sputum (even if asymptomatic) or features of an exacerbation (see → p. 246). Treatment should be for 14 days with either oral or IV antibiotics. IV antibiotics are indicated for severe infection or failure to eradicate organisms with oral antibiotics. Choice of antibiotics is based on clinical response more than *in vitro* resistance patterns, but recent sputum culture results will also guide therapy.

- In practice, it is usually appropriate to give the patient the same regime they had during their last exacerbation, provided there was a good clinical response, taking into account the patient's antibiotic allergies (desensitization may be required; see → p. 248)
- Recent sputum culture results can be helpful, although note that sputum cultures lack sensitivity. Have a low threshold for including anti-pseudomonal cover if *P. aeruginosa* has previously been isolated (even if assumed to have been eradicated). Results of *in vitro* antibiotic susceptibility testing do not always correlate with clinical response to antibiotics
- CF centres will have written management protocols; seek expert advice from your local CF centre if unsure.

Pseudomonas aeruginosa

Pseudomonas aeruginosa infection is associated with a more rapid decline in lung function. Most CF patients are chronically infected with *P. aeruginosa* by their teens: non-mucoid species colonize initially, which may be asymptomatic or intermittent and can be eradicated, and mucoid species then follow and permanent eradication is rare. The aims of treatment are prompt eradication of new isolates and maintenance therapy to reduce the bacterial load in colonized patients.

- *First isolates of P. aeruginosa* in patients who were previously *Pseudomonas*-free or who have never had *P. aeruginosa* should lead to prompt treatment with an eradication regimen (even if asymptomatic). Failure to treat may lead to the development of chronic airway infection. There is no clear evidence favouring a specific eradication regimen. An initial treatment protocol combining nebulized colistin 2 MU bd for 3 months with oral ciprofloxacin 750 mg bd (avoid in epilepsy; reduce dose in severe renal impairment; warn patient to stop if ankle pain as risk of Achilles tendon rupture) for 3 months is widely used. Consider a 2-week course of IV anti-pseudomonal antibiotics (Box 24.1) before starting treatment with nebulized colistin and oral ciprofloxacin in patients with a new *P. aeruginosa* isolate in the context of a respiratory exacerbation. Failure of eradication with oral and nebulized antibiotics should also prompt IV therapy
- *Maintenance treatment for chronic P. aeruginosa infection* comprises long-term nebulized anti-pseudomonal therapy, typically either nebulized colistin 1–2 MU bd or alternate months of nebulized tobramycin 300 mg bd (the alternate month can either be medication-free or the patient may nebulize colistin). Alternative, maintenance inhaled anti-pseudomonals are dry powder inhaler colistin and tobramycin, which

may be associated with improved adherence. Nebulized aztreonam lysine is the third-line inhaled anti-pseudomonal for patients who have not tolerated colistin or tobramycin, and nebulized levofloxacin has recently been approved in the UK as a fourth-line option

• *Treatment of exacerbations in patients with chronic P. aeruginosa infection* Mild exacerbations (e.g. following a viral upper respiratory tract infection (URTI)) should be treated with a 2-week course of oral ciprofloxacin, alongside usual maintenance nebulized antibiotics. IV anti-pseudomonal antibiotics (Box 24.1) for a minimum of 2 weeks are indicated for moderate and severe exacerbations as well as for first *P. aeruginosa* isolates not cleared by ciprofloxacin and colistin.

Box 24.1 Two-week course of IV antibiotic treatment of *Pseudomonas aeruginosa* in CF

Combinations of two drugs are typically used to achieve a synergistic effect—select one drug from the left-hand column alongside one drug from the right-hand column:

Ceftazidime 2–3 g tds	Tobramycin 7 mg/kg/day
Piperacillin/tazobactam 4.5 g tds	Amikacin 15 mg/kg/day
Aztreonam 2 g tds	Colistin 2 MU tds
Meropenem 2 g tds	

Notes:

• Intravenous (IV) tobramycin, amikacin, and colistin all require *therapeutic drug monitoring*; follow local policy. Use previous treatment doses (if available) as a guide to starting doses in individual patients, adjusted for current weight. Ensure adequate hydration and normal renal function at the start of therapy. Reduce dosage in renal impairment
• Symptoms of dizziness, hearing loss, or tinnitus during IV aminoglycosides (tobramycin, amikacin) suggest *oto- or vestibulo-toxicity*. The aminoglycoside should be stopped and ENT referral made for pure tone audiogram. Previous oto- or vestibulo-toxicity is an absolute contraindication to further IV aminoglycosides
• Note that IV gentamicin is no longer recommended in CF patients, and once-daily aminoglycoside dosing (rather than tds) is recommended
• Use of *nebulized* antibiotics in conjunction with IV administration of the same antibiotic may result in toxic drug levels, and many clinicians will stop nebulized antibiotics while the patient is receiving IV antibiotics
• IV fosfomycin may also be useful in the treatment of resistant *P. aeruginosa* infections.

CF antibiotics 2

Staphylococcus aureus

Staphylococcus aureus is a significant pathogen causing exacerbations. Prevention and eradication are important, even if the patient is asymptomatic. In adults, a minimum of 2 weeks of treatment (e.g. with flucloxacillin – follow local protocol) should be given when *S. aureus* is cultured. If *S. aureus* continues to grow, despite treatment with flucloxacillin, check that the *S. aureus* isolate is not multiple-resistant *Staphylococcus aureus* (MRSA), and add in a second anti-staphylococcal antibiotic (e.g. sodium fusidate or rifampicin) for 2 weeks. More prolonged oral antibiotics (e.g. further 4 weeks) or a course of IV antibiotics may be required. There is some evidence to support long-term flucloxacillin prophylaxis in infants, but this is not widely practised in adults, reflecting a lack of evidence of benefit in this age group as well as concerns regarding the development of MRSA.

Haemophilus influenzae

Haemophilus influenzae in sputum should be treated (e.g. with co-amoxiclav or doxycycline for 2 weeks) even if the patient is asymptomatic. More prolonged oral antibiotics or a course of IV antibiotics (e.g. co-amoxiclav or ceftriaxone) may be required. Resistance to amoxicillin and macrolides is common.

Burkholderia cepacia complex

Burkholderia cepacia complex comprises at least ten different subspecies (genomovars) of *B. cepacia*. These organisms are often resistant to many antibiotics and display inherent resistance to colistin. Some genomovars are highly transmissible, and patients colonized with *B. cepacia* should be segregated (including separate clinics and spirometers, and side rooms on a different ward) from non-colonized patients. Clinical consequences of infection are highly variable, ranging from asymptomatic to severe worsening of pulmonary infection with septicaemia ('cepacia syndrome'), which can be rapidly fatal. *B. cenocepacia* (genomovar III) is particularly associated with cepacia syndrome and is usually considered an absolute contraindication for lung transplant due to poor outcomes. Treat exacerbations with combination antibiotic therapy, directed by *in vitro* sensitivities where available. Meropenem appears to be a particularly useful antibiotic, and other options often include ceftazidime, piperacillin-tazobactam, aminoglycosides, and temocillin.

MRSA

MRSA has been associated with increased mortality in CF and leads to difficulties in antibiotic choice and delivery of care. Follow local guidelines for topical eradication in patients with MRSA skin carriage. 4-week long courses of oral rifampicin with sodium fusidate are useful for sputum eradication; other options include linezolid or nebulized vancomycin. IV teicoplanin or vancomycin are required for MRSA pulmonary exacerbations.

Non-tuberculous mycobacteria

Mycobacterium avium complex (MAC) and *Mycobacterium abscessus* are the most frequently encountered non-tuberculous mycobacteria (NTM) in CF (see ⊃ p. 620). In general, consider and treat other causes of deterioration (e.g. *P. aeruginosa*) prior to initiating anti-mycobacterial therapy. The clinical and radiological features of NTM may be difficult to distinguish from other infections, particularly *P. aeruginosa*, and both long-term antibiotics (e.g. macrolides, tobramycin) and bacterial overgrowth may inhibit NTM culture. Recent studies have suggested that the *M. abscessus* subspecies *massiliense* may be spread between patients within CF centres, although the transmission route and infection control measures required to control this organism are currently unknown. Furthermore, isolation of *M. abscessus* pre-transplant appears to be a risk factor for the development of post-transplant NTM disease and a poor outcome, and active *M. abscessus* infection is considered an absolute contraindication to transplant in many units.

Stenotrophomonas maltophilia

The clinical significance of *S. maltophilia* colonization in CF remains unclear. Address other causes of clinical deterioration in colonized patients prior to considering antibiotic treatment directed at *S. maltophilia*. *S. maltophilia* is inherently resistant to carbapenems, and most strains are also resistant to anti-pseudomonal drugs. Co-trimoxazole is the usual antibiotic of choice; other options include doxycycline, ticarcillin-clavulanic acid, or tigecycline.

Achromobacter xylosoxidans

The clinical significance of *A. xylosoxidans* infection is uncertain; consider treatment in chronically colonized patients with evidence of clinical deterioration in the absence of other causes. *A. xylosoxidans* is often multi-resistant, and antibiotic choice should be on the basis of susceptibility testing results; useful agents often include minocycline, meropenem, piperacillin-tazobactam, and chloramphenicol.

Management of exacerbations

Pulmonary exacerbations are the most common reason for hospital admission of CF patients. Patients are usually adept at recognizing a deterioration in their condition requiring treatment, and treatment is usually required if they present acutely, even if they appear fit and healthy.

Signs and symptoms of an exacerbation include:

- Increase in productive cough or dyspnoea
- Change in appearance or volume of sputum
- New signs on auscultation (often absent)
- New CXR changes (often absent)
- Weight loss >1 kg or 5% of body weight, associated with anorexia
- Fall in FEV$_1$ >10%
- Fever.

Persistent, low-grade symptoms, such as cough alone, are an indication for IV antibiotics if oral antibiotics have failed to bring about an improvement. IV antibiotics should also be considered if a new positive sputum culture fails to clear with appropriate oral antibiotics.

Investigations

- Baseline spirometry for FEV$_1$
- Weight
- O$_2$ saturation and, if <92%, blood gas
- CXR (exclude pneumothorax)
- Sputum (microscopy, culture, and sensitivity (MC&S), including specific testing for *P. aeruginosa* and *B. cepacia*, and acid-fast bacilli (AFB))
- Bloods, including C-reactive protein (CRP) (note that not all patients exhibit high inflammatory markers, even during severe exacerbations)
- Monitor blood sugars.

Treatment

Treatment is with appropriate antibiotics (see ➔ p. 242), O$_2$ therapy, increased physiotherapy and nutritional support, and control of hyperglycaemia. Many patients will self-administer IV antibiotics at home (see ➔ p. 248). Indications for inpatient treatment include: too unwell for home therapy; significant weight loss; poor response to recent home IVs; poor compliance or unable to self-administer IV therapy; patient preference; other complications (e.g. significant haemoptysis or pneumothorax; ➔ p. 252).

If *failing to improve* with empirical antibiotics:

- Review microbiology; repeat sputum MC&S and AFBs, and consider empirical change in antibiotics, including anti-pseudomonal cover (➔ p. 243)
- Consider hospital admission if failing to improve with home-based treatment
- Optimize airway clearance with intensive physiotherapy, and review mucolytics (➔ p. 250)
- Optimize nutritional support and glycaemic control (➔ p. 256)
- Assess adherence to treatment
- Exclude allergic bronchopulmonary aspergillosis (ABPA) (➔ p. 253)

- Review and repeat CXR imaging, and consider CT chest, followed by bronchoscopic lavage targeted to area of nodularity/consolidation on imaging (?NTM or fungal infection); stopping all antibiotics (including long-term macrolides and nebulized anti-pseudomonals) may increase bronchoscopic yield
- Consider empirical oral prednisolone in severely unwell patients who are failing to improve with appropriate antibiotics.

Non-invasive ventilation (NIV) may assist with airways clearance, in addition to providing ventilatory support. Consider the appropriateness of intensive care unit (ICU) admission as well as resuscitation status in severe exacerbations—liaise with CF consultant.

Intravenous antibiotic administration

- The majority of IV antibiotic courses can be administered at home, after an initial assessment and with home support from nursing staff. Many patients are relatively well during courses of IV antibiotics and are able to continue attending work or college, although it can take them considerable extra time to administer the antibiotics
- Most antibiotic regimes involve 14 days of IV antibiotics, administered via a peripheral long line or implantable venous access device (see ➲ Implantable venous access devices (IVADs))
- Prior to starting IV antibiotics, clinical assessment, including spirometry, should be performed. Patients should be reviewed at day 7 to ensure satisfactory clinical progress (and to consider changing antibiotics if little or no improvement) and at end of the course in outpatients to ensure clinical improvement
- Courses of IV antibiotics are often administered prophylactically before surgery, and regular elective courses of IV antibiotics may be useful for patients who have experienced a rapid and progressive increase in the decline of their lung function or who suffer frequent exacerbations.

Implantable venous access devices (IVADs)

- Inserted in patients with difficult IV access or those needing frequent courses of IV antibiotics
- Usually accessed by a trained nurse, patient, or family member. Access only with a gripper needle of the appropriate length; do not use standard needles, which may damage the IVAD; do not attempt to access IVADs unless you have been trained
- Flush with 5–10 mL of 100 U/mL heparin monthly and with 5 mL of 10 U/mL heparin at the end of each IV dose
- Avoid taking blood from IVAD, if possible, as this increases the risk of blockage and infection. Other complications include venous obstruction (including SVC obstruction), thrombosis, tip dislocation, and leakage
- If pain or swelling around IVAD site, arrange a portagram/linogram to look for occlusion or damaged catheter. If IVAD blocks: injection of 20–50 mL heparinized saline, gently alternating between irrigation and aspiration, may clear small occlusions. If this fails, consider urokinase 25,000 U in 3 mL 0.9% saline instilled into IVAD
- Infected or fractured lines need removal surgically or by interventional radiology.

Antibiotic desensitization

Antibiotic sensitivity is a major problem in CF, as repeated antibiotic courses are associated with the development of allergic reactions, especially to β-lactams. Rashes are common, but anaphylaxis (➲ p. 706) can occur. Always give first doses of a new antibiotic in hospital with resuscitation facilities at hand. Desensitization regimes can enable treatment with antibiotics that have previously caused an allergic reaction. Such regimes need to be given at the start of the antibiotic course each time it is used and during the course if doses are missed for >1 day. Depending on local policy, give a dilute antibiotic dose over 20 min, followed by slightly stronger concentration, and repeat for seven concentration strengths until full antibiotic strength is given. Takes 3–4 h. Stop infusion if any side effects develop.

Pulmonary interventions

Physiotherapy

Specialized CF physiotherapists teach effective airway clearance with the aim that patients perform this themselves twice daily on a long-term basis. This improves secretion clearance, decreases airflow obstruction, and improves ventilation. Several techniques are used: active cycle of breathing control (tidal volume breathing, then deep inspiration, and passive expiration, followed by forced expiration to mobilize secretions prior to coughing/huffing), autogenic drainage, Acapella® or flutter devices, positive expiratory pressure mask, and use of NIV for airway clearance. More intensive physiotherapy is administered during exacerbations. Physiotherapists also have key role in assessment of functional ability with exercise testing, evaluating treatments, and supporting exercise.

Mucoactive agents

- Recombinant rhDNase (recombinant human deoxyribonuclease; dornase alfa) is a nebulised mucolytic that cleaves DNA from dead neutrophils, decreasing sputum viscosity and aiding its clearance. It is the first choice mucoactive agent in CF. Used once daily 2500 U nebulized and should be taken at least 30min prior to doing airway clearance
- Hypertonic (7%) saline nebulised appears to increase mucociliary clearance and improves QoL and reduces exacerbations in trials. Consider if secretions are thick, tenacious, and difficult to expectorate. It is used immediately before or during usual airway clearance regime. Bronchospasm is a relatively common side effect: patients should receive a test dose, and pre-dosing with bronchodilators is often required
- Mannitol dry powder for inhalation has been approved for use in CF patients with rapidly declining lung function (defined as fall in FEV_1 >2%/y) who cannot use DNase or hypertonic saline because of ineligibility, intolerance, or inadequate response.

Macrolides

Macrolides have anti-inflammatory and immunomodulatory effects, in addition to their antimicrobial activity, and improve FEV_1 and decrease exacerbations in a subset of CF patients. They do not exhibit intrinsic antipseudomonal activity, but the macrolide azithromycin decreases sputum viscoelasticity and disrupts *P. aeruginosa* biofilms. Consider a 6-month trial of oral azithromycin (250 mg taken three times per week if <40 kg, or 500 mg three times per week if >40 kg) in patients who are deteriorating on conventional therapy. Checklist when considering macrolide therapy:
- Check LFTs after 1 month; use with caution if pre-existing liver disease
- Warn patient to stop immediately if symptoms of ototoxicity (hearing loss, disequilibrium, tinnitus), and omit macrolide while receiving IV aminoglycosides
- Macrolides may prolong QT interval—check baseline corrected QT interval is <440 ms (♂) or <450 ms (♀) on ECG, and use with caution alongside other QT-prolonging drugs (e.g. citalopram, domperidone, moxifloxacin, antifungals, etc.)
- Care with drug interactions, e.g. warfarin, itraconazole
- Avoid in patients with evidence of NTM infection and screen sputum for NTM prior to starting macrolides and while on treatment.

CFTR modulators

- Unlike standard therapies which address the downstream consequences of CFTR dysfunction, CFTR modulators directly target the basic defect underlying CF. They are orally bioavailable drugs which are effective in patients with specific mutations
- Check drug interactions and local protocols for monitoring recommendations
- Ivacaftor (Kalydeco®) is a CFTR potentiator and the first CFTR modulator to be used in clinical practice. Ivacaftor treatment results in sustained and significant improvements in lung function, exacerbation rate, weight gain, and QoL, and notably a halving of sweat chloride, in patients with a G551D or other gating mutation (5% of CF patients)
- Tezacaftor-Ivacaftor (Symkevi®/Symdeko®) is available in the UK for patients homozygous for F508del or heterozygous for F508del and a residual function mutation. In trials it led to a modest improvement in lung function and reduction in pulmonary exacerbations. Lumacaftor-Ivacaftor (Orkambi®) is a combination therapy which has been shown to slow decline in lung function in patients homozygous for F508del. Severe breathlessness has been reported within hours of initiating Lumacaftor-Ivacaftor. In practice Tezacaftor-Ivacaftor is currently first line modulator therapy for F508del homozygous patients in the UK
- Additional new modulators are under development and appear to be highly effective in clinical trials (➔ p. 259). Trials of the triple combination regimen of Elexacaftor, Tezacaftor, and Ivacaftor (called Kaftrio® in the UK, Trikafta® in the US) for patients with one F508del mutation and one minimal function mutation and for F508del homozygous patients (that is 90% of CF patients overall) report marked (10-14%) improvements in lung function and falls in sweat chloride. Kaftrio® has very recently been approved for NHS use and is awaiting a European licence.

Respiratory support

Respiratory failure and cor pulmonale can occur with later stage disease. Home O_2 may be required. Nocturnal NIV may be necessary as a 'bridge to transplant' in chronic respiratory failure and may also be useful in the palliation of symptoms of hypercapnia.

Steroids

Short oral courses may improve lung function, but side effects, such as growth impairment, osteoporosis, and diabetes, are significant. They are used in ABPA and severe unresponsive exacerbations.

Pulmonary complications

Pneumothorax

- Pneumothorax is more common in patients with advanced lung disease and is associated with a poor prognosis (48% 2 y mortality). Presentation is typically with breathlessness and chest pain and interestingly often also haemoptysis
- Manage according to standard pneumothorax guidelines (➋ p. 440). Consider IV antibiotics and physiotherapy (with modification of airway clearance as necessary). Withhold positive pressure techniques if the pneumothorax is undrained. Avoid spirometry
- The collapsed lung can be stiff and take longer to reinflate and require prolonged drainage and suction. Persistent air leaks may require surgical input, ideally with a limited procedure such as local abrasion. Pleurodesis is no longer considered a contraindication to later lung transplantation. Liaise with transplant centre if surgery is required.

Haemoptysis

- Small-volume haemoptysis is common, especially with concurrent infection and advanced disease. Massive haemoptysis (➋ p. 47) typically reflects bronchial artery bleeding and can be fatal
- Management of haemoptysis: correct clotting (e.g. vitamin K 10 mg od) and platelets; stop NSAIDs; low threshold for IV antibiotics; oral or IV tranexamic acid 1 g every 6–8 h (contraindications include renal failure, ischaemic arterial disease)
- For massive haemoptysis, anaesthetist may be required for airway management; sit patient upright, and give an ice-cold drink (reduces pulmonary pressures and vasoconstricts bronchial arteries); cross-match blood; consider nebulized adrenaline (1 mL of 1:1,000 made up to 5 mL with NaCl 0.9%); consider IV terlipressin (vasopressin analogue, increases systemic arterial pressure and reduces PAP; follow local guidelines for administration, typically 2 mg IV and then 1–2 mg every 4–6 h if continued bleeding). Physiotherapy review: airway clearance is usually stopped during active bleeding and then modified and recommenced as bleeding subsides
- Many clinicians temporarily stop NIV in patients with massive haemoptysis; nebulized drugs may also provoke further bleeding (particularly hypertonic saline); we recommend weighing their benefit against risk on an individual patient basis
- Bronchoscopy is rarely of value, instead perform CTPA to look for bronchial artery hypertrophy; bronchial artery embolization is the gold standard treatment of massive haemoptysis or recurrent bleeding, discuss with interventional radiology.

Allergic bronchopulmonary aspergillosis

ABPA (→ p. 562) may be difficult to diagnose in CF, as hypersensitivity (with positive *Aspergillus* skin prick tests and precipitins) and sputum culture of *Aspergillus* are both common. ABPA is screened for annually and should be considered when exacerbations respond poorly to appropriate antibiotics. Guidelines define a 'classic case' of ABPA in CF as:

* Acute or subacute clinical deterioration (cough, wheeze, exercise intolerance, exercise-induced asthma, decline in pulmonary function, increased sputum) not attributable to another cause
* Serum total IgE concentration >1,000 IU/mL (unless receiving systemic corticosteroids, which will suppress IgE)
* Presence of serum IgE antibody (RAST) to *A. fumigatus*
* Precipitating antibodies to *A. fumigatus*
* Infiltrates or mucus plugging on CXR or chest CT that have not cleared with antibiotics and physiotherapy.

Blood eosinophilia is also a common finding, and ABPA may occur with intermediate serum IgE concentrations of 500–1,000 IU/mL.

Treatment is with oral prednisolone 0.5–1.0 mg/kg (non-enteric-coated; maximum dose 60 mg) for 2 weeks, and, if there is a clinical improvement, continue at decreasing doses for 2–3 months. Intensive physiotherapy is an important part of the treatment regime, and hypertonic saline may be useful. Add antifungal therapy with itraconazole for 3–6 months if there is a slow or poor response to corticosteroids, relapse of ABPA, and in corticosteroid-dependent cases. Itraconazole checklist:

* Initial itraconazole dose is 5 mg/kg/day; give od, unless dose exceeds 200 mg/day, in which case it should be given bd; maximum daily dose 400 mg/day
* H_2 antagonists and proton pump inhibitors (PPIs) reduce absorption of itraconazole—take itraconazole with an acidic drink (e.g. orange juice or cola) if also taking antacids
* Check LFTs at baseline, after 1 month, and then every 3 months if therapy continues
* Review concomitant medications to avoid a drug-drug interaction.

In addition to ABPA, other forms of *Aspergillus*-related lung disease described in CF include aspergillomas (→ p. 566) and '*Aspergillus* bronchitis' (defined as positive respiratory cultures for *A. fumigatus* and radiological infiltrates in symptomatic patients who do not fulfil the above diagnostic criteria for ABPA but respond to antifungal therapy).

Asthma

Some CF patients have coexisting asthma, and some have asthma-like symptoms of prolonged exhalation, wheeze, and crackles due to underlying lung inflammation. This is difficult to diagnose, as these symptoms and a variable PEFR are found in many CF patients due to airway hyperresponsiveness. There may be bronchodilator responsiveness or bronchoconstriction after exercise or nebulized hypertonic saline. Treat with the standard asthma stepwise treatment: short-acting bronchodilator, inhaled corticosteroid, LABA, theophyllines (which may aid mucociliary clearance), leukotriene receptor antagonist (limited evidence in CF but may decrease eosinophilic inflammation), oral steroids.

Nutrition and gastrointestinal disease

Nutritional management

- The maintenance of good nutrition correlates with survival in CF, and specialist dietician input is crucial. Nutrition is more problematic as respiratory disease progresses (raised basal metabolic rate, increased work of breathing, ongoing infection, and inflammation)
- High-calorie, high-protein diets are encouraged. Patients may need nutritional supplements ± supplemental overnight enteral (nasogastric or gastrostomy) tube feeding. Weigh patients at every review; aim for body mass index (BMI) >19 kg/m²
- Pancreatic enzyme supplementation to avoid high faecal fat/energy loss is essential if pancreatic-insufficient (85% of patients). Use the smallest dose of pancreatin-containing lipase, required to control steatorrhoea. Typical preparations are Creon® (contains lipase, protease, and amylase) 10,000, 25,000, or 40,000, taken pre-meals. Typically, patients take 10–20 tablets/day and are educated to adjust the dosage, according to the fat and protein content of each meal. High-strength pancreatic enzyme preparations have been linked to fibrosing colonopathy; maximum lipase levels of 10,000 U/kg/day are recommended
- Fat-soluble vitamins are poorly absorbed in most patients with CF (particularly if pancreatic-insufficient) and require supplementation.

Gastrointestinal disease

- *Distal intestinal obstructive syndrome* (DIOS, previously termed meconium ileus equivalent) comprises bloating, abdominal pain, possible palpable right lower quadrant mass, and complete or incomplete intestinal obstruction by viscid faecal material in terminal ileum and proximal colon. Abdominal X-ray characteristically shows 'foamy' gas pattern in the right flank ± dilated small bowel loops/fluid levels. Can occur spontaneously or secondary to dehydration or intercurrent infection. Treatment is medical. Mild cases may respond to high doses of regular polyethylene glycol (Movicol®). Correct hydration using IV fluids, if necessary. More severe cases may be relieved by oral Gastrografin® (50 mL mixed with 200 mL of water or cordial tds for up to 5 days) or Klean-Prep® (can be given orally but usually via NG, and not nocturnally as risk of aspiration). If this is unsuccessful, patients will require a Gastrografin® enema (under radiological guidance) to determine the site of obstruction and for therapeutic benefit. Treatment is complete when clear fluid is passed from the rectum and symptoms have resolved. If not resolving, consider further imaging and surgical opinion (differential diagnosis includes acute small bowel obstruction, e.g. 2° to adhesions, and intussusception)
- *Gastro-oesophageal reflux* is common and may worsen lung disease. Combinations of PPIs, H₂ receptor antagonists, and prokinetics are usually required
- *Coeliac disease* appears to be more common in CF

- *Pancreatitis* occurs in pancreatic-sufficient patients, presenting as acute attack or chronic recurrent abdominal pain. Treat with bowel rest, PPI, IV rehydration
- *GI and pancreatic cancer* is significantly more common in CF. Colon cancer is five- to tenfold more common in CF than the general population; this risk increases to 25- to 30-fold higher in adult CF patients after lung transplantation. Symptomatic patients should be investigated promptly. Screening colonoscopy is recommended in the US for asymptomatic CF patients at age 40 y, or within 2 y of transplant for transplant-recipients over age 30 y; similar guidelines may be adopted in the UK.

Liver and biliary disease

- *Focal biliary cirrhosis* affects 5–10% of CF patients and leads to portal tract fibrosis, often with preserved hepatic architecture. Cirrhosis is frequently asymptomatic and develops insidiously in childhood. Annual screening liver US is performed, as blood tests can be unhelpful. Biopsy unhelpful as patchy disease. Treatment with ursodeoxycholic acid improves biochemical indices of liver function, although its long-term clinical benefits are unproven. Established cirrhosis can lead to portal hypertension and variceal bleeding; annual screening endoscopies are performed in patients with cirrhosis.

Other extrapulmonary disease

CF-related diabetes

- *CF-related diabetes (CFRD)* affects at least one-third of adult CF patients and is associated with a higher mortality. Pancreatic damage in CF (due to fibrosis) causes decreased insulin secretion. CFRD is a distinct type of diabetes but shares certain clinical features of both type I and type II diabetes. Unlike type I diabetes, onset of CFRD is usually insidious, and patients may be asymptomatic at diagnosis or present with a decline in pulmonary function or weight; ketoacidosis is very rare in CFRD. CFRD differs from type II diabetes in that weight loss is often an early feature and reactive hypoglycaemia is not unusual. Some patients exhibit overt diabetes during an infective exacerbation but return to normal glucose tolerance later. Early identification and treatment of CFRD improves health status, even in the absence of fasting hyperglycaemia; screening oral glucose tolerance tests are currently performed annually, although may be superseded by continuous glucose monitoring which is increasingly used for screening and monitoring CFRD. Management is with insulin (usually as basal bolus regimen), with blood glucose targets of 4–7 mmol/L; there is no role for oral hypoglycaemics or a hypoglycaemic diet. Microvascular complications can occur after 5–10 y of CFRD.

Bone and joint disease

- *Low bone mineral density* and increased fracture risk is common in CF. Risk factors include malabsorption of vitamin D and calcium, low BMI, decreased physical activity, delayed puberty, steroid use, diabetes. Screen with dual-energy X-ray absorptiometry (DEXA) scans. Treatment is with calcium and vitamin D supplements to ensure vitamin D-sufficient, bisphosphonates
- *Arthropathy and CF vasculitis* Acute or subacute arthritis occurs in around 5% of patients and often responds to NSAIDs. Sometimes arthritis is associated with skin lesions such as purpura or erythema nodosum.

Fertility

- *Women* with CF may be subfertile but should always be offered contraception if of reproductive age. If planning a pregnancy, their physical state should be optimized with antibiotics and nutrition. The outcome of pregnancy is improved by optimizing and maintaining pulmonary function and weight gain during the pregnancy, and close monitoring is required. Women with CF are also at risk of developing diabetes during pregnancy. Pregnancy does not affect survival when compared with the entire adult ♀ CF population, but impaired pulmonary function with FEV_1 <60% predicted and BMI <18 are likely to be the main predictors of worse maternal and foetal outcome, and some patients do experience an accelerated decline after pregnancy. Pulmonary hypertension (PHT) is considered an absolute contraindication to pregnancy. Breastfeeding is possible but intensifies the nutritional strain put on the mother. Many CF antibiotics are safe to use in pregnancy, but avoid ciprofloxacin, chloramphenicol, metronidazole, and IV colistin, and, if possible, avoid IV aminoglycosides. Ceftazidime at a reduced dose of 2 g tds is a safe first-line choice for patients infected with *P. aeruginosa*

- *Men* are usually infertile due to failure of the normal development or blockage of the vas deferens, seminal vesicle, ejaculatory duct, and body and tail of epididymis. Testicular histology is normal, and hence one option is surgical sperm retrieval for intracytoplasmic sperm injection (ICSI) into an egg, performed by fertility clinics
- Genetic counselling and screening should be offered to patients with CF and their partners.

Other manifestations

- *Chronic rhinosinusitis* is often troublesome and may worsen lung disease. Consider sinus CT. Treatment with topical steroids and decongestants is often unhelpful, and surgery may be required
- *Acute kidney injury* is more common in CF and associated with IV aminoglycosides, NSAIDs, dehydration, and pulmonary exacerbations
- *Electrolyte abnormalities* include hyponatraemia, hypokalaemia, hypochloraemia, and metabolic alkalosis. Salt tablets are required in hot weather due to excessive losses in sweat
- *Stress incontinence* is very common in women; treat with pelvic floor exercises.

Supportive care and future developments

Psychosocial support

Psychologists offer personal and family support regarding education, employment, burden of treatment, and adapting to progressive disease. Pre-transplant psychological assessment is carried out, as well as terminal care and bereavement counselling. Consider and treat depression, anxiety, and emotional difficulties, with referral to psychiatric services if necessary. Social worker involvement may help with benefit entitlements, travel insurance, disabled car badge, etc.

Immunization

Annual influenza as well as pneumococcal vaccination are recommended.

Lung transplantation

Lung transplantation (➔ p. 760) has a well-established role in CF, and patients should be considered for referral when their risk of death within 2 y is high. Predicting prognosis in CF is difficult; historically, an FEV_1 ≤30% predicted was associated with a poor prognosis and used as a trigger to consider transplantation, but, in the modern treatment era, this low level of lung function is associated with a median survival of 5.3 y and should not usually constitute the sole criterion for referral. Additional factors should be considered, e.g. evidence of rapid progressive deterioration (e.g. ↑ number of admissions/exacerbations, rapid fall in FEV_1), recurrent major haemoptysis not controlled by embolization, and recurrent or refractory pneumothorax; hypoxia (PaO_2 <7.3 kPa) and hypercapnia ($PaCO_2$ >6.7 kPa) are associated with <50% survival at 2 y and remain useful guidelines for transplantation. Young female patients with rapid deterioration have a poor prognosis and should be considered for early referral. *B. cenocepacia* infection is an absolute contraindication to transplant and active *M. abscessus* disease is also a contraindication in most UK centres. While on the transplant waiting list, the patient should have optimal nutrition and physical care, including treatment of low bone mineral density and gastro-oesophageal reflux, and maintenance of good diabetes control and BMI >17 kg/m². Following transplantation, the main immediate problems are infection and acute rejection, with bronchiolitis obliterans the predominant late complication (➔ p. 768).

Care of the dying CF patient

When all acknowledge that there are no further active treatment options, the focus of care should adjust to being palliative, with an emphasis on symptom relief, at home or in hospital or a hospice. The transition from active treatment to palliative care is often difficult in CF, as many end-of-life events begin as an exacerbation, and it may be difficult to predict or define when patients are entering a terminal phase. There is often an overlap between active and palliative care, e.g. some 'active' treatments (such as gentle physiotherapy and even NIV) may have a palliative role in symptom control, and, for this reason, most deaths occur in hospital. A particular challenge is palliative care of patients on an active transplant waiting list when unrealistic hopes about the availability of a last-minute transplant may delay discussion of end of life and compromise symptom control. Open and sensitive discussion about end-of-life care is encouraged, but approaches should be dynamic and tailored to the needs of individual patients. Effective communication among the CF team and ward staff is essential.

Future developments

- **Small molecule CFTR modulators** aim to correct the basic CFTR defect by increasing CFTR channel opening at the cell surface ('potentiators') or increasing the amount of cell surface CFTR protein ('correctors'); they are designed to be effective in patients with specific *CFTR* mutations. Several CFTR modulators are already in widespread clinical use (➲ p. 251), although pricing in the UK has proven controversial. CFTR modulators are likely to transform clinical outcomes in CF and become standard care for most patients
- **Gene therapy** aims to restore CFTR function by inserting a normal copy of the CFTR gene into epithelial cells to prevent progressive airways disease. This will theoretically be of benefit to patients with any mutation class, in contrast to mutation-specific small molecule-based therapies. A major challenge has been finding a suitable vector for delivery, with recent interest in adeno-associated viruses and liposomes. A placebo-controlled phase 2b trial of a nebulized CFTR gene-liposome complex reported encouraging results.

Further information

UK CF Trust. http://www.cysticfibrosis.org.uk.

CF Trust consensus documents on aspects of cystic fibrosis care. http://www.cysticfibrosis.org.uk/about-cf/publications/consensus-documents.aspx.

CF mutation database. http://www.genet.sickkids.on.ca.

Chapter 25

Drug and toxin-induced lung disease

Drug-induced lung disease: clinical presentations 262
Drug-induced lung disease: examples 264
Paraquat and organophosphate poisoning 270
Radiation-induced pulmonary disease 272
Inhalational lung injury 274
Carbon monoxide (CO) poisoning 278
Immunotherapy 280

Drug-induced lung disease: clinical presentations

Introduction

A vast number of drugs can damage the respiratory system, from nose to alveoli (see Box 25.1). The most up-to-date, complete, useful, and recommended list (plus references) is kept at ♒ http://www.pneumotox.com and can be searched by either drug (or drug type) or nearly 20 different clinical/radiological presentations; all agents have equal prominence but are coded with a star rating to indicate likely prevalence. This chapter describes the commoner drugs that produce respiratory problems. Often the clinical problem is to differentiate drug toxicity from other causes of interstitial lung disease (ILD).

> **Box 25.1 More common presentations of drug-induced lung disease and examples of causative agents**
>
> - ILD, pneumonitis, fibrosis
>   - Acute hypersensitivity pneumonitis (HP) (nitrofurantoin, methotrexate)
>   - Interstitial pneumonitis ± eosinophilia (amiodarone, ACE inhibitors, immunotherapy, sulfasalazine)
>   - Chronic organizing pneumonia (OP) (amiodarone, bleomycin)
>   - Pulmonary fibrosis (bleomycin, amiodarone, nitrofurantoin, β-blockers)
> - Airways disease
>   - Bronchospasm (β-blockers, contrast media)
>   - Obliterative bronchiolitis (busulfan, penicillamine)
>   - Cough (ACE inhibitors)
> - Pleural changes
>   - Pleural effusion/thickening (β-blockers, nitrofurantoin, methotrexate, dopamine agonists)
>   - Pneumothorax (bleomycin)
> - Vascular changes
>   - Thromboembolic disease (phenytoin)
>   - Pulmonary hypertension (PHT) (dexfenfluramine, other appetite suppressants)
>   - Vasculitis (nitrofurantoin, L-tryptophan)
> - Mediastinal changes
>   - Node enlargement (bleomycin, phenytoin)
>   - Sclerosing mediastinitis (ergot)
> - Pulmonary oedema (methotrexate, contrast media)
> - Pulmonary haemorrhage (methotrexate, nitrofurantoin, penicillamine, contrast media).

Drug-induced lung disease: examples

Amiodarone

Iodinated benzofuran used to suppress supra- and ventricular tachycardias. Lung toxicity correlates loosely with total dose and therefore usually occurs after a variable number of months. Seen in 10% of subjects on >400 mg/day. Rare if <300 mg/day.

Risk factors

- Daily dose >400 mg
- Increasing age of patient
- Use for >2 months, some reactions can occur within days
- Pre-existing lung disease (although not a contraindication to its use)
- Recent surgical intervention or lung infection.

Diagnosis

Usually one of exclusion and response to cessation of drug (which can take months). Infiltrative lung disease varying from acute respiratory distress (rare) through to organizing pneumonia (OP) (cough, pleuritic pain, fever, dyspnoea, asymmetric patchy infiltrates, effusion), and the most indolent—chronic interstitial pneumonitis (cough, dyspnoea, weight loss, diffuse, and/or focal opacities).

On computed tomography (CT), the liver, thyroid, and lungs will usually show increased attenuation, indicating a significant amiodarone load. A baseline chest radiograph (CXR) is useful.

Lung biopsies

These exclude other diagnoses and provide compatible findings, but there is dissent as to how diagnostic they are (except for the finding of foamy macrophages in the airspaces, filled with amiodarone–phospholipid complexes, but may occur in absence of lung toxicity). Mechanisms of toxicity are unclear, and there are features to suggest hypersensitivity and direct toxic damage.

Treatment

Steroids are effective and required in severe disease. The half-life of amiodarone in the tissues is in excess of a month, and response to stopping the drug may be slow. Prognosis is good in the majority.

Anti-TNF agents

Infliximab and etanercept, for example, represent a large step forward in the treatment of rheumatoid arthritis (RA) and Crohn's disease. However, there is a small, but important, risk of reactivating tuberculosis (TB), commonly extrapulmonary (see Э p. 610). Pneumonia and development of antibodies are also more common; SLE develops only rarely.

Azathioprine

Extensively used as an immunosuppressant but has remarkably little pulmonary toxicity other than via opportunistic lung infection. Case reports of pneumonitis only.

Bleomycin

DNA-damaging glycopeptide used in the treatment of lymphomas, germ cell tumours, squamous carcinomas (cervix, head, neck, and oesophagus). Pulmonary toxicity occurs in about 45%, with fatal pulmonary toxicity in 1–3%

Risk factors

- Older age
- Those receiving total dose of >400 IU
- Increased FiO2, probably via increased superoxide/free radical formation. Pneumonitis may be precipitated by supplementary O_2 for some time after drug administration—warn anaesthetist if surgery planned in patients who have received bleomycin in previous 6–12 months
- Smoking
- Pulmonary irradiation, not just in the irradiated field
- Renal failure decreases drug elimination and thus increases toxicity
- Associated use of cyclophosphamide.

Symptoms

Symptoms (cough, dyspnoea, chest pain, fever) develop 1–6 months after bleomycin. There is hypoxia and a restrictive defect. Progressive basal subpleural shadowing, small lungs, and blunting of costophrenic angles.

Diagnosis

Histological diagnosis is not normally necessary but is based on excluding other possible causes. High-resolution CT (HRCT) most commonly shows ground-glass (GG) opacities, but other appearances include bronchiolitis obliterans, organizing pneumonia, pleural effusions, pneumothorax, and subpleural pulmonary nodules. Diffusing capacity for carbon monoxide (DLCO) is the most sensitive early sign of bleomycin lung with a restrictive pattern being common. Bronchoscopy and BAL are helpful in excluding infection.

Treatment

- Bleomycin must be stopped on suspicion of damage, and some units use lung function tests (kCO) to detect early damage
- Prednisolone 1 mg/kg is used, and these improve radiological appearance (particularly HP and bronchiolitis obliterans organizing pneumonia)
- Use the minimum FiO2 to maintain an adequate SaO_2 (85–90%)
- Smoking cessation.

Busulfan

DNA alkylating, myelosuppressive agent mainly used to treat chronic myeloid leukaemia and prior to bone marrow transplantation, with a low rate of lung toxicity (4–10%) due to fibrosis.

Risk factors

- Cumulative doses >500 mg (mostly over 120 days)
- Concurrent administration of other alkylating agents
- Pulmonary irradiation.

Presents with cough and progressive shortness of breath (SOB), often years after exposure (usually about 4 y). CXR is typically unremarkable. Reduced kCO and restrictive defect. Diagnosis is usually by exclusion. The place of steroids is unproven.

Chlorambucil

DNA alkylating agent mainly used to treat chronic lymphocytic leukaemia (CLL), lymphomas, and ovarian cancer. It has additional immunosuppressive actions and is also used in conditions such as RA. Low risk (1%) of pulmonary toxicity and confined to those who have received >2 g. Similarly to busulfan, presentation may be many years later. Presents with cough, dyspnoea, weight loss, and basal crackles. CXR shows diffuse basal reticular shadowing. Non-specific histology. On suspicion, chlorambucil should be stopped; use of steroids is unproven. Prognosis is poor (50% fatal).

Cyclophosphamide

DNA alkylating agent mainly used to treat CLL, small cell lung cancer (SCLC), and other solid tumours. Particularly useful as an immunosuppressive agent in certain vasculitides and nephropathies. Lung toxicity is rare.

Risk factors
- Pulmonary irradiation
- O_2 therapy
- Concurrent drugs causing pulmonary toxicity, e.g. bleomycin.

Clinical presentation
Usually within 6 months, with a short duration of fever, cough, and fatigue. Reticular shadowing with GG appearance on CT. Later-onset progressive pulmonary fibrosis can also develop insidiously in those on therapy for many months with progressive SOB and dry cough. The histology of the more acute type can be similar to any of the acute interstitial pneumonias (e.g. OP, diffuse alveolar damage), whereas the more chronic form is indistinguishable from UIP. Cyclophosphamide is not itself toxic to the lung, but its metabolites are. There appears to be genetic variation to susceptibility, as there is no obvious dose–response relationship. Cessation of drug and steroid therapy is used successfully in the acute form, but the chronic form seems to progress inexorably, in a similar manner to UIP. Lung transplantation is an option. Note increased risk of *pneumocystis jirovecii* pneumonia (PCP) while taking cyclophosphamide.

Gold

Used in RA (historically), >500 mg cumulative dose can produce pneumonitis (possibly COP, obliterative bronchiolitis), with cough, dyspnoea, and basal crackles. Rare (1%) but associated with certain HLA types and distinctive histological feature of alveolar septal inflammation. Good prognosis following drug cessation; poor evidence for steroids.

Methotrexate

Folic acid derivative, inhibiting cell division by blocking dihydrofolate reductase and nucleic acid production. Mainly used in leukaemia and as an immunosuppressive, e.g. RA and psoriasis. Commonly (4–10%) causes a variety of lung pathologies, not associated with folic acid deficiency.

Risk factors
- Hypoalbuminaemia
- Diabetes
- Previous use of drugs that modify disease progress in RA
- Rheumatoid or other lung/pleural disease
- Not particularly dose-related; can occur at doses of <20 mg/week
- Daily, rather than intermittent (weekly), therapy
- >60 y.

Presentation
Both acutely (interstitial pneumonitis, fever, and eosinophilia) and over very long time periods; however, the subacute form (within a year, dyspnoea, fever, cough, hypoxia, basal crackles, restrictive defect, and reduced kCO) is commoner. Bilateral diffuse pulmonary infiltrates or mixed pattern with alveolar shadowing on CXR, occasional effusions.

Histology
More useful than in other drug toxicities, shows alveolitis, interstitial pneumonitis, epithelial cell hyperplasia, eosinophilic infiltration, and granuloma formation in the more acute hypersensitivity form and more UIP-like changes in indolent form. Mechanism of damage unknown but likely to be multifactorial.

Treatment
Consists of drug withdrawal and unproven use of steroids. Anecdotal reports support use of steroids in the more acute hypersensitivity form. Other methotrexate-related lung diseases include opportunistic lung infection (including PCP) and non-Hodgkin's B-cell lymphoma, which may regress with drug withdrawal and may be associated with Epstein-Barr virus.

Nitrofurantoin

Used commonly for long-term prophylaxis against urinary tract infections (UTIs). Acutely, nitrofurantoin causes a hypersensitivity vasculitis and, much less frequently, a chronic interstitial fibrosis. Most patients are women due to their much higher prevalence of chronic UTIs. The acute form presents abruptly with fever, dyspnoea, dry cough, rash, chest pain, hypoxia, crackles, and eosinophilia within a week or two of starting and is dose-independent. Lower zone diffuse patchy infiltrates and sometimes unilateral effusions on CXR. Lung biopsy reveals vasculitis, eosinophilia, reactive type II pneumocytes, focal haemorrhage, and some interstitial inflammation. Treatment consists of discontinuation, and improvement begins rapidly. Prognosis is good, with or without steroids.

O$_2$

Prolonged 80–100% O$_2$ therapy can provoke lung damage.

Penicillamine

Used in the treatment of RA, penicillamine may increase the prevalence of obliterative bronchiolitis. This is dose-related but rare, with a subacute onset (after several months) of dyspnoea and cough. There is a progressive obstructive pattern without bronchodilator response; 50% mortality.

Sulfasalazine

Used extensively in treatment of inflammatory bowel disease (IBD) (mainly ulcerative colitis). Rarely causes side effects but can cause new-onset dyspnoea and pulmonary infiltrates after any period of use. Cough, fever, lung crackles, and blood eosinophilia are the usual presentation. Prior allergy history, rash, and weight loss also seen with eosinophilic pneumonia as the usual pathology. Withdrawal of drugs is usually successful within weeks, and recovery can be hastened by steroids. Rare deaths when the histology is more like usual interstitial pneumonitis and may be more related to the condition than the sulfasalazine toxicity.

Talc

Commonly used for pleurodesis (see ➔ p. 878). Talc particles may be small enough to enter the circulation after intrapleural instillation, being found throughout the body at post-mortem. They appear to provoke a systemic reaction with fever, raised inflammatory markers, and hypoxia, suggestive of an acute respiratory distress syndrome (ARDS)-like pathology. Occasional deaths after talc pleurodesis have been reported. Refined talc with fewer smaller particles seems less toxic and is now commonly used for this reason.

Vaping

Recent case series show patients presenting with probable vaping related pneumonitis in the US. These patients presented with respiratory symptoms (dyspnoea, chest pain, cough, and rarely haemoptysis), GI upset, and constitutional symptoms. They had new pulmonary infiltrate which was clinically not explainable by infection alone. Patients were young (median age 19 y) and 80% of patients reported use of either THC (tetrahydrocannabinol) or CBD (cannabidiol) in addition to nicotine. Pneumonitis in one case series required hospitalization in 94%, intubation and mechanical in 32%, and has resulted in at least two deaths. The editorial covering these very recent case series now recommends physicians discourage patients from vaping.

Further information

Christiani et al. Vaping-induced lung injury. *NEJM* 2019 Sep 6 *ePub*.

Layden et al. Pulmonary illness related to e-cigarette use in Illinois and Wisconsin – preliminary report. *NEJM* 2019 Sep 6 *ePub*.

Henry et al. Imaging of vaping-associated lung disease. *NEJM* 2019 Sep 6 *ePub*.

Maddock et al. Pulmonary lipid-laden macrophages and vaping. *NEJM* 2019 Sep 6 *ePub*.

Paraquat and organophosphate poisoning

Paraquat

Widely used in much of the world as contact herbicides, although it is now banned in the UK and much of Europe. It kills plants by inhibiting NADP reduction during photosynthesis, which involves the production of superoxide radicals. Most of the toxicity of paraquat in animals is also believed to be due to the production of damaging superoxides. Most cases of poisoning are deliberate, and the treatment should be commenced as soon as possible. Serious poisoning is usually by ingestion (although paraquat is absorbed through the skin and mucous membranes, including the conjunctiva and bronchial mucosa).

- >6 g is always fatal
- <1.5 g is rarely fatal
- Between 1.5 and 6 g, the mortality is 60–70%
- Usually fatal if blood level >0.2 mg/mL at 24 h.

Clinical features

- Oral and oesophageal ulceration shortly after contact, with later formation of a pseudomembrane
- Renal failure (reversible) within a few days, but delayed excretion of paraquat prevents falls in blood levels
- Pulmonary oedema early on, evolving into ARDS
- Hepatic damage, jaundice, and raised transaminases
- Metabolic acidosis
- Death usually occurs within 1–2 weeks
- Pulmonary fibrosis if the patient survives, with varying degrees of recovery.

Organophosphate poisoning

An increasingly important topic due to high profile, albeit isolated, cases of organophosphorus nerve agent poisoning. Previously organophosphate poisoning presented due to ingestion of pesticides but can also be caused by inhalation/cutaneous exposure to nerve agents (including Sarin, VX, Novichok). These agents work by inhibiting AChR and causing widespread central, peripheral, and autonomic cholinergic activation. Carbamate poisoning causes similar effects. Cases my present in large clusters (such as in Sarin terrorist attacks in Japan and suspected nerve agent attacks in Syria) or in isolated cases (such as in the Novichok attack in Salisbury, UK). Presentation can be rapid with nerve agents, or delayed (days to weeks) with agents such as malathion. Symptoms include miosis, salivation, bronchorrhea, wheeze, dyspnoea, agitation, nausea, urination, lacrimation, vomiting, diarrhoea, and sweating. They can cause pinpoint pupils, either brady- or tachy-arrhythmia, hypotension, bronchospasm, loss of consciousness, seizures, and loss of respiratory drive leading to hypercapnic respiratory failure.

Management should focus on:
- PPE for staff
- Decontamination – removal and double bagging of clothing, wiping down excess liquid (clinic rolls 'blue towels')

- If nerve agent suspected seek specialist advice
- Involve intensive care unit (ICU) early
- Supportive management
- Often naloxone is trialled initially given the presentation with pinpoint pupils, but will be ineffective
- Atropine—initial 1–3 mg bolus and may be followed by infusion
- There may be roles for steroids, bronchodilators, and oxiomes following specialist advice.

Further information

Hulse et al. Organophosphorus nerve agent poisoning: managing the poisoned patient. *Br J Anaesth* 2019;**123**: 457–463.

Radiation-induced pulmonary disease

Manifestations of lung injury following radiotherapy include:

Radiation pneumonitis

- Often asymptomatic although may cause dyspnoea and chronic ventilatory failure, normally 6–12 weeks after treatment
- Radiographic abnormalities more common than clinical disease. Characteristically straight margins on CT infiltrate
- Pathological feature is of diffuse alveolar damage, with vascular intimal fibrosis
- Typically follows lung radiotherapy (breast and haematological mediastinal malignancy are rarer causes)
- Treatment of symptomatic disease is with steroids (1 mg/kg daily), although minimal evidence to support their use
- Risk of pulmonary fibrosis with or without acute illness
- Chemotherapy can increase the risk.

Radiation-induced organizing pneumonia

- Often presents with cough (rather than breathlessness, which is more suggestive of radiation pneumonitis)
- Characterized by migratory patchy consolidation, which always extends beyond radiation field on CT
- Typically follows breast radiotherapy
- Treatment is with steroids; often long courses are needed. Macrolides may have a role.

Radiation-induced chronic eosinophilic pneumonia

Possible association; few cases reported.

Inhalational lung injury

Definition

Agents damaging the lung and airways through direct toxicity. Much of the acute damage is common to many toxic agents, including pneumonitis/pulmonary oedema, mucosal damage/sloughing/airway debris. 2° infection is common due to breached defences.

Examples of toxic agents, listed alphabetically

Aldehydes (acetaldehyde, formaldehyde)
- Chemical and plastics industry, used for disinfection
- Highly irritant to mucosal membranes
- Acute damage—Pneumonitis and pulmonary oedema
- Chronic effects—Rhinitis/asthma.

Ammonia
- Fertilizer and plastics production, used in many chemical industries
- Highly irritant to mucosal membranes
- Acute damage
  - Upper airway obstruction from secretions and mucosal oedema
  - Lung damage and 2° infection
- Chronic effects—Airways obstruction and bronchiectasis described.

Chlorine
- Extensive use in the chemical industry, bleaching agent
- Acute damage
  - Overwhelming toxicity, producing rapid hypoxia
  - Pneumonitis and pulmonary oedema
- Chronic effects (e.g. from repeated accidental exposure)—Airways obstruction; sometimes reversible.

Cocaine (when smoked)
- Pneumothorax/pneumomediastinum
- Pulmonary haemorrhage
- Pulmonary oedema
- Allergic responses (asthma, pulmonary eosinophilia, HP).

Metals and metal compounds (as fumes or nebulized solutions)
- Mainly used in the chemical industry
- Acute damage
  - Mucosal irritation
  - Pulmonary oedema
- Chronic effects—Pneumoconiosis
- Some specific effects such as:
  - Sarcoid-like reaction to beryllium
  - Asthma from cobalt, chromium, nickel, vanadium
  - Fibrosing alveolitis from cobalt and zinc fumes.

Methyl isocyanate (Bhopal disaster: 3,800 dead, 170,000 injured)
- Chemical industry, carbamate pesticides
- Acute damage
  - Pneumonitis and pulmonary oedema
  - 2° infection
- Chronic effects
  - Airways obstruction
  - Bronchiolitis obliterans
  - Pulmonary fibrosis.

Hydrocarbons/mineral oils
- Used as lubricant and cooling agent
- Acute damage—Pneumonitis
- Chronic effects
  - Pneumonitis
  - Fibrosis
  - Asthma.

Nitrogen dioxide (NO_2)
- Chemical industry (explosives)
- Agricultural silos
- Odourless and therefore high doses inhaled without knowing
- Acute damage (several hours after exposure)—Silo-fillers lung
  (pneumonitis/pulmonary oedema)
- Later effects
  - 2° pulmonary oedema 2–8 weeks after exposure
  - Steroid-responsive, needs 2 months therapy after exposure.

Ozone
- Bleaching agent
- Product of welding
- Similar to NO_2
- Both immediate and late effects of pneumonitis/pulmonary oedema.

Phosgene
- Chemical warfare, chemical industry, chlorination
- Released from heated methylene chloride (paint stripper)
- Acute damage
  - Pneumonitis and pulmonary oedema
  - Produces carboxyhaemoglobin (COHb); breath CO therefore
    reflects degree of exposure.

Smoke
- Most smoke injury is due to heat damage to upper airway
- Hypoxia, vaporized toxins (e.g. formaldehyde, chlorine), systemic agents
  (e.g. CO and cyanide)
- Acute damage—Mucosal oedema and sloughing with airway blockage
- Look out for:
  - Peri-oral burns
  - Black sputum
  - Altered voice
  - Respiratory distress
  - Stridor (rapid inspiration to accentuate)
  - Additional CO and/or cyanide poisoning.

Sulphur dioxide
- Used as a fumigant, and bleaching agent in the paper industry
- Very irritant as dissolves to form sulfuric acid
- Acute damage
  - Sloughing of airway mucosa
  - Pneumonitis and haemorrhagic pulmonary oedema
- Chronic effects—Airways obstruction.

Welding fumes
- Many agents released
- Specific examples:
  - Cadmium—pneumonitis
  - Zinc—'metal fume fever'
  - Several agents may cause airways obstruction/COPD
- Siderosis (welder's lung), non-fibrogenic pneumoconiosis; results in iron deposits in lung, producing small rounded opacities.

Carbon monoxide (CO) poisoning

Definition and epidemiology

- CO is a colourless and odourless gas formed when carbon compounds burn in limited O_2
- It accounts for about 75 deaths per year in the UK, ~10% of which are accidental
- Accidental poisonings are commoner in the winter when faulty heating systems are in use
- Non-accidental deaths are mainly from car exhaust fumes
- Methylene chloride (industrial solvent, paint remover) is converted to CO in the liver and may present as CO poisoning
- Up to one-third die following acute high-level exposure, and another third may be left with permanent neurological sequelae
- Chronic low-grade CO exposure may present as non-specific ill health and may affect thousands of individuals.

Pathophysiology and related conditions

- CO competes avidly with O_2 (250 times greater) to bind with the iron in Hb, making it less available for O_2 carriage
- The Hb molecule is also distorted by combination with CO, making it bind more tightly to O_2, shifting the O_2 dissociation curve to the left. The PaO_2 at which the Hb is 50% saturated (P50) moves from about 3.5 down to 2 kPa. This further reduces O_2 delivery to the tissues: a 50% COHb level is vastly more dangerous than a 50% anaemia
- CO also binds to extravascular molecules, such as myoglobin and some of the cytochrome chain proteins, interfering with energy production, and, in this respect, is like cyanide
- Normal levels of COHb can be up to 3%, and up to 15% in heavy smokers
- Foetal Hb combines even more avidly with CO; thus, the foetus is especially vulnerable to CO poisoning of the mother.

Methaemoglobin

- Methaemoglobin is due to oxidation of $Fe2+$ to $Fe3+$ in Hb, thus preventing O_2 carriage. This is due either to inherited deficiencies of enzymes (cytochrome b5 reductase) that reduce the $Fe3+$ back to $Fe2+$, or toxic agents (e.g. nitrites (in 'poppers'), chloroquine) that overwhelm this reversal mechanism
- Methaemoglobin is slightly left-shifted, but a 40% methaemoglobinaemia may be asymptomatic, apart from the typical grey/blue colour of the patient, often mistaken for cyanosis.

Clinical features of CO poisoning

Immediate

- Nausea, headache, malaise, weakness, and unsteadiness
- Loss of consciousness, seizures, cardiac abnormalities (ischaemia, arrhythmias, pulmonary oedema)
- No cyanosis, healthy-looking 'cherry red' colour
- Suspect if several members of household present with these features.

Delayed (~1–3 weeks, can be longer)
- Cognitive defects and personality changes
- Focal neurology and movement abnormalities.

Investigations

- Pulse oximetry will appear *normal* due to COHb having similar absorption spectra to oxyhaemoglobin. Recent developments in multiwave pulse oximetry may allow rapid COHb detection
- Arterial PaO_2 levels may be *normal*
- COHb blood levels can be measured on a co-oximeter
- Breath CO measured with devices used for smoking cessation work well
- Routine tests to rule out other diagnoses.

Future developments

Isocapnic hyperpnoea may further raise the PaO_2. Alkalosis must be avoided though to prevent further left shift of the Hb dissociation curve. Can be done voluntarily with 5% CO_2 in O_2 or during intubation. Can double rate of CO elimination.

Further information

Kreck TC et al. Isocapnic hyperventilation increases carbon monoxide elimination and O_2 delivery. *Am J Respir Crit Care Med* 2001;**163**: 458–462.

Roth D et al. Accuracy of noninvasive multiwave pulse oximetry compared with carboxyhemoglobin from blood gas analysis in unselected emergency department patients. *Ann Emerg Med* 2011;**58**: 74–79.

Immunotherapy

Definition and epidemiology

Immunotherapy is now being used to treat many different cancer types either instead of chemotherapy or in addition to chemotherapy. Anti-CTLA4 (ipilimumab) and anti-PD1/PDL1 (nivolumab and pembrolizumab) monoclonal antibodies are now widely used in many different cancer tumour sites including malignant melanoma, non-small cell lung cancer, triple negative breast cancer, head and neck cancer, and bladder cancer. Immunotherapy can cause a range of immune mediated complications including pneumonitis. Pneumonitis is more common with anti-PD1/PDL1 immunotherapy than with anti-CTLA4 immunotherapy. Pneumonitis occurs in 2–4% of patients receiving anti-PD1/PDL1 monotherapy, with 1–2% of the reactions being severe (Grade 3 or 4). Severe pneumonitis is >3 times more likely with combination immunotherapy, such ipilimumab and nivolumab.

Diagnosis

- Presentation can be within days to months with cough, dyspnoea, and chest pain
- HRCT is recommended and has varied patterns including; GG only, organizing pneumonia, hypersensitivity pneumonitis
- Bronchoscopy and broncho-alveolar lavage are helpful in excluding infection, but biopsy is often unnecessary.

Treatment

- Depends on severity of reaction. Grade 1, with only radiological changes, continued therapy with close monitoring may be used
- Involving the patient's own oncologist is crucial as steroid therapy may compromise the effectiveness of further immunotherapy and potentially impact patient prognosis
- Grade 2 reactions are defined by the presence of symptoms. With more severe reactions (≥ Grade 2) treatment should be held
- Prednisolone 1 mg/kg/day should be considered if no response to stopping therapy at 48 h (Grade 2)
- IV methylprednisolone 1–4 mg/kg/day should be given for Grade 3 or 4 reactions (any of severe symptoms, worsening hypoxia, life-threatening reactions, difficulty in breathing, or ARDS)
- Empiric antibiotics are recommended for Grade 3 and 4 reactions and infection should be considered as a cause in all cases
- If there is no response to IV methylprednisolone at 48 h in Grade 3–4 reactions, then infliximab 5 mg/kg or mycophenolate mofetil should be considered while continuing steroids
- Before using infliximab, testing should be performed for latent TB (Serum Ellispot or Quantiferon) or CMV (Serum PCR)
- For Grade 3–4 reactions ICU should be involved as appropriate

- Once patients have improved to baseline, steroids should be weaned over 6 weeks (Grade 2) or 8 weeks (Grade 3–4) with frequent monitoring of the patient's condition
- Given this slow wean of steroids PCP prophylaxis should be considered (co-trimoxazole 480 mg bd M/W/F) along with considering calcium/Vitamin D and bisphosphonates.

Further information

Haanen J et al. Management of toxicities from immunotherapy: European Society for Medical Oncology Clinical Practice Guidelines. *Ann Oncol* 2017;**28**(**suppl 4**): iv119–iv142.

Chapter 26

Dysfunctional breathing

Definition 284
Pathophysiology 284
Clinical features 284
Diagnosis 285
Management 286
Prognosis 286
Nijmegen hyperventilation score 287

Definition

Dysfunctional breathing encompasses a range of breathing pattern abnormalities with breathlessness and overbreathing in the absence or in excess of any physiological abnormality. Hyperventilation syndrome is a form of dysfunctional breathing and the terms are often used interchangeably.

Dysfunctional breathing may occur as part of a spectrum of physical symptoms (e.g. chest pain, palpitations/tachycardia, fatigue, dizziness, paraesthesiae, headache, diarrhoea, inappropriate sweating, etc.) from anxiety or panic disorder. Other specialities may have been consulted due to the mixed symptomatology.

Pathophysiology

Dysfunctional breathing can occur *de novo* or follow a respiratory disorder that has resolved—such as a respiratory tract infection, or as a result of a chronic respiratory condition such as asthma. It appears to be based on a heightened awareness of breathing and concerns as to what the shortness of breath (SOB) signifies. The $PaCO_2$ is intermittently low, with a respiratory alkalosis. Recordings of breathing pattern often show a rather chaotic pattern.

Clinical features

- Intermittent episodes of breathlessness largely unrelated to exercise, although can be worsened by exercise
- May be associated with symptoms of respiratory alkalosis, such as numbness, tingling of the extremities, feelings of impending doom, and light-headedness, occasionally to the point of losing consciousness (cerebral vasoconstriction due to the hypocapnia)
- Sensation of not being able to take a satisfactory breath
- No history suggestive of an alternative current respiratory disorder, although there may have been one previously
- History of some stressful situation in the patient's life
- Previous episodes.

Diagnosis

Is essentially one of exclusion, but with additional confirmatory findings.
- No evidence of a respiratory cause, i.e. normal lung function, normal chest radiograph (CXR), and normal SaO_2 at rest and on exercise to the point of breathlessness (SaO_2 may even rise on exercise)
- No evidence of a cardiac cause for the breathlessness
- Irregular breathing pattern at rest and on exercise (watching the patient exercise often reveals the almost instant SOB and chaotic breathing)
- No evidence of pulmonary hypertension (PHT)
- No evidence to support thromboembolic disease
- No evidence of hyperthyroidism
- Low $PaCO_2$, raised pH on blood gases (and a normal A–a gradient)
- No metabolic acidosis on blood gases (e.g. ketoacidosis, lactacidosis)
- Unresolved psychological issues or social phobia/agoraphobia.
- The Nijmegen questionnaire (Table 26.1) has a good positive and negative predictive value for diagnosing hyperventilation syndrome.

Differential diagnosis

Important pathological causes to exclude are:
- Subtle interstitial lung disease (ILD) with a normal CXR: consider high-resolution computed tomography (HRCT)
- Mild asthma with normal basic pulmonary function tests (PFTs) at the time of testing: consider peak expiratory flow rate (PEFR) monitoring, exercise provocation, or bronchial reactivity testing
- PHT/thromboembolic disease: consider cardiac echo or computed tomographic pulmonary angiogram (CTPA)
- Hyperthyroidism
- Unexpected acidosis, e.g. renal failure, lactacidosis, ketoacidosis.

Management

It is important not to dismiss the patient's symptoms, implying it is 'all in the mind'. The patient has a real symptom, which requires a real explanation. There are no controlled trials of management, but most clinicians will offer an explanation based on an 'over-awareness' of respiratory sensations (occasioned by some previous respiratory illness), heightened by anxiety. It is important to explain that the associated symptoms of tingling and light-headedness are well recognized and harmless.

Review by an experienced respiratory physiotherapist and control-of-breathing exercises may be useful. Careful and convincing explanation without over investigation may be enough, stressing the normality of the investigations. A short period on an anxiolytic (e.g. diazepam 2–5 mg bd) may be helpful to demonstrate that the symptoms can be controlled. Management of the psychological problem may be possible.

Failure to respond should always prompt a reconsideration of whether an underlying disorder is gradually progressing to the point where an investigation becomes abnormal. On the other hand, repeated investigations will confirm the patient's concern that 'the doctors think there is something wrong.'

Prognosis

Some patients improve quickly with explanation of the underlying condition. Some tend to relapse at times of stress. Some prove resistant to any treatment and probably should be seen in the clinic regularly, but infrequently, to reduce their likelihood of involving other medical services with another pointless round of investigations.

Further reading

Boulding et al. Dysfunctional breathing: a review of the literature and proposal for classification. *ERJ* 2016;**25**.

Nijmegen hyperventilation score

Filled in by a patient (see Table 26.1).
 A score of ≥22 is highly suggestive of hyperventilation syndrome.

Table 26.1 Example of Nijmegen hyperventilation score

Before treatment	Never	Rare	Sometimes	Often	Very often
	0	1	2	3	4
Chest pain			✓		
Feeling tense				✓	
Blurred vision		✓			
Dizzy spells			✓		
Feeling confused			✓		
Faster/deeper breathing					✓
Shortness of breath				✓	
Tight feeling in the chest					✓
Bloated feeling in the stomach			✓		
Tingling fingers	✓				
Unable to breathe deeply				✓	
Stiff fingers or arms			✓		
Tight feeling around mouth	✓				
Cold hands or feet	✓				
Heart racing (palpitations)				✓	
Feeling anxious				✓	
Total score	34				

Eosinophilic lung disease

Eosinophilic lung disease *290*
Causes of eosinophilic lung disease 1 *292*
Causes of eosinophilic lung disease 2 *294*

Eosinophilic lung disease

Definition

Pulmonary eosinophilias are disorders classically associated with chest radiograph (CXR) infiltrates and a raised blood eosinophil count, although eosinophilic infiltration of the lung can occur *without* blood eosinophilia. Eosinophilia is found on lung biopsy or bronchoalveolar lavage (BAL).

- Eosinophils are granulocytes that are produced in bone marrow under the control of IL-5 and circulate for up to 10 h before localizing in tissues
- Their blood levels are usually tightly regulated
- In health, around 90% of body eosinophils are found in the gastro-intestinal (GI) tract mucosa, but they may be attracted to other tissues by local chemoattractant mechanisms, including mast cell activation and complement activation
- Eosinophils can survive in the tissues for weeks if appropriate cytokines are present
- Normal eosinophil counts are below 0.4×10^9/L (1–3% of peripheral white cell count (WCC))
- Counts of 0.4×10^9/L upwards can be seen in pulmonary eosinophilia
- Persisting high eosinophil levels ('hypereosinophilia') cause tissue damage, due to their pro-inflammatory effects, whatever the cause
- Eosinophils accumulate in allergic or hypersensitivity disease, parasitic infections, and cancer
- Steroids and severe sepsis both decrease eosinophil levels
- Asthma can cause a raised eosinophil count, especially if there is associated eczema, but an absolute eosinophil count of $>1 \times 10^9$/L is unusual and raises the possibility of an alternative diagnosis such as Churg–Strauss syndrome (now known as eosinophilic granulomatosis with polyangiitis, EGPA)
- Blood eosinophilia can occur in a variety of conditions. 1° eosinophilia occurs in haematological malignancies; 2° eosinophilia is a response to a stimulus, such as a parasite or allergy, and third, idiopathic eosinophilia, with no identifiable cause, is also known as the hypereosinophilic syndrome
- Possible causes of CXR infiltrates ± blood eosinophilia are shown in Table 27.1.

Table 27.1 Causes of CXR infiltrates ± blood eosinophilia

Condition	Characteristic points
Asthma with ABPA	Known asthma, with worsening symptoms, over weeks to months. Associated systemic symptoms. Raised blood eosinophil count, positive *Aspergillus* skin test, raised IgE, raised *Aspergillus* precipitins
Simple pulmonary eosinophilia (Löffler's syndrome)	Foreign travel. Symptoms for days to weeks. Cough, malaise, anorexia, rhinitis, night sweats, fever, dyspnoea, wheeze. Sputum contains eosinophils and larvae. Low-level blood eosinophilia. Occurs due to an allergic response to the passage of larvae through the lungs
Tropical pulmonary eosinophilia	Foreign travel. Symptoms for weeks to months, with remissions and relapses. Cough, wheeze, sputum, dyspnoea, chest pain, fever, weight loss, fatigue. Sputum contains eosinophils. Raised blood eosinophil count, high IgE. Occurs in response to filaria in blood and lymphatics
Chronic eosinophilic pneumonia	Symptoms for weeks to months, with associated systemic symptoms. Cough, sputum, haemoptysis, dyspnoea, recent-onset asthma, fever, weight loss, night sweats. Sputum eosinophilia, but blood levels can be normal
Acute eosinophilic pneumonia	Short duration of symptoms, <5 days. Fever, cough, dyspnoea, and myalgia. Unwell, hypoxic. High BAL eosinophil count, no blood eosinophilia
Hypereosinophilic syndrome	Symptoms for weeks to months. Associated systemic symptoms and other organ involvement. Fever, weight loss, cough, night sweats, pruritus. High blood eosinophil count
Churg–Strauss syndrome/EGPA	Rhinitis, past history of asthma. Other organ involvement. Associated systemic symptoms. Longer duration of symptoms, weeks to months. Blood eosinophilia and eosinophilic tissue infiltration
Drug-induced pulmonary eosinophilia	Recent new drug. Possible associated skin reaction. Symptoms within hours to days. Spectrum of illness, from mild to severely unwell, with cough, dyspnoea, fever, and hypoxia. Eosinophilic tissue infiltration, but blood eosinophilia not universal

Causes of eosinophilic lung disease 1

Asthma and allergic bronchopulmonary aspergillosis (ABPA)

(See ➔ p. 562)

- Fever or worsening asthma symptoms may be caused by type I and II hypersensitivity reactions to airway colonization by *Aspergillus fumigatus*
- Untreated, can cause central bronchiectasis
- CXR shows fleeting shadows
- Blood eosinophilia
- *Aspergillus* skin prick test is positive, and serum *Aspergillus* IgG precipitins are positive. Total and *Aspergillus* specific IgE levels are raised
- Treatment is with steroids, and antifungal agents may be necessary.

Simple pulmonary eosinophilia (Löffler's syndrome)

- Caused by parasitic infection, usually *Ascaris lumbricoides*, but also *Strongyloides* and hookworm (e.g. Ancylostoma)
- Occurs worldwide, especially in SE Asia, Africa, Central and South America
- The eggs of the parasite are found in the soil and are ingested. After 10–14 days, larvae migrate from the intestine via lymph and blood to the liver and lung. From the lung, they pass up the bronchial tree to be swallowed, to develop into roundworms in the gut
- The passage of larvae through the lung causes an allergic reaction. This may be asymptomatic but may cause cough, malaise, anorexia, rhinitis, night sweats, low-grade fever, occasional wheezing, and dyspnoea. The illness lasts around 2 weeks
- CXR shows transient bilateral shadows that are discrete and perihilar. They disappear usually between 6 and 12 days but can take up to 1 month
- Sputum also contains eosinophils and larvae
- Blood eosinophilia at a low level
- Stool examination reveals parasites, but only 2–3 months later when the adult worms are passed
- Treatment is with an antihelminth agent, such as albendazole or mebendazole, for 3 days. Steroids may be necessary if the pulmonary manifestations are severe.

Tropical pulmonary eosinophilia

- Hypersensitivity to migrating larvae of filarial worms *Wucheria bancrofti*, *Brugia malayi*, and *Brugia timori*, similar to Löffler's syndrome
- Occurs in the Indian subcontinent, SE Asia, and the South Pacific islands
- Insidious onset of cough, wheeze, sputum, dyspnoea, and chest pain, with associated fever, weight loss, and fatigue. Symptoms last for weeks to months, with remissions and relapses
- Examination reveals crepitations
- *CXR* shows bilateral uniform mottling of the lung fields, especially in the middle and lower zones. There may be cavitation and pleural effusion
- *Sputum and BAL* contain eosinophils
- *Pulmonary function tests (PFTs)* may be obstructive initially but can become restrictive in long-standing untreated cases
- *Histology* shows eosinophilic bronchopneumonia and eosinophilic abscesses
- *Blood eosinophil count* is raised. IgE is raised
- *Filarial complement test* is positive
- *Treatment* is with a filaricide diethylcarbamazine for 3 weeks. This rapidly improves symptoms.

Drug-induced pulmonary eosinophilia

- Pulmonary shadowing develops within hours to days of starting the drug and resolves usually within 1 week of stopping it
- It is due to an allergic reaction in the pulmonary vessel wall, caused by the drug, and occurs again on drug re-challenge
- There may be an associated skin reaction
- The drug should be avoided in the future and steroids given if necessary
- Severity of illness varies from mild to severely unwell, with cough, dyspnoea, fever, hypoxia. May occur in those with concomitant asthma
- Tissue eosinophilia, but may not have blood eosinophilia
- Possible drugs include ampicillin, carbamazepine, chlorpropamide, cocaine (inhaled), daptomycin, inorganic chemicals such as nickel, methotrexate, minocycline, NSAIDs, nitrofurantoin, penicillin, phenytoin, sodium aminosalicylate, sulphonamides, tetracycline. There are case reports of others (ℬ http://www.pneumotox.com).

Causes of eosinophilic lung disease 2

Chronic eosinophilic pneumonia

- Unknown cause
- $\female:\male$ = 2:1. Occurs in middle age, non-smokers
- Insidious onset over weeks to months, with cough, sputum, possibly haemoptysis, dyspnoea, recent-onset asthma, weight loss, night sweats, and high fever. Differential diagnosis includes tuberculosis
- *Diagnosis* is usually clinical and radiological but may need BAL or open lung biopsy
- *CXR* shows peripheral dense opacities with ill-defined margins (photographic negative of pulmonary oedema)
- *Computed tomography (CT)* shows peripheral airspace infiltrates
- *Sputum* eosinophilia
- *BAL* eosinophil count high
- *Blood* eosinophilia may not occur. Erythrocyte sedimentation rate is raised
- *Treatment* is with steroids, such as prednisolone 30–40 mg/day, and improvement is usually rapid, with the CXR clearing within 2–3 days and normal in 2 weeks. Decrease steroid dose once stable, but continue for 6 months
- Relapses common when steroids stopped, and they may need further courses.

Acute eosinophilic pneumonia

Unknown cause, occurs in any age or sex. Presents with fever, dry cough, dyspnoea, and myalgia.
Diagnostic criteria:
- Acute febrile illness of <7 days' duration
- Hypoxic respiratory failure
- Interstitial or alveolar CXR infiltrates
- BAL eosinophils >25%
- No parasitic, fungal, or other infection
- Prompt and complete response to steroids (oral prednisolone or IV methylprednisolone if respiratory failure)
- Failure to relapse after stopping steroids.

May be unwell and hypoxic, requiring ventilatory support. No peripheral blood eosinophilia. High-dose steroids should be given until the respiratory failure resolves, and then the dose can be tapered over 2–4 weeks. It possibly represents an acute hypersensitivity reaction to an unidentified inhaled antigen; case series of recent-onset smoking in some.

Hypereosinophilic syndrome

- Unknown cause. Rare
- Most common in men aged 30–40
- Present with fever, weight loss, night sweats, cough, and pruritus
- *Diagnosis* based on:
  - Marked blood eosinophilia of >1.5 × 10^9/L for 6 months or more
  - Signs and symptoms of eosinophilic tissue infiltration on histology
  - No evidence of another cause of eosinophilia
- Pulmonary involvement with interstitial infiltrates and pleural effusions on CXR. Cardiovascular involvement also occurs, with myocarditis, endocardial fibrosis, restrictive cardiomyopathy, valvular damage, and mural thrombus formation. These may cause considerable morbidity and mortality. Skin may be involved with urticaria and angio-oedema; central nervous system (CNS) involved with encephalopathy, arterial and venous embolism, peripheral neuropathy, or mononeuritis multiplex; GI tract with gastritis, nausea, diarrhoea, alcohol intolerance, and hepato- or splenomegaly; joints with effusions and Raynaud's. Kidney and muscles can also be infiltrated by eosinophils. Can be fatal
- *Blood* eosinophil levels may be as high as 70% of the peripheral WCC. IgE levels are often high
- *Treatment* is with high-dose steroids (e.g. 60 mg prednisolone), which improves about 50% of cases. May need to use other immunosuppressants such as cyclophosphamide, hydroxycarbamide, azathioprine, or interferon-alfa. Treatment should be tapered, according to falling eosinophil counts and end-organ improvement.

EGPA (Churg–Strauss syndrome)

(See ⮕ p. 722)
- Severe asthma, blood eosinophilia, and pulmonary infiltrates occur as part of a small- and medium-vessel vasculitis
- Also can affect GI tract, CNS, skin, and cardiovascular system
- There may be eosinophilic tissue infiltration
- ANCA usually, but not always, positive
- Treatment with steroids and immunosuppression.

Extreme environments— flying, altitude, diving

Lung disease and flying *298*
Altitude sickness *300*
Diving *302*

Lung disease and flying

Problems

Flying presents potential physiological challenges:
- Modest hypoxia
- Gas expansion/ contraction with ascent/ descent
- Recirculation of air with increased risk of air-borne infection

Hypoxia

Many modern passenger aircrafts are pressurized to the equivalent of around 5,000 ft (1,500 m), e.g. the Airbus 380. This equates to an atmospheric pressure of 85 kPa, compared to 101 kPa at sea level. Since FiO_2 remains constant, atmospheric oxygen (PiO_2) is reduced from 21 kPa to 18 kPa. In health this causes inconsequential falls in PaO_2 and SaO_2. Many companies pressurize to the minimum permitted of equivalent of 8,000 ft, e.g. Boeing 767—7,900 ft (2,400 m, the same as some of the lower ski resorts in Colorado). Lower pressurization saves fuel and extends aircraft fuselage life-span. At 8,000 ft the PiO_2 is 16 kPa, which is the same as breathing FiO_2 of 15% at sea level; even in health SaO_2 may fall to 90% or so.

Patients with pre-existing hypoxia due to lung disease sit nearer the steep part of the oxygen–haemoglobin dissociation curve, so small reductions in PiO_2 can result in greater desaturation than in health, and thus a greater fall in oxygen carriage by the blood. The extent of desaturation will vary considerably from patient to patient, particularly due to differences in hypoxic ventilatory drive.

Hypoxia challenge test

It is recommended patients with SaO_2 ≤94% at sea level have a hypoxic challenge test with measurement of PaO_2 or SaO_2 while breathing a 15% hypoxic gas mixture, equivalent to the PiO_2 at 8,000 ft, for 15 min. This is most easily achieved by using a 40% Venturi mask and nitrogen as the driving gas. There is no evidence this predicts whether a patient will, or will not, run into trouble, but aids decision making regarding safety to fly and supplementary oxygen. Hypoxic challenge testing in patients with moderate to severe chronic obstructive pulmonary disease (COPD) does not predict symptoms during a flight, although the pre-flight MRC dyspnoea score does. Supplemental O_2 reduces symptoms, regardless of the simulated hypoxia testing.

Empirically, as recommended in the British Thoracic Society (BTS) guidelines, O_2 is often prescribed if the approximated in-flight PaO_2 at 8,000 ft (2,400 m), is <6.6 kPa or 85% SaO_2 following a hypoxic challenge test. Further information such as how disabled the patient is already by shortness of breath, their previous flight experience, length of proposed flight, time since last exacerbation, and importance of the trip to the patient, should be used alongside hypoxic challenge tests.

Recommendations for supplemental O_2 are summarized in Box 28.1, and are adapted from the BTS guidelines.

Many airlines can provide supplementary oxygen at a flow rate of 2 or 4 L/min, with varying charges; the patient may need to bring their own oxygen concentrator on board. Patients should make enquiries regarding oxygen prior to booking their flight, allow at least a month to arrange it, and ensure they have adequate travel insurance. A MEDIF form or equivalent will require completion by the GP or specialist. Some airlines prohibit using O_2 during take-off and landing.

Box 28.1 Simple recommendations for O_2 when flying

Sea level SaO_2

>94% No supplementary oxygen required in flight

≤94% Perform 15% hypoxic challenge test

Hypoxic challenge test

PaO_2 >6.6 kPa or SaO_2 >85% No supplementary O_2 required

PaO_2 <6.6 kPa or SaO_2 <85% Supplementary O_2 required

Those with LTOT 2 L/min are advised to increase to 4 L/min. Those with a sea level requirement for >4 L/min oxygen to maintain adequate oxygenation are not recommended to fly.

If using a pulsed oxygen delivery system, they must be able to generate sufficient inspiratory flow to trigger the oxygen supply.

Volume changes in gas compartments

Ascent to the equivalent of 5,000 ft (1,500 m) increases the volume of gas trapped in compartments by 20%, ascent to 8,000 ft (2,400 m) by nearly 40%. A pneumothorax or non-communicating bullae therefore increases by this amount; patients with current pneumothorax should not fly. The BTS recommends that patients do not fly until at least 1 week after full radiographic resolution, or 2 weeks in the case of a traumatic pneumothorax. It is worth recommending that patients contact their airline and travel insurance if travelling within a month of a pneumothorax as some airlines require specific clearance. Patients having had recent thoracic surgery (for whatever reason) are now advised they can fly once recovered from the surgery itself (previously advised to wait 2 weeks). None of this is evidence-based, and the true risks of ignoring these guidelines are not known. Patients who have had a pneumothorax without definitive management (pleurodesis or surgery) should be warned about the risks of recurrence, which could be more serious in the presence of pre-existing lung disease. Through specialist consultation, patients with a chronic pneumothorax may be allowed to fly.

Ear pain may be caused during take-off and landing if nasal congestion prevents adequate pressure equilibration through the Eustachian tube.

Closed environment

Patients with infectious respiratory diseases, for example in certain situations with tuberculosis (TB), should not fly. There is a significant risk of infecting others due to the recirculation of air throughout the cabin and close proximity of passengers. Those with smear-positive TB should not fly until two weeks after they are smear negative and those with multidrug-resistant- or extensively drug-resistant TB should not fly until they have had two culture negative samples.

Altitude sickness

Hypoxia of high altitude may lead to high altitude illness, comprising acute mountain sickness, which is generally minor and self-limiting, and high altitude pulmonary or cerebral oedema, which is serious and even life threatening. High altitude illness can be prevented in the majority of people by adopting a slow ascent profile, allowing more time for acclimatization, typically increasing sleeping altitude by no more than 300 m/night above 3,000 m with a rest day every third day. This is often not practical, and so acetazolamide can be used to aid acclimatization. Travelers should be familiar with prevention, recognition, and treatment of altitude illness, and can download a free booklet at ℘ http://www.medex.org.uk.

Acute mountain sickness (AMS)

Symptoms include:
* Headache
* Nausea and anorexia
* Light-headedness, dizziness and fatigue
* Numbness/tingling of extremities
* Insomnia/sleep disturbance.

These symptoms are common, develop over 6–12 h after arrival, and affect at least a quarter of those flying to Colorado for a skiing holiday (altitude ~10,000 ft, 2,400–3,400 m, barometric pressure 70 kPa, PiO$_2$ tension 14.5 kPa, average SaO$_2$ on arrival 89–90%). Most of the symptoms are due to a respiratory hypocapnic alkalosis and resolve as the kidney retains [H$^+$] and excretes [HCO$_3^-$], normalizing the pH. This allows further hyperventilation, and the rise in SaO$_2$ helps resolve any of the symptoms due to the hypoxia itself. This scenario tends to be common in those with a higher hypoxic drive (as it encourages greater hypocapnia and alkalosis). Confusingly, these symptoms may also indicate the early development of the more major category.

High altitude pulmonary oedema (HAPE)

HAPE is serious and can be life threatening. It can develop rapidly, and some individuals are particularly susceptible. It is thought hypoxia provokes a non-uniform pulmonary vasoconstriction, so some pulmonary capillaries are exposed to high pulmonary pressures, causing stress-failure of the endothelium and exposing the basement membrane of the pulmonary capillaries. Fluid and high molecular weight proteins leak into the alveolar space, and an inflammatory response ensures. Symptoms/signs are:
* Extra breathlessness/cough
* Cyanosis
* Blood-tinged frothy sputum.

High altitude cerebral oedema (HACE)

Hypoxia also causes cerebral vasodilatation with increased cerebral blood flow, cerebral oedema, retinal haemorrhages, cerebral thrombosis, and petechial haemorrhages. Symptoms/signs are:
* Severe headache, nausea and vomiting
* Ataxia (may be the first sign)

- Confusion/disorientation/hallucinations/behavioural change/↓Glasgow Coma Scale
- Papilloedema.

Management

Acute mountain sickness is likely to resolve spontaneously over a few days with simple symptomatic treatment, analgesics, and avoiding dehydration. However, prophylaxis, or early treatment on symptom appearance, with *acetazolamide* is very effective, as are further ascent and encouraging descent. Acetazolamide provokes a mild metabolic acidosis (by reducing [H+] availability for excretion in the distal tubule) and 'preacclimatizes' the subject to allow greater hyperventilation in response to hypoxia without the usual alkalosis. It is recommended when rapid ascent to altitudes ≥2,500 m (8,200 ft) is unavoidable. 500 mg/day (slow release) for the 2 days prior to ascent is probably adequate for most subjects (or as treatment after symptoms develop). The commonest side effects are a harmless and reversible tingling of the extremities and loss of taste, particularly with fizzy drinks.

Temazepam has been shown to reduce the periodic breathing at night (by reducing the arousals that help maintain the periodicity) and does not appear to worsen the hypoxia or reduce vigilance levels the following day.

The best predictor of severe altitude sickness is a prior episode.

The management of the more severe forms of altitude sickness that tend to occur with rapid ascent to over 4,000 m (13,000 ft), pulmonary and cerebral oedema, is urgent.

Management of severe altitude sickness

Increase inspired O_2 tension by urgent rapid descent; do not wait until morning for evacuation! Supplemental oxygen, or a local pressurized environment (e.g. a portable hyperbaric chamber such as the Gamow bag: ⌖ https://www.youtube.com/watch?v=sJΛzu2ZHUuE).

HAPE

- Sit upright, and keep warm
- Nifedipine (20 mg bd up to qds + loading dose, 10 mg sublingually) to reduce PAP
- Acetazolamide may help by also reducing PAP as well as increasing the effective ventilatory response to altitude hypoxia.
- Consider salbutamol.

HACE

Dexamethasone (4 mg qds + loading dose, 8 mg) to reduce cerebral oedema.

Improvement is usually rapid once inspiratory O_2 tension is raised. Prophylaxis for this severe form of altitude sickness is controversial, but graded ascent is important; acetazolamide probably helps, and nifedipine is used by some, particularly if there is a history of a previous episode.

Diving

Problems

Increased recreational diving has raised the awareness of respiratory problems at depth. These can essentially be divided into five conditions:

- Barotrauma, e.g. ruptured bullae and pneumothorax
- Worsening of pre-existing disorder while at depth, e.g. asthma
- Nitrogen gas evolved from solution in body fluids (the 'bends')
- Breath-hold diving and ascent hypoxia
- Pulmonary oedema.

Pathophysiology

Barotrauma (second commonest cause of death in SCUBA divers after drowning)

During descent, any air-containing cavity in the body will be compressed by the rise in external pressure. If there is any communication with the airways (e.g. middle ear, lung bullae), then gas will slowly move into the airspace. On ascent, the airspace will expand and, if air cannot escape quickly enough, may lead to rupture of the eardrum or the bullae. *A tension pneumothorax can be rapidly fatal in this situation.* Obstructive lung diseases in general can predispose to ruptured alveoli. In addition to pneumothoraces, the escaped air can produce a pneumomediastinum, causing chest pain, and a radiolucent band (air in the pericardium) along the cardiac border on CXR. Breathing 100% O_2 will clear this air more quickly. Air emboli can also occur and produce a wide range of symptoms; hyperbaric O_2 may be required.

Pre-existing lung disease

The onset of an asthma attack during a dive can be disastrous and may be provoked by the dry gases breathed from SCUBA (self-contained underwater breathing apparatus) gear. See *British Sub-Aqua Club (BSAC) recommendations on asthma and diving* (see Box 28.2). Many lung diseases, e.g. cystic fibrosis (CF), COPD (unless FEV_1 ≥80% predicted), fibrotic lung disease, previous pneumothorax (with no pleurodesis), and lung bullae, are considered contraindications to diving. However, recently, BSAC has adopted the pragmatic approach of accepting that, in individuals with a history of spontaneous pneumothorax, who have had no pneumothorax for 5 y, the risk of pulmonary barotrauma is small and not significantly greater than for many in the general population, e.g. smokers. Such individuals may dive, provided that a CT scan of the chest and lung function tests (including flow–volume loops) show no reason to suggest that there is significant residual lung disease.

The bends or caisson disease

A caisson is an underwater air chamber in which people work. During periods of high pressure, extra nitrogen dissolves into the blood and other tissue fluids. This takes many minutes. On ascent, this nitrogen literally bubbles off. If the amount coming out of solution is too great, nitrogen bubbles act as emboli and limit blood flow. This produces micro-infarction, with activation of inflammatory and clotting cascades and damage to several organs, e.g. joints, spinal cord, brain. Limited diving times and slow ascents reduce this problem, as do breathing mixtures containing helium, rather than nitrogen. Severe cases require treatment in hyperbaric chambers.

Breath-hold diving

During breath-hold diving, increased pressure on the chest elevates alveolar and arterial PO_2. This extends breath-hold time, particularly with prior hyperventilation to reduce $PaCO_2$. During the dive, O_2 is used and PO_2 falls. On ascent, with rarefaction of the thoracic gas, PO_2 falls quickly, with possible loss of consciousness and drowning.

Pulmonary oedema

Reported while SCUBA diving in cold water, but the mechanism is not clear.

Box 28.2 BSAC recommendations on asthma

- Asthma may predispose to air trapping, leading to pulmonary barotrauma and air embolism, which may be fatal. An acute asthma attack can also cause severe dyspnoea that may be hazardous or fatal during diving
- These theoretical risks should be explained fully to the asthmatic diver. There is little, if any, evidence that the mildly controlled asthmatic that follows the guidelines below is at more risk
- Asthmatics may dive if they have allergic asthma, but not if they have cold-, exercise-, or emotion-induced asthma
- All asthmatics should be managed in accordance with BTS guidelines
- Only well-controlled asthmatics may dive
- Asthmatics should not dive if needed a therapeutic bronchodilator in the last 48 h or have had any other chest symptoms.

Control of asthma
- The asthmatic should not need more than occasional bronchodilators, i.e. daily usage would be a disqualifying factor, but inhaled steroids/cromoglicate/nedocromil are permissible
- During the diving season, he/she should take bd peak flows. A deviation of 10% from best values should exclude diving until within 10% of best values for at least 48 h before diving
- The medical examiner should perform an exercise test such as the 18 in (43 cm) step test for 3 min or running outside (not a bicycle ergometer) to increase the heart rate to 80% (210 minus age). A decrease in peak expiratory flow rate (PEFR) of 15% at 3 min post-exercise should be taken as evidence of exercise-induced bronchoconstriction and hence disbars. The patient should be off all bronchodilators for 24 h before the test
- A β2 agonist may be taken pre-diving as a preventative, but not to relieve bronchospasm at the time.

Further information

Individual airline guidance: ℘ https://europeanlung.org/en/lung-disease-and-information-airtravel/

Edvardsen A et al. COPD and air travel: does hypoxia-altitude simulation testing predict in flight respiratory symptoms? *Eur Respir J* 2013;**42**: 1216–1223.

Edvardsen A et al. High prevalence of respiratory symptoms during air travel in patients with COPD. *Respir Med* 2011;**105**: 50–56.

Cottrell JJ. Aircraft cabin pressures. *Chest* 1988;**98**: 81.

British Thoracic Society guidelines are currently awaited and will be published in 2020: ℘ https://www.brit-thoracic.org.uk/quality-improvement/clinical-statements/air-travel/

British Thoracic Society archived diving guidelines: ℘ https://www.brit-thoracic.org.uk/quality-improvement/guideline-archive/

BLF information on oxygen and airlines. ℘ http://www.blf.org.uk/Page/Airline-oxygen-policies.

MEDIF form for oxygen available at ℘ http://www.iata.org/

Information for doctors/patients. ℘ https://www.thebmc.co.uk/downloads/Mountaineering/Medical.

Information for patients. ℘ http://familydoctor.org/familydoctor/en/diseases-conditions/high-altitude-illness.html.

Information for patients and doctors. ℘ http://www.high-altitude-medicine.com.

Luks AM et al. Wilderness Medical Society consensus guidelines for the prevention and treatment of acute altitude illness. *Wilderness Environ Med*. 2010;**21**: 146–155.

Aberdeen emergency number for hyperbaric chambers. ☎ 07831 151 523 (☎ 0845 4086008 in Scotland). ℘ http://www.hyperchamber.com and ℘ http://www.ukdiving.co.uk/information/hyperbaric.htm.

Plymouth Diving Disease Research Centre. ℘ http://www.ddrc.org/ (24 h helpline and register of hyperbaric chambers). ☎ +44 (0)1752 209999. Email info@ddrc.org

Diving and medical conditions. ℘ https://www.bsac.com/safety/medical-matters-and-medical-forms/

British Thoracic Society archived diving guidelines can be found: https://www.brit-thoracic.org.uk/quality-improvement/guideline-archive/

Cochard G et al. Pulmonary oedema in scuba divers. *Undersea Hyperb Med* 2005;**32**: 39–44.

Gastrointestinal disease and the lung

Hepatic hydrothorax and hepatopulmonary syndrome *306*
Porto-pulmonary hypertension (POPH) *308*
Inflammatory bowel disease, coeliac disease, and
  pancreatitis *310*

Hepatic hydrothorax and hepatopulmonary syndrome

Hepatic hydrothorax

Predominantly right-sided pleural effusion occurring in patients with liver cirrhosis and no cardiorespiratory cause for the effusion, often with minimal ascites. The ascitic fluid accumulates in the chest as a result of diaphragmatic defects. Occurs in 5–10% of patients with cirrhosis and portal hypertension. Spontaneous bacterial empyema can occur and is associated with mortality of 20%.

Management includes:

- Patients should be encouraged to abstain from alcohol
- Salt restriction and diuretics
- Therapeutic pleural aspiration can be performed for symptomatic relief
- Chest drains should be avoided for hepatic hydrothorax due to the high rate of complications in this group
- Transjugular intrahepatic portosystemic shunt (TIPS)
- Liver transplantation.

Hepatopulmonary syndrome (HPS)

The triad of:

- Chronic liver disease and portal hypertension
- Arteriovenous (AV) shunting in the lungs, predominantly at the bases and subsequent ventilation-perfusion abnormalities
- Arterial hypoxia.

It occurs in 5–30% of patients with chronic liver disease. Enhanced pulmonary production of nitrous oxide (NO) is the key priming factor for pulmonary vasodilatation. Although levels of NO are increased in exhaled air, consistent with lung origin, levels normalize after liver transplantation. The mechanism is thought to be related to the release of vasoactive mediators from portal hypertension causing altered bowel perfusion, which, in turn, leads to pulmonary vascular dilatation, with decreased pulmonary vascular resistance (right-to-left shunt). HPS carries a worse prognosis in patients with cirrhosis.

Presentation

Progressive dyspnoea and cyanosis. Examination reveals clubbing and telangiectasia, with associated stigmata of chronic liver disease.

Diagnosis

- *Hypoxia* on blood gases: <8.6 kPa on air, at rest, and upright. Platypnoea and orthodeoxia are present, i.e. breathlessness and desaturation on sitting upright, caused by preferential perfusion of basal pulmonary vasculature where the arteriovenous malformations (AVMs) will be, and arteriovenous (AV) shunting is therefore increased. Lying flat relieves this. These changes may be seen in other lung diseases and can been seen in cardiac shunt but, in the presence of liver disease, is suggestive of HPS. Hypoxia is only partially corrected by 100% O_2 due to the pulmonary shunting

- *Contrast-enhanced echo* is positive. Contrast/saline bubbles are injected peripherally and are normally seen only in the right heart and are then filtered by the pulmonary bed. In the presence of intrapulmonary shunts, these are seen in the left atrium within 3–6 cardiac cycles after opacification in the right atrium. (False positive results occur if right-to-left cardiac shunt present, which can be excluded during echo.) This is the most practical method of detecting pulmonary vascular dilatation. This qualitative method is more sensitive and less invasive than technetium-labelled albumin scan
- *Pulmonary technetium-99 perfusion scan* assesses the shunt fraction. Normally, the radiolabelled albumin is trapped in the pulmonary capillary bed. In the presence of intrapulmonary or cardiac shunts, there is significant uptake of radiolabelled albumin in the brain or spleen. A shunt index fraction of >20% indicates severe HPS (normal uptake <6%)
- *Computed tomography (CT) chest* is performed to rule out other pulmonary comorbid disease
- *Single breath diffusion capacity for CO* is consistently abnormal in HPS. This is not specific and may not normalize after transplant.

Treatment
- O_2 if PaO_2 <8 kPa
- Avoid vasodilators. There is minimal evidence for pharmacological intervention
- Mainstay of treatment is liver transplantation, which cures the condition in 80%. Hypoxia may take up to 14 months to improve. Severe hypoxia (PaO_2 <6 kPa) is associated with increased mortality post-transplant, as there is increased risk of hepatic ischaemia
- Transjugular intrahepatic portosystemic shunt (TIPS) is ineffective
- Coil embolization can be tried in selected cases with AV communications.

Prognosis
Poor, with a mortality of 40% by 2.5 y.

Porto-pulmonary hypertension (POPH)

Pulmonary arterial hypertension (PAH) occurring in association with liver cirrhosis and portal hypertension. It occurs in an estimated 2–5% of patients with cirrhosis and is present in around 16% of those referred for liver transplant. The mechanism is unclear but probably relates to a hyperdynamic circulation, high cardiac output, cytokine release, and possible PE.
Defined as:
- Elevated pulmonary artery pressure (PAP) (>25 mmHg at rest, >30 mmHg during exercise)
- Increased pulmonary vascular resistance due to pulmonary vasoconstriction and obliterative vascular remodelling (≥3 Wood units)
- Abnormal LV end diastolic/wedge pressure (<15 mmHg)
- In the setting of portal hypertension (portal pressure >10 mmHg).

Presentation

Dyspnoea on exertion, possibly syncope, chest pain, fatigue, palpitations, haemoptysis, and orthopnoea. There may be signs of volume overload with raised JVP and pedal oedema. Loud second heart sound, with pulmonary and tricuspid regurgitation, as well as stigmata of chronic liver disease. It is usually diagnosed 4–7 y after the diagnosis of portal hypertension.

Diagnosis

- *Hypoxia* on blood gases, but less so than in HPS. Worse on exertion
- *Chest radiograph (CXR)* may be normal or show prominent pulmonary arteries and enlarged right heart
- *ECG* shows right ventricular hypertrophy, right bundle branch block, right axis deviation, and sinus tachycardia
- *kCO* may be decreased
- *Echo* is the main screening test and is diagnostic of PHT if the right ventricular pressure is >50 mmHg
- Exclude other causes of PHT
- *Right heart catheterization (RHC)* with vasodilator studies can be performed
- The changes in the vessels in POPH are the same histologically as those seen in PAH (see ➲ p. 449).

Treatment

Options are the same as for patients with PAH with vasodilators, prostacyclin, and endothelin antagonists (see ➲ p. 460). Avoid β-blockers, so manage varices with banding. Anticoagulation is not advised due to the risk of variceal bleeding. Long-term oxygen therapy if PaO₂ <8 kPa. If mean PAP <40 mmHg, can undergo liver transplantation, which may reverse mild to moderate POPH, although symptoms may take weeks to months to resolve. Severe POPH is not reversed and is associated with significant intra- and postoperative morbidity and mortality. A few cases of heart–lung–liver transplants have been reported.

Prognosis

Poor in severe POPH, with a median survival after diagnosis of 6 months without transplant.

Further information

Porres-Aguilar M et al. Portopulmonary hypertension and hepatopulmonary syndrome: a clinician orientated overview. *Eur Respir Rev* 2012;**21**: 223–233.

Rodriguez-Roisin R, Krowka MJ. Hepatopulmonary syndrome—a liver-induced lung vascular disorder. *N Engl J Med* 2008;**358**: 2378–2387.

Inflammatory bowel disease, coeliac disease, and pancreatitis

Inflammatory bowel disease (IBD)

Pulmonary involvement tends to occur after the onset of the IBD but can predate it. Pulmonary involvement is found in up to a quarter of patients, but this is usually subclinical. Patients can develop a variety of clinical syndromes, including airway inflammation, subglottic stenosis, chronic bronchitis, bronchiectasis, and chronic bronchiolitis. Bronchoscopy may reveal inflammatory tissue within the large airway walls, which, on biopsy, shows mucosal ulceration, basal cell hyperplasia, basement membrane thickening, and submucosal inflammatory cell infiltration. IBD is also associated with the development of ILD, such as cryptogenic organizing pneumonia (COP), pulmonary infiltrates with eosinophilia, or neutrophilic necrotic parenchymal nodules. Pulmonary involvement tends to be steroid-responsive. Inhaled steroids can be tried for chronic bronchitis, but oral or IV steroids may be required for worsening lung involvement. Note that drugs used in the treatment of IBD may also cause lung disease such as sulfasalazine (alveolitis), mesalazine, or infliximab (both: pulmonary infiltrates and eosinophilia; infliximab: reactivation of latent tuberculosis).

Ulcerative colitis

Pulmonary involvement is usually asymptomatic or may be associated with dry cough. Minimal interstitial change may be suggested by abnormal pulmonary function tests. Airway inflammation causing bronchitis and bronchiectasis may be seen. Restrictive, obstructive, or reduced kCO defects may be seen. Usually normal CXR and CT. No specific treatment indicated.

Crohn's disease

Pulmonary involvement less common than in ulcerative colitis, but similar changes found.

Coeliac disease

May be associated with idiopathic lung fibrosis, causing restrictive defect. Also may be at increased risk of asthma, bird fancier's lung, and hemosiderosis. Increased risk of lymphoma and malignancy in GI tract.

Pancreatitis

Acute pancreatitis is frequently associated with exudative pleural effusion. Raised amylase in the pleural fluid is suggestive (see ➲ p. 49). Acute respiratory distress syndrome may develop, which requires supportive care and mechanical ventilation (see ➲ p. 115).

Further information

Mahadeva et al. Clinical and radiological characteristics of lung disease in inflammatory bowel disease. *Eur Respir J* 2000;**15**: 41–48.

Hypersensitivity pneumonitis

Causes *312*
Diagnosis *314*
Management *316*

Causes

Definition

Group of lung diseases typically caused by inhalation of organic antigen to which the individual has been previously sensitized. Disease following inhalation of inorganic antigens and drug ingestion is also reported. Hypersensitivity pneumonitis (HP; previously termed extrinsic allergic alveolitis) is often divided into 'acute' and 'chronic' forms, based on the time course of presentation. Acute HP often follows a short period of exposure to a high concentration of antigen and is usually reversible. Chronic HP typically follows a period of chronic exposure to a low antigen dose and is less reversible. These two presentations may overlap, and 'subacute' forms of the disease are recognized.

Epidemiology

Exact prevalence unknown. At least 8% of budgerigar and pigeon keepers and up to 5% of farmers may develop HP. HP is thought to be more common in non-smokers (mechanism unclear; may reflect inhibition of alveolar macrophage function by smoke).

Causes

Many different antigens have been reported to cause HP, ranging from the relatively common (bird fancier's lung and farmer's lung in the UK; summer-house HP in Japan) to the more unusual and exotic (shell lung—proteins on mollusc shells; pituitary snuff-taker's disease; sericulturist's lung—silkworm larvae proteins; sax lung—yeast on saxophone mouthpieces). Important examples are listed in Table 30.1.

Table 30.1 Causes of HP—examples

Antigen	Sources	Diseases
Organisms		
Thermophilic actinomycetes (*Micropolyspora faeni*, *Thermoactinomyces vulgaris*), *Aspergillus* spp.	Mouldy hay; sugar cane; compost; mushrooms; contaminated water in humidifiers and air conditioners	Farmer's lung; bagassosis; compost lung; mushroom worker's lung; humidifier lung
Aspergillus clavatus	Mouldy barley	Malt worker's lung
Trichosporon cutaneum	House dust	Summer-house HP (Japan)
M. *avium* complex	Hot tub mist, ceiling mould	Hot tub lung
Animal protein		
Bird proteins	Bloom on bird feathers and droppings	Bird fancier's lung
Rat proteins	Rat droppings	Rat lung
Chemical		
Toluene diisocyanate	Paints	Isocyanate HP

Pathophysiology

Pathogenesis of HP is not fully understood and may involve T-cell-mediated immunity and granuloma formation (type IV hypersensitivity) and/or antibody–antigen immune complex formation (type III hypersensitivity). It is not an atopic disease and is not characterized by a rise in tissue eosinophils or IgE (type I hypersensitivity); this may, in part, be due to the small particle size of offending antigens, which tend to be deposited more distally in the airspaces than the larger particles associated with asthma. Lung histology specimens typically reveal an interstitial inflammatory infiltrate, often with accompanying bronchiolitis and OP. Non-caseating granulomata are often present and typically are ill-defined and single (compared with sarcoidosis where granulomata are well defined and are grouped subpleurally or near bronchi). Chronic HP is characterized by fibrosis and often by the absence of granulomata and airways involvement, particularly if antigen exposure has ceased.

Diagnosis

Clinical features

Acute HP
- Breathlessness, dry cough, and systemic symptoms (fever, chills, arthralgia, myalgia, headache) occur 4–8 h after exposure to antigen
- Examination: crackles and squeaks on auscultation, fever; wheeze may occur, leading to a misdiagnosis of asthma
- In the absence of ongoing exposure, symptoms settle spontaneously within 1–3 days. Episodes may be recurrent.

Chronic HP
- Slowly progressive exertional breathlessness, dry cough, sometimes systemic symptoms (weight loss) over the course of months to years. May be history of acute episodes
- Examination: crackles and squeaks on auscultation, clubbing rare; may be features of cor pulmonale.

Investigations
- *Imaging: acute HP*
  - *Chest radiograph (CXR)* Diffuse, small (1–3 mm) nodules or infiltrates, sometimes ground-glass (GG) change, apical sparing. Normal in up to 20% of cases
  - *High-resolution computed tomography (HRCT)* Patchy or diffuse GG change and poorly defined micronodules. Areas of increased lucency/mosaic attenuation (enhanced on expiratory HRCT) occur due to air trapping from bronchiolar involvement
  - Both CXR and HRCT appearances may quickly normalize following removal from antigen exposure
- *Imaging: chronic HP*
  - *CXR* Typically upper and mid-zone reticulation, reduced lung volumes
  - *HRCT* Diffuse centrilobular nodules, GG change, mosaic attenuation from air trapping, may be honeycombing and traction bronchiectasis (may mimic appearance of UIP, although upper lobe predominance is typical in HP)
- *Pulmonary function tests (PFTs)* Typically restrictive pattern with reduced gas transfer and lung volumes; mild obstruction is also sometimes observed. May be normal. Hypoxia may occur
- *Bloods* Acute HP associated with neutrophilia but not eosinophilia. Inflammatory markers often increased
- *Serum antibody (IgG) precipitin* Results are presented either as an ELISA or as a number of precipitin lines, referring to the number of different epitopes to which an individual responds. Precipitins to organic antigens are found in 90% of patients but are also present in up to 10% of asymptomatic farmers and 50% of pigeon breeders. Precipitin levels often fall in the absence of ongoing antigen exposure
- *Bronchoalveolar lavage (BAL)* Lymphocytosis (often >50%) is a characteristic finding, particularly in the setting of ongoing antigen exposure but is not, in itself, diagnostic and may be found in asymptomatic exposed individuals

- *Transbronchial (TBB) or surgical lung biopsy* may be required in cases of diagnostic uncertainty. TBB often fails to provide sufficient tissue for adequate histological analysis
- *Inhalation antigen challenge* may be unpleasant and is not recommended routinely.

Diagnosis

Based on the combination of history of antigen exposure and typical clinical and HRCT features. Atypical presentations require further investigation to support the diagnosis such as BAL lymphocytosis or characteristic histological features on lung biopsy (a bronchiolocentric granulomatous lymphocytic pneumonitis). The underlying causative antigen cannot be identified in up to 40% of cases.

Differential diagnosis

- Atypical pneumonia
- Idiopathic interstitial pneumonias (IIPs) (particularly idiopathic pulmonary fibrosis, non-specific interstitial pneumonia, respiratory bronchiolitis-associated interstitial lung disease)
- Sarcoidosis
- Vasculitis
- Occupational asthma (e.g. from isocyanates)
- Drug-induced lung disease (including pesticides)
- Organic dust toxic syndrome (follows very high levels of exposure to agricultural dusts; symptoms transient; benign course)
- Silo-filler's disease (variable respiratory manifestations following exposure to nitrogen dioxide in silos; ranges from mild bronchitis to fatal bronchospasm).

Management

Centres on antigen avoidance, which is frequently difficult. If complete removal from antigen is unrealistic (e.g. farmers), measures to reduce exposure may be of benefit (such as respiratory protection with high-performance, positive-pressure masks; avoidance of particularly heavy exposure; improved ventilation and use of air filters; drying of hay prior to storage).

In acute HP, symptoms typically resolve following cessation of antigen exposure, and treatment is usually not required. Removal from exposure may also result in symptomatic and physiological improvement in chronic HP, although this is less certain and established pulmonary fibrosis is often irreversible.

When treatment is required, corticosteroids are frequently used, although there is a lack of randomized controlled evidence to support this. Steroids may hasten the resolution of impaired pulmonary function in acute HP, although their effect on long-term outcome is unclear; they appear to be of benefit in some cases of chronic HP. A typical regimen is prednisolone 0.5 mg/kg until symptoms and radiological changes have resolved, and then slowly reduce dose over several months to a maintenance dose of approximately 10 mg daily. Courses of 3–6 months may be sufficient in subacute HP, although more prolonged courses are usually required for progressive or chronic disease.

Prognosis

Highly variable. Prognosis is usually excellent following removal from antigen exposure in acute HP, although progression to respiratory failure and death may very rarely occur after short-term exposures of very high intensity. Recurrent episodes of acute HP do not necessarily progress to chronic HP and fibrosis, and chronic HP may develop in the absence of previous acute HP episodes. Development of chronic HP with ongoing exposure may eventually lead to cor pulmonale and death, although again this is variable and many patients do not exhibit disease progression despite chronic exposure. Persistent low-dose exposure (e.g. budgerigar in the house) may be more likely to progress to the chronic fibrotic form of HP than intermittent high-dose exposure (e.g. pigeon fanciers), which predisposes more to episodes of acute HP.

Chapter 31

Idiopathic interstitial pneumonias

Overview *318*
Idiopathic pulmonary fibrosis (IPF): diagnosis *320*
IPF: management *324*
IPF: prognosis and future developments *326*
Non-specific interstitial pneumonia (NSIP) *328*
Cryptogenic organizing pneumonia (COP) *330*
Acute interstitial pneumonia (AIP) *332*
Respiratory bronchiolitis-associated interstitial lung disease (RB-ILD) *334*
Desquamative interstitial pneumonia (DIP) *335*
Lymphoid interstitial pneumonia (LIP) *336*

Overview

Definition

The idiopathic interstitial pneumonias (IIPs) comprise a group of diffuse lung diseases of unknown aetiology that primarily involve the pulmonary interstitium—the area between the alveolar epithelium and capillary endothelium, as well as the septal and bronchovascular tissues that make up the fibrous framework of the lung. These primarily interstitial processes, however, frequently also involve the airways, vasculature, and alveolar airspaces. The underlying pathological process is one of varying degrees of inflammation and fibrosis.

The terminology used to describe the IIPs may be confusing; these conditions have been subject to much reclassification, reflecting the lack of understanding of their underlying aetiology and pathogenesis. Idiopathic pulmonary fibrosis (IPF; previously termed cryptogenic fibrosing alveolitis) is the commonest IIP and is characterized by the radiological and histological pattern of usual interstitial pneumonia (UIP). The other IIPs are distinct disease entities and are all rare. They all represent a subgroup of interstitial (or diffuse parenchymal) lung diseases.

Diagnosis

Made using a multidisciplinary approach, taking into account the combination of clinical, high-resolution computed tomography (HRCT), and histological features—distinguish from other causes of diffuse lung disease (see ● p. 31). Histological patterns are often considered to be the most specific but must be interpreted in the context of clinical and radiological features. Surgical lung biopsy is recommended for some cases of suspected IIP, with the notable exception of patients exhibiting typical clinical and HRCT features of IPF. Transbronchial biopsies (TBBs) have a very limited role due to the generally patchy distribution of the IIPs, although they may be useful in the diagnosis of acute interstitial pneumonitis (AIP) and organizing pneumonia (OP), as well as the exclusion of other causes of diffuse lung disease (e.g. sarcoidosis).

The conditions currently included within the classification of IIPs, together with their key clinical, imaging, and histological features and prognosis, are presented in Table 31.1 (in order of frequency) and discussed in detail in the remainder of this chapter.

Further information

British Thoracic Society. Interstitial lung disease guideline. *Thorax* 2008;**63**(suppl. V): v1–58.

Travis et al. An Official American Thoracic Society/European Respiratory Society Statement: Update of the International Multidisciplinary Classification of the Idiopathic Interstitial Pneumonias. *AJRCCM* 2013; **188**(6)

NICE. *Idiopathic pulmonary fibrosis in adults: diagnosis and management.* 2013 ℘ http://www.nice.org.uk/guidance/cg163

Table 31.1 Idiopathic interstitial pneumonias: summary of key features

Idiopathic pulmonary fibrosis (IPF) (historically cryptogenic fibrosing alveolitis (CFA))	*Onset* Over months to years *HRCT* Fibrosis, honeycombing, subpleural, basal distribution, minimal ground glass (GG) *Histology* Usual interstitial pneumonia (UIP): areas of interstitial fibrosis (made up of foci of proliferating fibroblasts) interspersed with normal lung (temporal and spatial heterogeneity), minimal inflammation *Prognosis* Poor
Non-specific interstitial pneumonia (NSIP)	*Onset* Over months to years *HRCT* GG, fine reticulation, often basal distribution, minimal honeycombing *Histology* Varying degrees of inflammation and fibrosis, more uniform appearance than UIP *Prognosis* Variable, can be good
Cryptogenic organizing pneumonia (COP) (historically idiopathic bronchiolitis obliterans organizing pneumonia, BOOP)	*Onset* Over months *HRCT* Areas of consolidation, basal, subpleural, peribronchial predominance *Histology* Alveolar spaces 'plugged' with granulation tissue ± extension into bronchioles *Prognosis* Generally good
Acute interstitial pneumonia (AIP)	Many similarities to ARDS *Onset* Over days *HRCT* Diffuse GG and patchy consolidation *Histology* Diffuse alveolar damage: interstitial oedema, intra-alveolar hyaline membranes, followed by fibroblast proliferation and interstitial fibrosis *Prognosis* Poor
Respiratory bronchiolitis-associated interstitial lung disease (RB-ILD)	*Onset* Over years Symptoms usually mild *HRCT* Centrilobular nodules, GG, thick-walled airways *Histology* Pigmented macrophages in bronchioles *Prognosis* Good
Desquamative interstitial pneumonia (DIP)	*Onset* Over weeks to months *HRCT* GG *Histology* Pigmented macrophages in alveolar airspaces (perhaps a more extensive form of RB-ILD), temporally uniform appearance *Prognosis* Good
Lymphoid interstitial pneumonia (LIP)	*Onset* Over years *HRCT* GG, often reticulation, cysts *Histology* Diffuse interstitial lymphoid infiltrates *Prognosis* Variable

Idiopathic pulmonary fibrosis (IPF): diagnosis

Definition

Chronic interstitial pneumonia of unknown cause characterized histologically by temporal and spatial heterogeneity, with areas of fibrosis and architectural distortion interspersed with areas of normal lung. This occurs as different areas of lung are in varying stages of evolution of the pathological process. The term UIP refers to the radiological (HRCT) and histological appearance of IPF (previously known as CFA). Note that the UIP pattern is non-specific and can be seen in other conditions, e.g. connective tissue disease, asbestosis.

Epidemiology

Prevalence figures vary from 6 to 14/100,000, although prevalence may be 175/100,000 in patients >75 y. Slightly more common in ♂. Median age at presentation 66 y. Familial form well described but very rare.

Causes and pathophysiology

The development of fibrosis was previously thought to reflect a response to chronic inflammation, although this has been questioned in light of the observations that inflammation is not a major feature of pathological specimens and that responses to 'anti-inflammatory' treatment with steroids are poor. An alternative, currently favoured theory is that repeated alveolar epithelial injury leads directly to aberrant wound healing, with activation of mesenchymal cells and the formation of fibroblastic and myofibroblastic foci that secrete excessive extracellular matrix, primarily collagens. The nature of the lung injury remains obscure. Epidemiological studies suggest that triggers include inhalation of metal dust and wood dust, smoking, gastro-oesophageal reflux (GORD), or exposure to herpesviruses. Cytokine production (e.g. plasminogen activator inhibitors, matrix metalloproteinases, transforming growth factor-β) by alveolar epithelial cells may play an important role in the development of fibrosis. Host genetic factors are also likely to be important in the pathogenesis of fibrosis, e.g. *MUC5B* gene polymorphisms and telomerase mutations.

Clinical features

- Typically presents with gradual-onset exertional breathlessness and cough; average of 9 months of symptoms prior to presentation
- 5% of patients are said to be asymptomatic, although this is likely to be an underestimate
- Fine basal late inspiratory crackles
- Clubbing may be present
- Cyanosis and cor pulmonale in severe disease.

Investigations

- *Blood tests* Raised ESR and CRP and mild anaemia may occur; positive RhF and/or ANA may occur at low titres in the absence of associated connective tissue disease
- *Pulmonary function tests (PFTs)* Typically restrictive pattern with reduced VC and transfer factor; reduced gas transfer with preserved lung volumes is suggestive of pulmonary hypertension (PHT) or coexisting emphysema. O_2 saturations are frequently reduced, particularly on exertion; ABGs may demonstrate type I respiratory failure
- *Chest radiograph (CXR)* Peripheral and basal reticular shadowing, may extend to other zones, sometimes with honeycombing; rarely may be normal
- *HRCT* Features include bilateral, peripheral, and subpleural reticulation, with honeycombing, traction bronchiectasis, architectural distortion, and minimal or no GG change. Predominantly basal initially, more extensive later in disease course. Extent of disease on CT correlates with physiological impairment. Predominant GG appearance suggests an IIP other than IPF—consider lung biopsy
- *Bronchoalveolar lavage (BAL)* is not routinely required and is rarely helpful. Typically shows neutrophilia, sometimes mild eosinophilia. Marked eosinophilia (>20%) or lymphocytosis (>50%) should raise possibility of alternative diagnosis
- *Lung biopsy* (via video-assisted thoracoscopic surgery (VATS) or thoracotomy) If there is diagnostic doubt
- *Transthoracic echo* to estimate the pulmonary artery pressure in selected patients.

Histology

UIP, a fibrosing pattern characterized by temporal and spatial heterogeneity: patches of active fibroblastic foci (reflecting acute injury) are interspersed with honeycombing/architectural distortion (reflecting chronic scarring) and areas of normal lung, reflecting varying stages of evolution of the disease process in different areas of lung. Interstitial inflammation is minimal. Significant inter-observer disagreement between expert pathologists regarding the presence of a UIP pattern on lung biopsy has been reported, and an overall diagnosis taking into account clinical, radiological, and histological features is recommended.

Diagnosis

Can be confidently made in most cases on the basis of clinical and HRCT findings. Lung biopsy is not generally recommended in patients with typical clinical and HRCT features of IPF but should be considered in the presence of unusual features (e.g. predominant GG /nodules/consolidation/upper lobe involvement on HRCT, or young patient). When required, biopsies should be obtained at VATS or thoracotomy; TBBs are not recommended, as they provide smaller samples, which are rarely diagnostic.

Differential diagnosis

- Left ventricular failure (a common clinical misdiagnosis in IPF, and patients are often prescribed inappropriate diuretics)
- Fibrotic NSIP and other IIPs
- Asbestosis (may mimic clinically and radiologically, with UIP pattern on histology; occupational history and presence of pleural plaques may suggest this diagnosis)
- Connective tissue disease (may mimic clinically and radiologically, with UIP pattern on histology—particularly in rheumatoid arthritis (RA); lung involvement may precede extrapulmonary manifestations of disease)
- Chronic hypersensitivity pneumonitis (HP) (suggested by typically upper/mid-zone predominance, micronodules, GG, areas of reduced attenuation, lymphocytic BAL fluid; uncommonly, it may be associated with a UIP pattern)
- Chronic sarcoidosis
- Drug-induced lung disease (refer to ॐ http://www.pneumotox.com).

IPF: management

Clinical trials in IPF

These are particularly challenging. Older studies were hindered by inclusion of a heterogeneous patient group, but, even within groups of patients with well-defined IPF, there remains significant heterogeneity in clinical course. Furthermore, some large studies of IPF have been poorly designed, e.g. failing to include a placebo group.

Drug treatments that are *not* recommended, based on previous studies, include: corticosteroid monotherapy, combination 'triple therapy' (with prednisolone, azathioprine, and acetylcysteine), azathioprine, cyclophosphamide, colchicine, ciclosporin, imatinib, interferon gamma-1b (INSPIRE study), bosentan (BUILD-3 study), ambrisentan, etanercept, and warfarin. Specific points of note from these studies include:

• Prior to the reclassification of IIPs, studies suggested that *corticosteroids* might improve lung function and symptoms. However, these studies almost certainly included patients with conditions other than IPF that are associated with a better treatment response and prognosis (e.g. NSIP)

• Combination of oral *prednisolone*, *azathioprine*, and *acetylcysteine* was initially reported to confer a small improvement in lung function when compared with prednisolone and azathioprine alone (IFIGENIA trial, 2005), and, despite the lack of a placebo arm, this study led to widespread use of such 'triple therapy'. Interim analysis of the PANTHER-IPF study in 2012 demonstrated that this combination was, however, associated with higher mortality and hospitalization rates than placebo, and consequently the use of azathioprine or triple therapy is no longer recommended.

Management

Treatment options should be considered in the context of the individual patient's clinical condition, comorbidity, and wishes, particularly in view of the often-unpredictable disease course and high frequency of treatment side effects. Principles of treatment are as follows:

• *Pulmonary rehabilitation* Should be tailored to the needs of the patient following assessment which may include a six-minute walk test (6MWT) and quality of life assessments. Can be repeated at 12-month intervals

• *Supportive treatment* Consider use of home O_2 concentrator if limited by breathlessness and persistent resting PaO_2 <7.3 kPa or <8 kPa in the setting of clinical features of PHT. Use of ambulatory O_2 may improve exercise tolerance. GORD is common in IPF and may drive lung fibrosis; symptomatic patients should be treated with proton pump inhibitors (PPIs) ± pro-motility agents (e.g. domperidone). Cough may be troublesome; consider oral codeine. Opioids are frequently required for palliation of severe breathlessness. Thalidomide may be used under specialist interstitial lung disease multidisciplinary team (MDT) for intractable cough related to IPF. Ensure patients and their families have access to the palliative care team if required.

- *Anti-fibrotic dugs* Consideration of starting these drugs should be undertaken by a specialist interstitial lung disease MDT. Pirfenidone (inhibits collagen synthesis, and reduces fibroblast proliferation) has been associated with a small beneficial effect on rate of forced vital capacity (FVC) decline (CAPACITY trials 1 and 2) but is often limited by side effects, mainly gastrointestinal. Further meta-analysis including further studies (ASCEND, SP3) have suggested an improvement in lung function, exercise tolerance and mortality. It has been approved by the National Institute for Health and Care Excellence (NICE) for use in the UK for patients with FVC between 50% and 80% predicted although should be discontinued if there is evidence of ongoing disease progression (decrease in FVC by 10% or more within 12 months). Nintedanib, a tyrosine kinase inhibitor, has also been shown to slow disease progression to a similar extent and is approved by NICE under the same restrictions as pirfenidone. *Both pirfenidone and nintedanib can cause derangement of liver function tests (LFTs).* LFTs and full blood count should be monitored monthly for the first 6 months of treatment and 3-monthly if stable after this. Clinically significant changes in LFTs should be discussed with the specialist centre.
- Monotherapy with oral *acetylcysteine* (an antioxidant and antifibrotic) at a dose of 600 mg tds is of unproven but unlikely to cause significant harm, and it is widely used. Uncertainty over benefits should be discussed with patients before starting therapy. Studies do not support treatment with *steroids* in IPF, and NICE guidance recommends that steroids should not be used in an attempt to modify disease progression (except in acute exacerbations where benefit is possible but unproven; see Box 30.1).
- *Monitoring* Disease progression and response to treatment are best assessed by serial measurements of FVC and total lung carbon monoxide transfer factor (TLCO); document them at each clinic attendance. Absolute changes in FVC or TLCO of 10–15% or more are considered significant in terms of assessing disease progression. Note that a realistic aim of disease-modifying treatment in IPF is to slow progression, rather than improve lung function. Changes in symptoms, such as exercise tolerance and cough frequency/severity, may also be useful. Most departments also use 6MWTs to monitor disease progression.
- *Lung transplantation* Patients with IPF are often referred for consideration of transplantation too late, and many die while on the waiting list (which is around 12 months in the UK). Guidelines recommend referral of all suitable patients with histological or radiographic evidence of UIP, irrespective of VC and without delaying for trials of treatment. These are not widely applied in the UK, and, in practice, referral is usually considered in symptomatic patients aged <65 y, with TLCO <40% predicted, fall in FVC ≥10%, or in TLCO ≥15% over 6 months, O_2 desaturation <88% on 6MWT or acute, rapid deterioration preceding diagnosis (see ➲ p. 759).

IPF: prognosis and future developments

Prognosis

Highly variable; many patients remain stable or decline slowly over years, while a subgroup declines more quickly ('accelerated variant', mainly male smokers), and 5–20% experience a very rapid decline after a period of relative stability ('acute exacerbation' of IPF; see Box 31.1); prognosis is difficult to predict in individual patients. Mean survival from diagnosis is 2.9–5 y. Poor prognostic factors include TLCO <40% at presentation, O_2 desaturation <88% during 6MWT, and fall of ≥10% in FVC or ≥15% in TLCO in the first 6–12 months. The presence of PHT is associated with a particularly poor prognosis. More extensive fibroblastic foci on lung biopsy have also been shown to correlate with shorter survival. Death is commonly due to respiratory failure and/or infection. Increased risk of developing lung cancer, particularly in peripheral fibrotic areas of lung.

Future developments

There is significant current interest in clinical trial design for IPF and specifically the development of robust outcome measures. Only relatively few trials to date have included patients with advanced disease. The development of biomarkers to identify subgroups of patients with differing responses to treatment or outcomes is another area of interest. Therapeutic agents currently under evaluation include:

- Clinical trials of the use of pirfenidone and nintedanib in combination are underway.
- Silent *GORD* appears to be common in IPF, and episodes of micro-aspiration may drive lung fibrosis; clinical trials of treatment of asymptomatic GORD are in progress
- A trial of *co-trimoxazole* reported no effect on lung function but a possible mortality benefit, which may be partly explained by attenuation of increased mortality related to immunosuppression; side effects were common, particularly nausea and rash
- Trials of a number of agents targeting the inflammatory pathways such as the *CCL2-specific monoclonal antibody* CNTO 888 and the IL-4 and IL-13 pathways are underway
- *Stem cell therapy* aimed at repairing lungs injured by fibrosis is an area of future research.

Box 31.1 Acute exacerbations of IPF

Acute exacerbations of IPF are otherwise unexplained acute worsening of dyspnoea or new development of dyspnoea in patients with known IPF.
- Usually defined as onset <30 days, although some patients experience apparent exacerbations over the course of 10–12 weeks.
- *HRCT* typically shows extensive GG and/or consolidation superimposed on a background UIP pattern of reticulation or honeycombing.

Consider other exacerbants, in particular, infection (including *pneumocystis jirovecii* pneumonia (PCP), pneumothorax, left heart failure, PE, and other causes of lung injury (e.g. drug-induced).
- CTPA, with HRCT slices, is usually the radiological investigation of choice, as PEs may coexist with ILD.
- *BAL* is helpful in excluding atypical infection (particularly PCP), but patients are often too hypoxic to safely undergo this procedure.
- Treatment is usually attempted with *high-dose steroids* (e.g. intravenous (IV) methylprednisolone 750 mg–1 g on 3 consecutive days, followed by maintenance therapy with 0.5–1 mg/kg/day of prednisolone).

In practice, infection is difficult to confidently exclude, and treatment with broad-spectrum antibiotics, alongside steroids, is usual.

Acute exacerbations are increasingly recognized as an important cause of death in mild to moderate, apparently stable, IPF, and also appear to occur in the setting of other forms of fibrotic lung disease such as connective tissue disease-associated pneumonitis, chronic HP, and fibrotic NSIP.
- The *mechanism* is poorly understood, although viral infection may act as a trigger and some exacerbations occur post-operatively, including after surgical lung biopsy.
- The *histological* pattern is of diffuse alveolar damage associated with UIP, although a minority of cases have features of OP.
- Inpatient *mortality* is >60%, rising to >90% within 6 months of discharge.
- The outcome of invasive ventilation in patients with known IPF is very poor (mortality approaching 100%), and ICU admission is not usually appropriate in the setting of underlying IPF/extensive fibrotic change.

Non-specific interstitial pneumonia (NSIP)

Definition
- The term NSIP is a description of a histological pattern, rather than a specific clinical entity.
- This form of IIP is particularly poorly understood, and the histological pattern of NSIP probably encompasses several distinct clinical/radiological conditions—indeed, a proposed subclassification divides NSIP into three clinicoradiological syndromes; the clinical utility of this subclassification is uncertain:
  - NSIP with an IPF-like profile/overlap (NSIP/IPF),
  - NSIP with an organizing pneumonia profile (NSIP/OP), and
  - NSIP with a hypersensitivity profile (NSIP/HP).
- Patients with NSIP on lung biopsy have a generally better prognosis and greater response to steroids when compared with patients with IPF.
- NSIP may be idiopathic or occur in association with other systemic conditions, most notably connective tissue diseases.

Epidemiology
Typically affects younger patients than IPF, with age of onset 40–50 y. May rarely affect children.

Causes/associations
- Idiopathic
- Connective tissue disease (NSIP may be the first manifestation of disease)
- Drugs
- Infection
- Immunodeficiency (including HIV, post-bone marrow transplant, chemotherapy).

Clinical features
There are few specific clinical features that help distinguish NSIP from other IIPs. Described features include:
- Breathlessness, cough
- Weight loss is common
- Onset gradual or subacute; typical symptom duration before diagnosis varies 0.5–3 y
- Crackles at lung bases, later more extensive
- Clubbing in a small proportion of patients.

Investigations
- *HRCT* frequently shows GG change, often in a basal distribution, with or without reticulation and traction bronchiectasis. The appearance is usually more confluent and homogeneous than the patchy heterogeneous distribution seen in IPF. Honeycombing is usually absent (occasionally seen in fibrotic NSIP)
- *PFTs* Typically restrictive pattern, but impaired gas transfer in only 50%. Desaturation on exertion is common

- *BAL* Lymphocytosis common
- *Lung biopsy* is often required
- Investigations to exclude underlying disease (see under Causes/associations).

Histology

- Variable, ranging from a predominantly 'cellular' pattern (mild to moderate interstitial inflammation, no fibrosis) to a 'fibrotic' pattern (interstitial fibrosis, more homogeneous appearance than in UIP and lack of fibroblastic foci or honeycombing; lung architecture may be relatively preserved).
- NSIP may be subclassified, based on the relative proportions of inflammation and fibrosis:
  - NSIP 1 (primarily inflammation, termed 'cellular')
  - NSIP 2 (inflammation and fibrosis)
  - NSIP 3 (primarily fibrosis).
- Features of both NSIP and UIP are sometimes seen on biopsies from the same individual—in such cases, the diagnosis is considered to be IPF (indicating a poor prognosis).

Diagnosis

Clinical and HRCT features are non-specific, and surgical lung biopsy is often required for diagnosis. An exception is NSIP in the setting of connective tissue disease, when histological confirmation is not usually required. Biopsy evidence of NSIP should be interpreted in the context of clinical and radiological findings, using a multidisciplinary approach in order to assign to the 'best fit' NSIP syndrome (NSIP/IPF, NSIP/OP, or NSIP/HP).

Management

Treatment is with corticosteroids, with a typical prednisolone dose of 0.5 mg/kg. Bone protection is recommended in patients while on high dose corticosteroids. Consider PPI, and co-trimoxazole prophylaxis (960 mg three times/week) against PCP. As with IPF, disease progression and response to treatment are best assessed by serial measurements of FVC and TLCO, with absolute changes of 10–15% or more considered significant. Additional immunosuppressive treatments (usually azathioprine or mycophenolate mofetil) are used in patients who fail to respond to corticosteroids alone.

Prognosis

Variable. Most patients improve or remain stable on treatment. 'Cellular' pattern on biopsy is associated with a good prognosis. Fibrotic NSIP is associated with a markedly better prognosis than IPF (5 y survival >50% in fibrotic NSIP, compared with 10–15% in IPF).

Cryptogenic organizing pneumonia (COP)

Definition

COP is a disease of unknown cause, characterized by 'plugging' of alveolar spaces with granulation tissue that may also extend up into the bronchioles. In addition to the 'cryptogenic' form, OP may also occur in the context of other diseases (see under Causes of OP). Use of the term 'bronchiolitis obliterans organizing pneumonia (BOOP)' is no longer recommended, as it erroneously suggests a primarily airways disease and is easily confused with bronchiolitis obliterans, a distinct disease entity.

Epidemiology

More common in non-smokers. Mean age of onset 55 y although can affect any age. ♂ = ♀.

Causes of organizing pneumonia

- Cryptogenic (COP)
- Organizing pneumonia secondary to:
  - Infection (including pneumonia, lung abscess, bronchiectasis)
  - Drug reaction or radiotherapy
  - Connective tissue disease (particularly myositis, RA, Sjögren's)
  - Diffuse alveolar damage
  - Inflammatory bowel disease
  - Haematological malignancy
  - Post-bone marrow transplant
  - Lung malignancy or airways obstruction
  - Pulmonary infarction.

Clinical features

- Typically short (<3 months) history of breathlessness and dry cough, often with malaise, fevers, weight loss, and myalgia. Often presents as a 'slow-to-resolve chest infection', frequently after several courses of antibiotics
- Breathlessness is usually mild, although a minority of patients experience severe breathlessness with rapid onset of respiratory failure and sometimes death ('fulminant COP')
- Examination may be normal or reveal crackles. Clubbing is absent.

Investigations

- *Blood tests* Raised CRP and ESR, neutrophilia
- *PFTs* Mild to moderate restrictive pattern is typical, although mild airways obstruction may also be seen in smokers. Mild hypoxaemia is common
- *CXR* classically shows patchy consolidation, sometimes with nodular shadowing. May present as a solitary mass on CXR
- *HRCT* Areas of consolidation with air bronchograms, sometimes with associated GG or small nodules. Often basal, subpleural, and peribronchial. May migrate spontaneously. Reticulation may suggest poor response to treatment. Less common appearance is as a solitary mass that may cavitate and that is often mistaken radiologically for a lung cancer. Septal thickening may occur

- *TBB* may confirm diagnosis, but there is concern that the relatively small samples may not effectively exclude associated diseases. TBB may be adequate in patients with typical clinical and HRCT features who are subsequently followed up closely. If a tissue diagnosis is required, surgical lung biopsy (at VATS) is the investigation of choice
- *Trial of treatment* may be used to help confirm the diagnosis, without biopsy
- *BAL*, if performed, shows lymphocytosis, neutrophilia, and eosinophilia.

Histology

- Alveolar spaces 'plugged' with granulation tissue (fibrin, collagen-containing fibroblasts, often with inflammatory cells), sometimes with extension up into the bronchiolar lumen.
- Patchy.
- Lack of architectural distortion.
- Examine for evidence of underlying cause, e.g. infection, vasculitis.

Diagnosis

Usually made on the basis of clinical and HRCT features and biopsy histology. Remember that the histological finding of 'OP' is non-specific, and search for 2° causes (see under Causes of OP). Lung cancers may be surrounded by patches of OP, and biopsy of these areas in patients with a solitary lung mass may give misleading results.

Differential diagnosis

- Infective consolidation
- Connective tissue disease, vasculitis
- Lymphoma, alveolar cell carcinoma
- Lung cancer (when OP presents as lung mass).

Management

Steroids are the mainstay of treatment. Optimal dose and duration unknown. Typical initial dose of oral prednisolone is 0.5–1.5 mg/kg daily for 1–3 months, before slowly weaning the dose over a total period of 6–12 months based on clinical, radiological, and lung function response. In fulminant disease, use pulsed IV methylprednisolone 750 mg–1 g on 3 consecutive days, followed by maintenance therapy with 0.5–1 mg/kg/day of prednisolone. Additional treatment with azathioprine or cyclophosphamide may be considered in patients with minimal response to steroids; IV pulses of cyclophosphamide may be tried in critically ill patients if failure to respond 5–7 days after steroid treatment.

Prognosis

Generally good. Most patients respond to steroids and improve within a week of starting treatment. Consider alternative diagnosis (e.g. lymphoma) if no improvement on steroid doses >25 mg/day. Relapse is common on reduction of steroid dose, and treatment courses of 6–12 months are usually required. A minority improve spontaneously. Lack of steroid response and progressive respiratory failure and death are rare but well documented.

Acute interstitial pneumonia (AIP)

Definition
Rapidly progressive form of interstitial pneumonia characterized histologically by diffuse alveolar damage. May be considered as an idiopathic form of ARDS. Formerly known as Hamman–Rich syndrome.

Epidemiology
Poorly described. Mean age of onset is 50 y but may occur at any age. Patients often previously healthy.

Clinical features
- Often preceded by 'viral'-type illness, with systemic symptoms, e.g. fevers, tiredness, myalgia, arthralgia
- Rapid onset (over days) of breathlessness; usually presents <3 weeks after symptom onset
- Widespread crackles on examination.

Investigations
- *CXR* Bilateral diffuse airspace shadowing with air bronchograms, progressing to widespread reticulation and GG; often spares costophrenic angles, heart borders, and hila
- *HRCT* Bilateral diffuse GG and patchy airspace consolidation in early stages; later traction bronchiectasis, cystic change, reticulation
- *PFTs* Restrictive, reduced gas transfer. Often profound hypoxia and respiratory failure
- *BAL* Increased total cells, red blood cells, and hemosiderin. Non-diagnostic but may be useful in excluding infection
- *Lung biopsy* required for diagnosis. TBB may be diagnostic; the risk of pneumothorax is higher in mechanically ventilated patients (about 10%). Surgical lung biopsy is otherwise required.

Histology
Diffuse alveolar damage: hyaline membranes, oedema, interstitial inflammation, and alveolar septal thickening, progressing to organizing fibrosis and sometimes honeycombing.

Diagnosis
Based on lung biopsy and exclusion of causes of ARDS.

Differential diagnosis
See Ɔ p. 27. Consider, in particular, the possibility of drug-induced pneumonitis or AIP occurring as a manifestation of antisynthetase syndrome (see Ɔ p. 220).

Management

No treatment demonstrated to be of benefit. In practice, treat infection (including consideration of unusual organisms), and consider high-dose steroids (e.g. IV methylprednisolone 750 mg–1 g on 3 consecutive days, followed by maintenance therapy with 0.5–1 mg/kg/day of prednisolone). There is a suggestion that outcome may be better following early use of high-dose steroids, although robust evidence is lacking. Clinical and radiological features may be indistinguishable from fulminant COP, which is likely to be more steroid-responsive. High-flow O_2. ICU admission and mechanical ventilatory support usually required.

Prognosis

Overall mortality at least 50%, although difficult to predict outcome in individuals. Survivors may stabilize, develop chronic progressive ILD, or experience recurrent exacerbations.

Respiratory bronchiolitis-associated interstitial lung disease (RB-ILD)

Definition
'Respiratory bronchiolitis' is a pathological term referring to the accumulation of bronchiolar pigmented macrophages in cigarette smokers and is asymptomatic in nearly all cases. A minority of smokers with respiratory bronchiolitis, however, develop a form of ILD known as RB-ILD. The exact relationship between RB-ILD and DIP is unclear—they may be considered as different forms of the same underlying disease, with DIP associated with a more extensive accumulation of macrophages throughout alveolar spaces.

Epidemiology
Invariably occurs in current or previous smokers, typically >30 pack years. ♂:♀ ≈ 2:1. Usual age of onset 30–40 y.

Clinical features
- Usually mild breathlessness and cough
- Small proportion have severe dyspnoea and respiratory failure
- Often crackles on examination.

Investigations
- *PFTs* Often show restrictive or combined obstructive and restrictive picture, with mildly impaired gas transfer
- *CXR* Thick-walled bronchi, reticular or GG change, may be normal
- *HRCT* Centrilobular nodules, GG change, thick-walled airways, often with associated centrilobular emphysema
- *BAL* Typically reveals pigmented alveolar macrophages.

Histology
Accumulation of pigmented brown macrophages in terminal bronchioles. Patchy bronchiolocentric distribution. These findings are frequently incidental in healthy smokers, and the diagnosis of RB-ILD is usually made on the basis of clinical and HRCT features; BAL and lung biopsy may be of value in excluding other conditions.

Management
Smoking cessation is the mainstay of treatment. Corticosteroids are occasionally used, with uncertain benefit.

Prognosis
Available data are limited; prolonged survival is common, although improvements in symptoms or physiology appear to occur in only a minority of patients.

Desquamative interstitial pneumonia (DIP)

Definition
ILD that occurs in smokers and is associated with the pathological finding of abundant pigmented macrophages located diffusely throughout alveolar airspaces. It may represent a more extensive form of RB-ILD, in which macrophages are restricted to peribronchiolar regions. The term DIP is misleading, as desquamation of epithelial cells is not responsible for the histological findings, as previously thought; a more accurate term is 'alveolar macrophage pneumonia', although this is not in widespread use.

Epidemiology
Very rare. Majority of patients are smokers, although may also occur following inhalation of inorganic dusts, including passive inhalation of cigarette smoke. Typically occurs aged 30–50.

Clinical features
Onset of breathlessness and cough over weeks to months is typical. Clubbing is present in up to 50% of patients.

Investigations
- *PFTs* Mild restrictive pattern common, sometimes with reduced gas transfer
- *CXR* May be normal or may demonstrate reticular or GG pattern, particularly affecting lower zones
- *HRCT* GG seen in all cases, typically lower zone or peripheral predominance. Reticulation and honeycombing may be present although tend to be mild
- *BAL* Increase in pigmented macrophages.

Histology
Diffuse accumulation of pigmented macrophages in alveolar airspaces. Changes are uniform.

Diagnosis
Clinical and HRCT features are non-specific, and surgical lung biopsy is often required for diagnosis.

Management
Smoking cessation. Corticosteroids are often used, with high response rates reported in retrospective cohorts.

Prognosis
Usually good prognosis. Improvement in GG on HRCT may correlate with response to treatment. Survival 70% after 10 y. Fluctuating course with remissions, and relapses may occur.

Lymphoid interstitial pneumonia (LIP)

Definition

Interstitial pneumonia characterized by diffuse lymphoid infiltrates and often lymphoid hyperplasia. Previously considered to be a precursor to pulmonary lymphoma and difficult to distinguish from lymphoma histologically; it is now considered a distinct entity and is thought to only rarely undergo malignant transformation. Only a minority of cases are idiopathic; actively investigate for an underlying cause (see under Causes/associations).

Epidemiology

Very rare. Commoner in women. May occur at any age.

Causes/associations

- Idiopathic
- Connective tissue disease—particularly Sjögren's syndrome, also RA, systemic lupus erythematosus
- Immunodeficiency, particularly HIV and common variable immunodeficiency
- Infection, e.g. PCP, hepatitis B
- Autoimmune disease, e.g. haemolytic anaemia, Hashimoto's thyroiditis, pernicious anaemia, chronic active hepatitis, primary biliary cirrhosis, myasthenia gravis
- Drugs, e.g. phenytoin.

Clinical features

Gradual-onset breathlessness and cough over several years. Fever, weight loss may occur. Crackles may be heard on examination.

Investigations

- *Blood tests* Mild anaemia may occur; poly- or monoclonal increase in serum immunoglobulins is common
- *CXR* Lower zone alveolar shadowing or diffuse honeycombing
- *HRCT* Predominant GG change, often with reticulation and cysts, and sometimes honeycombing and nodules. The presence of cysts is probably most helpful in differentiating from NSIP
- *BAL* Non-clonal lymphocytosis
- Investigations to identify underlying cause (see under Causes/associations).

Histology

Diffuse interstitial lymphoid infiltrates, predominantly involving alveolar septa, sometimes with lymphoid hyperplasia or honeycombing. Cellular NSIP, follicular bronchiolitis, and lymphoma may give similar appearances.

Management

Steroids are frequently used and often appear to improve symptoms.

Prognosis

Progression to extensive fibrosis occurs in around one-third of patients.

Chapter 32

Lung cancer

Epidemiology and types 338
Clinical features 340
Investigations 342
Diagnostic procedures 344
Staging 348
Non-small cell lung cancer (NSCLC): surgery 350
NSCLC: systemic anti-cancer therapy 354
NSCLC: radiotherapy 356
Small cell lung cancer (SCLC): treatment 358
Lung cancer: emerging areas 359
Superior vena caval obstruction (SVCO): aetiology, clinical
    assessment, and management 360
Hypercalcaemia 364
Syndrome of inappropriate secretion of antidiuretic hormone
    (SIADH) 365
Spinal cord compression 366
Pulmonary carcinoid tumours 368
Pulmonary nodules 1 372
Pulmonary nodules 2 376
Lung cancer screening 378

Epidemiology and types

Epidemiology

- >47,000 new cases diagnosed per annum in the UK
- More women die from lung cancer than from any other cancer, including breast
- ♂:♀ ≈ 2:1, but numbers ↓ in men, ↑ in women, because of ↑ smoking
- 90% are smoking-related
- Stopping smoking ↓ risk, but remains higher than in non-smokers
- Risk of lung cancer may be increased by asbestos exposure, arsenic and heavy metal exposure, pulmonary fibrosis, radiation exposure, and in patients with HIV.

Types of lung cancer

See Box 32.1. In practical terms, lung cancer is divided into two groups, which influence management and treatment decisions.

Non-small cell lung cancer (NSCLC)

- Accounts for ~80% of all lung cancers
- *Squamous cell carcinoma* is the commonest histological type. Usually presents as a mass on chest radiograph (CXR) but may cavitate and look radiologically like a lung abscess. Rarely, there may be multiple cavitating lesions. Hypercalcaemia may be a feature
- *Adenocarcinoma* may not necessarily be smoking-related. Can occur in scar tissue or sites of fibrosis. Can be a lung 1° or a 2° from adenocarcinomas at other sites, especially if causing pleural infiltration and subsequent pleural effusion. Adenocarcinomas have been reclassified (see Box 32.2)
- *Bronchioloalveolar/bronchoalveolar cell carcinoma* (BAC) is rare and has now been reclassified mostly as either *invasive mucinous adenocarcinoma* or *lepidic adenocarcinoma* (see Box 32.2). It can rarely cause copious sputum production (bronchorrhoea). Typically causes fluffy airspace shadowing on CXR and may be multifocal, sometimes in both lungs.

Small cell lung cancer (SCLC)

- Accounts for ~15% of all lung cancers
- Most aggressive of lung cancer subtypes
- Usually disseminated by the time of diagnosis (haematogenous spread)
- Frequently *metastasizes* to liver, bones, bone marrow, brain, adrenals, or elsewhere
- Syndrome of inappropriate secretion of antidiuretic hormone (SIADH) with hyponatraemia is common in SCLC
- Surgery usually not appropriate due to extent of disease. Rarely, small cell is an unexpectedly histology finding in a resected nodule.
- Chemo- and radiosensitive
- Untreated extensive stage SCLC is rapidly progressive and has a median survival of 6 weeks.

Box 32.1 World Health Organization (WHO) histological classification of epithelial lung tumours, 2015

- Adenocarcinoma
- Squamous cell carcinoma
- Neuroendocrine carcinoma (small cell, large cell neuroendocrine and carcinoid)
- Preinvasive (diffuse idiopathic pulmonary neuroendocrine cell hyperplasia (DIPNECH))
- Large cell carcinoma
- Adenosquamous carcinoma
- Sarcomatoid carcinoma
- Salivary gland-type
- Papillomas
- Adenomas

Box 32.2 World Health Organization (WHO) histological classification of lung adenocarcinomas, 2015

- Lepidic adenocarcinoma
- Acinar adenocarcinoma
- Papillary adenocarcinoma
- Micropapillary adenocarcinoma
- Solid adenocarcinoma
- Invasive mucinous adenocarcinoma
- Mixed invasive mucinous and nonmucinous adenocarcinoma
- Colloid adenocarcinoma
- Foetal adenocarcinoma
- Enteric adenocarcinoma
- Minimally invasive adenocarcinoma
- Nonmucinous
- Mucinous
- Preinvasive lesions
- Atypical adenomatous hyperplasia
- Adenocarcinoma in situ
- Nonmucinous
- Mucinous

Further information

Travis WD et al. The 2015 World Health Organization classification of lung tumors: impact of genetic, clinical and radiologic advances since the 2004 classification. *J Thorac Oncol* 2015;**10**(9): 1243–1260.

Clinical features

Smokers and ex-smokers with chest symptoms, especially those aged over 40, need investigation.

Symptoms and signs

These may be due to local tumour effects, metastatic tumour effects, or paraneoplastic manifestations. Many patients have no specific signs. In some, the lung cancer may be an incidental finding on CXR or computed tomography (CT) performed for another reason.

Local tumour effects
- Persistent cough or change in usual cough
- Haemoptysis
- Chest pain (suggests chest wall or pleural involvement)
- Unresolving pneumonia or lobar collapse
- Unexplained dyspnoea (due to bronchial narrowing or obstruction)
- Wheeze or stridor
- Shoulder pain (due to diaphragm involvement)
- Pleural effusion (due to direct tumour extension or pleural metastases)
- Hoarse voice (tumour invasion of the left recurrent laryngeal nerve)
- Dysphagia
- Raised hemidiaphragm (phrenic nerve paralysis)
- SVCO (see ➲ p. 360)
- Horner's syndrome (miosis, ptosis, enophthalmos, anhidrosis) due to apical or Pancoast's tumour damaging sympathetic chain
- Pancoast's tumours can also directly invade the rib and brachial plexus, causing C8–T1 dermatome numbness, shoulder pain, and weakness of small muscles of the hand.

Metastatic tumour effects
- Cervical/supraclavicular lymphadenopathy (common, present in 30%, and may be an easy site for diagnostic biopsy)
- Palpable liver edge
- Bone pain/pathological fracture due to bone metastases
- Neurological sequelae 2° to cerebral metastases (median survival of NSCLC with brain metastases is 2 months)
- Hypercalcaemic effects (due to bony metastases or direct tumour production of parathyroid hormone (PTH)-related peptide or PTH); see ➲ p. 364
- Dysphagia (compression from large mediastinal nodes).

Paraneoplastic syndromes
Endocrine syndromes are due to the ectopic production of hormones or hormonally active peptides. Neurological syndromes are due to antibody-mediated CNS damage.
- Cachexia and wasting
- Clubbing (up to 29% of patients; any cell type, more common in squamous and adenocarcinoma)
- Hypertrophic pulmonary osteoarthropathy (HPOA), often in association with clubbing, any cell type; more common in squamous and adenocarcinoma. Periosteal bone proliferation with symmetrical painful arthropathy (predominantly large joints, but hands and feet also affected)

- Gynaecomastia
- SIADH (mainly SCLC) in up to 10% of patients; see ➜ p. 365
- Ectopic adrenocorticotropic hormone (ACTH) (Cushing's syndrome, but due to rapid development; biochemical changes predominate, mainly SCLC) in 2–5% of patients
- Lambert–Eaton myasthenic syndrome (LEMS)—with SCLC. Affects proximal limbs and trunk, with autonomic involvement (dry mouth, constipation, erectile failure) and hyporeflexia (although reflexes return on exercising the affected muscle group), and only a slight response to edrophonium. Symptoms may predate diagnosis of lung cancer by up to 4 y. Caused by autoantibodies against P/Q-type voltage-gated calcium channels (VGCC). Decreased acetylcholine release at motor nerve terminals leads to the proximal weakness. Diagnosis made by VGCC autoantibody detection. EMG shows increased amplitude of muscle action with high-frequency repetitive stimulation, and repeated muscle contraction may lead to increasing strength and reflexes. Treatment of underlying SCLC may cause neurological improvement. If weakness is severe, IV immunoglobulin (or plasmapheresis) may give short-term benefits. 3,4-diaminopyridine may increase muscle strength in 85% of patients. Prednisolone alone or with azathioprine or ciclosporin can increase muscle strength and provide long-term control in non-responders
- Cerebellar syndrome (usually SCLC)
- Limbic encephalitis (SCLC, also breast, testicular, other cancers). Occurs within 4 y of diagnosis of cancer. Personality change, seizures, depression, subacute-onset confusion, and short-term memory loss. Diagnosed by pathological or radiological involvement of limbic system. Anti-Hu antibodies positive in 50% if associated with lung cancer
- Dermatomyositis/polymyositis
- Glomerulonephritis.

Lymphangitis carcinomatosis

Infiltration of pulmonary lymphatics by tumour. May be due to lung cancer or breast, prostate, stomach, or pancreatic malignancies. Causes SOB, cough, and is often associated with systemic signs of advanced malignancy. May be visible on CXR as fine linear shadowing throughout both lung fields. Septal lines present. May look like pulmonary oedema. Easily diagnosed on CT. Oral steroid treatment and diuretics can give symptomatic relief, but it is usually a short-lived response. Often part of a rapid decline.

Further information

Keogh M et al. Treatment for Lambert–Eaton myasthenic syndrome. *Cochrane Database Syst Rev* 2011;**2**:CD003279.

Investigations

Patients should be referred under the '2-week wait' cancer scheme and should be seen within 14 days of referral. The aim of investigations is to reach a histological diagnosis and tumour stage in order to determine the most appropriate treatment. Current UK government guidelines recommend patients should receive treatment within 31 days of the decision to treat and within 62 days of their urgent referral. New NHS England Faster Diagnosis Standard (FDS), mandated from April 2020, requires a diagnosis by 28 days. The National Optimal Lung Cancer Pathway (NOLCP), produced in 2017 by an NHS Clinical Expert Group, sets out a model by which this can be achieved.

In outpatients

- *History and examination*, including smoking and occupational histories
- *Spirometry* pre-biopsy or surgery
- *Review imaging*—location and size of lesion(s), mediastinal and cervical lymphadenopathy, pleural involvement, rib destruction, intrathoracic and extrathoracic metastases. CXR can be normal
- *Blood tests*, including full blood count, renal and bone profile, and liver function tests (LFTs). Check clotting if biopsy planned
- *Sputum cytology* rarely indicated (only considered in patients who are unfit for bronchoscopy or biopsy)
- *Diagnostic pleural tap*, if effusion present
- *FNA* of enlarged supraclavicular or cervical lymph nodes.

Radiology

- *CT neck, chest, liver, adrenals (contrast-enhanced) to assess tumour site and size* Lung cancers frequently metastasize to the mediastinal lymph nodes, liver, and adrenals. CT can locate lesions amenable to biopsy (either the 1° tumour or a metastasis). Assesses size of local and regional lymph nodes. Poor at assessing whether enlarged nodes are reactive (inflammatory) or represent metastatic spread (79% sensitive, 78% specific). Can assess tumour invasion to mediastinum and chest wall
- *Ultrasound (US)* of neck or liver may provide information about enlarged lymph nodes or metastases suitable for biopsy
- *Magnetic resonance imaging (MRI)* Used to answer specific questions relating to tumour invasion/borders. Good for assessing brachial plexus involvement. No role in nodule assessment
- *Positron emission tomography (PET)* Metabolically active tissues, such as tumours, show increased uptake of radiolabelled 18-fluorodeoxyglucose (FDG). Patients fast 4 h before the test, and, if they have diabetes, glucose should be within the normal range. Improves rate of detection of local and distant metastases. Useful for risk stratifying nodules, assessing regional lymph nodes (88% sensitive, 93% specific) and for seeking metastatic spread. Usually performed with a non-breath-hold CT as a PET/CT. Perform in:
  - All patients considered for radical therapy (including radical radiotherapy) to look for involved lymph nodes and distant metastases

- Patients with apparent N2–3 disease on CT of uncertain significance, who are otherwise surgical candidates
- Limited stage SCLC, staged by standard staging methods to identify metastases, as SCLC avidly takes up FDG.

FDG avid nodes that would exclude a patient from surgery if malignant should be confirmed as malignant with a biopsy. PET may reveal a distant abnormality, other than the 1° lung cancer, which could be a solitary metastasis or a second cancer. It is important therefore to biopsy isolated PET abnormalities before determining that a cancer is not resectable.

PET false negatives Occur in tumours with a low metabolic activity (typical carcinoids), small/ground-glass (GG) nodules, and hyperglycaemic patients. *False positives* occur in patients with benign pulmonary nodules with a high metabolic rate such as infective granulomata/rheumatoid nodules.

- *CT head* Indicated if any neurological evidence of metastatic disease such as persistent vomiting, fit, focal neurological signs, headache, unexplained confusion, or personality change. Also undertaken routinely in patients having curative intent treatment for stage II disease.
- *MRI head* NICE recommended for those with stage III disease being treated with curative intent
- *Bone scan* Now infrequently undertaken given widespread use of PET. Potential indications – bony pain, pathological fracture, hypercalcaemia, raised ALP. Highly suggestive of bony metastases if multiple areas of increased uptake. Solitary lesion may require further evaluation.

Multidisciplinary team

- Should include a chest physician, radiologist, thoracic surgeon, oncologist, pathologist, lung cancer nurse, and palliative care specialist who meet regularly in order to discuss patients and plan the most appropriate course of management.
- The Department of Health and NICE in the UK have produced guidelines for performance in lung cancer care. These encourage access to the multidisciplinary team (MDT) in decision making for the treatment and investigation of all patients with lung cancer.

Further information

NICE lung cancer guidelines (NG122) 2019. ℬ http://www.nice.org.uk
NHS guidance on implementing a timed lung cancer diagnostic pathway 2018. ℬ http://www.england.nhs.uk/wp-content/uploads/2018/04/implementing-timed-lung-cancer-diagnostic-pathway.pdf

Diagnostic procedures

Investigations are performed to obtain a tissue diagnosis and to stage cancer in order to determine the most appropriate treatment. Aim to achieve diagnosis and staging with as few procedures as possible. Establishing diagnosis and presence of metastatic spread at a single test is desirable, if possible.

Critical to obtain enough tissue to enable accurate histology and, importantly now, *molecular profiling* for advanced lung cancers to look for targetable mutations (e.g. *EGFR* and *ALK* driver mutations in adenocarcinomas and tumour expression of PD-L1; see ➲ p. 354). Aspects of further investigation may be inappropriate if the patient has advanced disease, is frail with comorbid conditions, or does not want to pursue diagnosis. This should be documented in their notes to aid audit and cancer service evaluation.

Bronchoscopy

Method of obtaining histological and cytological specimens. Suitable for central tumours. Tumours can be washed, brushed, and biopsied. Bronchoscopic samples are more likely to be histologically positive if there is:

• An endobronchial component to the tumour
• Tumour <4 cm from the origin of the nearest lobar bronchus
• A segmental or larger airway leading to the mass.

Always perform *after* CT scan to help plan and target bronchoscopy. Tumour position bronchoscopically may contribute to operative decisions: tumour confined to a lobar bronchus may be resectable with lobectomy; tumour <2 cm from the main carina requires pneumonectomy; left vocal cord paralysis indicates inoperability due to tumour infiltration of the left recurrent laryngeal nerve; and a splayed carina occurs 2° to enlarged mediastinal nodes. Advanced bronchoscopic techniques (e.g. endobronchial ultrasound (EBUS), CT-guided navigation bronchoscopy, or fluoroscopically-guided bronchoscopy) may help obtain diagnostic samples.

Transbronchial needle aspiration (TBNA)

Of lymph nodes (almost always combined with EBUS). Can be performed to obtain tissue and allow staging at the time of bronchoscopy and reduces need for mediastinoscopy (see ➲ p. 345). May also be combined with EUS-FNA (endoscopic ultrasound-guided fine-needle aspiration) via the oesophagus. If required for staging purposes, PET FDG avid lymph nodes and nodes >10 mm in short axis on CT should be sampled.

CT/US-guided biopsy

Of tumour or of an enlarged lymph node, especially in the neck, or of a metastasis (see Box 32.3). 85–90% sensitivity when sampling primary lesions >2 cm. Where possible, biopsy of a metastasis should be the investigation of choice, simultaneously giving staging and diagnosis.

DIAGNOSTIC PROCEDURES 345

Mediastinoscopy

Surgical biopsy of mediastinal lymph nodes to determine whether they are inflammatory or have malignant invasion. Suprasternal notch incision under general anaesthetic, blunt dissection, palpation, and endoscopic visualization and biopsy of nodes: paratracheal, prevascular, tracheobronchial, and anterior subcarinal. 93% sensitivity, 96% specificity. Technically more difficult if SVCO. Bleeding in <0.3%, left recurrent laryngeal nerve injury in 1%, pneumothorax, mediastinal emphysema, infection, oesophageal perforation (all rare). Repeat mediastinoscopies have lower positive yield and higher complication rate.

Mediastinotomy

Performed infrequently. Biopsy of aorto-pulmonary, sub-aortic, phrenic, or hilar nodes. Also can assess direct tumour invasion of central pulmonary artery or thoracic aorta, which would preclude curative surgery. Right or left parasternal incision, blunt dissection, palpation, and endoscopic visualization and biopsy of nodes.

Thoracoscopy

May be required to determine whether a pleural effusion contains malignant cells or is inflammatory, e.g. due to pneumonia caused by an obstructing lesion. Malignant effusions are evidence of M1a disease and hence are a contraindication to surgery/radical treatment.

Operative

It is sometimes difficult to obtain definitive cytology or histology preoperatively. If there is a high suspicion of malignancy, surgery can be performed regardless. After surgery, patients are given a pathological stage, which is sometimes different to the clinical stage (after histologically examining resection margins, lymph nodes, and pleura).

Box 32.3 Radiologically guided lung biopsy

Indications
- Radiologically-suspicious mass/nodule(s), not amenable to bronchoscopy, without distant sites of disease (which would be more informative for staging and easier to biopsy)
- Multiple chest nodules in patient not known to have malignancy
- Persistent undiagnosed single or multiple focal infiltrates.

Pre-biopsy preparation
- Discuss with Radiologist/MDT
- No absolute spirometry cut-offs, but FEV_1 >1L (or 35% predicted) is usually felt to be lower risk. Careful discussion about higher risk patients
- Check APTT and PT ratios <1.4 and platelets >100×10^9/L. If not, discuss with haematologist to determine whether it is safe to proceed
- High-risk patients should have overnight admission following biopsy
- Written information for patient, with informed signed consent.

Biopsy preparation
- Perform without sedation, if possible
- Use US, if possible (more straightforward than CT)
- Local anaesthetic to skin and subcutaneous tissue
- Perform at least two passes, may use FNA or cutting needle. FNA high diagnostic yield for malignant lesions (95%) but less for benign (10–50%). Cutting needles are as good for malignancy and better for benign diagnoses; also, more likely to provide enough tissue for molecular profiling. Operator decision.

Post-biopsy
- Observation by staff for 1 h in case of complications
- Erect CXR 1 h after biopsy and review by doctor
- Manage any pneumothorax, according to BTS guidelines (see ➔ p. 446). Increasing use of ambulatory drainage devices and daily outpatient review. Small pneumothoraces often resolve spontaneously but may need inpatient admission if there are concerns.

Complications
- Rates vary, but ~20% pneumothorax risk, ~3% require chest drain
- Haemoptysis 5%, death 0.15%.

See Manhire A et al. Guidelines for radiologically guided lung biopsy. *Thorax* 2003:**58**: 920–934.

Staging

Clinical and radiological tools categorize tumour size, location, regional and distant spread, and aid determination of most appropriate treatment. They can also therefore give prognostic information.

- *SCLC* is staged as limited or extensive but now also staged using the 8th edition of the tumour, node, metastasis (TNM) staging system (see Box 32.4):
  - *Limited* Confined to ipsilateral hemithorax and supraclavicular lymph nodes. Median survival with treatment, 15–20 months; without treatment, 12 weeks
  - *Extensive* Everything else. Median survival with treatment, 8–13 months; without treatment, 6 weeks
- *NSCLC* is commonly classified using TNM staging system (see Box 32.4 and Table 32.1). Frequency of patient stage at diagnosis: I and II, 42%; III, 34%; IV, 24%.

Table 32.1 Lung cancer clinical staging and survival

Stage	TNM classification	Survival	
		Median (months)	5y (%)
0	Tis		
IA1	T1mi or T1a N0 M0		92
IA2	T1b N0 M0		83
IA3	T1c N0 M0		77
IB	T2a N0 M0		68
IIA	T2b N1 M0		60
IIB	T1a–2b N1 M0	66	53
	T3 N0 M0		
IIIA	T1a–2b N2 M0	29	36
	T3 N1 M0		
	T4 N0–1 M0		
IIIB	T1a–2b N3 M0	19	26
	T3–4 N2 M0		
IIIC	T3–4 N3 M0	13	13
IVA	M1a–1b	12	10
IVB	M1c	6	0

Box 32.4 8th edition of the TNM staging system for lung cancer (IASLC/UICC/AJCC)

Extent of 1° tumour (T)

Tx 1° tumour cannot be assessed
T0 No evidence of 1° tumour
Tis Carcinoma *in situ*
T1 Tumour ≤3 cm, within lung but not in main bronchus
    T1a(mi)—minimally invasive adenocarcinoma
    T1a—tumour ≤1 cm
    T1b—tumour >1 cm but ≤2 cm
    T1c—tumour >2 cm but ≤3 cm
T2 Tumour >3 cm but ≤ 5 cm, or in main bronchus (not carina) or invading visceral pleura, or with atelectasis extending to the hilar region
    T2a—tumour >3 cm but ≤4 cm
    T2b—tumour >4 cm but ≤5 cm
T3 Tumour >5 cm but ≤7 cm or further nodule(s) in same lobe or invading: chest wall, phrenic nerve or parietal pericardium
T4 Tumour >7 cm or further nodule(s) in different ipsilateral lobe or invading: diaphragm, mediastinum, heart, great vessels, trachea, oesophagus, recurrent laryngeal nerve, carina, spine or carina.

Regional lymph nodes (N)

Nx Cannot be assessed
N0 No nodes
N1 Ipsilateral peribronchial/hilar nodes
N2 Ipsilateral mediastinal/subcarinal nodes
N3 Contralateral mediastinal/hilar nodes or any scalene/supraclavicular nodes.

Distant metastasis (M)

Mx Cannot be assessed
M0 No distant metastasis
M1 Distant metastasis present
    M1a—separate tumour nodule in contralateral lobe, pleural/pericardial involvement
    M1b—single metastasis
    M1c—multiple metastases

Further information

Goldstraw P et al. The IASLC Lung Cancer Staging Project: Proposals for Revision of the TNM Stage Groupings in the Forthcoming (Eighth) Edition of the TNM Classification for Lung Cancer. *J Thorac Oncol* 2016;11(1): 39–51

Mountain CF, Dresler CM. Regional lymph node classification for lung cancer staging. *Chest* 1997;111: 1718–1723.

Non-small cell lung cancer (NSCLC): surgery

Much of the investigation of lung cancer is to determine whether a patient has disease that is potentially curable by surgery. Other treatment options include chemotherapy, radiotherapy, and best supportive care, i.e. symptom-based conservative management. The MDT proposes the most appropriate choice(s) of treatment which is then discussed with the patient.

Surgery

The aims of surgery for lung cancer are to completely excise the tumour and local lymphatics, with minimal removal of normal functioning lung parenchyma.

- Stages I and II NSCLC are usually amenable to surgery if the patient is fit enough (see Fitness for surgery). This has a high chance of cure in stage I (>70% in IA), and a reasonable chance in stage II. 10–20% of NSCLC patients undergo resection. When standard lobectomy not possible, consider sublobar resection, stereotactic ablative radiotherapy (SABR), or other ablative treatments. Adjuvant chemotherapy is advocated for stage II tumours
- For resectable stage IIIA-N1 tumours, surgery is followed by adjuvant chemotherapy to improve survival rates. Induction chemoradiotherapy followed by surgery may be considered for patients with stage IIIA–N2
- Stages IIIB to IV are not usually resectable. If stage III disease can be treated within a radical radiotherapy field, radical concurrent chemoradiotherapy may be considered. Patients with good PS with a small primary and low volume oligometastatic disease (e.g. ≤3 metastases), may be considered for radical treatment to all sites with surgery/ablative therapies and chemotherapy
- Stages 0/tumour *in situ* often will have no defined 1° lesion amenable to resection. The natural progression of these tumours is still unknown; they may progress or regress with time.

Resectability of a tumour implies likelihood of complete removal by surgery; this is different from patient operability, which is determined by the patient's fitness for surgery.

Fitness for surgery

- *Global risk score* May be useful for estimating risk of death (e.g. Thoracoscore)
- *Age* is not a contraindication, but increasing age is associated with an increased perioperative morbidity. Higher mortality risk if over 80 and if pneumonectomy, rather than lobectomy (14% mortality vs 7%, respectively). Right pneumonectomy has higher mortality than left pneumonectomy (more lung removed). 2y post-operative survival similar to that of other age groups
- *Lung function* Approaches vary but include measurement of FEV_1 and lung carbon monoxide transfer factor (TLCO) in all, with calculation of predicted post-operative (PPO) values.

PPO = (pre-operative FEV_1 or TLCO) x (19 – number of segments resected)/19)

- ACCP 2013 guidelines – PPO FEV_1 and PPO TLCO both >60% suggest low risk for death and complications and no further tests required
  - For values <60% but >30%, stair climb or SWT recommended
  - For values <30% (or SWT of <25 shuttles or <400m, or climb test <22m), full CPET recommended.
  - If VO_2max <35% predicted (or <10 mL/kg/min) consider patient for lung-conserving procedures or non-operative treatment.
  - LVRS may be considered if a cancer is within an area of upper lobe emphysema
- NICE 2019 guidelines – PPO FEV_1 or TLCO <30% does not necessarily outrule radical treatment but patients should be counselled about increased risks and likely dyspnoea.
  - SWT >400m represents good function for those with moderate/high risk dyspnoea
  - VO_2max >15 mL/kg/min is cut off for good function on CPET
- *Cardiovascular* Postpone surgery if patient has had MI within 30 days. Cardiology opinion if patient has had MI within 6 months. Echo if they have heart murmur. Preoperative ECG for all
- *Central nervous system (CNS)* If any history of transient ischaemic attacks, strokes, or carotid bruits, need carotid Doppler studies and vascular surgeon opinion, if necessary
- *Smoking* Do not delay surgery to stop smoking, but counsel patients and offer NRT
- *Nutritional* Requirements should be optimized, with advice from a dietician, if necessary. Patients presenting with a preoperative weight loss of 10% or more ± PS≥2 are more likely to have advanced disease or comorbidities. Therefore, require careful staging and search for evidence of comorbidity.

Types of surgery

- *Lobectomy* or bi-lobectomy for localized tumour, or pneumonectomy for tumour involving >1 or 2 lobes. If hilar nodes are infiltrated by tumour, a more radical lobectomy or a pneumonectomy is required. The local lymph nodes are removed in each procedure for pathological staging.
- *Segmentectomy* removes part of a lobe (supplied by a segmental bronchus) along the intersegmental planes and may be performed for a localized peripheral lesion with clear regional lymph nodes, especially if the post-operative respiratory function is predicted to be borderline.
- *Wedge resection* is another lung-preserving operation that removes only the tumour, with minimal surrounding lung parenchyma, but there is a higher local recurrence rate (up to 23%). Both segmentectomy and wedge resection should have ≥2 cm clear margins around a tumour.
- *Sleeve resections* involve a lobectomy and the removal of a section of bronchus affected by tumour, forming an anastomosis between the airway proximal and distal to it. This may avoid a pneumonectomy. Resection margins should be macroscopically free from tumour. If there is limited local tumour invasion to the chest wall, this can be resected with a 5 cm margin. Reconstruction with prosthetic material may be necessary if two or more ribs are resected, aiming to preserve the chest wall function.

Post-operative complications
- Bronchopleural fistula
- Respiratory failure
- Infection
- Phrenic nerve damage causing diaphragmatic paralysis
- Recurrent laryngeal nerve damage causing hoarse voice
- Prolonged chest wall pain
- Mortality: 1–3.5% for wedge resection, 2–4% for lobectomy, 6–8% for pneumonectomy.
- Risk increases with increasing age, associated ischaemic heart disease, impaired respiratory function, and poor PS.

Following surgery
Patients are usually followed up on a 6–12-monthly basis for CT review for 5 y (although optimal follow-up unclear). This is to ensure they are radiologically clear of tumour recurrence, and there is not a second 1° tumour. They should also be advised to seek earlier review if they have symptoms of persistent haemoptysis or new cough, weight loss, new chest pain. If histology shows incomplete resection margins, post-operative chemoradiotherapy given to try and improve local disease control.

NSCLC: systemic anti-cancer therapy

Previously, systemic treatment for advanced lung cancer was with cytotoxic chemotherapy only. The addition of personalized therapy, based on tumour genetics and gene expression, has led to a significant increase in response rates, progression free survival and tolerability of treatment. The term 'systemic anti-cancer therapy' (SACT) is therefore more accurate than chemotherapy and includes chemotherapy, inhibitors against tyrosine kinases (which have been activated in some cancers, e.g. 'driver mutations' seen with *EGFR* mutations and *ALK/ROS1* rearrangements), and molecularly targeted therapy (e.g. checkpoint inhibitors targeting PD-1 or PD-L1 (see Box 32.5)).

- Consider SACT in patients with advanced disease as a palliative intervention (to prolong life and minimize symptoms) for those with WHO PS0–2 (see ⟳ p. 357).
- With the advent of targeted treatment, essential to obtain adequate tissue for molecular characterization to choose correct SACT. For advanced disease, biopsy samples are tested for the following;
  - **For non-squamous NSCLC**:
    - *EGFR-TK* (epidermal growth factor receptor tyrosine kinase) mutations
    - *ALK* (anaplastic lymphoma kinase) tyrosine kinase gene rearrangement
    - *ROS1* (c-ROS oncogene 1) receptor tyrosine kinase gene rearrangement
    - Tumour PD-L1 expression
  - **For squamous NSCLC**
    - Tumour PD-L1 expression

Box 32.5 'Checkpoint inhibitor' immunotherapy against PD-1 and PD-L1

Programmed death protein-1 (PD-1) is a transmembrane protein expressed on T cells, B cells, and NK cells. Binds to programmed death ligand 1 (PD-L1) expressed on the surface of some tumour cells. PD-1:PD-L1 interaction perpetuates cancer by inhibiting apoptosis of the tumour cell, promotes peripheral T effector cell exhaustion, and promotes conversion of T effector cells to Treg cells.

- Anti-PD-1 and anti-PD-L1 antibodies are inhibitors that disrupt this 'checkpoint' and allow the immune system to act against cancer cells.
- Anti-PD-1 antibodies include pembrolizumab and nivolumab.
- Anti-PD-L1 antibodies include atezolizumab, avelumab, and durvalumab.
- These can cause toxicities (immune-related adverse events – irAEs), which are usually transient but can be severe – skin, colitis, hepatotoxicity, hypothyroidism/hyperthyroidism, pituitary inflammation and uveitis; usually treated with treatment cessation ± steroids.

- SACT treatment regimens are complex and fast-changing but the following is an overview.
  - For non-squamous NSCLC, usual initial treatment;
    - *EGFR-TK* mutations (17% of NSCLC in UK; typically affecting never-smoking women ± Asian ethnicity): Treat with tyrosine kinase inhibitors (TKI) – afatinib, dacomitinib, erlotinib or gefitinib. Toxicities include GI, LFT derangements, pneumonitis, dry eyes, corneal erosions
    - *ALK* gene rearrangements ('fusion oncogene' created when *EML4* and *ALK* genes are fused, creating *EML4-ALK*; typically younger patients with light/no smoking history): Treat with TKI – alectinib, crizotinib, or ceritinib. Toxicities – GI, LFT derangements, pneumonitis, bradycardia, visual disturbances
    - *ROS-1* gene rearrangement: Treat with TKI – crizotinib
    - *If no mutation and PD-L1 expression ≥50%*: Treat with pembrolizumab (anti-PD-1 antibody)
    - *If no mutation and PD-L1 expression <50%*: Treat with atezolizumab (anti-PD-L1 antibody)+bevacizumab (VEGF inhibitor)+carbo platin+paclitaxel OR pembrolizumab+pemetrexed+(carbo/cisplatin) OR pemetrexed+carboplatin or other platinum doublet chemotherapy
  - **For squamous NSCLC, usual initial treatment**;
    - *PD-L1 expression ≥50%*: Treat with pembrolizumab monotherapy
    - *PD-L1 expression <50%*: Treat with pembrolizumab+paclitaxel+car boplatin if tolerated, otherwise (gemcitabine/vinorelbine)+(carbo/cisplatin).
- Combined chemoradiotherapy may be given with curative intent for some patients with stage III disease (or lower stages, not suitable for surgery). Cisplatin+etoposide is a common choice of chemotherapy in this context.
- *Side effects of chemotherapy* Nausea, myelosuppression, ototoxicity, peripheral neuropathy, nephropathy if dehydrated. Alopecia with taxanes
- Patients are monitored during SACT with repeat CT to establish whether they have partial response, stable disease, or progressive disease, despite treatment. This influences decisions regarding further treatment.

Adjuvant therapy

The use of radiation or chemotherapy (or both) following complete sur-gical resection to improve survival. Adjuvant chemotherapy has been found to confer approx. 5% increase in 5 y survival, compared with sur-gery alone in trials. Cisplatin-based combination treatment is now offered post-operatively to patients with PS0–1 and stage II/III disease NSCLC (i.e. N1/2 nodal disease or tumours >4 cm). Adjuvant radiotherapy trials have shown no evidence of a survival benefit, except possibly in those with N2 disease.

NSCLC: radiotherapy

May be given for:
- Curative intent (high dose)
- Palliative control (high dose)
- Symptom relief (low dose).

Radiotherapy has no benefit following complete 1° tumour surgical resection.

Radical radiotherapy is high-dose radiotherapy given with curative intent.
- Recommended for patients with localized chest disease, stages I–III with PS0–1 (see Box 32.6), who are either resectable (but unfit for surgery or do not want surgery) or unresectable but can be treated within a radical radiotherapy field without undue toxicities
- SABR/stereotactic body radiation therapy (SBRT) allows the delivery of very high radiation doses to small early stage lung cancers (tumours ≤5 cm, up to and including stage IIA (T2b N0 M0)), with good local control outcomes. Increasingly used in early stage patients unfit for surgery. The treatment course is shorter than conventional radiotherapy (typically given in 3–5 fractions) and is usually associated with an acceptable toxicity profile. If SABR not possible, conventional/ hyperfractionated radiotherapy may be given
- Conventional radiotherapy is used when SABR not possible. Various regimes are used in different centres (e.g. 55 Gy in 20 fractions over 4 weeks or 60–66 Gy in 30–33 fractions over 6.5 weeks).
- Need PFTs, including TLCO before radiotherapy. FEV_1 should be ≥1.5l.

High-dose palliative radiotherapy is given to patients with symptomatic disease, good PS, no evidence of metastases, and who will be able to tolerate a high-dose regime. An example of such a regime would be 36–39 Gy in 12–13 fractions over 6 weeks. Improves median survival by 2 months.

Low-dose radiotherapy is given for symptom relief in patients who would be unable to tolerate high-dose palliative radiotherapy or those with evidence of metastases. Symptoms palliated include pain, haemoptysis, breathlessness, or cough.

Urgent radiotherapy is used in combination with oral steroids for relief of SVCO by tumour, although stenting performed interventional radiology is now the treatment of choice, where possible. Radiotherapy takes ~10 days to be effective.

Prophylactic cranial irradiation is not recommended for NSCLC outside a clinical trial.

Chemoradiotherapy is used to improve tumour radiosensitization for localized disease. There may be some additional advantages with treatment of potential distant micrometastases. Should be considered for stages II–III disease in patients who are not fit for surgery.

Box 32.6 World Health Organization (WHO)/Eastern Cooperative Oncology Group (ECOG) performance status (PS)

0 = Fully active, able to carry on all pre-disease performance without restriction

1 = Restricted in physically strenuous activity but ambulatory and able to carry out work of a light or sedentary nature, e.g. light house work, office work

2 = Ambulatory and capable of all self-care but unable to carry out any work activities. Up and about >50% of waking hours

3 = Capable of only limited self-care, confined to bed or chair >50% of waking hours

4 = Completely disabled. Cannot carry on any self-care. Totally confined to bed or chair.

See Oken MM et al. Toxicity and response criteria of the Eastern Cooperative Oncology Group. *Am J Clin Oncol* 1982;**5:** 649–655.

Small cell lung cancer (SCLC): treatment

Surgery

Limited stage SCLC may be appropriate for surgical resection if there is no evidence of metastases (T1–2a N0 M0). This is rare. The patient should also be considered for post-operative combination chemotherapy for treatment of micro-metastases, especially if histology was only determined at operation.

Chemotherapy

Combination chemotherapy is used for limited and extensive SCLC.
- Etoposide with either cisplatin or carboplatin is the standard regime
- Given 3-weekly, commonly for 4–6 cycles
- Different regimes are selected, according to PS
- Patients with PS3 may benefit from less intensive outpatient chemotherapy on a 3-weekly basis
- Patients are carefully assessed, and, if there is no sign of a response to treatment, based on CT scan, they may be switched to second-line agents, although there is limited evidence of benefit
- Patients with relapsed SCLC but good PS may be offered anthracycline-containing regimes or further platinum-based treatment for a maximum of six cycles. Oral topotecan is an option if they are unable to tolerate IV chemotherapy. Response rates to second-line chemotherapy are low (~10%)
- 80–90% response if limited disease; 60–80% if extensive disease
- Chemotherapy may increase median survival to 15–20 months in limited disease and 8–13 months for extensive disease.

Radiotherapy

- Patients with limited stage disease (which is encompassable in a radical radiotherapy volume, broadly equivalent to T1–4 N0–3 M0)) with PS0/1 should have consolidation radiotherapy to the chest disease, with the first or second cycle of chemotherapy. If unfit for combination treatment, give after chemotherapy completion if they have a response or partial response
- Prophylactic cranial radiotherapy (25 Gy over 10 fractions) is advised at completion of chemotherapy for those with limited disease or those with extensive disease and good prognostic factors. This improves three-year survival for limited stage SCLC by 5%
- In patients with extensive disease, including cerebral metastases, or poorer PS, chemotherapy is given first. If there is a good response, palliative thoracic radiotherapy may be given
- Of benefit to symptomatic bone metastases, cord compression, SVCO.

Lung cancer: emerging areas

Radiofrequency ablation (RFA)/Microwave ablation (MwA)

* Applied via a probe inserted into a nodule/tumour under CT guidance with general anaesthesia
* Causes tissue death by thermal necrosis
* Lesions initially increase in size and density, and may cavitate, but then become fibrotic scar tissue
* May become a tool to treat patients with 1° lung cancer unsuitable for curative surgery/radiotherapy due to comorbid disease
* The size of the cancer that can be treated is limited (maximum 5 cm, best results with <3 cm)
* Peripheral lesions are easier to access
* Side effects of therapy:
  * Pleuritic chest pain
  * Pneumothorax
  * Empyema
  * Haemoptysis
  * Haemorrhage
  * Low-grade fever
* FEV_1 should ideally be >1L
* Tumour follow-up with contrast-enhanced imaging, as ablated tissue does not enhance
* Used currently mainly in pulmonary metastases from GI or renal cell cancers, or sarcomas, which are not suitable for surgical resection, but also some data for 1° NSCLC. No long-term RCT reported.

Targeted molecular therapy

In addition to the currently-treated molecular targets, further gene driver mutations are under investigation including *HER2*, *NTRK*, *MET*, and *RET*.

Liquid biopsies

Increasing interest in testing blood for circulating tumour DNA (ctDNA) to genotype cancer without invasive biopsies. Potential utility when biopsy impossible/dangerous or in monitoring tumour genotype evolution as disease progresses (to allow selection of further SACT). Sensitivity likely lower than direct tumour biopsy.

Further information

NICE lung cancer guidelines (NG122) 2019. ♂ http://www.nice.org.uk

Detterbeck FC et al. Executive summary. Diagnosis and management of lung cancer, 3rd edition: American College of Chest Physicians Evidence-Based Clinical Practice Guidelines. *Chest* 2013;**143**: 7S–37S.

♂ http://www.cancerresearchuk.org

♂ http://www.macmillan.org.uk/information-and-support/lung-cancer, information for patients

♂ http://www.roycastle.org, patient network, ☎ 0333 323 7200.

Superior vena caval obstruction (SVCO): aetiology, clinical assessment, and management

Obstruction of the flow of blood in the superior vena cava (SVC) results in the symptoms and signs of SVCO. It is caused by two different mechanisms (which may coexist): *external compression or invasion* of the SVC by tumour extending from the right lung (four times more common than the left lung), lymph nodes, or other mediastinal structure; or due to *thrombosis* within the vein.

Aetiology

The commonest cause (~85%) is malignancy. Lung cancer and lymphoma together cause 95% of malignant SVCO.

Malignant causes

- *Lung cancer* Up to 4% of lung cancer patients will develop SVCO at some point during their disease. Up to 10% of SCLC present with SVCO
- *Lymphoma* Up to 4% of lymphoma patients will develop SVCO, most commonly in non-Hodgkin's lymphoma. This usually occurs due to extrinsic compression of the SVC by enlarged lymph nodes
- *Other malignant causes* Thymoma, mediastinal germ cell tumours, tumours with mediastinal metastases (commonest is breast cancer).

Benign causes

Include granulomatous disease, intrathoracic goitre, and central venous lines, Port-A-Cath®, and pacemaker wires (causing thrombosis). In the past, SVCO was commonly due to untreated infection, e.g. syphilitic thoracic aortic aneurysm or fibrosing mediastinitis (due to actinomycosis, TB, blasto-mycosis, or *Aspergillus*). These are all now rare.

Clinical features

- Facial and upper body oedema, with facial plethora, often with increased neck circumference, and a cyanotic appearance
- Venous distension of the face and upper body. SVCO due to malignancy usually develops over days to weeks, so an adequate collateral circulation does not have time to develop. Pemberton's sign—facial plethora, distress, and sometimes stridor after lifting the arms above the head for a few minutes—may suggest the diagnosis
- Breathlessness
- Headache—worse on bending forwards or lying down
- Cough/haemoptysis or other signs of an underlying lung malignancy
- Hoarse voice
- Dysphagia
- Syncope/dizziness (reduced venous return)
- Confusion.

Diagnosis

Usually made clinically from the signs of facial and upper body swelling, with distension of superficial veins across the chest wall, neck, and upper arms.

Investigations

The investigation and treatment of SVCO was previously considered a medical emergency. SVCO is now not considered to be immediately life-threatening, making treatment less urgent and allowing a definitive diagnosis to be made prior to treatment. The exception to this rule is the patient who presents with stridor or laryngeal oedema, which is a medical emergency.

- *CXR* Up to 85% have an abnormal CXR (as lung malignancy is the commonest underlying disorder). Mediastinal widening is common
- *CT chest with contrast* can stage the underlying malignancy and image the venous circulation and collateral blood supply
- *Histological diagnosis* Usual practice is to obtain a tissue diagnosis of the underlying disease before starting treatment, as the underlying diagnosis can alter treatment markedly. Symptomatic obstruction will have been developing for some weeks prior to presentation, and, in the clinically stable patient, a delay of 24–48 h while the correct underlying diagnosis is obtained is warranted. Radiotinoscopy prior to biopsy can lead to problems making a subsequent histological diagnosis, and, similarly, high-dose steroids can make the diagnosis of lymphoma difficult. Diagnostic samples may be obtained using:
  - Pleural fluid cytology
  - US-guided biopsy of an extrathoracic lymph node (e.g. supraclavicular or cervical nodes—low risk)
  - Bronchoscopy, or mediastinoscopy if no endobronchial disease, may be needed, depending on CT features. There may be increased risk of bleeding post-biopsy because of venous congestion, and anaesthesia is theoretically riskier because of possible associated tracheal obstruction or pericardial effusion (potentially leading to haemodynamic compromise due to cardiac tamponade), though these can be anticipated from the CT scan
  - Sputum.

Management

See Box 32.7.

▶▶ Box 32.7 SVCO: management

This is usually in two phases:
- Initial general treatment: O_2, analgesia, sitting the patient up (to reduce venous pressure), and steroids (in some)
- Followed by treatment of the underlying disease causing the SVCO, dependent on the tissue diagnosis. The major differential in terms of treatment is small cell carcinoma (initial chemotherapy), non-small cell carcinoma (initial radiotherapy), and lymphoma (chemotherapy). The presence of SVCO usually means that surgical resection of a NSCLC is not possible.

Steroids
- Limited trial data to support the use of steroids in SVCO, prior to definitive treatment; most would start them fairly promptly (e.g. dexamethasone 8 mg bd; avoid in the evening, as affects sleep).
- They may reduce oedema and improve symptoms.
- Ideally, a tissue diagnosis should be obtained before commencing steroids but may not always be possible.
- Problematic if the underlying diagnosis is lymphoma as steroids may alter the histology, making a definitive diagnosis more difficult.
- In an older smoker, with an obvious CXR mass (in whom the diagnosis is likely to be lung cancer), steroids can probably be started without risk to the underlying histology.

Radiotherapy
- 90% of patients are oedema-free by 3–4 weeks. In those with a poor response to radiotherapy, only 25% survive 1 y.

Intraluminal stents
- Used for malignant SVCO and may be a first-line treatment while radiotherapy is planned.
- Successful in 90% of cases, with relief of symptoms in most patients within 48 h.
- They do not preclude subsequent radiotherapy or chemotherapy.
- In SCLC, however, chemotherapy will improve SVCO rapidly, so stent insertion may not be necessary.
- Unclear if post-procedure anticoagulation is required. Some centres advocate the use of low-dose warfarin anticoagulation (i.e. 1 mg/day), aiming for an INR of <1.6.
- Thrombosis in the SVC is not a contraindication to the procedure, as clot can be dispersed mechanically or with thrombolysis at the time of the procedure.
- *Stent complications* Stent migration is the major complication, but most patients do not live long enough for this to be a major problem.

Anticoagulation
Some recommend prophylactic anticoagulation in the presence of SVCO. Small increased risk of intracerebral bleeding, but the benefits of SVCO treatment may be limited by subsequent SVC thrombus if anticoagulation is not started. This is controversial.

SVCO due to thrombosis
Usually in association with central venous lines or pacemaker wires. If the clot is <5 days old (as judged by symptoms), thrombolysis is warranted. Subsequent oral anticoagulation may reduce recurrence.

Prognosis

Depends on the underlying disease and is unrelated to the duration of SVCO at presentation. The majority of SVCO is due to mediastinal spread of carcinoma of the lung, so the overall prognosis is generally poor but depends on the patient's PS, stage and extent of disease, and the cell type.

Further information

Rowell NP, Gleeson FV. Steroids, radiotherapy, chemotherapy and stents for SVCO in carcinoma of the bronchus: a systematic review. *Clin Oncol (R Coll Radiol)* 2002;**14**: 338–351.

Hypercalcaemia

Definition and aetiology

A serum calcium level over 2.75 mmol/L is considered abnormal; borderline values need repeating. In malignancy, a raised calcium is due to increased osteoclast activity, either from bony metastases or the production of PTH-related protein. A serum level over 3.25 mmol/L is rare outside malignancy although can occur in sarcoidosis.

Clinical features

Values over 3 mmol/L are usually symptomatic. Common symptoms are confusion, weakness, nausea, reduced fluid intake, and constipation. There may be a short QT interval on ECG and renal failure.

Investigations

Exclude other causes of hypercalcaemia, and identify the tumour, although in most patients with malignant hypercalcaemia, the diagnosis of malignancy will already be known. The PTH will be suppressed in malignant hypercalcaemia but raised in hyperparathyroidism. The phosphate will tend to be low in hyperparathyroidism and hypercalcaemia due to ectopic PTH, and normal/high in sarcoidosis, metastatic bone disease, and with excess vitamin D. Check for renal failure.

Management

See Box 32.8.

▶▶Box 32.8 Management of hypercalcaemia

- Isotonic saline infusion (250 mL/h initially, to reverse dehydration, but avoid fluid overload, reducing to 150 mL/h) (± furosemide to increase calcium excretion)
- Steroids help, but less so than in sarcoid-associated hypercalcaemia, partly through reduced intestinal absorption.

In addition to this initial management:

- Reduce bone reabsorption with bisphosphonates (takes a few days for maximum effect). The bisphosphonates can also reduce the pain of 2° bony deposits and may reduce pathological fracture rate.
  - *IV preparations* Disodium pamidronate, 15–60 mg infused over 2 h. Works for several weeks. Zoledronic acid, 4 mg over ≥15 min, repeated monthly, if required
  - *Oral preparations* Sodium clodronate, one 800 mg tablet bd.

Syndrome of inappropriate secretion of antidiuretic hormone (SIADH)

Definition and aetiology

Excessive retention of water relative to electrolytes due to inappropriate production of antidiuretic hormone (ADH). Hence, there is hyponatraemia (<135 mmol/L), hypo-osmolality, a urine osmolality >100 mosmol/kg, a urine sodium concentration usually above 40 mmol/L, normal acid–base (and potassium), and usually a low plasma urea concentration. Diuretic-induced hyponatraemia will be accompanied by evidence of dehydration, e.g. raised urea. Causes of SIADH include:

- Drugs, e.g. carbamazepine, fluoxetine, high-dose cyclophosphamide
- Post-major surgery
- Pneumonia
- HIV infection
- CNS disorders, e.g. stroke, infection, psychosis
- SCLC, either ectopic ADH production or stimulation of normal ADH production (poor prognostic factor).

Clinical features

Lethargy and confusion often when sodium levels fall below 130 mmol/L and nearly always when below 120 mmol/L.

Investigations

Low sodium in the presence of a low urea and an appropriate clinical setting may be adequate to make a diagnosis. If sodium depletion/water overload are a possible alternative cause of hyponatraemia, they should be accompanied by a urine osmolarity <100 mosmol/kg (or a specific gravity <1.003 or a urine sodium <40 mmol/L). Therefore, values increasingly above this are suggestive of SIADH (unless the patient is on loop diuretics when, of course, the urinary sodium concentration will be higher).

Management

See Box 32.9.

> ▶▶**Box 32.9 Management of inappropriate ADH secretion**
> - Fluid restriction (0.5–1.0 L/day) will help but is often unpleasant for the patient
> - Salt tablets/extra-dietary salt
> - May resolve over a few weeks following chemotherapy
> - Hypertonic saline is rarely indicated and can provoke brainstem damage (demyelination) through rapid changes in osmolality
> - Drugs (not routinely used but may be useful): demeclocycline (450 mg bd, tetracycline derivative; blocks ADH action at the distal renal tubules and can be used long term) or tolvaptan (15 mg od, V2 ADH receptor antagonist; monitor sodium concentration every 6 h during first 2 days of treatment; watch LFTs).

Spinal cord compression

This is a medical emergency requiring prompt treatment within 24h to prevent irreversible paraplegia and loss of bowel and bladder function.

Definition and aetiology

Spinal cord compression occurs commonly in patients with metastatic cancer (in about 5% of all cancer patients, particularly breast, lung, and prostate cancer). It may be the first presentation of cancer but often occurs in patients with a known 1° tumour. Cord compression is commonly caused by direct spread from a vertebral metastasis into the extradural space (most commonly, thoracic spine) or, less commonly, from pressure on the cord from a 1° tumour in the posterior mediastinum or the retroperitoneum, or by pressure from a mass of retroperitoneal nodes. It is unusual to have a metastasis within the cord itself, although meningeal spread can occur. Spinal cord compression causes interruption of the arterial supply to the cord and subsequent infarction.

Clinical features

- Patients frequently experience back pain initially, due to associated vertebral collapse. This precedes any neurological signs. Pain is not, however, universal
- Neurological signs may be non-specific:
  - Weak legs
  - Constipation
  - Urinary incontinence
- Leg weakness develops over hours to days, with associated sensory loss
- Loss of bladder and bowel sensation is a late sign and usually heralds irreversible paraplegia within hours or a few days
- Examination reveals bilateral upper motor neurone signs in the legs, with increased tone, weakness, brisk reflexes, and extensor plantars
- There may be sensory loss in the legs, particularly with a loss of proprioception and a sensory level on the trunk
- Sensory loss in the saddle area, with decreased rectal tone, suggests a cauda equina lesion. The bladder may be palpable.

Investigations

Have a low threshold for investigating a patient with known cancer with back pain.

- *MRI* of the spine is the investigation of choice to demonstrate the level of the cord compression
- *CT* is less reliable but can also be helpful, if MRI is not available
- *Plain spine X-ray* may show vertebral metastases, but this is usually unhelpful, as there is no imaging of the spinal cord. Time should not be wasted in obtaining a plain X-ray
- *Bone scan* shows vertebral metastases but again does not image the spinal cord. Earlier scans showing bony metastases may alert the physician to the possibility of future cord compression
- If patient is not known to have underlying malignant disease, a search for a 1° tumour should be performed but must not delay treatment of the spinal cord compression. Take full history (weight loss, anorexia, specific symptoms), and perform full examination, CXR, blood tests, PSA, and myeloma screen.

Management

See Box 32.10.

▶▶Box 32.10 Management of spinal cord compression

Management depends on tumour type and overall prognosis. Discuss with oncologist and/or neurosurgeon to determine which definitive treatment(s) are the most appropriate for the patient.

- High-dose steroids (dexamethasone IV 4 mg/6h). These should be started while waiting for MRI scan, if the clinical picture suggests cord compression
- Radiotherapy to the metastasis or tumour causing cord compression, particularly if there are multiple sites of cord compression or if surgery is not advised
- Surgical decompression of the cord, reconstruction, and stabilizing the spinal column
- Catheter, if in urinary retention
- Care for pressure areas
- Deep vein thrombosis prophylaxis
- Consider chemotherapy, if appropriate, for underlying cancer causing the spinal cord compression, once the initial treatment has taken place
- Rehabilitation, ideally in unit with spinal cord expertise.
- Early referral to physiotherapists and occupational therapists with oncology expertise.

A Dutch study showed 66% of patients with metastatic cord compression (from all cancers) admitted to rehabilitation centres were discharged and the average survival post-discharge was 808 days. 52% were alive at 1 y.

Prognosis

Patients who are mobile at presentation have the best prognosis and are likely to have preserved neurological function following treatment. If there is some preserved motor function, 30% will be able to walk post-treatment. If paraplegia is present pre-treatment, <10% will be able to walk afterwards. Loss of bladder function for >24–48 h cannot be reversed.

Further information

Conway R et al. What happens to people after malignant cord compression? Survival, function, quality of life, emotional well-being and place of care 1 month after diagnosis. *Clin Oncol* 2007;**19**: 56–62.

Eriks IE et al. Epidural metastatic spinal cord compression: functional outcome and survival after in-patient rehabilitation. *Spinal Cord* 2004;**42**: 235–239.

Pulmonary carcinoid tumours

These are uncommon 1° lung tumours, comprising 1–2% of all tumours. More common in women; typical age 40–50 y. A form of neuroendocrine tumour and can have similar histology to SCLC. Occasionally associated with multiple endocrine neoplasia type 1 (MEN1).

Pathophysiology

Although typically slow-growing benign tumours, more aggressive subtypes exist, with metastatic potential. Commonly, located endobronchially but can also be located peripherally in the lung.

Clinical features

- Endobronchial carcinoids can cause isolated wheeze, dyspnoea, infection, haemoptysis, or persistent lobar collapse
- Parenchymal carcinoids are often asymptomatic, being detected on routine CXR
- Carcinoid syndrome, with flushing, tachycardia, sweats, diarrhoea, wheeze, and hypotension, occurs in 2–5% of pulmonary carcinoid tumours, predominantly when there are liver metastases
- Carcinoid tumours can also be associated with Cushing's syndrome, due to ectopic ACTH production (occurs in 1–2%).

Investigations

- *CXR* may reveal a well-defined tumour, which should be further characterized on CT. *Tumourlets* are multiple endobronchial or parenchymal carcinoid tumours <0.5 cm. PET has decreased sensitivity for detecting carcinoid tumours, compared with NSCLC (75% in one study), but is frequently used, particularly for more aggressive atypical carcinoids. Octreotide scan or Ga^{68}-DOTA-Octreotate PET have a role in staging, particularly for typical carcinoids
- *Baseline bloods* including renal, bone profile, and plasma chromogranin A levels. For Carcinoid syndrome, measure 24 h urine 5HIAA levels. For Cushing's syndrome, measure serum cortisol and ACTH, and 24 h urine cortisol levels
- *Bronchoscopy* is performed for endobronchial carcinoid tumours. They typically appear intraluminal, cherry red, and covered with intact epithelium. Brushings may be adequate for diagnosis. Biopsy had been previously thought to be associated with risk of significant bleeding, although case series suggest risk likely low. Some avoid biopsy altogether and proceed to surgical resection, based on clinical diagnosis. CT-guided biopsy for peripheral tumours
- *Histological diagnosis* can be difficult, as appearances can be similar to SCLC. Special stains and immunohistochemistry are used to help differentiate. Clinically, however, these tend to be quite different conditions, and clinical details can aid pathological diagnosis. Carcinoid tumours are characterized as being *typical* or *atypical*. They each have a characteristic pattern:

- *Typical carcinoids* have no necrosis, occasional nuclear pleomorphism, and <2 mitoses/2 mm² (10 HPFs). Distant metastases are rare, and metastasis to lymph nodes occurs in 5–20% of cases. The 5-y survival is 87–100%, and 10 y survival is 82–87%
- *Atypical carcinoids* may show focal necrosis and often have nuclear pleomorphism. Increased mitotic activity – 2 to 10 mitoses/2 mm² (10 HPFs). Increased levels of Ki-67 expression (Ki-67 'labelling index', an immunohistochemical marker of cell proliferation) is used by some, but this does not reliably distinguish from typical carcinoids. Distant metastases in ~20% and metastasize to the lymph nodes in 30–70% of cases. The 5-y survival is 30–95%, and 10-y survival is 35–56%
- Association with *DIPNECH* (diffuse idiopathic pulmonary neuroendocrine cell hyperplasia). Extremely rare widespread neuroendocrine cell hyperplasia and tumourlets. It is regarded as a pre-invasive lesion, including for carcinoid tumours.

Management

- Should be coordinated by a neuroendocrine tumour MDT
- Isolated pulmonary carcinoid tumours should be considered for surgical resection, usually lobectomy with nodal dissection. Resection is ideally limited, removing minimal amounts of normal lung parenchyma (e.g. a sleeve resection is favoured over pneumonectomy). Tumour resection is associated with resolution of any features of the carcinoid syndrome
- Endobronchial resection may be rarely possible in highly selected patients with an intraluminal polypoid tumour with no CT evidence of an extraluminal component. Careful bronchoscopic and imaging follow-up is essential
- Tumour size does not relate to the presence of lymph node metastases, and, therefore, local lymph nodes should be systematically sampled perioperatively

Metastatic carcinoid

- QoL and disease trajectory are primarily used to determine treatment for metastatic carcinoid
- Isolated liver metastases can be treated with resection, arterial embolization, or radiofrequency ablation
- **Hormonal overproduction** (30% of advanced carcinoids) can be controlled with somatostatin analogues (SSA), e.g. octreotide/ lanreotide (for Carcinoid syndrome) and ketoconazole/metyrapone (for Cushing's syndrome). Other options include liver debulking/ embolization, SSA with interferon and peptide receptor radiotargeted therapy (PRRT) (see next point)

- **Bulk of disease** may be stabilized with an SSA, local ablative treatments (radiological embolization/radiotherapy/surgical) or PRRT, e.g. ^{90}Yttrium-DOTA octreotide and ^{177}Lutetium DOTA octreotide, is considered when a Gallium or Octreotide scan is positive (suggesting likely benefit to PRRT). For advanced unresectable progressive carcinoid, chemotherapy may be given, although limited trial efficacy data mean there is no standard regime. Typical regimes - 5-fluorouracil, dacarbazine, and temozolomide alone or in combination, but also combinations of 5-FU with streptozotocin or oxaliplatin. Role for other drugs, such as mTOR inhibitors (e.g. everolimus), with a possible benefit associated with addition of everolimus to long-acting octreotide therapy.

Further information

Caplin ME et al. Pulmonary neuroendocrine (carcinoid) tumors: European Neuroendocrine Tumor Society expert consensus and recommendations for best practice for typical and atypical pulmonary carcinoids. *Ann Oncol.* 2015;**26**(8): 1604–1620.

Pulmonary nodules 1

Definition

Focal, round, or oval areas of increased opacity in the lung, measuring ≤3 cm in diameter. Divided into solid and sub-solid nodules (SSN). SSN are subdivided into pure GG nodules (pGGN) and part solid nodules (PSN). Greater use of CT and thinner slice spiral CT scanning has led to increased detection rates. CT allows localization of a nodule and determination of its features. Use of maximum intensity projection (MIP) with CT images assists detection of nodules. Volumetric analysis using CT-aided software aids nodule characterization and assesses whether its volume has increased over time.

Table 32.2 Causes of pulmonary nodules

Benign	Malignant
Intrapulmonary lymph node	Lung cancer
Infectious granulomata	Solitary metastasis
Non-infectious granulomata	
Bronchial adenoma	
Benign hamartoma (developmental abnormality, containing cartilage, epithelium, and fat. Can contain smooth muscle. Slow-growing. Can be seen at any age, especially 40+; often calcify)	

- Table 32.2 lists causes of nodules, many of which are benign
- 20–30% of patients with lung cancer present with a solitary nodule
- Of the nodules detected on CT in smokers with a normal CXR, 1–2.5% will be malignant
- Nodule prevalence in a 55–74 yo screening population with a significant smoking history is 26% with lung cancer prevalence of 1%
- The Early Lung Cancer Action Project screening programme in the USA used CT scans in over-60-year-olds, with at least a 10-pack year history of smoking, and found non-calcified nodules in 23%, which were seen on CXR in 7%. Of these nodules, 11% were malignant
- Early detection of these malignant nodules might alter the management of the patient, with surgical resection of a stage I cancer
- There is increasing recognition of premalignant/minimally invasive adenocarcinomas and their CT features. Atypical adenomatous hyperplasia (AAH; premalignant) is typically a pGGN <5mm on CT; adenocarcinoma in situ (AIS; premalignant) is a pGGN 5–30 mm; minimally invasive adenocarcinoma (MIA; premalignant) is a PSN with solid area <5 mm.

Management of patients with pulmonary nodules

- Various different algorithms for management of pulmonary nodules, including BTS and Fleischner Society guidelines
- Always look for previous CT imaging, including from other hospitals. These may confirm stability of nodules for many years, rendering further imaging unnecessary
- Differentiate between solid and subsolid nodules—subsolid nodules require longer follow up
- Volumetric analysis of nodules is preferable to linear measurements
- Brock and Herder models are used to calculate risk of malignancy. See ♒ http://www.brit-thoracic.org.uk/quality-improvement/quality-standards/pulmonary-nodules/

For solid pulmonary nodules

- Follow-up nodules which are ≥5 mm or ≥80 mm³. Smaller nodules do not need follow-up unless history of malignancy
- For nodules ≥8 mm or ≥300 mm³, undertake Brock model assessment of malignancy. When malignancy risk <10%, imaging following-up (at 3 mo then 12 mo unless 5–6 mm, in which case 12 mo). If malignancy risk ≥10%, undertake PET/CT then further Herder model risk assessment. If this shows risk <10%, continue ongoing CT follow-up. For risk 10–70%, consider biopsy or CT follow-up. For risk >70%, consider excision (±biopsy)
- When interval CT demonstrates growth/volume doubling time (VDT) ≤400 days, consider treatment (±biopsy). For VDT 400–600 days, consider biopsy/ongoing surveillance. For VDT >600 days, CT surveillance or discharge reasonable.

For SSN nodules

- Follow-up nodules ≥5 mm. Smaller nodules do not need follow-up unless history of malignancy
- Repeat CT at 3 mo. If enlarging size or enlarging/new solid component, consider treatment. If stable, undertake Brock model risk of malignancy and also consider morphology (adverse = solid component, pleural indentation, bubble-like appearance)
- For malignancy risk <10%, interval CT at 1, 2, and 4 y from baseline if stable. For risk >10%, consider biopsy/resection/observation.

PET/CT scan

Useful in lesions >7 mm. Malignancy sensitivity >95%, specificity >80%. False positives with granulomatous, infectious, and inflammatory nodules. False negatives with low metabolic activity tumours (e.g. bronchoalveolar cell carcinomas).

Biopsy

Difficult on small nodules <7 mm and those behind a rib or scapula.

Resection

For confirmed cancer, enlarging nodules, and those with high clinical/radiographic likelihood of malignancy consider lobectomy, or anatomical segmentectomy if borderline fitness. Nodule may need to be localized with CT preoperatively, using a radiographically placed hook wire or injection of methylene blue.

Radiotherapy (e.g. SABR)

This or CT guided microwave/radiofrequency ablation (under general anaesthetic) if nodule proven to be malignant, but surgical treatment is not indicated due to PS.

Pulmonary nodules 2

Factors that suggest a pulmonary nodule is malignant

- Size >1 cm
- Smokers, older age
- Increasing volume with time (volume doubling time 30–480 days, although low grade tumours may have doubling time up to 900 days)
- Enhancement with contrast, suggesting increased vascularity (>15 Hounsfield units)
- Increased FDG uptake with PET, compared with normal tissue. Estimated sensitivity of PET is 97% for identifying cancer
- Occult extrathoracic disease identified on PET scanning
- Irregular or spiculated margin, with distortion of adjacent vessels—the 'corona radiata' sign. Pleural indentation with nodule
- Associated GG shadowing
- Cavitation with thick irregular walls
- Upper lobe location.

Factors that suggest a pulmonary nodule is benign

- Stable or decreasing size for 2 y
- Nodule resolves during follow-up
- Non-smoker
- Lack of enhancement with contrast
- Smooth, well-defined margins (although 21% of smooth nodules may be malignant)
- Benign pattern of calcification: central, diffuse solid, laminated, or 'popcorn-like'—related to prior infections or calcification in a hamartoma. Follow-up not required
- Small perifissural and subpleural nodules with triangular or lentiform shape—these are intrapulmonary lymph nodes. Follow-up not required
- Intranodular fat—likely hamartoma
- Cavitation with thin smooth walls
- Younger age
- Resident in histoplasmosis endemic areas such as North America.

Pulmonary nodule with extrathoracic malignancy

In a patient with pre-existing malignancy, a pulmonary nodule could be a metastasis, new lung cancer, or benign disease. The histology of the extrapulmonary neoplasm and the patient's smoking history influence this. These cases need discussion within the cancer MDT to determine whether nodule biopsy or treatment of the underlying 1° cancer would be the most appropriate management.

One study determined the likelihood of a pulmonary nodule being a new 1° or metastasis, based on the site of the original cancer.

* *New lung 1° more likely* if the 1° tumour is head and neck, bladder, breast, bile ducts, oesophagus, ovary, prostate, stomach
* *Metastasis more likely* if the 1° tumour is melanoma, sarcoma, testes
* *Either new 1° or metastasis possible* if the 1° tumour is salivary gland, adrenal, colon, parotid, kidney, thyroid, thymus, uterus.

Further information

Callister ME et al. British Thoracic Society guidelines for the investigation and management of pulmonary nodules. *Thorax* 2015;**70**(Suppl 2): ii1–ii54.

MacMahon H et al. Guidelines for management of incidental pulmonary nodules detected on CT Images: From the Fleischner Society 2017. *Radiology* 2017;**284**(1): 228–243.

Lung cancer screening

This is an area that is currently under investigation. Screening programmes are based on the premise that the early detection of lung cancer and any subsequent intervention will improve the patient's survival. To be detectable on CXR, a lung cancer needs to be 1 cm diameter and 3–4 mm diameter to be detectable on CT. Low-dose CT (LDCT) has been used for screening studies, delivering an average dose of 1.5 mSv, compared with 8 mSv for a standard CT. LDCT finds nodules in 10–50% of those screened, and these have a significant false positive rate of 96% (CXR, 95%). These false positives may be associated with morbidity from biopsy/unnecessary treatment or psychological harm. Uncertain overdiagnosis rate, i.e. cancers that would not progress in a patient's lifetime if not treated. Other changes also detected on LDCT, including emphysema and coronary artery calcification.

There is no evidence of reduction in lung cancer mortality from CXR or sputum cytology screening studies. Mortality benefits associated with LDCT in defined populations.

Screening studies

- Four previous CXR screening studies in the 1970s were negative, of which the *Mayo Lung Project* has been the most studied. This compared 4-monthly CXR and sputum cytology for 6 y in smokers 45 y old or older of 20+/day, with infrequent or no screening in a control group. 206 cancers were found in the study group and 160 in the control group, but all-cause mortality was not affected by screening, even at 20 y
- More recent studies have used low-dose spiral CT scanning. The *Early Lung Cancer Action Project (ELCAP)* in New York recruited 1,000 symptom-free volunteers aged 60+ with a 10-pack year history of smoking, who would be fit for a thoracotomy. There was no control group. Baseline CXR and CT were performed. Non-calcified nodules were present in 23% of patients at baseline on CT. Repeat CT was performed for nodules <5 mm; nodules >6 mm were biopsied, and nodules >11 mm received standard care. 2.7% of all the patients entered had malignant nodules with stage I disease in 2.3%. All but one patient had their cancer surgically resected
- *International ELCAP* screened 31,567 asymptomatic over-40-year-olds at risk for lung cancer between 1993 and 2005. The median age was 61. Of these, 13% had a positive result, requiring follow-up at baseline CT and 5% at annual CT. Lung cancer was diagnosed in 1.5% of people (85% stage I), with 411 having resection and 57 having radiotherapy ± chemotherapy. There was no non-treatment randomized control group, so it is still difficult to interpret whether the earlier diagnosis and intervention led to longer survival

- The *National Lung Screening Trial (NLST)* evaluated annual LDCT vs CXR screening in 53,454 patients aged 55–74 y with a 30-pack year smoking history (including those who quit within 15 y), showing a 20% reduction in lung cancer and 6.7% reduction in all-cause mortality in the CT arm. 320 patients would need to be screened to prevent one lung cancer death. Notably, the trial was delivered in specialist centres, with low complication rates, and such mortality benefits may not be reproducible in other centres
- The *NELSON* European RCT included 15,822 current/former smokers evaluated LDCT screening at increasing screening intervals (1, 2, and 2.5 years), compared with no screening. Final publication of peer-reviewed results awaited but presented data suggests male mortality reduction of 26% at 10 y, female mortality reduction of 39% at 10 y
- Given the results of NLST, American organizations, including the ACCP, have recommended high-risk smokers aged 55–74 should be offered annual LDCT screening, but only if provided in the same care environment as was provided in NLST. CXR and sputum cytology are not recommended. Such screening recommendations are contentious, given ongoing clinical trials, the radiation exposure associated with screening, and lack of evidence for optimal screening duration
- In the UK, there are several pilot studies of LDCT screening and counselling for smoking cessation, but this is not currently nationwide
- The role of PET in screening also needs to be evaluated.

Further information

Detterbeck FC et al. Executive summary. Diagnosis and management of lung cancer, 3rd ed: American College of Chest Physicians Evidence-Based Clinical Practice Guidelines. *Chest* 2013; **143**: 7S–37S.
National Lung Screening Trial Research Team. Reduced lung-cancer mortality with low-dose computed tomographic screening. *N Engl J Med* 2011; **365**: 395–409.

Chapter 33

Mediastinal abnormalities

Introduction 382
Anatomy 384
Mediastinal abnormalities 1 386
Mediastinal abnormalities 2 390

Introduction

The mediastinum is the area within the centre of the chest containing the heart, great vessels, nerves, lymph nodes, trachea, oesophagus, and thymus. Two-thirds of mediastinal masses are benign. Age 20–40 y; presence of symptoms and anterior location of a mass are all associated with an increased likelihood of malignancy. Common symptoms of mediastinal disease include cough, chest pain, and dyspnoea, as well as symptoms relating to any structure being compressed or disrupted such as dysphagia, stridor, superior vena caval obstruction (SVCO), or Horner's syndrome. Systemic effects (night sweats, weight loss in lymphoma) and paraneoplastic effects (e.g. myasthenia with thymoma) may be seen. Mediastinal disorders can also be asymptomatic. They may be found incidentally following a chest radiograph (CXR).

Anatomy

Divided into three or four compartments to aid diagnosis. The 2017 ITMIG (International Thymic Malignancy Interest Group) statement favours a three-compartment paradigm (in which the superior compartment is omitted) based on cross-sectional anatomy.

Prevascular (anterior) mediastinum

The area behind the body of the sternum and in front of the fibrous pericardium and great vessels. Contains thymus, fat, lymph nodes and left brachiocephalic vein.

Paravertebral (posterior) mediastinum

The area adjacent to the vertebral bodies containing the thoracic spine, neurovascular bundles, spinal ganglia, sympathetic chain and lymphatic tissue.

Visceral (middle) mediastinum

Anterior to a vertical line connecting a point on each thoracic vertebral body 1 cm posterior to its anterior margin. Contains heart and pericardium, great vessels, thoracic duct, trachea, carina, oesophagus, and lymph nodes. These compartments and structures are represented in Fig. 33.1.

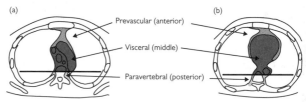

Fig. 33.1 Mediastinal compartments at level of (a) aortic arch and (b) left atrium.

Likely nature of mediastinal mass according to anatomical site

Anterior mediastinal mass
- Thymus (thymoma, thymic cyst, thymic hyperplasia, thymic carcinoma)
- Lymphoma
- Thyroid goitre
- Parathyroid adenoma
- Germ cell tumour (GCT; teratoma, seminoma, non-seminomatous GCT)
- Lipoma
- Morgagni anterior diaphragmatic hernia (see ⊃ p. 398).

Middle mediastinal mass
- Bronchogenic cyst
- Pericardial cyst
- Lymphadenopathy (lymphoma, sarcoid, metastatic carcinoma)
- Foregut duplication/cyst
- Oesophageal cancer
- Vascular abnormalities.

Posterior mediastinal mass
- Neural tumour (incl. neurofibroma, neurosarcoma)
- Meningoceles
- Spinal lesions.

Approach to the patient with a mediastinal mass
- Full history
- Examination, including skin, lymphadenopathy (neck, axillae, groins), and testes
- Look for fatigability: ptosis, ophthalmoplegia, inability to maintain upward gaze
- Look for signs of SVCO or stridor
- Blood tests, including alpha-fetoprotein (AFP), beta human chorionic gonadotrophin (βHCG), anti-acetylcholine receptor (AChR) antibody
- CXR
- Computed tomography (CT) chest (± magnetic resonance imaging (MRI)/positron emission tomography (PET)/CT in some cases)
- Locate previous imaging.

Mediastinal abnormalities 1

Neural tumours

Mostly occur in the posterior mediastinum. 75% are benign in adults. MRI often helpful in assessment.

- *Schwannomas and neurofibromas* are benign peripheral nerve sheath tumours. They may be multiple. Usually asymptomatic, although can cause segmental pain. Slowly enlarge and rarely can cause cord compression, with dumbbell-shaped tumours straddling the intervertebral foramen. Can be surgically excised
- *Malignant peripheral nerve sheath tumours or neurosarcomas* include new malignant growths and benign neurofibromas that have undergone malignant change. They may cause systemic features of malignancy and can invade locally and metastasize.
- *Autonomic nervous system tumours*, including neuroblastomas and ganglioneuromas, range from benign to malignant. Surgical removal is the treatment of choice, with radiotherapy and chemotherapy if the tumour is malignant.

Thymoma

Tumour of epithelial origin arising in the thymus. May contain functioning thymic tissue. $\male = \female$. Rare below age 20. Myasthenia gravis is present in 30–40% of patients with a thymoma; this is often unimproved after thymectomy and may even develop after the thymoma is removed. 20% of patients presenting with myasthenia gravis are found to have a thymoma, particularly if patients are over 50 and $\male$. This group is likely to have positive AChR autoantibodies, which bind to AChRs at the post-synaptic motor endplate, decreasing available acetylcholine binding sites, causing nerve fatigability.

Patients with thymomas are usually symptomatic with pain, dyspnoea, dysphagia, or myasthenia gravis symptoms. Many other associated paraneoplastic syndromes have been noted including pure red cell aplasia and Good syndrome (acquired hypogammaglobulinaemia and thymoma associated with recurrent infections, diarrhoea, and lymphadenopathy).

Thymomas contained within the thymic capsule tend to be benign, although they do have malignant potential; those that have extended outside the capsule are malignant and may involve local structures or metastasize. Widely staged using Masaoka–Koga staging system (Box 33.1), but 8th AJCC/UICC/IASLC tumour, node, metastasis (TNM) staging now recommended (Box 33.2). World Health Organization histology classification system defines type based on morphology into A, AB, B1, B2, and B3 with relevance to prognosis (B3 worse).

Diagnose with CT, and treat with surgical excision of the thymus, avoiding prior FNA or biopsy, as this may cause tumour seeding outside the capsule.

Consider post-operative radiotherapy and chemotherapy for invasive tumours, especially those not completely excised. Thymectomy is often indicated in patients with myasthenia gravis, even without thymoma, as it may lead to symptomatic improvement. This gives best results in those with detectable AChR antibody levels and younger patients early in the disease course, particularly those with severe disease.

Box 33.1 Masaoka–Koga thymoma staging system

Stage I	Encapsulated without invasion
	Treated with surgical resection
Stage II	Invasion beyond capsule

Stage II Invasion beyond capsule

     IIa–Microscopic capsular invasion

     IIb–Macroscopic capsular invasion into fat or stuck to (without extension through) mediastinal pleura or pericardium

Treated with surgical resection and post-operative radiotherapy (PORT)

Stage III Invasion into other organ (lung, pericardium, vessel)

Treated with surgical resection and PORT

Stage IV Metastatic

     IVa–Pleural / pericardial metastasis

     IVb–Metastasis elsewhere

Treated with debulking surgery, chemotherapy, radiotherapy.

Box 33.2 8th edition of the TNM staging system for thymoma (IASLC/UICC/AJCC)

Extent of 1° tumour (T)
Tx   1° tumour cannot be assessed
T0   No evidence of 1° tumour
T1   Encapsulated/involving fat (T1a) or mediastinal pleura (T1b)
T2   Pericardial involvement
T3   Lung, brachiocephalic vein, SVC, phrenic nerve, chest wall, pulmonary artery, or vein involvement
T4   Aorta (+ branches), intrapericardial pulmonary artery, myocardium, oesophagus, or trachea involvement.

Regional lymph nodes (N)
Nx   Cannot be assessed
N0   No regional lymph node metastasis
N1   Anterior mediastinal nodes
N2   Other intrathoracic or cervical nodes

Distant metastasis (M)
Mx   Cannot be assessed
M0   No distant metastasis
M1   Pleural, pericardial or other metastases present
        M1a–Pleural/pericardial nodules
        M1b–Pulmonary nodule or distant metastases

Stage	TNM classification
I	T1 N0 M0
II	T2 N0 M0
IIIA	T3 N0 M0
IIIB	T4 N0 M0
IVA	Any T, N1, M0
	Any T, N0-1, M1a
IVB	If any N2 disease
	If any M1b disease

Thymic cyst

- May be congenital or acquired 2° to inflammation
- Asymptomatic unless large and causing symptoms of compression
- Benign but usually treated with surgical excision, as diagnostic certainty may be difficult.

Thymic carcinoid

- Not associated with myasthenia gravis and behaves aggressively, with local recurrence and metastasis
- May be associated with Cushing's syndrome
- Treatment with surgery, chemotherapy, radiotherapy or octreotide
- *Also:* thymic carcinoma, thymic lipoma, and thymic hyperplasia.

Germ cell tumours

Arise from immature germ cells, which fail to migrate during development. Tend to be in an anterior and midline location.

- *Mature cystic teratomas* represent 80% of germ cell tumours. These are benign and occur in young adults. ♂=♀. Often asymptomatic but can erode surrounding structures and cause symptoms. Serum AFP is normal. CXR shows well-defined mass, which may contain flecks of calcification. Potential for malignant degeneration. Treatment is by surgical excision
- *Seminoma* occurs in men age 20–40 y. Mediastinal seminomas are malignant and almost always arise within the thymus and are histologically indistinguishable from those occurring in the testes. Can be 1° mediastinal tumour or metastasis from testicular tumour; therefore, always examine testes and perform US. Patients frequently present with chest pain. CXR shows non-calcified lobulated anterior mediastinal mass, confirmed with CT. Serum AFP is normal, and this aids diagnosis. Diagnose with biopsy. Up front surgical excision is not recommended as is usually incomplete. Treatment is with cisplatin-based chemotherapy initially, which can cause infertility, and therefore patients may wish to consider sperm banking before treatment. Tumours are radiosensitive, so radiotherapy used if they are bulky. Long-term survival expected in 80%. Better prognosis than non-seminomatous germ cell tumours
- *Non-seminomatous germ cell tumours* (including choriocarcinoma, teratocarcinoma, and yolk sac tumours) are all malignant and occur in men in their 30s. They are symptomatic due to local invasion, and they metastasize. CXR shows mediastinal mass, and diagnosis is with biopsy. βHCG and AFP are raised and fall with tumour response. Treatment is with cisplatin-based chemotherapy. Radiological residual disease is usually subsequently resected.

Thyroid

Retrosternal goitre occurs, especially in older women. Usually asymptomatic unless large and compressing the trachea, causing dyspnoea and stridor. May be seen on plain CXR. CT and radioactive iodine isotope scans are helpful in diagnosis. Flow–volume loops are abnormal if there is tracheal compression. Surgery is recommended if there is airway compromise but can lead to tracheomalacia afterwards.
Also: parathyroid adenoma.

Mediastinal abnormalities 2

Lymphoma

The mediastinum is frequently involved in patients with Hodgkin's lymphoma. CT scan is necessary to assess the extent of this and to assess response to treatment. To establish the histological diagnosis of lymphoma, an adequate tissue sample is required; this should be from a biopsy, rather than a fine-needle aspirate (which is not usually enough for diagnosis). This may be best achieved surgically via mediastinoscopy. Examine patient for peripheral lymph nodes, as these may be easier to biopsy. Treatment is with chemotherapy initially.

Enlarged lymph nodes

- *Metastases* from breast, lung, and oesophageal cancer
- *Castleman's disease* (CD; angiofollicular lymph node hyperplasia) Giant lymph node hyperplasia. Rare. Two forms:
  - *Unicentric CD (UCD)* involves a single region of the body. In the chest, can cause mediastinal or hilar lymph node mass. Often asymptomatic or may cause cough or wheeze due to localized compression. Non-progressive. May have fever and raised ESR. Nodal biopsy shows follicles of pericapillary lymphocytes and proliferation of the plump and eosinophilic capillary endothelial cells. Removal of node(s) may improve symptoms and be curative. May not require treatment. Can also occur on pleura
  - *Multicentric CD (MCD)* involves multiple regions of the body. More aggressive disease that has two subtypes: (a) human herpesvirus 8 (HHV-8) associated MCD in immunosuppressed (usually HIV) and (b) idiopathic MCD (iMCD). MCD is a lymphoproliferative disorder with prominent systemic symptoms (night sweats, fatigue, weight loss) as well as generalized lymph node enlargement, hepatosplenomegaly, paraproteinaemia, and skin rash. Biopsy shows prominent plasma cell infiltration. Related to IL6 overproduction. Treatment for HHV-8-MCD is with rituximab first line, which induces remission in a high percentage of patients. For HHV-8-MCD patients with aggressive disease or poor performance status, rituximab ± steroids ± chemotherapy may be preferred first line, but prognosis is poor. Treatment for iMCD is complex but may include IL-6 blockade (siltuximab) ± steroids ± chemotherapy. MCD can progress to lymphoma and is rapidly fatal without treatment
- *Also:* lymphangioma.

Cysts

- *Enteric or bronchogenic cysts* can be related to the oesophagus or the airways, especially near the carina. Lined by intestinal/gastric or respiratory epithelium. Often diagnosed in childhood, as they cause dyspnoea, stridor, or cough due to limited space to expand. Seen on CXR and CT and treated with surgical excision
- *Pleuropericardial cysts* mostly occur at the cardiophrenic angles and can measure up to 25 cm diameter. ♂=♀. Usually asymptomatic but may cause chest pain. CXR shows smooth, round shadow abutting the heart. Excision can be carried out at thoracoscopy, but conservative management is favoured. Also known as springwater cysts.

Inflammation

- *Mediastinitis* occurs after oesophageal perforation or rupture, due to malignancy, instrumentation, or vomiting (Boerhaave's syndrome). Patients are ill, with pain and fever. CXR may show widened mediastinum or air in the mediastinum. Pneumothorax or pleural effusion may also be seen. Treatment includes repairing the defect, parenteral feeding, and antibiotics. High morbidity and mortality
- *Mediastinal fibrosis* Rare idiopathic condition that occurs in middle age. Symptoms depend on which aspects of the mediastinum are involved but may include dyspnoea, wheeze, haemoptysis, hoarse voice, dysphagia, PHT, SVCO. CXR shows a widened mediastinum. Diagnosis made on biopsy, particularly to exclude malignancy. Treatment is supportive; steroids and surgical debulking ineffective. Prognosis variable, depending on sites involved. May be associated with retroperitoneal fibrosis, radiotherapy, methysergide, autoimmune disease, or infection with TB, histoplasmosis, *Aspergillus*, or *Nocardia*.

Mediastinal emphysema

Pneumomediastinum. Can be caused by sneezing, straining, Valsalva man-oeuvres, vomiting, substance abuse, parturition, positive pressure ventilation, instrumentation, or TBB. Usually symptomless but occasional pain. Hamman's sign may be present (click with each heartbeat on auscultation over lung). Treat with high-flow O_2. Resolves spontaneously.

Vascular

Aortic aneurysms are usually asymptomatic, but symptoms relate to compression of adjacent structures. May diagnose on CXR as a widened mediastinum. This is best imaged via CT or MRI. Surgery should be considered to prevent death from rupture.

Further information

Duwe BV et al. Tumors of the mediastinum. *Chest* 2005;**128**: 2893–2909.

Carter BW et al. ITMIG classification of mediastinal compartments and multidisciplinary approach to mediastinal masses. *Radiographics* 2017;37(2):413–436.

⌘ http://www.iaslc.org/Research-Education/IASLC-Staging-Project/Staging-Educational-Materials

Paediatric lung disorders

Chronic lung disease of prematurity *394*
Virus associated wheeze (VAW) *396*
Congenital abnormalities *398*
Transition *400*

Chronic lung disease of prematurity

Chronic lung disease of prematurity (CLD)

Formerly (and still in the USA) known as bronchopulmonary dysplasia (BPD). Advances in neonatal medicine have led to improved survival of premature babies with immature lungs and respiratory disease. Babies born at lower gestational ages are surviving into adulthood, due to therapy with antenatal steroids to prevent respiratory distress syndrome and the use of artificial surfactant to decrease the surface tension of the neonatal alveolar membrane. There have also been improvements in ventilatory techniques, and CLD usually occurs in babies who have been mechanically ventilated. Most long-term studies have been on patients before these improvements in management.

Usual causes

- Volutrauma from prolonged ventilation
- High-pressure ventilation
- Ventilation with high O_2 concentrations.

Typical presentation

Premature baby remaining O_2-dependent after 36 weeks post-conceptional age. Infrequent in those born at 32+ weeks and weighing >1,500 g. May require prolonged home O_2 therapy, up to 1 y or beyond. 50% of infants will need hospital re-admission during their first year with respiratory infection. Some have significant pulmonary sequelae during childhood and adolescence: airways hyperreactivity, persistent wheeze, chronic hypoxaemia, and pulmonary hypertension (PHT). Duration of O_2 dependence predicts long-term sequelae. May also have additional disabilities associated with prematurity such as cerebral palsy or learning difficulties.

Pathology

Cytokine-mediated scarring and repair.

- *Early inflammatory phase*: bronchial necrosis, alveolar destruction, capillary permeability, and associated obliterative bronchiolitis.
- *Subacute fibroproliferative phase*: type II pneumocyte hyperplasia, bronchial and bronchial smooth muscle hypertrophy, and interstitial and perialveolar fibrosis.
- *Chronic fibroproliferative phase*: airway remodelling for up to 1 y and bronchial wall thickening. Prior to surfactant use, these changes were more severe.

Pulmonary function tests (PFTs)

Functional respiratory abnormalities persist with increased airway resistance and airway hyperresponsiveness. Residual volume (RV) and RV/total lung capacity (TLC) are raised, indicative of air trapping. Air trapping improves over 3–4 y as lung growth occurs; however, small airway abnormalities persist, at least until the age of 10 y. A cohort will not achieve expected normal lung volumes and therefore may have fixed-airway obstruction/chronic obstructive pulmonary disease (COPD) in adult life without accelerated lung function decline or smoking. Expired nitrous oxide (NO) levels are usually not raised, indicating a non-eosinophilic-driven process.

Chest radiology

Persisting mild to moderate abnormalities, multifocal areas of reduced lung attenuation and perfusion, bronchial wall thickening, and decreased bronchus/pulmonary artery diameter ratios on computed tomography (CT). Radiological abnormalities correlate with physiological evidence of air trapping.

PHT

Occurs commonly when persistent lung disease; complex pathophysiological factors. Tends to improve with age.

Adulthood

Few longitudinal studies beyond adolescence. Longitudinal studies show airflow obstruction without eosinophilia. Common high-resolution computed tomography (HRCT) findings include subpleural opacities and expiratory gas trapping but not emphysematous change. It is likely that individuals, even without smoking, will have significant fixed airflow obstruction in later adult life, similar to individuals with COPD. There are no evidence-based consensus guidelines for management and individual disease traits (such as fixed/variable airflow obstruction, airway inflammation and hypoxaemia) should be considered and treated as appropriate.

Further information

Tracy and Berkelhamer. Bronchopulmonary dysplasia and pulmonary outcomes of prematurity. *Pediatric Ann* 2019;**48**: e148–e153.

Bolton et al. Lung consequences in adults born prematurely *Thorax* 2015,**70**. 574–500.

Caskey et al. Structural and functional lung impairment in adult survivors of bronchopulmonary dysplasia *Ann Am Thorac Soc* 2016;**13**: 1262–1270.

Virus associated wheeze (VAW)

A controversial area. Wheezing is common in infants and toddlers and is often due to viral respiratory tract infections (particularly respiratory syncytial virus or human rhinovirus), causing VAW. VAW is associated with maternal smoking, contact with other children, and not being breastfed. This transient early wheezing is common, affecting 50% of pre-school children, and is distinct from childhood asthma. Children affected by VAW are often not atopic and may have no family history of atopy, and usually have no symptoms in the interval between viruses. VAW usually resolves by the age of 6 y. VAW without interval symptoms usually does not respond to bronchodilators.

Childhood asthma

Children who develop asthma will usually have a history of VAW. Children with asthma may have a family history of asthma, eczema or atopic dermatitis, may have episodes of wheeze unrelated to viruses, may have food allergies, and may have peripheral blood eosinophilia (≥4%). Half have mild symptoms, which regress by puberty. Those with more severe disease, requiring regular inhaled steroids, often have disease that persists into adult life. Children with asthma are treated similarly to young adults with asthma using a stepwise management approach. In those <5 y oral leukotriene receptor antagonists can be used instead of ICS.

Further information

Miller et al. Wheezing exacerbations in early childhood: evaluation, treatment, and recent advances relevant to the genesis of asthma *J Allergy Clin Immunol Pract* 2014;**2**: 537–543.

Martinez et al. Asthma and wheezing in the first six years of life. The Group Health Medical Association. *NEJM* 1995;**332**: 133–138.

Gough et al. General and respiratory health outcomes in adult survivors of bronchopulmonary dysplasia: a systematic review. *Chest* 2012;**141**: 1554–1567.

Dogaru et al. Breastfeeding and childhood asthma: systematic review and meta-analysis *Am J Epidemiol* 2014; **179**: 1153–1167.

Lodge and Dharmage. Breastfeeding and perinatal exposure, and the risk of asthma and allergies. *Curr Opin Allergy Clin Immunol* 2016;**16**: 231–236.

BTS SIGN Guideline (158) of the management of asthma 2019 ℘ https://www.brit-thoracic.org.uk/quality-improvement/guidelines/asthma/

Congenital abnormalities

Tracheomalacia

Floppy trachea, can be associated with oesophageal atresia, and rarely associated with CLD of prematurity. Rarely will require intubation or tracheostomy. For further information see ⊃ p. 712.

Congenital lobar emphysema

Often idiopathic but overinflation of a lobe can be due to localized bronchomalacia or bronchial obstruction. May cause wheeze or produce chest deformity. Rarely resolves spontaneously.

Diaphragmatic hernia

A diaphragmatic defect, causing abdominal contents to be present in the chest (e.g. bowel, liver). This may cause respiratory distress soon after birth and may have been detected during the antenatal period by US, or occasionally when the defect is small can be completely asymptomatic and found incidentally on chest radiograph (CXR), with bowel seen in the chest. There are two types:

- *Bochdalek hernia* The congenital absence of posterolateral part of diaphragm, with associated hypoplastic lung due to bowel limiting growth. Treatment is with surgical repair of the diaphragmatic defect, but survival rate is only 50% due to underlying lung problems
- *Morgagni hernia* Anteromedial herniation through the foramen of Morgagni, which is more commonly found in adulthood. It may be asymptomatic or cause symptoms of fullness, tightness, or pain in the anterior chest; it does not cause intestinal obstruction. CXR shows a cardiophrenic angle density. Surgical repair is difficult and is usually not necessary.

Cystic adenomatoid lung

Cystic and adenomatous abnormalities arising from defective branching morphogenesis in the lung. Can affect any lobe. Presentation is variable. Can be diagnosed antenatally and often newborns are asymptomatic. Can cause neonatal respiratory distress or can present later in childhood with recurrent infection. May be mistaken for diaphragmatic hernia. Treatment is by resection of the affected lobe for symptomatic patients. Surgical resection in asymptomatic patients is more controversial.

Pulmonary sequestration/sequestrated segment

Segment of lung parenchyma with no bronchial connection that is unventilated. May be supplied by aberrant artery from the aorta and have anomalous pulmonary drainage to the right atrium. Can be intra-lobar, sharing pleura with the rest of the lung, or extra-lobar, which is separated from the lung by a lining of pleural tissue. Mostly left-sided; 75% are situated between the diaphragm and left lower lobe. Often associated with other congenital abnormalities. Can be a chance finding on CXR at any age, when cystic change may be seen in this area. Contrast CT or magnetic resonance imaging may aid diagnosis. Surgical resection may be necessary if there is repeated infection in this segment.

MacLeod's (or Swyer–James or Brett's) syndrome

A rare disease characterized by hyperlucency of lung or lobe, due to loss of parenchymal and vascular structure which may following childhood post infective obliterative bronchiolitis. CXR shows a hypertranslucent lung with reduced vascular markings and a small pulmonary artery. Commonly associated with recurrent lung infections and bronchiectasis.

Pectus

Pectus excavatum (depression of the anterior chest wall) and pectus carinatum (anterior protrusion of the sternum) are chest wall morphological deformities that are usually recognized during early childhood. The pathogenesis is unknown. They can be part of syndrome including; Marfan's, Noonans', Poland, and Turner's. They can be associated with kyphoscoliosis. Pectus may progress to cause more issues in adult-life including restricted lung volumes (particularly if associated kyphoscoliosis), respiratory infections and bronchiectasis, and heart disease (particularly mitral prolapse). Some cases require surgical treatment.

Transition

Overview

Transition in medical terms describes the process of adolescent patients with chronic health conditions moving under the care of adult services. All chronic respiratory disease patients needing long-term follow-up are likely to transition to adult services but several conditions have formal local transition pathways (muscular dystrophies, spinal muscular atrophy, cerebral palsy, cystic fibrosis—for specific CF transition see ⊃ p. 238). Careful multidisciplinary team handover from paediatric to adult teams is important. Medical transition often coincides with other forms of transition possibly including:

- patient taking responsibility for their own treatments and treatment choices
- leaving full-time education and entering employment
- living independently
- moving away from their childhood home
- financial responsibilities
- forming new relationships
- family planning.

Transition needs careful planning and should take place over several years, probably starting from ~14 y. Toolkits can be a helpful aid to transition.

Further information

Trout et al. A transition toolkit for Duchenne muscular dystrophy. *Pediatrics.* 2018;**142**(**Suppl 2**): S110–S117.

Information about transition for muscular dystrophies: ℅ http://www.musculardystrophyuk.org/assets/0001/6223/Transition_guide_factsheets_web.pdf.

Pleural effusion

Clinical features and imaging 402
Malignant pleural effusion: causes and investigations 404
Malignant pleural effusion: management 408
Parapneumonic effusion and empyema: definition and clinical features 412
Parapneumonic effusion and empyema: bacteriology and investigations 414
Parapneumonic effusion and empyema: management and outcome 416
Tuberculous pleural effusion 420
Other causes of pleural effusion 422

Clinical features and imaging

A pleural effusion results from the accumulation of abnormal volumes (>10–20 mL) of fluid in the pleural space. Pleural effusions are common and are associated with many different diseases; see Chapter 8 for a step-by-step approach to the diagnosis of a patient with a pleural effusion, differential diagnosis of effusions, and details of pleural fluid analysis.

Clinical features

- May be asymptomatic or associated with breathlessness, dry cough, pleuritic chest pain (suggesting pleural inflammation), chest 'heaviness', and sometimes pain referred to the shoulder or abdomen
- Signs on examination include reduced chest expansion, reduced tactile vocal fremitus, a stony dull percussion note, quiet breath sounds, and sometimes a patch of bronchial breathing above the fluid level. A friction rub may be heard with pleural inflammation.

Imaging

Chest radiograph (CXR)

- Sequential blunting of posterior, lateral, and then anterior costophrenic angles are seen on radiographs as effusions increase in size
- Posteroanterior (PA) CXR will usually detect effusion volumes of 200 mL or more; lateral CXR is more sensitive and may detect as little as 50 mL pleural fluid
- Classical CXR appearance is of basal opacity obscuring hemidiaphragm, with concave upper border. Massive effusion may result in a 'white-out' of the hemithorax, with mediastinal displacement away from the effusion; lack of mediastinal shift in such cases raises the possibility of associated volume loss due to bronchial obstruction from a lung cancer
- Other CXR appearances include rounded or lentiform shadowing in loculated interlobar effusions and diffuse shadowing throughout the hemithorax on supine films
- CXR appearance may suggest the underlying diagnosis, e.g. bilateral effusions with cardiomegaly in cardiac failure; massive effusions are most commonly seen due to malignancy.

Ultrasound (US)

See ⊃ p. 895. Has a much higher sensitivity than CXR at detecting and localizing pleural fluid and is useful for distinguishing pleural fluid from pleural masses or thickening. Sonographic appearances can be useful at predicting exudates (echogenic or septated fluid) and for predicting malignancy. Its use for pleural procedures increases success at fluid aspiration and reduces risk of complications.

Computed tomography (CT) chest

With pleural contrast (images acquired 60–90 s post contrast injection) is useful in distinguishing benign and malignant pleural disease: nodular, mediastinal, or circumferential pleural thickening and parietal pleural thickening >1cm are all highly specific for malignant disease. Scans are best performed prior to complete drainage of fluid. CT may also reveal evidence of extrapleural disease, e.g. lymphadenopathy or parenchymal change, which may suggest, e.g. cancer or tuberculosis (TB).

Magnetic resonance imaging (MRI)
Role is unclear; it may have increasing role in distinguishing benign from malignant pleural disease.

Positron emission tomography (PET)/CT
Does not have an established role in evaluating pleural effusions – both benign and malignant aetiologies can cause 18-fluorodeoxyglucose (FDG) avidity. A role in targeting guided biopsies to FDG avid areas is under investigation.

Malignant pleural effusion: causes and investigations

Epidemiology

Most common cause of exudative pleural effusion in patients older than 60 y. About 40,000 cases of malignant effusion each year in the UK.

Causes

Most malignant effusions are metastatic, with lung and breast the most common primary sites (see Table 35.1).

Table 35.1 Primary sites and frequency

Primary site	Approximate frequency (%)
Lung	38
Breast	17
Lymphoma	12
Mesothelioma	10
Genitourinary tract	9
Gastro-intestinal (GI) tract	7
Unknown 1°	11

Other rarer tumours include sarcoma, melanoma, leukaemia, and mye-loma; almost any malignant tumour may spread to the pleural cavity. *Mesothelioma* is an important cause of malignant effusions. For discussion see Ɔ p. 130.

Clinical features

Breathlessness is the main symptom; chest pain, cough, weight loss, and an-orexia may also be present. A small proportion of patients are asymptom-atic. Effusions may be unilateral or bilateral and are frequently large volume.

Differential diagnosis

Consider other potential causes of pleural effusion in patients known to have cancer, e.g. due to pneumonia, pulmonary embolus (PE), radiotherapy, pericardial disease, or drugs.

Investigations

For details of a strategy for investigating the patient with an undiagnosed pleural effusion Ɔ p. 52. Key investigations in patients suspected to have a malignant effusion are:

Pleural fluid cytology

Sensitivity for malignancy is about 60%. Immunostaining of malignant cells may provide clues as to the likely primary site. Visualization of monoclonal cells in fluid on flow cytometry may support a diagnosis of lymphoma.

CT chest, abdomen and pelvis (including pleural-phase contrast)
Nodular, mediastinal, or circumferential pleural thickening and parietal pleural thickening >1cm on CT are highly specific for malignant disease. May also demonstrate extrapleural disease, e.g. lymphadenopathy or suggest a primary.

Pleural biopsy histology
See ⊃ p. 869. Required in cytology-negative cases. Options:
- *CT-guided* cutting needle biopsy has been demonstrated to be a more effective diagnostic test for malignant pleural disease than Abrams' pleural biopsy (sensitivity 87% in CT-guided biopsy group vs 47% in Abrams' group)
- *US-guided* needle biopsies are also effective and relatively straightforward to perform
- *Thoracoscopy* (see ⊃ p. 907) is an extremely useful investigation allowing direct visualization of the pleural space, with a high sensitivity (>92%) for biopsies. Therapeutic talc poudrage (talc is 'puffed' directly on to the pleural surfaces) may be performed at same time, with a pleurodesis success rate >80%. Usually performed using conscious sedation and local anaesthesia. Complications (such as empyema) are rare.

Serum/pleural fluid tumour markers
For example, CEA, CA19-9, CA15-3, CA125, PSA, should not be routinely used for investigation of pleural effusions, having a poor combined sensitivity for malignant disease. Mesothelin has a low sensitivity of 48–84% and specificity 70–100% for mesothelioma and is therefore not routinely recommended.

Prognosis

Median survival 1–12 months from diagnosis; shortest in urological (not renal), melanoma, sarcoma, GI, and lung cancers, longest in mesothelioma, gynaecological, and haematological malignancies. Lower pleural fluid pH may be associated with shorter survival, but this is contentious. The LENT score places patients with malignant pleural effusions into low, moderate, and high-risk categories, with median survival of 319, 130, and 44 days respectively (Table 35.2)

Table 35.2 LENT score for pleural effusion prognostication

L	Pleural fluid LDH (IU/L)	Score
	<1500	0
	>1500	1
E	ECOG Performance Status	
	0	0
	1	1
	2	2
	3-4	3
N	Neutrophil:lymphocyte ratio in blood	
	<9	0
	>9	1
T	Tumour histology	
	Mesothelioma/haematological	0
	Breast/gynaecological/renal cell	1
	Lung/other	2

Total: 0-1 = low risk; 2-4 = moderate risk; 5-7 = high risk

Further information

Roberts ME et al. Management of a malignant pleural effusion: British Thoracic Society pleural disease guideline 2010. *Thorax* 2010;**65**(Suppl. 2): ii32–40.

Maskell NA et al. Standard pleural biopsy vs CT-guided cutting-needle biopsy for diagnosis of malignant disease in pleural effusions: a randomised controlled trial. *Lancet* 2003;**361**: 1326–1331.

Clive AO et al. Predicting survival in malignant pleural effusion: development and validation of the LENT prognostic score. *Thorax* 2014; **69**(12): 1098–1104.

Malignant pleural effusion: management

Key points influencing the management of malignant effusions are:
- Symptoms, performance status, and wishes of the patient
- Sensitivity of the 1° tumour to chemotherapy, e.g. small cell lung carcinoma, lymphoma, ovarian and breast carcinoma may respond to chemotherapy, although, in some cases, pleural effusions remain problematic and require additional treatment
- Extent of lung re-expansion following effusion drainage.

Treatment options

Observation and follow-up if asymptomatic.

Therapeutic pleural aspiration

Remove 1–1.5 L pleural fluid to improve breathlessness (see ➔ p. 891). Allows evaluation for possible non-expandable lung on post-procedure CXR (alternatively, use pleural manometry during aspiration). Can be performed at the bedside as a day-case procedure, avoiding hospital admission. Useful in the palliation of breathlessness in patients with a poor prognosis and in rare cases where effusion reaccumulates very slowly. Most effusions recur within 1 month of aspiration, and these patients should be considered for pleurodesis or indwelling pleural catheter (IPC) insertion; repeated aspiration may be inconvenient and uncomfortable for the patient and carries a risk of complications such as empyema, pneumothorax, and tumour seeding (in mesothelioma).

If the breathlessness does not improve following fluid aspiration, then there is little to be gained by repeated aspiration, and other causes of breathlessness should be considered, e.g. lymphangitis carcinomatosis, PE.

Intercostal chest drainage and pleurodesis

The aim of pleurodesis is to seal the visceral pleura to the parietal pleura with adhesions to prevent pleural fluid accumulating. The success of pleurodesis depends on the degree of apposition of the visceral and parietal pleura, which depends on the degree of lung re-expansion following drainage of the effusion. Non-expandable 'trapped' lung occurs when tumour encases the visceral pleura and prevents lung expansion. Lung expansion may also be inhibited by a proximal airway obstruction or by a persistent air leak (e.g. after tearing of a friable tumour-infiltrated lung on re-expansion). Trapped lung may also be caused by non-malignant, fibrotic processes, e.g. rheumatoid pleuritis, haemothorax, TB.

The patient should be admitted and the effusion drained with an intercostal tube. Provided lung fully re-expands on CXR, proceed to pleurodesis (see ➔ p. 875). A randomized controlled trial (RCT) suggested that smaller bore chest tubes (12F) were associated with higher pleurodesis failure than larger bore chest tubes (24F)—30% vs 24% respectively; however, effect size small and mechanism unclear—many continue to use smaller bore tubes. If lung fails to re-expand fully (trapped lung; CXR shows a pneumothorax or hydropneumothorax), consider chest drain suction, which may encourage lung expansion and allow pleurodesis.

Indwelling pleural catheter insertion

Increasingly used as primary therapy and may be inserted at time of diagnostic thoracoscopy to allow pure outpatient management. Spontaneous pleurodesis occurs later in 30–70% (may be increased with aggressive daily IPC drainage). For fully-expanded lung, day-case pleurodesis, via IPC, is well tolerated and increases pleurodesis rate (from 23% to 43% at day 35) without admission to hospital. Compared with standard chest tube drainage and talc pleurodesis, IPC usage reduces hospital length of stay by 2–3.5 days with no significant differences in breathlessness or quality of life. The most frequent complications are symptomatic loculations, catheter blockage and soft tissue/pleural infection. Can be inserted as a day-case procedure. Needs additional out-patient support (e.g. trained district nurse or respiratory specialist nurse), although some patients/family members perform the drainage themselves after education.

Treatment options for trapped lung or failed pleurodesis

- *Pleurodesis* may be successful, despite only partial lung re-expansion, and should still be considered if there is >50% apposition of lung against chest wall on CXR. It may be repeated if unsuccessful initially
- *Insertion of a long-term IPC* is likely to be the preferred treatment for patients with significantly trapped lung and avoids the need for recurrent pleural aspiration (see ➲ p. 858)
- *Repeated therapeutic pleural aspiration* should be avoided, unless prognosis is particularly limited (<1 month)
- *Intrapleural fibrinolytics* (e.g. tPA, urokinase or streptokinase) had previously been proposed to aid drainage of multiloculated effusions resistant to drainage and pleurodesis. An RCT of urokinase (TIME3), however, did not demonstrate improvement in dyspnoea or pleurodesis success over placebo (despite improvements in hospital stay, CXR, and survival). Case series have also reported use to attempt treatment of symptomatic loculations associated with IPC. Routine use not currently recommended
- *Thoracoscopy* enables the disruption of pleural adhesions and may have a role in facilitating pleurodesis in select patients with trapped lung
- *Pleuroperitoneal shunts* are effective in patients with trapped lung or failed pleurodesis, in the absence of multiple loculations. Now rarely used. Shunting of fluid may occur spontaneously, at high pressures, or may require manipulation of a percutaneous pump chamber, inserted at thoracoscopy or mini-thoracotomy. Main problem is shunt occlusion, which occurs in at least 10% of cases, and necessitates shunt removal. Malignant spread may also occur
- *Surgical pleurectomy* may be performed as video-assisted thoracoscopic surgery (VATS). The procedure is effective in the management of refractory malignant effusions. May be useful in a minority of patients with good performance status and prognosis. Not suitable for patients with heavily diseased visceral pleura and trapped lung; consider in patients who have failed pleurodesis
- *Palliative care team* involvement should also be considered.

Further information

Davies HE et al. Effect of an indwelling pleural catheter vs chest tube and talc pleurodesis for relieving dyspnea in patients with malignant pleural effusion: the TIME2 randomized controlled trial. *JAMA*. 2012;**307**(22): 2383–2389.

Rahman NM et al. Effect of opioids vs NSAIDs and larger vs smaller chest tube size on pain control and pleurodesis efficacy among patients with malignant pleural effusion: The TIME1 randomized clinical trial. *JAMA*. 2015;**314**(24): 2641–2653.

Thomas R et al. Effect of an indwelling pleural catheter vs talc pleurodesis on hospitalization days in patients with malignant pleural effusion: The AMPLE randomized clinical trial. *JAMA*. 2017;**318**(19): 1903–1912.

Bhatnagar R et al. Outpatient talc administration by indwelling pleural catheter for malignant effusion. *NEJM*. 2018;**378**(14): 1313–1322.

Mishra EK et al. Randomized controlled trial of urokinase versus placebo for nondraining malignant pleural effusion. *AJRCCM*. 2018;**197**(4): 502–508.

Parapneumonic effusion and empyema: definition and clinical features

Definition and pathophysiology

Pleural effusions occur in up to 57% of patients with pneumonia. An initial sterile exudate (simple parapneumonic effusion) may, in some cases, progress to a complicated parapneumonic effusion and eventually empyema (see Fig. 35.1).

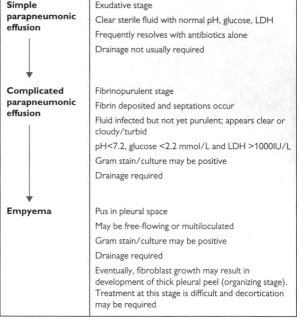

Simple parapneumonic effusion	Exudative stage
	Clear sterile fluid with normal pH, glucose, LDH
	Frequently resolves with antibiotics alone
	Drainage not usually required
Complicated parapneumonic effusion	Fibrinopurulent stage
	Fibrin deposited and septations occur
	Fluid infected but not yet purulent; appears clear or cloudy/turbid
	pH<7.2, glucose <2.2 mmol/L and LDH >1000IU/L
	Gram stain/culture may be positive
	Drainage required
Empyema	Pus in pleural space
	May be free-flowing or multiloculated
	Gram stain/culture may be positive
	Drainage required
	Eventually, fibroblast growth may result in development of thick pleural peel (organizing stage). Treatment at this stage is difficult and decortication may be required

Fig. 35.1 Parapneumonic effusion and empyema: definition and clinical features.

Pleural infection may also occur in the absence of a preceding pneumonic illness ('primary empyema').

Clinical features

Common

- Consider the diagnosis particularly in cases of 'slow-to-respond' pneumonia (e.g. failure of C-reactive protein (CRP) to fall ≥50% in first 3 days), pleural effusion with fever, or high-risk groups with non-specific symptoms such as weight loss
- Similar to clinical presentation of pneumonia: fever, sputum production, chest pain, breathlessness
- Anaerobic empyema may present less acutely, often with weight loss and without fever.

Rare

- Infected pleural fluid may spontaneously drain through the chest wall (*empyema necessitatis*) or into the lung, leading to a bronchopleural fistula and severe pneumonia
- History of atypical chest pain, vomiting, or oesophageal instrumentation suggests possible underlying oesophageal rupture (measure pleural fluid amylase)
- History of a recent sore throat may suggest Lemierre's syndrome (acute oropharyngeal infection with *Fusobacterium* species leads to septic thrombophlebitis of the internal jugular vein and subsequent metastatic infection and abscess formation, commonly in the lungs and pleura; consider US of internal jugular vein if suspected); see ➔ p. 544.

Risk factors for developing empyema

Include diabetes, alcohol abuse, gastro-oesophageal reflux, and IV drug abuse. Anaerobic infection is associated particularly with aspiration or poor dental hygiene. Empyema may rarely occur following bronchial obstruction from a tumour or foreign body. Many patients, however, have no apparent risk factors. One study identified clinical variables associated with development of pleural infection in those with pneumonia: albumin <30g/L, CRP >100mg/L, platelets >400 × 10⁹/L, sodium <130mmol/L, intravenous drug use, and chronic alcohol use.

Differential diagnosis

Includes malignancy, TB (when the pleural fluid is usually lymphocytic), and rheumatoid pleuritis.

Further information

Davies HE et al. Management of pleural infection in adults: British Thoracic Society pleural disease guideline 2010. *Thorax* 2010;**65**(Suppl. 2): ii41–ii53.

Maskell NA et al. UK controlled trial of intrapleural streptokinase for pleural infection. *N Engl J Med* 2005;**352**: 865–874.

Rahman NM et al. Intrapleural use of tissue plasminogen activator and DNase in pleural infection. *N Engl J Med* 2011;**365**: 518–526.

Parapneumonic effusion and empyema: bacteriology and investigations

Bacteriology

- *Community-acquired infection* (% of cases):
  - *Streptococcus 'milleri'* group (~30%)
  - Anaerobes (~15–30%)
  - *Streptococcus pneumoniae* (~15%)
  - *Staphylococcus aureus* (~10%)
  - Other less common organisms include other streptococci, enterobacteriaceae, *H. influenzae*, *Pseudomonas*, TB, and *Nocardia*
- *Hospital-acquired infection* (% of cases):
  - Methicillin-resistant *Staphylococcus aureus* (MRSA) (~25–30%)
  - *Staphylococcus aureus* (~10–20%)
  - Enterobacteriaceae (~20%)
  - Enterococci (~10%)
  - Others include streptococci, *Pseudomonas*, and anaerobes.

Pleural infection is frequently polymicrobial.

Investigations

- *Diagnostic pleural tap* using US is essential if pleural infection is possible and fluid depth is >10 mm (smaller effusions can usually be monitored). Frankly purulent or turbid/cloudy pleural fluid, organisms on pleural fluid Gram stain or culture, or pleural fluid pH <7.2 are all indications for chest tube drainage. Of pleural infections, 40% are culture-negative. Identification of anaerobes is improved following inoculation of blood culture bottles with pleural fluid. US typically shows an echogenic effusion that may be septated, but absence of these features does not rule out pleural infection
- *Contrast-enhanced pleural-phase CT* may be useful both in supporting the diagnosis and visualizing the distribution of fluid, although CT is poor at demonstrating septations. Empyema is associated with pleural enhancement and increased attenuation of extrapleural subcostal fat. The displacement of adjacent lung by empyema may help to distinguish from a parenchymal lung abscess. Empyemas frequently appear lenticular and may exhibit the 'split pleura' sign of enhancing separated visceral and parietal pleura. Absence of pleural thickening on CT is unusual in empyema. CT may also sometimes identify a proximal endobronchial obstructing lesion
- *Blood cultures* positive in only 14% of cases, but, in these cases, they are often the only positive microbiology
- *Bronchoscopy* is only indicated if a bronchial obstructing lesion is suspected.

Parapneumonic effusion and empyema: management and outcome

Management

Antibiotics

All patients with pleural infection should be treated with antibiotics; refer to local hospital prescribing guidelines. Typical choices:

- *Community-acquired* empyema—β-lactam/β-lactamase inhibitor (e.g. co-amoxiclav) or second-generation cephalosporin (e.g. cefuroxime), combined with metronidazole for anaerobic cover. Ciprofloxacin and clindamycin together may be appropriate
- *Hospital-acquired* empyema—cover Gram-positive and Gram-negative organisms and anaerobes. MRSA infection is common. Consult with microbiology team. One option is meropenem and vancomycin.

Rationalize with culture and sensitivity results (although note that anaerobes are frequently difficult to culture and may coexist with other organisms). Avoid aminoglycosides, which penetrate the pleural space poorly. 'Atypical' coverage is not usually indicated for community-acquired pleural infection.

Switch to oral antibiotics when apyrexial and improving clinically. Co-amoxiclav is a useful single agent with anaerobic cover (not if penicillin-allergic). Optimal duration of antibiotic treatment unclear, although likely to be at least 3 weeks.

Chest tube drainage

> **Indications for chest tube drainage**
> - Purulent pleural fluid
> - Organisms on pleural fluid Gram stain or culture
> - Pleural fluid pH <7.2.*
>
> * *This is not an absolute cut-off*, as pH values vary between pockets of a multiseptated effusion and drainage may be still indicated for higher pH values. Also note that Proteus spp. infection gives pH >7.6.

Drain insertion should be carried out under US or CT guidance. Ideal chest tube size remains subject to debate. Small (10–14 F), flexible tubes are more comfortable and have been demonstrated to be as effective as large drains in the management of empyema. Usually apply suction (–20 cmH$_2$O), and flush regularly (e.g. 20 mL normal saline every 6 h) to prevent occlusion. Consider drain removal when clinical improvement occurs. If there is no indication for drainage, give antibiotics and monitor closely. If slow to improve or deteriorate, re-sample the effusion and consider chest drain.

Intrapleural fibrinolytics

A 2011 RCT (MIST2) showed that the combination of intrapleural tPA and DNase significantly improved CXR appearances for patients with pleural infection (1° outcome) and reduced surgical referral and hospital stay with a similar adverse event profile (2° outcomes). Lone tPA or DNase did not confer such benefits (and there was an increased rate of surgical referral for DNase alone). The effects of tPA/DNase combination treatment need further investigation to determine the appropriate circumstances for its use.

The 2005 MIST1 RCT showed that intrapleural streptokinase had no effect on mortality and need for surgery or hospital stay, and is therefore not recommended.

Nutritional support
Dietician review; consider supplementary NG feeding.

Thromboprophylaxis
Given a high risk for developing venous thromboembolism, all patients should receive low molecular weight heparin unless contraindicated.

Surgery
Consult with thoracic surgeon if there are ongoing features of sepsis and residual pleural collection after 5–7 days despite tube drainage and treatment with antibiotics. Surgical techniques include:
- *VATS* allows the breakdown of adhesions and drainage of residual collection, but it is frequently unsuccessful in chronic empyema with very thickened visceral pleura
- *Thoracotomy and decortication* Removal of fibrinous and infected tissue from the pleural space—a major surgical procedure
- *Open thoracic drainage* Resection of segments of several ribs adjacent to the empyema and insertion of large-bore drains into the cavity: a more minor procedure that can be performed under local anaesthesia but results in open chest wound for long period (typically around 5 months).

Difficulties in management

Chest drainage ceases despite residual pleural collection
- Attempt to flush drain with normal saline
- Ensure that drain is not kinked at skin insertion site or lying subcutaneously
- Consider CT to assess extent of residual collection and drain position
- Remove drain if persistently blocked
- Consider further image-guided chest drain(s), surgery
- If there has been significant clinical improvement, with falling CRP and white cell count, further drains may not be warranted despite residual fluid.

Failure to clinically improve despite antibiotics and chest drain
- Review microbiology results, and ensure appropriate antibiotics
- CT to assess extent of residual collection and drain position
- Surgical referral (at days 5–7)
- Options if unfit for surgery:
  - Consider use of tPA/DNase if not already used
  - Further image-guided small-bore drains into loculated effusions
  - Large-bore drain
  - Surgical rib resection and open drainage under local anaesthesia.

Outcome

About 15% of patients require surgery. Empyema 1 y mortality is about 15%. Increased age, renal impairment, low serum albumin, hypotension, and hospital-acquired infection are associated with a poor outcome. Most of these factors are considered in the RAPID score, which stratifies patients into low, medium, and high-risk groups (associated with increasing mortality at three months). CXR may remain abnormal despite successful treatment of empyema, with evidence of calcification or pleural scarring or thickening.

Further information

Rahman NM et al. A clinical score (RAPID) to identify those at risk for poor outcome at presentation in patients with pleural infection. *Chest*. 2014;**145**(4): 848–855.

Tuberculous pleural effusion

Definition and epidemiology

Tuberculous pleural effusion usually develops from a delayed hypersensitivity reaction to mycobacteria released into the pleural space. It is a common manifestation of 1° TB in regions with a high prevalence, affecting children and young adults; it may also be associated with reactivation of TB in older individuals. May occur more commonly in the setting of HIV co-infection.

Rarely, TB may present as pseudochylothorax or tuberculous empyema.

Clinical features

- Clinical features are similar to those of pulmonary TB, i.e. fever, sweats, weight loss, and dyspnoea, although it may present acutely with pleuritic chest pain and fever, mimicking pneumonia
- Effusions are typically small to moderate in volume although can be massive.

Investigations

- Associated parenchymal infiltrate on *CXR* in less than one-third of cases
- *Tuberculin skin tests* positive in two-thirds of cases
- *Interferon G release assays* (IGRAs) reported to have high sensitivity (~90%) but fail to distinguish between latent and active TB
- *Pleural fluid* Lymphocytosis, exudative effusion, pH and glucose moderately depressed, mesothelial cells rare. Pleural fluid acid-fast bacillus (AFB) smears are positive in around 5–10% of cases; pleural fluid cultures are positive in 25% of cases and take 2–6 weeks
- Blind *Abrams' pleural biopsy* alone has a sensitivity of 79%
- *Thoracoscopic biopsies* have a sensitivity of nearly 100%
- Measurement of *adenosine deaminase* (an enzyme released by macrophages after phagocytosis of *Mycobacterium*) in pleural fluid may be of benefit in regions where TB is highly prevalent; a raised value is very sensitive for pleural TB but is non-specific and may also occur in empyema and malignancy. May have a role as a 'rule-out' test
- *Polymerase chain reaction (PCR)* for mycobacterial DNA in the pleural fluid may be useful diagnostically but is not widely available
- *Induced sputum* for AFB may have a diagnostic role in high-risk patients with lymphocytic effusions, even in the absence of parenchymal disease on CXR.

Treatment and outcome

- Tuberculous pleural effusions resolve spontaneously in the majority of cases, but two-thirds of untreated patients go on to develop pulmonary TB within 5 y, and so treatment is recommended
- Treatment is the same as for pulmonary TB (see ➜ p. 592)
- Pleural fluid volumes may increase during effective treatment, and therapeutic thoracentesis may be required
- Meta-analysis shows that steroids may reduce speed of resolution of pleural fluid, but no clear evidence of benefit on long term respiratory function and evidence of side effects associated with steroid usage
- Pleural thickening and calcification are common long-term consequences of tuberculous pleural effusion.

Further information

Ryan H et al. Corticosteroids for tuberculous pleurisy. *Cochrane Database Syst Rev.* 2017;**3**: CD001876.

Other causes of pleural effusion

Pleural effusion due to PE

- Fourth commonest cause of pleural effusion in the USA
- Consider in all patients with undiagnosed pleural effusion, particularly if there is a history of pleuritic chest pain or of breathlessness/hypoxia out of proportion to the size of the effusion
- Frequently complicates other disease processes, e.g. occurs in 1/5 of patients with cardiac failure and pleural effusions
- Effusions are usually small (<1/3 of hemithorax) and unilateral although may be bilateral
- Pleural fluid analysis is non-diagnostic; appearance varies from clear to bloody; 80% are exudates and 20% transudates. Bloodstained pleural fluid is not a contraindication to anticoagulation
- Imaging investigations, e.g. computed tomographic pulmonary angiogram (CTPA), are required to make the diagnosis; these should be performed prior to thoracentesis if PE is strongly suspected.

Rheumatoid arthritis (RA)-associated pleural effusion

- Pulmonary changes may be the first manifestation of RA
- Rheumatoid pleurisy is more common in men (70% are in men)
- Pleural fluid may be yellow-green, serous, turbid, or bloody
- Unilateral or bilateral
- Pleural fluid glucose level frequently low (<1.6 mmol/L) and progressively falls in chronic effusions
- Pleural fluid pH commonly reduced (<7.3)
- Low pleural fluid complement levels (C4 <0.04 g/L) may also favour the diagnosis
- Pleural fluid RhF titre is not more diagnostically helpful than serum RhF
- Typically persist for months to years, although duration may be several weeks
- Some cases may respond to treatment with steroids.

Haemothorax

- Haemothorax is defined as a pleural effusion with a haematocrit >50% of peripheral blood haematocrit
- Causes include trauma, iatrogenic, malignancy, pulmonary infarction, pneumothorax, thoracic endometriosis, and aortic rupture
- Massive haemothorax defined as >1,500 cm³ of blood in hemithorax and is most commonly due to trauma. Traumatic haemothorax requires a chest drain and sometimes thoracotomy; all cases should be discussed immediately with the cardiothoracic surgical team
- Large volumes of residual blood in the pleural space will clot and may lead to pleural thickening, empyema, or trapped lung. Tube drainage may be ineffective, and thoracoscopy or thoracotomy with decortication is often needed.

Pleural effusion after coronary artery bypass graft (CABG)

- Small, typically left-sided pleural effusions occur in the majority of patients post-CABG, and most resolve spontaneously
- Larger (>25% of hemithorax) effusions can be subdivided:
  - Pleural effusions occurring *within 30 days* of surgery. Classically bloody and eosinophilic exudate, with high LDH; probably related to post-operative bleeding into pleural space
  - Pleural effusions *>30 days* after surgery. Typically clear and lymphocytic exudate; cause unknown, perhaps immunological or a form of post-cardiac injury syndrome
- Main symptom in each case is breathlessness; chest pain and fever are unusual
- Management consists of repeated therapeutic thoracentesis to alleviate breathlessness. Recurrent effusions after 1 y are rare and may be difficult to treat; non-steroidal anti-inflammatories (NSAIDs), prednisolone, or thoracoscopy and pleurodesis may be considered
- Differential diagnosis of pleural effusion post-CABG includes PE, cardiac failure, pleural infection, post-cardiac injury syndrome, chylothorax.

Pleural effusion following asbestos exposure

The main differential diagnosis is between benign asbestos pleural effusion (see ➲ p. 126) and mesothelioma (see ➲ p. 130).

Pleural thickening

- Pleural fibrosis and thickening may follow previous episodes of pleural inflammation. Causes include previous empyema, tuberculous pleuritis, rheumatoid pleuritis, haemothorax, thoracotomy, and asbestos exposure (diffuse pleural thickening; see ➲ p. 127)
- May be asymptomatic or cause breathlessness
- CXR features include blunting of the costophrenic angle or apices, sometimes with associated calcification
- US or CT may be required to distinguish from a pleural effusion
- Treatment is difficult and usually unnecessary; decortication may be considered.

Pneumoconioses

Overview and causative mineral dusts 426
Coal-worker's pneumoconiosis 428
Silicosis 430
Berylliosis 432

Overview and causative mineral dusts

- Pneumoconioses are non-neoplastic pulmonary diseases caused by the reaction of the lung to the inhalation of mainly mineral, but also organic, dusts (see Table 36.1)
- Inhaled particles of dust size <5 micron reach the terminal airways and alveoli and settle on the epithelial lining. From here, they are slowly cleared by macrophages or alveolar cells. They may pass into the lymphatic system, be cleared via the airway, or remain in the alveolus
- The dust particles can lead to an inflammatory reaction within the lung, depending on their physical and chemical properties
- The inflammation causes characteristic alterations in pulmonary structure and radiological abnormalities
- Of the diseases caused by inhalation of mineral dusts, many are becoming less common in the UK, due to improved protection of workers from dusts and decreasing levels of mining. Newer industrial nations may see increasing numbers of cases of pneumoconiosis
- Organic dusts causing hypersensitivity pneumonitis (HP) and allergic asthma are discussed on ➔ p. 311 and ➔ p. 158. Asbestos-related diseases are discussed separately on ➔ p. 123.

Table 36.1 Causative mineral dusts

Mineral dust	Disease	Examples of exposure
Coal dust	Simple pneumoconiosis Progressive massive fibrosis Caplan's syndrome	Coal mining, especially hard coal
Silica	Silicosis Caplan's syndrome	Foundry work, sandblasting, stone cutting, hard rock mining, ceramics
Asbestos	Asbestosis Benign asbestos-related pleural disease Mesothelioma Lung cancer	Mining, milling, and fabrication Installation and removal of insulation
Beryllium	Acute berylliosis Beryllium granulomatosis	Mining, fabrication of electrical and electronic equipment, workers in nuclear and aerospace industry
Iron oxide	Siderosis	Welding
Barium sulphate	Baritosis	Mining
Tin oxide	Stannosis	Mining
Aluminium	Like silicosis (bauxite worker's lung, Shaver's disease)	Mining, firework, painting, and armament manufacture

Types of mineral dust exposure
Non-fibrous mineral dusts
- Silica
- Coal dust
- Mixed mineral dusts containing quartz: slate, kaolin, talc, non-fibrous clays.

Fibrous mineral dusts
- Asbestos
- Other mineral fibres.

Metal dusts and fumes
- Iron, aluminium, beryllium, cobalt

Chest disease in coal miners

It was recognized many years ago that coal miners had higher levels of respiratory disease than the general population. Coal miners can get any, or all, of:
- Chronic bronchitis
- Chronic obstructive pulmonary disease (COPD)
- Pneumoconiosis.

They may be eligible for compensation for all of these. It can be difficult to establish the independent effects of coal dust due to high smoking rates among miners. However, it is now thought that coal dust contributes to the COPD and bronchitis caused by smoking, because:
- Miners have an increased prevalence of cough, sputum, and decreased FEV_1 when compared with non-miners. The risk of cough increases with increasing dust exposure
- FEV_1 declines in proportion to the amount of dust exposure
- In smokers, the response to dust is probably different to that of non-smokers, with worse disease at a given level of exposure.

In the past, tuberculosis (TB) has also been a major problem among miners and their families, relating to their socio-economic conditions.

SWORD is the Surveillance of Work-related and Occupational Respiratory Disease scheme run in the UK to monitor the numbers of patients with occupational lung diseases. Patients with a clinical diagnosis of an occupational lung disease are confidentially reported by respiratory or occupational health physicians.

Coal-worker's pneumoconiosis

This is the condition caused by the deposition of coal dust within the lung and its associated inflammatory reaction.

There are two types:
- Simple pneumoconiosis, which can progress to
- Complicated pneumoconiosis, also known as progressive massive fibrosis (PMF).

These diseases are common among coal miners who work in poorly ventilated conditions. The risk of pneumoconiosis varies with different compositions of coal from different geographical areas, but the larger the amount of dust to which the miner is exposed, the greater the risk of developing pneumoconiosis.

Pathology

Simple pneumoconiosis

Coal dust is inhaled into the alveolus and is engulfed by macrophages, forming a black stellate lesion, the coal macule. This causes cytokine release and subsequent inflammatory cell recruitment, leading to fibroblast activation. These coal macules are found throughout the lung, especially in the upper zones of the upper and lower lobes and often associated with surrounding bronchiolar dilatation. They are not palpable. Regional lymph nodes also become blackened. In time, larger nodules develop, containing reticulin and collagen between the macrophages, and associated bronchiolar dilatation leading to focal emphysema is seen.

PMF

Occurs on this background but with aggregation of the fibrotic nodules to form larger lesions 2–10 cm diameter. Macroscopically, these look like large black scars, extending from the lung parenchyma to the chest wall. The central area of these nodules may be necrotic, and the outer rim is firm and collagenous. It is not understood what causes the progression of small nodules to PMF, although continued exposure to coal dust in the presence of simple pneumoconiosis makes this development more likely.

Clinical features

Simple pneumoconiosis

Usually asymptomatic, with no associated clinical signs. This is a relatively benign disease.

PMF

Usually associated with cough, productive of mucoid or blackened sputum, and breathlessness, particularly on exertion, and may, in time, lead to the development of cor pulmonale. Examination is unremarkable, with no clubbing and no crepitations audible (the presence of crepitations suggests a different diagnosis).

Investigations

- *Chest radiograph (CXR)* In *simple pneumoconiosis*, there is nodular shadowing, with nodules of varying size, up to 10mm, particularly in the upper and middle zones. Pneumoconiosis can be graded according to the number of different sized nodules: p = <1.5 mm, q = 1.5–3 mm, and r = 3–10 mm. Nodule numbers increase with increasing dust inhalation and usually stop forming when the miner has left the work environment. *PMF* is diagnosed when one or more opacities of >1 cm diameter are present, on the background of simple pneumoconiosis. These lesions are often located in the upper lobes and enlarge, becoming increasingly radiodense and clearly demarcated with time. They may distort the adjacent lung and cause emphysema. The lesions continue to progress out of the work environment
- *High-resolution computer tomography (HRCT)* of *simple pneumoconiosis* shows parenchymal nodules 1–10 mm in size, with upper zone predominance. In *PMF*, nodules of >1 cm are seen, with irregular borders and associated parenchymal distortion and emphysema. Larger lesions may have cavitation and necrosis. They may also have areas of calcification
- *Pulmonary function tests (PFTs)* Simple pneumoconiosis: FEV_1 and FVC are normal, although total lung carbon monoxide transfer factor (TLCO) may be slightly decreased. PMF: signs of airway obstruction due to emphysema, and restriction due to loss of lung volumes. TLCO is reduced.

Management

Minimization of dust exposure with improved mine ventilation, respirator provision, and monitoring of dust levels. Miners have CXR every 4 y and are moved to less dusty work, if they show signs of pneumoconiosis, to prevent the development of PMF. Miners with signs of coal-worker's pneumoconiosis are entitled to industrial injury benefits from British Coal (see ⊃ p. 138). No increased risk of lung cancer with pneumoconiosis or PMF.

Caplan's syndrome

Miners with seropositive rheumatoid arthritis (RA) or positive serum rheumatoid factor (RhF) can develop large well-defined pulmonary nodules. These occur on a background of simple pneumoconiosis and in those with a relatively low coal dust exposure. They may be multiple and may cavitate. They cause no significant functional impairment and have no malignant potential.

Silicosis

This is a chronic nodular, densely fibrosing pneumoconiosis, caused by the prolonged inhalation of silica particles.
- Long lag time of decades between exposure and clinical disease
- Insidious onset, progressive
- Larger radiological opacities than those seen in coal-worker's pneumoconiosis and more rapid progression
- The pattern of disease depends on the level and duration of the silicone dust exposure.

Silica is present mostly as crystalline quartz, which is mined and quarried, and used in industries such as ceramics, brick making, and stone masonry. It is becoming less prevalent in Western societies, due to changes in silica working conditions.

Pathology

Quartz and cristobalite forms of crystalline silica cause silicosis. When they accumulate within the airways, lymphocytes and alveolar macrophages engulf the particles and are removed into the lymphatic system. Any remaining silica dust causes focal aggregations of macrophages, which are, in time, converted into fibrosing nodules, the silicotic nodule. Silica dust can cause surfactant secretion from the alveolus due to local irritation. This leads to further macrophage recruitment. Large nodules are formed by the aggregation of smaller nodules.

Different types of silicosis

There are four types, and the distinction is often not clear.
- *Acute silicosis* is caused by intense exposure to fine dusts such as those produced by sandblasting. It may become apparent in workers within a few months to a year of starting work. Rapid deterioration over 1–2 y, with treatment being ineffective. Rare now, due to regulation of silica levels in the workplace
  - *Clinically* Dry cough, shortness of breath (SOB), and a feeling of tightness on breathing deeply. Rapid deterioration over a few weeks. Fine crepitations are heard over the lower zones bilaterally. Respiratory failure
  - *CXR* Patchy bilateral lower airspace consolidation, which may look like pulmonary oedema
  - *Pathology* Irregular fibrosis adjacent to alveolar spaces filled with a lipoproteinaceous exudate, similar to that found in alveolar proteinosis
- *Subacute silicosis* This is the classic picture of silicosis, which is now quite rare. Dry cough, gradual onset of SOB
  - *CXR* Upper and mid-zone nodules are present, measuring 3–5 mm in diameter. Initially indistinct but become clearer with time. Nodules coalesce and calcify and can progress to PMF where the centre may cavitate. Associated calcified hilar lymphadenopathy (eggshell calcification) and possible pleural thickening. Nodules continue to develop with continued exposure but, due to long lag time, will also develop when patient stops being exposed. In some cases with heavy exposure to silica, patients may develop progressive upper zone fibrosis with sparse nodularity

- *PFTs* Slow decline, including in TLCO, with mild restrictive pattern, unless the silicosis has caused emphysema when obstructive or mixed picture is seen
- *Pathology* Dust particles within the alveoli are phagocytosed by macrophages. They are removed to the lymphatics where they lodge and cause diffuse inflammatory change. Layers of collagen are deposited around the dust particle. Nodules are found within the 2° pulmonary lobule where they cause fibrosis
- *Chronic silicosis* occurs with lower dust concentrations than those seen in active silicosis; appears 10–30 y after first exposure
  - *CXR* A few upper- and mid-zone nodules occur, which become calcified after 10 y or so. There is no associated parenchymal distortion. There may be associated hilar lymphadenopathy.

If there is further silica exposure, this disease may progress, with coalescence of nodules.

- *Silicotuberculosis* Increased likelihood of active TB infection in people with silicosis, most likely due to the reactivation of quiescent lesions. Silica within the lung is thought to affect the efficacy of the macrophage at clearing *Mycobacterium tuberculosis*. TB can be difficult to diagnose, due to multiple pre-existing CXR nodules. Cavitation may occur. Haemoptysis, fever, worsening respiratory function, and new soft CXR opacities should prompt sputum examination and bronchoalveolar lavage (BAL). Confirmed TB should be treated with the usual three- or four-drug regime. non-tuberculous mycobacteria (NTM) infection is also more common.

Management

Prevention of silicosis by monitoring and minimizing dust levels with adequate ventilation. Masks can be useful for short-term use if the high levels of dust are transiently unavoidable. Silicosis diagnosed with: history of silica exposure (with amount of exposure and latency taken into account), compatible imaging, and lack of another diagnosis which would fit history and imaging better. Lung biopsy is usually not necessary if these three conditions are met, only if alternative diagnosis being considered. Prescribe bronchodilators if airflow limitation, O_2 if respiratory failure; consider lung transplant if severe. Disability benefits available from the Department for Work and Pensions (see ❥ p. 734). Small increased risk of lung cancer with silicosis and associated PMF.

Berylliosis

Beryllium is a light, strong industrial metal. It is mined and often used as an alloy in the manufacture of fluorescent tubes for lighting and televisions, radiological equipment, in atomic reactors, and in heat-resistant ceramics. Cases of berylliosis are now rare, as beryllium levels have been tightly regulated to avoid sensitization. However, due to the long latent period between exposure and granuloma formation, as well as accidental beryllium exposure, cases are still occurring. There are two types of disease.

- *Acute beryllium disease*
  - An acute alveolitis due to the direct effects of high-dose inhaled beryllium fumes
  - Subsequent widespread airway oedema and pulmonary oedema, which causes dyspnoea, cyanosis, and widespread inspiratory crepitations
  - CXR shows pulmonary oedema. It may be self-limiting if mild but, if severe, is usually fatal
  - Corticosteroids may prevent progression, but the patient is often left with residual pulmonary impairment
- *Subacute and chronic berylliosis*
  - A delayed hypersensitivity-type reaction due to beryllium, occurring long after beryllium exposure in a minority of individuals
  - Can be clinically indistinguishable from sarcoidosis
  - Also sometimes seen in the wives of beryllium workers and those who live near beryllium refineries.
  - Inhalation of beryllium or the exposure of beryllium to a skin abrasion causes initial sensitization in 2–19% of exposed individuals. Only low levels of exposure are required for this
  - There is a T-cell-mediated immune response, with the production of numerous inflammatory cytokines, which cause granulomatous inflammation
  - Following a long latent period, which may be months to 10 y plus after exposure, non-caseating granulomatous tissue reactions occur in the lungs or on the skin
  - There is a genetic predisposition to the response to beryllium exposure, and it is HLA-mediated (HLA-DPB1(Glu69)). HLA status could be used to identify workers at high risk of berylliosis (but is not routinely used at present).

Clinical features of chronic berylliosis

- *Symptoms* Dry cough, dyspnoea, fever, malaise, night sweats. Macular skin lesions, which do not spontaneously resolve
- *Signs* No clubbing or crepitations in early disease, but both occur with established fibrosis. Hepato/splenomegaly and macular skin lesions. Does not cause uveitis or erythema nodosum.

Investigations

- *CXR* Fine reticulonodular appearance throughout both lungs. Finer nodules than those seen in sarcoidosis. Progression to interstitial fibrosis, with irregular linear opacities diffusely or favouring upper lobes. Hilar lymphadenopathy can occur, but always in association with interstitial lung disease (ILD)
- *HRCT* Subpleural micronodular change, thickened interlobular septae, traction bronchiectasis, and honeycombing. There may be ground-glass shadowing
- *BAL* High levels of T-lymphocytes
- *PFTs* Restrictive defect, with decreased kCO
- *Pathology* Non-caseating granulomata. Endobronchial and transbronchial biopsies may be adequate, taken from area of abnormal lung on CT. *May be indistinguishable from sarcoidosis.* May develop irregular fibrosis with bulla and cyst formation
- *Beryllium lymphocyte proliferation test (BeLPT)* assesses if patient is sensitized to beryllium. This blood test has become the standard industry test to see which beryllium workers are sensitized and therefore part of the diagnostic work-up. Can also be performed on BAL fluid to increase diagnostic accuracy. False negative rate, so borderline and negative tests generally repeated.

Management

Corticosteroids are given to try and prevent disease progression. Continue indefinitely on the lowest dose that maintains symptom control, as few patients gain complete resolution of symptoms, CXR, or PFTs. Other immunosuppressants have been tried, but evidence limited. Annual screening of beryllium-exposed workers with CXR. If they develop breathlessness or skin rashes, this may be an indication to start oral steroids to delay progression to interstitial fibrosis. Avoid further beryllium exposure once evidence of berylliosis occurs and possibly when evidence of sensitization.

Prognosis

Progressive disease, although those with very low exposure who develop CXR changes may find they resolve. Associated delayed skin sensitivity (anergy) to tuberculin. Granulomata do not spontaneously resolve although can be excised if causing problems such as troublesome lesions on the skin. Interstitial fibrosis occurs in the lungs, which is progressive and leads to cyanosis and death. Other complications include pneumothorax, hypercalcaemia, hypercalciuria, and nephrocalcinosis.

Differential diagnosis

- Sarcoidosis
- TB.

In clinic

- Ask patients with suspected sarcoidosis about possible exposure to beryllium
- Monitor PFTs and CXR to assess disease response or progression.

Pneumothorax

Clinical features and investigations *436*
Initial management *440*
Further management *442*
Algorithm for treatment of spontaneous pneumothorax *444*
Specific situations *446*

Clinical features and investigations

Definition

A pneumothorax is air in the pleural space. May occur with apparently normal lungs (1° pneumothorax) or in the presence of underlying lung disease (2° pneumothorax). May occur spontaneously or following trauma.

Epidemiology

- Annual incidence of 1° pneumothorax is around 9 per 100,000
- 1° pneumothoraces occur most commonly in tall thin men aged between 20 and 40 y. They are less common in women ($\circlearrowleft$:$\circlearrowleft$ ≈ 5:1)—consider the possibility of underlying lung disease (e.g. lymphangioleiomyomatosis (LAM), catamenial pneumothorax)
- Cigarette or cannabis smoking is a major risk factor for pneumothorax, increasing the risk by a factor of 22 in men and 9 in women. The mechanism is unclear; a smoking-induced influx of inflammatory cells may both break down elastic lung fibres (causing bulla formation) and cause small airways obstruction (increasing alveolar pressure and the likelihood of interstitial air leak)
- Evidence of familial clustering in 10%. Sporadic and familial cases of gene mutation seen (e.g. mutations in folliculin gene (*FLCN*; Chr 17)).
- Syndromes related to tumour suppressor genes, including Birt–Hogg– Dubé (BHD) syndrome (autosomal dominant (AD) mutation in *FLCN*; causes skin hamartomas, renal tumours (in 1/3) and pulmonary lower lobe cysts) and tuberous sclerosis complex-associated LAM (TSC-LAM—15% of LAM cases, the rest are sporadic; autosomal dominant (AD) germline mutation in *TSC1* and *TSC2* causing loss of function of tumour suppression; causes pulmonary cysts and multi-system changes (skin, brain, abdomen, heart, eyes, mouth))
- Syndromes related to connective tissue disorders, including Marfan's (AD; mutation in fibrillin 1 gene *FBN1*), vascular Ehlers–Danlos (type IV; AD), Loeys-Dietz syndrome (AD), homocystinuria (AR).

Causes and pathophysiology

1°

- Pathogenesis is poorly understood; pneumothoraces are presumed to occur following an air leak from apical subpleural blebs and bullae, although small airway inflammation is often also present and may contribute by increasing airways resistance, causing 'emphysema-like changes' (ELC).

2°

- Underlying diseases include: COPD (60% of cases), asthma, interstitial lung disease (ILD), necrotizing pneumonia, tuberculosis (TB), *Pneumocystis jirovecii* pneumonia (PCP), cystic fibrosis (CF), Langerhans cell histiocytosis (LCH), LAM, Marfan's syndrome, oesophageal rupture, lung cancer, catamenial pneumothorax, and pulmonary infarction
- Pneumothorax may be the first presentation of the underlying disease.

Clinical features

- Classically presents with acute onset of pleuritic chest pain and/or breathlessness. Breathlessness is often minimal in young patients and is more severe in 2° pneumothorax
- Signs of pneumothorax include tachycardia, hyperinflation, reduced expansion, hyper-resonant percussion note, and quiet breath sounds on the pneumothorax side. These are frequently absent in small pneumothoraces. Hamman's sign refers to a 'click' on auscultation in time with the heart sounds, due to movement of pleural surfaces with a left-sided pneumothorax
- May feel 'bubbles' and 'crackles' under the skin of the torso and neck if there is subcutaneous emphysema
- Presents in ventilated patients with acute clinical deterioration and hypoxia or increasing inflation pressures.

Investigations

- *Chest radiograph (CXR)* is the diagnostic test in most cases, revealing a visible lung edge and absent lung markings peripherally. Blunting of the ipsilateral costophrenic angle due to low-volume bleeding into the pleural space may be seen. Pneumothoraces are difficult to visualize on supine films: look for a sharply delineated heart border, hemidiaphragm and costophrenic angle depression ('deep sulcus sign'), and increased lucency on the affected side
  - Width of the rim of air surrounding the lung on CXR may be used to classify pneumothoraces into small (rim of air measured at level of hilum ≤2 cm) and large (>2 cm). A 2 cm rim of air approximately equates to a 50% pneumothorax in volume
  - Tiny pneumothoraces that are not apparent on posteroanterior (PA) CXR may be visible on lateral chest or lateral decubitus radiographs
  - CXR appearance may also show features of underlying lung disease, although this can be difficult to assess in the presence of a large pneumothorax
- *Computed tomography (CT) chest* may be required to differentiate pneumothorax from bullous disease and is useful in diagnosing unsuspected pneumothorax following trauma and in looking for evidence of underlying lung disease
- *Ultrasound (US) chest* (● p. 895) is used by some, particularly in the context of resuscitation, acute trauma, and post-intervention. Operator dependent. Likely higher sensitivity than CXR. Does not reliably enable quantification of size of effusion and there are worrying mimics of pneumothorax with conditions of decreased pleural sliding (including post-pleurodesis, bullae, hyperexpansion with chronic obstructive pulmonary disease (COPD))
- *Arterial blood gases (ABGs)* frequently show hypoxia and sometimes hypercapnia in 2° pneumothorax.

Prognosis

- Untreated, pneumothoraces without an ongoing air leak resolve at rate of ~2% of volume of hemithorax every 24 h
- Average of 30% (wide range in studies) of 1° pneumothoraces recur, most within 2 y. Continued smoking, blebs/bullae on imaging, low body weight, female gender, being a taller male, and familial history increases the risk of recurrence. Risk of recurrence increases with each subsequent pneumothorax; risk of recurrence is around 30% after a first pneumothorax, about 40% after a second, and >50% after a third
- Mortality of 2° pneumothorax is 10%
- Recurrence of 2° pneumothorax occurs in 39–47% and is associated with age, pulmonary fibrosis, and emphysema. Recurrence rates may be as high as 80% in patients with LCH or LAM.

Further information

Sahn SA, Heffner JE. Spontaneous pneumothorax. *N Engl J Med* 2000;**342**: 868–874.
Boone PM et al. The genetics of pneumothorax. *Am J Respir Crit Care Med* 2019;**199**(11): 1344–1357.

Initial management

There is considerable variation among clinicians regarding optimal pneumo-thorax management. The treatment algorithm presented on → p. 444 (see Fig. 37.1) is taken from the BTS guidelines.

General management points

- Determine whether the pneumothorax is 1° or 2° (known lung disease/evidence of lung disease clinically or age >50 with significant smoking history)
- Management is determined by degree of breathlessness and hypoxia, evidence of haemodynamic compromise, presence and severity of any underlying lung disease, and, to a lesser extent, CXR pneumothorax size
- Severe breathlessness out of proportion to pneumothorax size on a prior CXR may be a feature of impending tension pneumothorax
- 2° pneumothorax has a significant mortality (10%) and should be managed more aggressively. Treat also the underlying disease
- For 2° pneumothorax, avoid non-invasive ventilation (NIV) and high flow nasal oxygen (HFNO) when feasible—positive pressure may worsen air leak. If absolutely essential, drain pneumothorax
- Randomized studies are ongoing evaluating the use of ambulatory management for both 1° and 2° pneumothorax using specific ambulatory drainage devices or Heimlich valves.

Aspiration

- Procedure described on → p. 881
- Halt the procedure if painful or if the patient coughs excessively; do not aspirate >2.5 L of air, as this suggests a large air leak and aspiration is likely to fail
- Aspiration is successful if the lung is fully or nearly re-expanded on CXR and patient feels symptomatically better with improved physiology
- If initial aspiration of a 1° pneumothorax fails, a chest drain is likely to be required if benefits outweigh risks.

Chest drainage

- Procedure described on → p. 854
- Associated with significant morbidity and even mortality, and not required in the majority of patients with 1° spontaneous pneumothorax
- Small (10–14F) drains are sufficient in most cases; consider large-bore (24–28F) drain in 2° pneumothorax with large air leak, severe subcutaneous emphysema, or in mechanically ventilated patients
- Never clamp a bubbling chest drain (risk of tension pneumothorax)
- When air leak appears to have ceased, clamping of the drain for several hours followed by repeat CXR may detect very slow or intermittent air leaks, thereby avoiding inappropriate drain removal; this is controversial, however, and should only be considered on a specialist ward with experienced nursing staff. Digital suction device can give similar information
- If water level in drain does not swing with respiration, the drain is either kinked (check underneath dressing as tube enters skin), blocked, clamped, or incorrectly positioned (drainage holes not in pleural space; check CXR)

- Heimlich flutter valves (or thoracic vents) are an alternative to underwater bottle drainage and are being used increasingly in some centres. They allow greater patient mobilization and sometimes outpatient management of pneumothorax.

O_2

- All hospitalized patients should receive high-flow (10 L/min) inspired O_2 (unless CO_2 retention is a problem). This reduces the partial pressure of nitrogen in blood, encouraging removal of air from the pleural space and speeding up resolution of the pneumothorax.

Persistent air leak

- Arbitrarily defined as continued bubbling of chest drain 48 h after insertion
- Leak can be quantified with digital suction devices. A significant (≥100 mL/min) leak on day 1 may predict ongoing leak on subsequent days
- Consider drain suction (–10 to –20 cmH$_2$O), insertion of large-bore drain, and/or thoracic surgical referral. If not fit for surgery, further considerations could include use of Heimlich valve or blood patch pleurodesis
- Check that persistent bubbling is not the result of 'outside' air being sucked down the drain, e.g. following drain displacement such that a hole lies outside the pleural cavity, or if enlargement of the drain track occurs, allowing outside air to enter and then be aspirated down the drain.

Discharge

- Prior to discharge, discuss flying and diving (see p. 299 and p. 302, respectively), and advise to return to hospital immediately if breathlessness worsens. Document this in medical notes.

Further management

Outpatient follow-up

- Repeat CXR to ensure resolution of pneumothorax and normal appearance of underlying lungs. Undertake CT if any suspicion of undiagnosed pulmonary pathology. Some propose low dose CT for most apparent 1° spontaneous pneumothorax to look for evidence of LCH, LAM, endometriosis, or BHD
- Discuss risk of recurrence, and emphasize smoking cessation, if appropriate
- Consider possible causes, including catamenial (peri-menstrual chest pain/haemoptysis), BHD (family history of pneumothorax, skin lesions, renal cancer), Marfan's syndrome (tall stature, pectus carinatum), and Ehlers Danlos syndrome (joint hypermobility, skin laxity)
- Ascent to altitude with a pneumothorax is potentially hazardous. Guidelines recommend that patients should not fly for at least 1 week from the resolution of spontaneous pneumothorax on CXR. This time interval is arbitrary, however, and patients should understand that there is a high initial risk of recurrence that falls with time, and they may wish to avoid flying for a longer period, e.g. 1 y
- Advise never to dive in the future, unless patient has undergone a definitive surgical procedure.

Surgical management

Indications for cardiothoracic surgical referral

- Second ipsilateral pneumothorax
- First contralateral pneumothorax
- Bilateral spontaneous pneumothorax
- Persistent air leak or failure of lung to re-expand (3–5 days of drainage)
- Spontaneous haemothorax
- Professions at risk (e.g. pilots, divers) after first pneumothorax.

Note that these are guidelines only, and patient choice will of course also influence the decision for surgical intervention.

Surgical treatments aim to repair the apical hole or bleb and close the pleural space. Options:

- *Video-assisted thoracoscopic surgery (VATS)* Recurrence rates are higher than for open thoracotomy (4% vs 1.5%) although less invasive procedure and shorter hospital stay. Apical blebs/bullae are stapled, and mechanical pleural abrasion and/or parietal pleurectomy (rather than talc poudrage, although recent European Respiratory Society (ERS) statement suggests talc safe) is usually favoured for closure of the pleural space. Often the procedure of choice in young patients with 1° pneumothorax
- *Open thoracotomy* Same range of operative interventions undertaken as for VATS but associated with longer recovery (albeit with marginally lower recurrence rates)
- *Transaxillary mini-thoracotomy* uses a relatively small axillary incision and may be a less invasive alternative to open thoracotomy.

Chemical pleurodesis
- Talc most commonly used; procedure described on ⊃ p. 878
- Can be performed via intercostal drain or at VATS
- Failure rates around 10–20% and some concern about the long-term safety of intrapleural talc; therefore, previously not recommended in younger patients although recent ERS statement suggests safe
- Consider pleurodesis via intercostal drain only as a last resort in older patients with recurrent pneumothorax in whom surgery would be high risk (e.g. patients with severe COPD)
- Likelihood of successful pleurodesis in the setting of an incompletely re-expanded lung with a persistent air leak remains uncertain, although it may be attempted if surgery is not an option. In this context, blood patch pleurodesis favoured by some in place of talc.

Algorithm for treatment of spontaneous pneumothorax

Fig. 37.1 is an adapted version of the BTS guidance for treatment of a spontaneous pneumothorax.

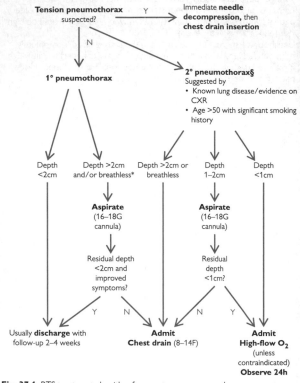

Fig. 37.1 BTS treatment algorithm for spontaneous pneumothorax.

* Disagreement exists regarding this point; in the setting of a relatively asymptomatic patient with a large 1° pneumothorax and no adverse physiology, there may be no justification for intervention. Indeed, the risk of intervention may well outweigh the risk of the pneumothorax, and conservative management is preferable.

§ In our opinion, breathlessness and the degree of physiological compromise are much more important in guiding management than absolute pneumothorax size on CXR. For example, it may be appropriate to insert a CT-guided chest drain in a patient with a <1 cm 2° pneumothorax who is particularly compromised while, conversely, an asymptomatic patient with >2 cm 2° pneumothorax may be best managed conservatively.

Further information

MacDuff A et al. Management of spontaneous pneumothorax: British Thoracic Society pleural disease guideline 2010. *Thorax* 2010;**65**(Suppl. 2): ii18–31.

Tschopp JM et al. ERS task force statement: diagnosis and treatment of primary spontaneous pneumothorax. *Eur Respir J* 2015;**46**(2): 321–335.

Specific situations

Tension pneumothorax

- Pneumothorax acts as a one-way valve, with air entering the pleural space on each inspiration and unable to escape on expiration. The progressive increase in pleural pressure compresses both lungs and mediastinum and inhibits venous return to the heart, leading to hypotension and potentially cardiac arrest
- Occurrence is not related to pneumothorax size, and tension can occur with very small pneumothoraces in the context of air trapping in the lung from obstructive lung disease
- Typically presents with acute respiratory distress, agitation, hypotension, raised jugular venous pressure (JVP), and tracheal deviation away from the pneumothorax side. Reduced air entry on affected side
- May present with cardiac arrest (pulseless electrical activity) or with acute deterioration in ventilated patients
- **Note**: CXR features of contralateral shift of trachea conventionally taught to represent tension but this is not necessarily the case. Physiological negative *contralateral* pleural pressure and 'less negative' *ipsilateral* pleural pressure as seen in non-tension pneumothorax often causes tracheal shift. Symptoms more relevant than imaging.

See Box 37.1.

Box 37.1 Management of a tension pneumothorax

- If strong clinical suspicion, give high-flow O_2 and insert large-bore cannula into second intercostal space in mid-clavicular line on side of pneumothorax
- Do not wait for a CXR if patient seriously compromised or cardiac arrest has occurred
- Do not wait for a CXR if the diagnosis is clinically certain
- Hiss of escaping air confirms diagnosis
- Aspirate air until the patient is less distressed, and then insert chest drain in safe triangle (see ➲ p. 854), leaving cannula in place until finished and the underwater seal is bubbling satisfactorily.

Iatrogenic pneumothorax

- Causes include transbronchial biopsy (TBB), transthoracic needle lung biopsy, subclavian line insertion, mechanical ventilation, pleural aspiration, pleural biopsy, external cardiac massage, and percutaneous liver biopsy
- Presentation may be delayed, even several days after procedure
- Most cases do not require intervention and improve with observation, although aspiration is sometimes required
- Drainage is seldom needed although is more commonly required in patients with COPD. The exception is mechanically ventilated patients, who will require an intercostal drain in the majority of cases.

Traumatic pneumothorax

- Up to half may not be clinically apparent or visible on CXR; chest CT is required for diagnosis
- Majority of patients require intercostal drain. Ensure adequate analgesia; intercostal nerve block may be required
- Consider VATS early if persistent air leak.

Subcutaneous (or 'surgical') emphysema

- Occurs as air tracks below skin under pressure from the pleural space
- May result from large air leaks, particularly in the presence of underlying lung disease, e.g. COPD. May also occur if chest drain is blocked or displaced so that holes lie subcutaneously
- Harmless in majority of cases although rarely may result in significant respiratory compromise from upper airway compression
- Treat with high-flow (10 L/min) inspired O_2 (unless CO_2 retention a problem). Check that the drain is patent (swinging, bubbling)
- Management if unwell: O_2, large-bore chest drain on suction. If the airway is compromised, consider anaesthetizing and incising areas of affected skin, and 'milking' out subcutaneous air; subcutaneous drains are sometimes used, and, in rare cases, tracheostomy is required.

Pneumothorax in pregnancy

- Increased risk of pneumothorax recurrence during pregnancy
- Standard 1° pneumothorax treatment is usually effective, but close liaison with obstetricians and thoracic surgeons
- Elective assisted delivery (forceps/ventouse) near term with epidural anaesthesia is advocated
- Consider VATS after pregnancy.

Pneumothorax in HIV

- Most commonly occurs as a result of PCP. Empirical treatment of PCP is advised (see ⊃ p. 572)
- Use of nebulized pentamidine may increase the risk of pneumothorax
- Consider early intercostal drainage and surgical referral.

Pneumothorax in CF

See ⊃ p. 252.

Catamenial pneumothorax

- Pneumothorax occurring at the same time as menstruation
- Usually recurrent
- Pathogenesis is unknown; possibilities include pleural endometriosis or transfer of air into pleural spaces through a diaphragmatic defect from the peritoneal cavity at menstruation
- Treatment options: VATS, pleurodesis, ovulation-suppressing drugs.

Re-expansion pulmonary oedema

- Occurs in up to 14% of cases following treatment and causes breathlessness and cough, with evidence of oedema in the re-expanded lung (and sometimes both lungs) on CXR
- More common in young patients with large 1° pneumothoraces and may be associated with late presentations to hospital
- May be precipitated by early use of suction (<48 h)
- Self-resolving in most cases although may rarely be fatal.

Further information

MacDuff A et al. Management of spontaneous pneumothorax: British Thoracic Society pleural disease guideline 2010. *Thorax* 2010;**65**(Suppl. 2): ii18–31.

Pulmonary hypertension (PHT)

Pulmonary hypertension (PHT) *450*
PHT: investigations *452*
PHT: features of clinical groups 1 *454*
PHT: features of clinical groups 2–5 *458*
PHT management 1 *460*
PHT management 2: general and surgical *464*

Pulmonary hypertension (PHT)

Definition

PHT is a haemodynamic and pathophysiological state that can be found in multiple clinical conditions (see Box 38.1). Normal resting mean pulmonary artery pressure (PAP) is around 14 mmHg and a pressure above 20 mmHg is roughly 2 standard deviation (SD) from the normal mean PAP. PHT is defined as a mean PAP ≥20 mmHg at rest, as assessed by right heart catheterization (RHC) (although this definition is lower than the current treatment threshold of >25 mmHg, clinical trials are ongoing at lower thresholds). In clinical groups 1, 3, and 4, the pulmonary artery wedge pressure (PAWP) is normal at ≤15 mmHg but the pulmonary vascular resistance is raised (>3 Wood Units). In group 2 PAWP is >15 mmHg and can be raised in group 5. Resting PHT is significant, as >70% of the vascular bed must be lost for the PAP to rise.

Pathophysiology

Each group has differing characteristic pathological features, but vasoconstriction, remodelling of the pulmonary vessel wall, medial hypertrophy of distal pulmonary arteries ± fibrotic change, and thrombosis lead to raised pulmonary vascular resistance and ultimately right heart failure. An imbalance between nitric oxide (NO) and prostacyclin (a potent vasodilator and platelet inhibitor) and thromboxane A2 (a potent vasoconstrictor and platelet agonist) has been identified in pulmonary arterial hypertension (PAH). Unfavourable imbalances between other regulators of vascular tone and smooth muscle cell growth, including endothelin-1, NO, and serotonin, have also been implicated.

Presenting features

- The symptoms of PHT are primarily due to right ventricle (RV) dysfunction. The symptoms are non-specific, often leading to a delay in diagnosis from first symptoms.
- Exertional breathlessness, due to the inability to increase cardiac output with exercise. World Health Organization (WHO) functional assessment classification used to quantify; see Box 38.2.
- Chest pain (right heart angina)
- Fatigue and weakness
- Syncope or pre-syncope, due to a fall in systemic blood pressure (BP) on exercise
- Palpitations
- Peripheral oedema and other signs of right-sided fluid overload.

Examination

Signs of right heart fluid overload and right ventricular hypertrophy (RVH) are associated with advanced disease and include:

- RV heave, RV third sound
- Wide splitting of S2 with loud P2
- Pansystolic murmur of tricuspid regurgitation (TR), diastolic murmur of pulmonary insufficiency
- Raised JVP, with giant V waves
- Hepatomegaly, ascites, peripheral oedema
- Cyanosis
- Possible telangiectasia, digital ulceration, and sclerodactyly in PHT associated with scleroderma

- Stigmata of chronic liver disease with portal hypertension
- Clubbing suggests interstitial lung disease (ILD) or congenital heart disease
- Lungs normally clear, unless underlying ILD in association with connective tissue disease or if pulmonary oedema associated with pulmonary veno-occlusive disease.

Box 38.1 Updated clinical classification of PHT

- 1. Pulmonary artery hypertension (PAH)
  - 1.1 Idiopathic
  - 1.2 Heritable (e.g. *BMPR2* mutation)
  - 1.3 Drug- and toxin-induced
  - 1.4 Associated pulmonary arterial hypertension (APAH—connective tissue disease, human immunodeficiency virus (HIV), portal hypertension, congenital heart disease, Schistosomiasis)
  - 1.5 PAH long-term responders to calcium channel blockers (CCB)
  - 1.6 Pulmonary veno-occlusive disease and/or pulmonary capillary haemangiomatosis
  - 1.7 Persistent PHT of the newborn
- 2. PHT due to left heart disease
  - 2.1 PHT due to heart failure with preserved ejection fraction
  - 2.2 PHT due to heart failure with reduced ejection fraction
  - 2.3 Valvular disease
  - 2.4 Congenital/acquired cardiovascular conditions leading to post-capillary PHT
  - 2.5 Congenital/acquired pulmonary vein stenosis
- 3. PHT due to lung diseases and/or hypoxia
  - 3.1 Chronic obstructive pulmonary disease (COPD)
  - 3.2 Interstitial lung disease (ILD)
  - 3.3 Other pulmonary diseases with mixed restrictive and obstructive pattern
  - 3.4 Sleep-disordered breathing
  - 3.5 Alveolar hypoventilation disorders
  - 3.6 Chronic exposure to high altitude
  - 3.7 Developmental abnormalities
- 4. Chronic thromboembolic PHT (CTEPH) and other pulmonary artery obstructions
  - 4.1 CTEPH
  - 4.2 Other pulmonary artery obstructions—angiosarcoma, other intravascular tumours, arteritis, congenital pulmonary artery stenosis, parasites (hydatidosis)
- 5. PHT with unclear and/or multifactorial mechanisms
  - 5.1 Haematological disorders: chronic haemolytic anaemia, myeloproliferative disorders, splenectomy.
  - 5.2 Systemic disorders: sarcoidosis, pulmonary histiocytosis, lymphangioleiomyomatosis (LAM), neurofibromatosis
  - 5.3 Metabolic disorders: glycogen storage disease, Gaucher's disease, thyroid disorders
  - 5.4 Others: pulmonary tumoural thrombotic microangiopathy, fibrosing mediastinitis, chronic renal failure (with/without dialysis), segmental pulmonary hypertension

Adapted from the 6th World Symposium on Pulmonary Hypertension (Galie et al. An overview of the 6th World Symposium on Pulmonary Hypertension. *Eur Respir J*. 2019;**53**: 1802148)

PHT: investigations

The investigations aim to make a diagnosis of PHT and investigate any possible underlying cause (see Box 38.1). In 85% of patients presenting with symptoms caused by established PHT, a CXR and *electrocardiogram* (ECG) will be abnormal.

- *Chest radiograph (CXR)* may show enlarged pulmonary arteries and an enlarged cardiac silhouette, with pruning (loss) of peripheral vessels
- *ECG* Right atrial dilatation, right axis deviation (RAD), RVH, and strain
- *Arterial blood gases (ABG)* Slight hypoxia and hypocapnia (correlating with disease severity), with a fall in O_2 saturation on exercise
- *Pulmonary function tests (PFTs)* The lung volumes may be normal or show a mild restrictive or obstructive defect with a reduced total lung carbon monoxide transfer factor (TLCO) (late in the disease course). Abnormal if PHT due to underlying lung disease
- *High resolution computed tomography (HRCT) chest* to exclude underlying lung disease
- *Ventilation-perfusion (V/Q) scanning/Computed tomographic pulmonary angiogram (CTPA)* to exclude chronic thromboembolic disease as a cause. V/Q is more sensitive than CTPA. Normal or low probability V/Q scan effectively excludes CTEPH
- *Echocardiogram (echo)* The most useful screening tool in PHT. Typically shows enlargement of right-sided cardiac chambers, with paradoxical interventricular septum movement and TR. The systolic PAP can be estimated from the peak velocity of the tricuspid regurgitant jet, using Doppler techniques, and the estimated right atrial pressure from the inferior vena cava (IVC) (assumed to be 5–10 mmHg). The echo probability of PHT can be categorized dependent on the velocity of the tricuspid regurgitant jet; low probability if ≤2.8 m/s (or not measurable) and no other PHT signs, intermediate if ≤2.8 m/s and other PHT signs, or if 2.9–3.4 m/s without other PHT signs, high if 2.9–3.4 m/s with other PHT signs or if >3.4 m/s. Pericardial effusions may be present and represent worse prognosis. Bubble echo can help to exclude an intracardiac shunt and also increases the Doppler signal, allowing easier measurement of peak TR velocity
- *Cardiac magnetic resonance imaging (MRI)* to evaluate RV size, morphology, and function
- *Abdominal ultrasound scan (USS)* if liver cirrhosis/portal hypertension suspected
- *RHC* The 'gold standard' test to confirm the diagnosis, assess the PAP, pulmonary capillary wedge pressure, and cardiac output (with a Swann–Ganz catheter, by thermodilution or Fick). Also can exclude a left-to-right intracardiac shunt. *Vasodilator responsiveness* is measured with incremental doses of a short-acting vasodilator such as inhaled NO or intravenous (IV) eoprostenol or adenosine. A positive vasodilator response is defined as a drop in mean PAP by >10 mmHg to <40 mmHg, with an unchanged or increased cardiac output. Only about 5–10% of patients are responders
- *6-minute walk test (6MWT)* for objective assessment of exercise capacity. Walking distances of <300 m and O_2 desaturation of >10% indicate worse prognosis in PAH. Increase in 6MWT distance following

treatment often used in assessment and in trials but may not be best
outcome measure for PHT subgroups
* *Cardiopulmonary exercise testing (CPET)* (see ➲ p. 976) O_2 uptake at the
anaerobic threshold and peak exercise are reduced in relation to disease
severity
* *Selective pulmonary angiography* is rarely required, as CTPA and V/Q
can detect nearly all cases of thromboembolic disease
* *Blood tests* Routine tests, including HIV test, thyroid-stimulating
hormone (TSH), angiotensin-converting enzyme (ACE), autoantibodies
(anti-centromere antibody, anti Scl-70, and ribonuclear protein (RNP))
if connective tissue disease suspected; thrombophilia screen in CTEPH
* *Brain natriuretic peptide (BNP/NT-proBNP) plasma levels* If elevated,
associated with worse prognosis in PAH.

A National Pulmonary Hypertension Service was established in the UK
in 2001 to coordinate diagnosis and treatment in five regional centres,
recognizing the need to provide best care (with complex interventions)
and optimize funding for expensive treatments. The five UK centres are:
* London—Hammersmith Hospital (general), Royal Brompton Hospital
(adult congenital heart disease), Royal Free Hospital (connective
tissue disease), Great Ormond Street Hospital for Children (children)
* Cambridge—Royal Papworth Hospital
* Sheffield—Royal Hallamshire Hospital
* Newcastle—Freeman Hospital
* Glasgow—Western Infirmary, Scottish Pulmonary Vascular Unit,
Golden Jubilee National Hospital.

Guidelines suggest referral to a specialist centre after CXR, ECG, simple
spirometry, and echo (but not cardiac catheterization, as this should be
done in parallel with a vasodilator study in a specialist centre).

PHT centre will: confirm/refine diagnosis, assess severity and prognosis, plan treatment, review progress 3–6-monthly, with appropriate
investigations repeated, and gather data for national database to facilitate
audit and research.

**Box 38.2 WHO functional assessment classification in
PAH (modified from New York Heart Association (NYHA)
heart failure classification)**
* Class I: No limitation of physical activity.
* Class II: Slight limitation of physical activity. They are comfortable at
rest. Ordinary physical activity does not cause undue dyspnoea or
fatigue, chest pain, or near syncope.
* Class III: Marked limitation of physical activity. They are comfortable
at rest. Less than ordinary physical activity causes undue dyspnoea or
fatigue, chest pain, or near syncope.
* Class IV: Inability to carry out any physical activity without symptoms.
Signs of right heart failure. Dyspnoea and/or fatigue may even be
present at rest. Discomfort is increased by any physical activity.

Modified from Galie N et al. Guidelines for the diagnosis and treatment of pulmonary hypertension. *Eur Heart J* 2009;**30**: 2493–2537, with permission from OUP.

PHT: features of clinical groups 1

Clinical group 1: PAH

Pathological lesions affect the distal pulmonary arteries, with medial hypertrophy, intimal proliferative and fibrotic changes, adventitial thickening with moderate perivascular inflammatory infiltrates, and thrombotic lesions. Pulmonary veins are unaffected.

Idiopathic

The incidence of IPAH in Europe and the USA is 1–2 cases per million population per year. The mean age at diagnosis is 36, with a ♀ preponderance of about 2:1. Although rare, it is important to diagnose, as it affects a young age group and has an extremely poor outcome without treatment

Heritable

A familial predisposition is seen in 6–10% of IPAH cases where the disease is transmitted in an autosomal dominant fashion. Incomplete penetrance and anticipation are seen, with presentation at a younger age in successive generations. The responsible gene has been localized to *Chr 2* (locus 2q 31–32). Abnormal cardiovascular responses to exercise have been demonstrated in asymptomatic carriers of *BMPR2*.

Bone morphogenetic protein receptor type II (BMPR2)

A receptor in the transforming growth factor beta (TGF-β) receptor superfamily and is an important regulator of apoptosis and proliferation. The identification of a mutation in *BMPR2*, present in 70% of familial PAH, has improved understanding. It is hypothesized that defective signalling via this pathway may result in abnormal endothelial proliferation and cell growth in response to various insults, with an inability to terminate the proliferative response to injury. Due to incomplete disease penetrance in the presence of a mutation in *BMPR2* (15–20%), it is thought that the genetic abnormality may have to be accompanied by some additional environmental factor, e.g. hypoxia, to cause PAH.

Other mutations:

ALK1 and endoglin (with or without HHT) PAH occurs in around 15% of patients with HHT, an autosomal dominant vascular dysplasia. Other recognized TGF-β receptor superfamily mutations include BMPR1B and SMAD9

Drug- and toxin-induced

Damage to the pulmonary artery endothelium can be caused by drugs. Some drugs are definitely associated with PAH, e.g. aminorex, fenfluramine, dexfenfluramine, benfluorex, methamphetamines, dasatinib, and toxic rapeseed oil. Others possibly cause PAH, e.g. cocaine, phenylpropanolamine, L-tryptophan, St John's Wort, amphetamines, interferon-α and -β, alkylating agents, bosutinib, direct-acting antiviral agents against hepatitis C, leflunomide, indirubin (Chinese herb Qing-Dai). A careful history must be taken. PHT can develop within 4 weeks of starting the drug, with increasing incidence with longer use.

PAH associated with (APAH)

Conditions which have a similar clinical presentation to IPAH, with identical histological findings. This group accounts for about half the patients looked after in specialist centres.

Connective tissue diseases

PAH develops in about 15% of patients with systemic sclerosis and is most frequently seen as an isolated phenomenon in patients with limited cutaneous disease. Also occurs 2° to ILD, with a very poor prognosis. Life expectancy is <1 y in patients with systemic sclerosis, isolated PHT, and a gas transfer of <25% of normal. Patients with systemic sclerosis should be screened annually with echo for PHT, even if no symptoms are present. Obliteration of the alveolar capillaries and arteriolar narrowing are induced by both the 1° vascular disease and any interstitial fibrosis. Other connective tissue diseases, including rheumatoid arthritis (RA), systemic lupus erythematosus (SLE), Sjögren's syndrome, dermatomyositis, can also lead to 2° PHT. There is a strong association with Raynaud's phenomenon, and a ♀ predominance is seen. Immunosuppressive therapy can improve PAH associated with SLE or mixed connective tissue disease.

HIV infection

PAH is found in up to 1 in 200 HIV-positive people, more common in men and intravenous drug users (IVDUs). The incidence is about 0.1%, 6–12 times higher than the general population. The development of PAH is independent of CD4 cell count but is associated with duration of infection. The mechanism is unclear. It is hypothesized that HIV-infected macrophages release vasoactive cytokines that lead to endothelial damage and proliferation.

Portal hypertension

PAH is seen in up to 5% of patients with portal hypertension of whatever cause, increasing with duration of liver disease. Porto-pulmonary hypertension is probably due to the failure of the liver to remove vasoactive substances from the portal circulation, with their resultant accumulation and presentation to the pulmonary arterial endothelium (see → p. 308).

Congenital heart disease

Pressure overload caused by systemic to pulmonary shunts. Includes large defects (Eisenmenger's syndrome), moderate to large defects, small defects (small ventricular and atrial septal defects). Smaller defects may not explain the degree of PHT and behave more like idiopathic PAH, here closing the defect may not help.

Schistosomiasis

Portal hypertension along with local vascular inflammation caused by *Schistosoma* eggs. A common cause worldwide.

Chronic haemolytic anaemia

Includes sickle cell disease, thalassaemia, hereditary spherocytosis, stomatocytosis, and microangiopathic haemolytic anaemia; may result in PAH. The mechanism is related to a high rate of NO consumption, leading to a state of resistance to NO bioactivity

PAH long-term responders to calcium channel blockers (CCB)

A minority of patients with PAH will show long-term response to calcium channel blockers.

Pulmonary veno-occlusive disease and/or pulmonary capillary haemangiomatosis

Difficult disorders to classify; share some characteristics with IPAH, but also a number of differences. HRCT helpful in diagnosis; characteristic interstitial oedema with diffuse central ground-glass opacification and thickening of interlobular septa. Possible lymphadenopathy and pleural effusion also. Pulmonary capillary haemangiomatosis suggested by diffuse bilateral thickening of interlobular septa and the presence of small, centrilobular, poorly circumscribed nodular opacities. While biopsy can help confirm the diagnosis it is not currently recommended as it is high risk. Can be idiopathic, inherited (consider genetic testing for *EIF2AK4*), drug and toxin related (industrial organic solvents, particularly trichloroethylene), associated with connective tissue disease (CTD), or associated with HIV.

Persistent PHT of the newborn

PHT: features of clinical groups 2–5

Clinical group 2: PHT due to left heart disease

Includes heart failure with preserved ejection fraction, heart failure with reduced ejection fraction, valvular heart disease, and some congenital heart disease.

Clinical group 3: PHT due to lung diseases and/or hypoxia

The majority of patients with PHT seen by a respiratory specialist will have PHT due to chronic hypoxic lung disease such as COPD. Chronic hypoxia causes pulmonary vasoconstriction and, in the longer term, vascular re-modelling. Inflammation, mechanical stress of hyperinflated lungs, loss of capillaries, and toxic effects of cigarette smoke all contribute to the patho-physiological mechanisms. Patients with 'out of proportion' PHT due to underlying lung disease should be referred to a specialist centre—that is dyspnoea insufficiently explained by mechanical disturbances, mean PAP ≥40–45 mmHg at rest.

COPD

PHT is often an incidental finding in a patient with a chronic respiratory disease.

- A significant proportion of COPD patients will develop PHT, possibly up to 25%. The level of PAP in these patients is much lower than that seen in patients with PAH
- COPD with PHT has a much poorer prognosis than COPD without PHT. In patients with a PAP <25 mmHg, the 5-y survival is >90%. In those with a PAP >45 mmHg, the 5-y survival is <10%. Whether this is due to the PHT itself or whether the PHT is a marker of worse hypoxia and disease severity is unclear.

PHT in COPD was thought to be due to hypoxia and emphysematous destruction of the vascular bed, but neither of these factors correlates well with PAP. Cigarette smoke may have a direct effect on the intrapulmonary vessels, with the upregulation of mediators leading to aberrant vascular structural remodelling and physiological changes in vascular function

Other causes:

- ILD
- Other pulmonary diseases with mixed restrictive and obstructive pattern
- Sleep-disordered breathing with the obesity hypoventilation syndrome, not just obstructive sleep apnoea (OSA) (see ➔ p. 702)
- Alveolar hypoventilation disorders, e.g. due to neuromuscular disease. Both alveolar hypoxia and hypercapnia produce pulmonary vasoconstriction, thereby increasing PAPs
- Chronic exposure to high altitude
- Developmental abnormalities.

Clinical group 4: Chronic thromboembolic PHT and other pulmonary artery obstructions

CTEPH

A frequent cause of PHT, with both proximal and distal clot. Recent data suggest that CTEPH occurs in up to 4% of cases of acute non-fatal PE, higher than previously thought.
- Pathogenesis is unclear, but abnormalities in the clotting cascade, endothelial cells, or platelets may all contribute.
- Natural history of pulmonary thromboemboli is resolution or near-total resolution of clot, with restoration of normal pulmonary haemodynamics within 30 days in 90% of patients.
- Right-sided pressures return to normal in most patients by 2 weeks.

In CTEPH, thromboemboli do not resolve, forming endothelialized fibrotic obstructions of the pulmonary vascular bed. *In situ* thrombosis and vascular remodelling of small distal pulmonary arteries also contribute. Peripheral PAH-like arteriopathic changes are also seen in the distal pulmonary arteries in non-obstructed areas. Collateral vessels from bronchial, intercostal, diaphragmatic, and coronary arteries can develop to partially reperfuse areas distal to complete obstruction.
The clinical deterioration parallels the loss of RV functional capacity.
- Risk factors for CTEPH include increasing age, idiopathic PE, and a larger perfusion defect.
- Splenectomy is associated possibly by inducing a pro-thrombotic state due to loss of filtering function of the spleen.
- Antiphospholipid antibodies are present in 10–20% of patients.

The diagnosis is not usually made until advanced PHT is present. Progressive PHT seems to result from changes in the small peripheral resistance vessels in the vascular bed, as opposed to being due to progressive pulmonary events. 2° hypertensive changes, probably induced by high PAPs, lead to incremental increases in RV afterload, with increasing PHT, ultimately leading to RV failure. Patients with CTEPH have a 5y survival of <10% if the PAP >50mmHg. CTPA helps determine whether there is any surgically accessible CTEPH.
Treatment options include:
- Central/distal pulmonary endarterectomy
- Catheter related balloon pulmonary angioplasty for inoperable disease, or
- Riociguat (licensed for inoperable distal disease or persistent PH following pulmonary endarterectomy).

Clinical group 5: PHT with unclear and/or multifactorial mechanisms

Heterogeneous conditions with different pathological pictures; aetiology unclear or multifactorial.
- Haematological disorders: myeloproliferative disorders, splenectomy
- Systemic disorders: sarcoidosis, pulmonary Langerhans cell histiocytosis (LCH), LAM, neurofibromatosis, vasculitis
- Metabolic disorders: glycogen storage disease, Gaucher's disease, thyroid disorders
- Others: tumoural obstruction, fibrosing mediastinitis, chronic renal failure on dialysis.

PHT management 1

Calcium channel blockers (CCBs)

- Vasoresponders at RHC should be considered for therapy with CCBs. They should not be used in those with a negative vasodilator challenge, as they may increase mortality
- Only a small number of patients with IPAH and vasodilator response at RHC do well with CCBs (now classified as 1.5). High-dose nifedipine (120–240 mg daily) and diltiazem (240–720 mg daily) are recommended in patients with IPAH with a positive vasodilator response. They should then be followed closely to determine if they are long-term CCB responders, with repeat RHC after 3–4 months of treatment. If their response is inadequate, further PAH therapy should be started
- Vasodilator responsiveness does not predict a favourable long-term response to CCB therapy in patients with APAH and connective tissue disease; high-dose CCBs are often not well tolerated in these patients
- Amlodipine has more selective vasodilating properties and, at doses of up to 20 mg daily, may be useful in those intolerant of the other agents or if RV function is impaired
- Calcium antagonists should be started in hospital and titrated with careful monitoring
- Verapamil is not used, because of its negative inotropic effects
- Side effects include hypotension and oedema, which may limit use.

Phosphodiesterase type-5 inhibitors (PDE-5),

For example, sildenafil and tadalafil. These augment the vasodilatory effects of NO, causing pulmonary vasodilatation, and improve exercise capacity and haemodynamics in PAH in patients in functional classes II and III.

- Common side effects: headache, flushing, epistaxis, nasal congestion
- *Sildenafil* is taken orally tds and has proven benefits in IPAH, APAH with connective tissue disease, congenital heart disease, and CTEPH
- *Tadalafil* oral, once a day.

Riociguat

Enhances cyclic GMP production and can be used in inoperable CTEPH PHT, IPAH, and PAH related to CTD. Results are favourable in terms of exercise capacity, haemodynamics, and disease progression.

Prostanoids

Prostacylin is produced predominantly by endothelial cells and is a potent vasodilator. It inhibits platelet aggregation and has antiproliferative and cytoprotective properties.

Side effects are usually dose-related and include:
- headache
- jaw pain
- diarrhoea
- flushing
- nausea
- arthralgia

Prostaglandin treatment doubles the time on the lung transplantation waiting list and improves transplantation outcomes. Improved haemodynamics may lead to some patients coming off transplant waiting lists. Tolerance develops to IV prostaglandin therapy, with increasing dose requirements over time. The mechanism for this is unclear.

• *Epoprostenol* A synthetic prostacyclin analogue potent vasodilator, acting via increasing intracellular cyclic adenosine monophosphate (cAMP). It is the only drug shown to improve survival in IPAH in randomized controlled trials (RCTs). It probably has its effects as a selective pulmonary vasodilator and potentially through vascular remodelling and platelet adhesion. It also improves symptoms, exercise capacity, and haemodynamics in IPAH and PAH associated with scleroderma. It is inactive in the circulation after 5 min and is given therefore by continuous IV infusion via a portable pump and tunnelled central venous catheter. Pump failure can be life-threatening

• *Treprostinil* is a prostacyclin analogue that can be given as a continuous subcutaneous or IV infusion, as it has greater *in vivo* stability than epoprostenol. It improves symptoms, exercise capacity, and pulmonary haemodynamics. Pain at the subcutaneous infusion site is the major side effect. Due to its current pricing structure, treprostinil is not routinely prescribed for new patients

• *Iloprost* is a prostacyclin analogue and is more potent than epoprostenol. It has a half-life of 25 min and can be given by continuous IV infusion or nebulizer (6–9 times a day). Side effects: headache, cough, mild diarrhoea, and nausea.

Selexipag

An oral prostacyclin IP receptor agonist. Shown to reduce a composite of death and disease progression on its own or when used in combination therapy.

Endothelin receptor antagonists (ERA)

Endothelin is a powerful vasoconstrictor and pro-inflammatory mediator and causes smooth muscle cell proliferation. Plasma levels raised in some forms of PHT.

• *Bosentan* is an oral endothelin receptor A and B antagonist shown to improve exercise capacity, haemodynamics, functional class, and time to clinical worsening in patients with IPAH, APAH with connective tissue disease, and Eisenmenger's syndrome. The first oral therapy approved for the treatment of PHT. Three-year survival for a cohort of mainly WHO functional class III patients starting on bosentan was >85%. The major side effect is reversible liver transaminitis, causing discontinuation in ~3%. Liver function tests (LFTs) should be monitored monthly during treatment. Other side effects include headache and peripheral oedema

• *Ambrisentan* is a selective type A blocker, with a better liver safety profile. Can improve symptoms, exercise capacity, haemodynamics, and time to clinical worsening in patients with IPAH and APAH with HIV and connective tissue disease.

• *Macitentan* is a dual endothelin receptor antagonist. Shown to reduce a composite endpoint of morbidity and mortality and increases exercise capacity.

Current practice

There are very clear nationally agreed guidelines on starting treatment for PHT. Drug therapies for PHT should only be commenced by a designated specialist PHT centre. Non-specialist clinicians should not routinely pre-scribe these therapies. These centres use CCBs in vasodilator responders, but only continue these if there is a sustained response. Otherwise:

- *First-line therapy:* dual therapy is started much sooner than previously recommended and may be started first line in selected patients. Usually PDE inhibitor is started followed by quickly adding an ERA to optimize patients
- *Triple therapy:* only for patients who have been accepted as suitable for transplant.

PHT management 2: general and surgical

General management

- *Anticoagulation* All patients with CTEPH and most with IPAH should be commenced on anticoagulation. There is no evidence for use in other subtypes unless otherwise indicated
- *Long-term O_2* Hypoxaemia is due to reduced cardiac output, V/Q mismatching, and right-to-left shunting through a patent foramen ovale. Added O_2 may reduce any further rise in PAP resulting from additional hypoxic pulmonary vasoconstriction. Supplemental O_2 should achieve a pO_2 of >8kPa during rest, exercise, and sleep
- *Diuretics and digoxin* Diuretics may be useful for the treatment of oedema, but excess pre-load reduction may limit their usefulness. Digoxin has been shown to improve cardiac output acutely in IPAH, though its longer-term effects are not known
- *Treatment of arrhythmias*
- *Identification and treatment of iron deficiency anaemia* Iron deficiency anaemia is common in PAH and may be associated with worse outcomes. Look for an underlying cause and consider IV iron replacement as oral iron absorption may be poor
- *Immunization* Annual influenza and one-off pneumococcal vaccination
- *Contraception* may be required, as pregnancy is poorly tolerated in IPAH, with a 30–50% mortality.

Surgical treatments

- *Pulmonary thromboendarterectomy* is the treatment of choice in CTEPH for proximal obstructive disease. This is the surgical removal of organized thrombotic material and aims to strip away the pulmonary arterial endothelium, starting proximally and extending out to remove all clots in the subsegmental levels. It is done on cardiopulmonary bypass with circulatory arrest. The PAP usually falls within 48 h of surgery. Operative mortality is <10% in experienced hands.
- *Atrial septostomy* Creation of a right-to-left shunt by balloon atrial septostomy aims to increase systemic blood flow by bypassing the pulmonary circulation, particularly in patients with syncope or severe right heart failure. It is a palliative procedure and can be used for symptom control prior to transplantation, with the defect being closed at the time of transplant. Also used in people receiving prostanoid therapy having syncope. Arterial desaturation occurs following the procedure but is normally offset by the increased cardiac output seen with increased O_2 delivery. It is not indicated in severe left heart failure or in patients with impaired left ventricle (LV) function
- *Balloon pulmonary angioplasty* is a relatively new procedure for distal CTEPH with web disease. This usually requires multiple catheter lab treatments and is only performed at the Royal Papworth Hospital in the UK.

- *Transplantation* Improves survival and quality of life in patients with PHT. In those with preserved LV function, lung transplant is the procedure of choice. Return of normal RV function is found after transplantation. As for all diseases needing transplantation, timing of referral and operation is crucial, as organ availability is limited. The incidence of obliterative bronchiolitis appears to be higher post-transplantation for PHT than in transplantation for other diseases, although the reason for this is uncertain.

Prognosis

Prognosis in PHT is variable, depending on functional class, haemodynamic compromise with cardiac index, right atrial pressure, and prognosis is linked to mean PAP at presentation. The clinical course is one of progressive deterioration with episodes of acute decompensation. The median survival in NYHA functional class III (symptomatic on mild exertion) is 2.8 y and 6 months in NYHA class IV (symptomatic at rest) without treatment.

End-of-life care

Palliative care by a multidisciplinary team (MDT) may be warranted to improve symptoms such as fatigue, breathlessness, abdominal bloating, nausea, and pain (see ➲ pp. 808–809).

Future developments

A number of agents are currently being investigated, including rho kinase inhibitors, vascular endothelial growth factor receptor inhibitors, angiopoietin-1 inhibitors, and elastase inhibitors. Animal studies have suggested a possible role for gene and stem cell therapies.

Further information

Galie et al. An overview of the 6th World Symposium on Pulmonary Hypertension. *Eur Respir J.* 2019;**53**: 1802148

2015 ESC/ERS Guidelines for the diagnosis and treatment of pulmonary hypertension. *Eur Respir J.* 2015;**46**: 903–975

Clinical year in review: Pulmonary Hypertension. *Eur Respir Rev.* 2016;**25**: 4–11.

Patient group. ♫ http://phauk.org

Pulmonary thromboembolic disease

Epidemiology and pathophysiology 468
Aetiology 470
Clinical features 472
Diagnosis of acute PE 474
Investigations 476
Treatment 478
Special circumstances 484
Rare causes 486

Epidemiology and pathophysiology

Definition

Pulmonary embolism (PE) is an obstruction of part of, or the entire, pulmonary vascular tree, usually caused by thrombus from a distant site.

Epidemiology

- The overall annual incidence is 60–70/100,000, with a UK annual death rate of 100/million. The estimated overall population incidence of deep vein thrombosis (DVT) is 0.5 per 1,000 person years
- PE may account for up to 15% of all post-operative deaths. It is the commonest cause of death following elective surgery, and the commonest cause of maternal death
- Post-mortem studies have consistently shown a frequency of 7–9%, and large inpatient studies have shown a frequency of around 1%, with a mortality of 0.2%. The mortality is much higher in patients with serious underlying comorbid disease
- The incidence is likely to be stable, but improved diagnostic methods mean that it is probably reported more frequently.

Pathophysiology

- 75% of thrombi are generated in the deep venous system of the lower limbs and pelvis, probably initiated by platelet aggregation around venous valve sinuses. Activation of the clotting cascade leads to thrombus formation, with Virchow's triad (venous stasis, injury to the vessel wall, and increased blood coagulability) predisposing to thrombus formation. Venous stasis is increased by immobility and dehydration. In addition, coagulation factors may be altered in various disease states, e.g. in the acute phase response, malignancy, and autoimmune disease
- 20% of leg thrombi embolize, with a higher incidence in above than below knee clots. Large clots may lodge at the bifurcation of the main pulmonary arteries, causing haemodynamic compromise. Smaller clots will travel more distally, infarcting the lung and causing pleuritic pain. These are more commonly multiple and bilateral and are found most often in the lower lobes where blood flow is greatest
- Thrombi can also develop in the right heart following myocardial infarction (MI)
- Paradoxical emboli start within the venous system and enter the arterial circulation, usually via a patent foramen ovale (causing right-to-left shunt). They typically present with features of cerebral ischaemia and these should be considered as the cause for a stroke in the young
- Septic emboli are found in endocarditis, in association with intraventricular septal defects/arteriovenous (AV) shunts or central venous access.

Haemodynamic effects of PE

Effects depend on the size of the clot and which area of the pulmonary vascular tree it subsequently obstructs, as well as the pre-existing state of the myocardium.

- As the pulmonary vasculature in a healthy lung has a large capacitance, the mean pulmonary arterial pressure (PAP) does not rise until at least 50% of the vascular bed has been occluded
- As the PAP rises, right ventricular (RV) afterload increases, with a resulting increase in RV end diastolic pressure. The RV will start to fail as the PAP reaches over 40 mmHg *acutely*
- This causes a reduction in pulmonary blood flow, leading to reduced left ventricle (LV) filling and a reduction in systemic blood pressure (BP)
- Adequate blood volume for right-sided heart filling is vital. The 2° effects are much worse if right-sided filling cannot be maintained, e.g. if the patient is dehydrated, hypovolaemic, or erect
- Arterial hypoxia results from several factors: reduced cardiac output, consequently a low mixed venous PaO_2, a higher perfusion to the remaining alveoli, resulting in inadequate oxygenation of this blood
- Hypoxia will be worse if there is a larger premorbid ventilation-perfusion (V/Q) spread, e.g. in the elderly and in those with pre-existing lung disease. The increased blood flow, with a lower mixed venous PaO_2 passing through low V/Q areas, overwhelms their oxygenating ability. It is therefore possible for a young person with healthy lungs to have a normal PaO_2 and A–a gradient following a significant PE
- Death is due to circulatory collapse from the inability of the right heart to acutely maintain an adequate cardiac output.

Aetiology

Risk factors can be divided into major and minor factors (see Table 39.1). This division is important for an assessment of clinical probability.

Table 39.1 Risk factors for venous thromboembolism (VTE)

Major risk factors (relative risk × 5–20)	
Surgery	Major abdominal/pelvic surgery
	Orthopaedic surgery (especially lower limb)
	Post-operative intensive care
Obstetrics	Pregnancy (higher incidence with multiple births)
	Caesarean section
	Pre-eclampsia
Malignancy	Pelvic/abdominal
	Metastatic/advanced
Lower limb problems	Fracture, varicose veins
Reduced mobility	Hospitalization
	Institutional care
	Long haul flight
Previous proven VTE	
Minor risk factors (relative risk × 2–4)	
Cardiovascular	Congenital heart disease
	congestive cardiac failure (CCF)
	Hypertension
	Central venous access
	Superficial venous thrombosis
Oestrogens	Oral contraceptive pill (OCP) (especially third-generation higher oestrogen-containing)
	Hormone replacement therapy (HRT)
Miscellaneous	Occult malignancy
	Neurological disability
	Thrombotic disorders
	Obesity
	inflammatory bowel disease (IBD)
	Nephrotic syndrome
	Dialysis
	Myeloproliferative disorders
	Behçet's disease

Risk of malignancy

Occult cancer will be present in 7–12% of patients presenting with idiopathic VTE. National Institute for Health and Care Excellence (NICE) guidance (2012) recommends considering further investigations for cancer with an abdominopelvic computed tomography (CT) and a mammogram for women in all those aged >40 with a first episode of unprovoked PE or DVT. No studies so far show that this strategy leads to a reduction in cancer-related mortality.

Inherited thrombophilias

- 25–50% of patients with VTE have an identifiable inherited thrombophilia, e.g. antiphospholipid syndrome, deficiency of antithrombin III, a prothrombin gene defect, protein C or protein S deficiency
- These usually need to interact with an additional acquired risk factor to cause VTE
- Factor V Leiden is present in 5% of the population and 20% of patients presenting with thrombosis
- If antiphospholipid syndrome is suspected at the time of PE diagnosis (young patient, no other obvious risk factors), this has implication for the anticoagulation choice; direct oral anticoagulants (DOACs) are not recommended because of the increased risk of thrombosis
- Current recommendations do not advocate routine screening for inheritable thrombophilias, unless in specific circumstances (see further text on thrombophilia testing), as the number needed to test to prevent an episode of VTE would be very high. In addition, detecting a heritable thrombophilia does not predict a significantly higher rate or earlier occurrence of VTE in the absence of a 2° risk factor.

Consider thrombophilia testing in:

- Patients with recurrent venous thrombosis
- Patients <40 with venous thrombosis with no obvious risk factors
- Thrombosis 2° to pregnancy, OCP, HRT
- Thrombosis at an unusual site—cerebral, mesenteric, portal, or hepatic veins
- Do not offer testing in those continuing lifelong anticoagulation or in those with provoked clot.

All except factor V Leiden deficiency and the prothrombin gene mutation, need to be tested for when the patient is *off* anticoagulants.

'Economy class syndrome'

Refers to thromboembolic disease associated with long-distance sedentary travel, with an increasing incidence of disease with increasing distance travelled. A 2001 study of >135 million passengers showed an incidence of PE of 1.5 cases/million for travel over 5,000 km, compared with 0.01 cases/million for travel under 5,000 km. For travel over 10,000 km, the incidence increased to 4.8 cases/million.

Clinical features

Acute PE

Typically presents in four main ways.

- *Pulmonary infarction and small volume haemoptysis* ± pleuritic pain. Arterial blood gases (ABGs) may be normal and electrocardiogram (ECG) changes uncommon. Localizing signs may be present, e.g. pleural rub
- *Isolated dyspnoea* (in 25%) Defined as acute breathlessness in the absence of haemorrhage or circulatory collapse. The thrombus is more likely to be central, with hypoxia on blood gases. The patient may have sudden-onset and unexplained breathlessness, in the presence of risk factors for VTE. There may also be angina from increased right heart work and inadequate O_2 delivery to its muscle
- *Collapse, poor reserve* (in 10%) May be due to a small PE, often in an elderly patient with limited cardiorespiratory reserve. These patients can rapidly decompensate with even a relatively small PE. The clinical findings may be non-specific and reflect more the underlying disease process and thus fail to arouse suspicion of a PE
- *Circulatory collapse in a previously well patient* Hypotension ± loss of consciousness in 1%. Usually due to extensive pulmonary artery occlusion from massive PE, causing marked hypoxia and hypocapnia (due to hyperventilation) and acute right heart failure, with chest pain due to right heart angina, raised jugular venous pressure (JVP), and fainting on sitting up. ECG may be normal, show sinus tachycardia or right heart strain. Echocardiogram shows pulmonary hypertension (PHT) and RV failure. These patients have the highest mortality, up to 30%.

Chronic thromboembolic disease

Typically presents with more insidious onset of breathlessness over the course of weeks to months due to increasing load of recurrent small-volume clots.

Dyspnoea and tachypnoea (respiratory rate (RR) >20) are the commonest presenting features and are absent in only 10% of patients.

Remember to consider PE in the differential diagnosis of:

- Unexplained shortness of breath (SOB)
- Collapse
- New-onset atrial fibrillation (AF)
- Signs consistent with acute right heart failure
- Pleural effusion.

Examination of a patient with PE

- May be normal
- Tachycardia and tachypnoea are common
- AF
- Reduced chest movement (due to pain)
- Pleural rub
- Classically loud P2 and splitting of the second heart sound, with a gallop rhythm (acute right heart strain)

- Hypoxia (with hypocapnia due to hyperventilation, and an increased A–a gradient), *but* PaO_2 may be in the normal range in young healthy individuals
- Low-grade fever
- Signs of DVT (common, in around 25%)
- Acute right heart failure—low cardiac output and raised JVP, with reduced BP and perfusion pressure
- Deterioration in cardiac output on sitting up, when filling pressure falls.

Diagnosis of acute PE

The diagnosis of a PE can be difficult and involves a clinical assessment of probability. This takes risk factors, clinical presentation, and clinical signs into account. Investigations performed may add weight to the clinical decision, rather than being stand-alone diagnostic tests. Therefore, the estimation of the pre-test clinical probability of DVT and PE is of vital importance in interpreting the results of the tests performed.

Pre-test clinical probability scoring systems

See Table 39.2 and Table 39.3.

Table 39.2 Wells' score for DVT

Clinical feature	Score
Active cancer (treatment ongoing, within 6 months, or palliative)	1
Paralysis, paresis, or recent plaster immobilization of the lower extremities	1
Recently bedridden for 3 days or more or major surgery within 12 weeks requiring general or regional anaesthesia	1
Localized tenderness along the distribution of the deep venous system	1
Entire leg swollen	1
Calf swelling at least 3 cm larger than asymptomatic side	1
Pitting oedema confined to the symptomatic leg	1
Collateral superficial veins (non-varicose)	1
Previously documented DVT	1
An alternative diagnosis is at least as likely as DVT	−2
Likelihood of DVT	
DVT *likely*	≥2 points
DVT *unlikely*	≤1 point

Local alternative scoring systems may be in place.
NB: These scoring systems should always be used with the D-dimer result.

D-dimer

Has an important role in diagnosing and excluding PE and should only be used with a pre-test clinical probability assessment following careful clinical evaluation by an experienced clinician. D-dimers are sensitive for DVT and thromboembolism, but not specific. They are rarely in the normal range in cases of acute thromboembolism but are not a valid screening test for PE alone. D-dimers are generated as a result of fibrinolysis, which occurs

Table 39.3 Wells' score for PE

Clinical feature	Score
Clinical signs and symptoms of DVT (minimum of leg swelling and pain with palpation of the deep veins)	3
An alternative diagnosis is less likely than PE	3
HR >100 bpm	1.5
Immobilization for >3 days or surgery in the previous 4 weeks	1.5
Previous DVT or PE	1.5
Haemoptysis	1
Malignancy (on treatment, treated in the past 6 months, or palliative)	1
Likelihood of PE	
PE *likely*	>4 points
PE *unlikely*	≤4 points

in many clinical situations, including sepsis, post-surgery, pneumonia, neoplasia, inflammatory disease, pregnancy, and advanced age; some laboratories will quote as 10× age as the upper limit normal (aged over 55)
- Only a normal result (which virtually excludes PE) is of clinical value
- An abnormal result (however high) does not necessarily imply a significantly increased probability of PE
- The sensitivity ranges from 87% to 99%, depending on the assay used; these should be known before incorporating into diagnostic algorithms
- D-dimer testing for excluding PE has been validated as an outpatient test but not in inpatient groups.

Assessment and documentation of pre-test clinical probability in PE is paramount. This enables accurate clinical assessment and may obviate the need for imaging.

An alternative explanation for the symptoms should be sought when a PE is excluded.

Investigations

- *ECG* Non-specific changes are frequent. Most commonly, sinus tachycardia. AF, right bundle branch block (RBBB), anterior T-wave inversion (indicating RV strain) are common. The $S_1Q_3T_3$ pattern is uncommon
- *Chest radiograph (CXR)* A good-quality departmental CXR is required. No specific features are characteristic in PE, but it may reveal another pathology. Small effusions are present in 40% (80% are exudates, 20% transudates). Focal infiltrates, segmental collapse, and a raised hemidiaphragm can also occur
- *ABGs* may be normal, especially in the young and healthy. Hypoxia and hypocapnia, due to hyperventilation, with an increased A–a gradient, are more common
- *D-dimer* (see ➜ p. 474)
- *Brain natriuretic peptide* (BNP) levels in acute PE reflect severity of RV strain and haemodynamic compromise, providing additional prognostic information to that of echo
- Elevated *cardiac troponin* levels are associated with worse short-term prognosis in acute PE. Heart-type fatty acid-binding protein (H-FABP), an early marker of myocardial injury, is reported to be superior to troponin or myoglobin measurements for risk stratification of PE on admission. There are currently no universally accepted criteria for the measurement of myocardial injury in acute PE
- *Computed tomographic pulmonary angiogram (CTPA)* is the gold standard investigation and is recommended as the initial imaging technique in suspected non-massive PE. It has a sensitivity of >95% and may enable an alternative diagnosis to be made if PE is excluded. Advances in imaging mean that a 16-slice multi-detector row scanner can image the entire chest with resolution approaching 1 mm, requiring a breath-hold of <10 s. Emboli can be detected in sixth-order pulmonary vessels, which are so small that their clinical relevance is uncertain. CTPA should be performed within 1 h in suspected massive PE and within 24 h of suspected non-massive PE. The sensitivity and specificity of CTPA depends on the location of the emboli, with lower sensitivity for clot confined to the segmental or subsegmental pulmonary vessels, compared with more central clot. CTPA needs specialist reporting
- In those with a high clinical probability, but negative CTPA, the options are:
  - PE has been excluded; stop anticoagulation, or
  - Perform further imaging (leg US, conventional pulmonary angiogram, venous phase CT to include the legs)

In one large prospective multicentre study, with all patients investigated with CTPA and leg US, those with negative tests and low or intermediate clinical probability were not anticoagulated. Only 0.2% had a definite PE after 3 months of follow-up. Those with negative tests, but high clinical probability, were investigated further, and PE was identified in 5% (Musset D et al. *Lancet* 2002;360: 1914).

A volume of 100–150mL contrast media is required for CTPA, which poses a substantial risk of nephropathy (in patients with renal insufficiency and diabetes) and sometimes fluid overload (patients with impaired LV function). In these patients, leg ultrasound (US) and/or isotope lung scanning might be safer first-line investigations.

Isotope lung scanning (V/Q scan)—mostly now superseded by CTPA. Some units may just perform the Q (perfusion) part of the scan. May be useful as a first-line imaging investigation in patients with a normal CXR and with no concurrent cardiopulmonary disease, in whom a negative scan can reliably exclude a PE. Scans are reported as low, intermediate, or high probability, and the report's meaning must be interpreted in light of the pre-test clinical probability score. Further imaging is necessary for those in whom:
• The scan is indeterminate
• There is a discordant scan result and clinical probability.

> *The clinical significance of the V/Q scan report is:*
> • Normal = no PE
> • Low or intermediate pre-test clinical probability *plus* low probability scan = PE excluded
> • High pre-test clinical probability *plus* high probability scan = PE diagnosed
> • Any other = need further imaging.

Other imaging techniques

• *Leg US* Around 70% of patients with a proven PE have a proximal DVT; hence, leg imaging can be used as an alternative to lung imaging in those with clinical DVT. A single examination is not adequate to exclude subclinical DVT (venography is more sensitive). It is safe to withhold anticoagulation in patients with suspected DVT and a single negative leg US, but these data cannot yet be extrapolated to those presenting with suspected PE. If a leg US is positive in a patient with clinical features of PE, this excludes the need for further imaging. Up to 50% of patients with a clinically obvious DVT will have a high-probability V/Q scan
• *Conventional pulmonary angiogram* is available in a few specialist centres only where catheter fragmentation of large clots may be of therapeutic benefit. Now mostly superseded by CTPA
• *CT venography* is an emerging area. It can be combined with CTPA to image the pelvic leg veins simultaneously
• *Echo* is diagnostic in submassive and massive PE. The transoesophageal route is more sensitive, enabling visualization of intrapulmonary and intracardiac clot. Gives prognostic information and aids risk stratification.
• *Transthoracic US* is used uncommonly. May show peripheral infarcts with peripheral PEs.

Treatment

Risk stratification

The PE severity index (PESI, see Table 39.4) is a validated score allowing stratification of immediate risk following PE, dividing patients into high-risk and non-high-risk groups, and clearly defines a low-risk population suitable for outpatient management. The simplified PE severity score (sPESI, see Table 39.5) uses 6 variables and is non-inferior to the PESI in predicting 30-day mortality.

- *High-risk (also known as massive, haemodynamically unstable) PE* Shock or hypotension, with positive biomarkers of RV dysfunction, is a life-threatening emergency and has a mortality of >15%. Usually caused by a very large clot burden, but can be seen with smaller volume clot in those with poor cardio-respiratory reserve
- *Non-high-risk PE* can be stratified with the use of cardiac biomarkers of RV dysfunction or myocardial injury into *intermediate high risk/sub-massive* - (one or more positive markers but no shock, mortality 3–15%, requires in-hospital management) and *low-risk* PE (negative markers, mortality <1%)
- Echocardiographic features of RV dysfunction occur in up to 25% of all patients with PE and are associated with a twofold increased risk of death. There is no agreed definition of the echo features of RV dysfunction. On CTPA, flattening of the intraventricular septum and an RV/LV ratio >0.9 suggests RV strain, correlating with echo findings and biomarkers.

Table 39.4 PESI

Clinical feature	Score
Age—add 1 point per year of age	Age
♂ patient	10
History of cancer	30
History of heart failure	10
History of chronic lung disease	10
HR ≥110	20
Systolic BP <100 mmHg	30
RR ≥30/min	20
Temperature <36°C	20
Altered mental status? (disoriented, lethargy, stupor, or coma)	60
SaO$_2$ on room air <90%	20
Totals:	
≤65 Class I: Very low risk	
66–85 Class II: Low risk	
86–105 Class III: Intermediate risk	
106–125 Class IV: High risk	
>125 Class V: Very high risk	

Table 39.5 sPESI

Parameter	Score	Risk Class	Total points
Age >80 y	1	low risk	0
Cancer*	1	high risk	≥1
Chronic			
cardiopulmonary disease 1			
Pulse ≥100 bpm	1		
SBP<100 mmHg 1			
Arterial O2 SaO2 <90%			
(with or without O2)	1		

*active cancer (diagnosed within last 12 m) or on active treatment. A score of 0 is classified as low risk

Anticoagulation

Low molecular weight heparin (LMWH)

As effective as standard unfractionated intravenous (IV) heparin and should be given to patients with intermediate or a high pre-test clinical probability immediately, prior to imaging.

Unfractionated heparin

Should be considered in massive PE (faster onset of action); first dose bolus prior to commencement of LMWH. Renal impairment (estimated glomerular filtration rate (eGFR) <30); use either unfractionated heparin or LMWH with anti-factor Xa monitoring. Use unfractionated heparin if risk of bleeding.

Oral anticoagulation

Direct oral anticoagulants (DOACs) are now the mainstay of treatment. Apixaban, dabigatran, edoxaban, and rivaroxaban are all licensed for the treatment of venous thromboembolism. Apixaban and rivaroxaban are preferable as they do not require 5 days of LMWH treatment first. A high-dose regimen is tailed off after 7 and 21 days, respectively. DOACs have a lower bleeding risk then warfarin/LMWH and are non-inferior in terms of efficacy.

Length of anticoagulation

- Temporary provoking risk factor: 3 months
- First episode of idiopathic PE—review anticoagulation at 3 months. Discuss with patient, including consideration of risk of bleeding and risk of recurrence. Some advocate 6 months' treatment or lifelong treatment—in which case this decision should be reviewed annually, as the relative risks and benefits of anticoagulation may change
- For patients with active cancer—6 months of LMWH before a decision as to whether to continue with a vitamin K antagonist (VKA) long term

- Recurrent idiopathic PE—no guidelines exist; length of treatment depends on individual circumstances, with risk of bleeding balanced with risk of recurrent event, and often long-term anticoagulation
- Persisting risk factors: lifelong anticoagulation may be recommended

Side effects
- The risk of bleeding increases with age and concurrent illness
- Higher bleeding rate with concomitant aspirin use and previous GI bleed

Additional treatments

IV Fluids
Required to maintain the blood pressure. Ionotropes may be required.

High-flow oxygen
If significant hypoxia, target saturation 94–98%. Significant hypoxia with haemodynamic instability should prompt early intubation and transfer to ICU.

Outpatient/ambulatory management
Low-risk PE (PESI I–II or sPESI 0) can be considered for outpatient management as long as there is a robust system in place and no social or other medical reasons requiring admission to hospital. Up to 44% of patients may meet criteria or ambulatory management. If RV dilatation is seen on echo or CT, a negative cardiac biomarker (troponin or BNP) can help to reassure that this is not clinically relevant. Advice on when to represent and follow-up plans to be provided pre discharge.

Thrombolysis

There is emerging evidence to support the use of thrombolysis in certain subgroups of patients with PE; however, this is a controversial area, and the risk/benefit analysis of this treatment must always be carefully considered.

High Risk PE
Causing circulatory collapse (systolic BP <90 mmHg or a pressure drop of 40 mmHg with no other explanation). Current NICE guidance (2012) recommends unfractionated heparin and subsequent systemic thrombolysis. In practice, thrombolysis is usually given to the acutely unwell/peri-arrest patient, when the history and physical findings are suggestive of massive PE, in the absence of another reasonable explanation. There is rarely time for imaging or investigations in this situation. See Box 39.1.

Intermediate risk PE
Those in PESI classes III and IV. If these patients have a high cardiac biomarker or evidence of RV dysfunction on CT or echo, they should be labelled as intermediate high risk and be considered for thrombolysis or reperfusion therapy. However, the PEITHO study demonstrated no mortality benefit at 7 or 30 d from thrombolysis with a higher bleeding rate. Systolic blood pressure (SBP) <110 mmHg, RR >20 bpm, active cancer, and heart failure were associated with a poorer outcome. No clear guidance exists for this patient group at present and senior clinicians must be involved early.

Contraindications
None absolute; rarely a consideration in the life-threatening situation. Risk
of major haemorrhage is 3–4 times that of heparin (around 13% in large
studies), with a higher incidence of bleeding in the elderly. Active bleeding
or recent intracerebral bleed are contraindications.

Catheter directed thrombolysis and half-dose thrombolysis
May improve outcomes and reduce bleeding rates but there is limited current data to support these.

Embolectomy
Rarely done, and only in life-threatening massive PE or if thrombolysis
is contraindicated. Options include surgical embolectomy (few regional centres only) and mechanical clot fragmentation via right heart
catheterization.

▶▶Box 39.1 Management of acute massive/high risk PE
Acute massive PE has a mortality of 20%; involve senior colleagues early,
and arrange transfer of the patient to a critical care area.
- O₂—100%, via non-rebreathe mask
- IV access. Send baseline bloods, including clotting. Perform ECG
- Analgesia, if required; consider opiates
- Management of cardiogenic shock—fluids and inotropes may be
  required in submassive or massive PE to maintain RV filling
- Start IV heparin unless active gastrointestinal (GI) bleeding or
  intracerebral haemorrhage:
  - Bolus dose 5,000–10,000 U or 80 IU/kg
  - Maintenance infusion of 1,300 IU/h or 18 U/kg/h
  - Adjust infusion rate until APTT is 1.5–2.5× control. Check APTT
    4–6 h after initial bolus and 6–10 h after any dose change. When
    APTT is in the therapeutic range, check it daily
- Investigation to confirm PE depends on the clinical state of patient.
  Ideally perform urgent echo, and, if this is non-diagnostic, perform
  a CTPA but not delaying for >1 h. It may, however, be unwise to
  move a sick patient to the radiology department for a CTPA. If
  there is circulatory collapse and the patient is peri-arrest and PE is
  the most likely cause, confirmation of the diagnosis should not be
  sought but treatment prioritized. Remember aortic dissection, cardiac
  tamponade, and acute MI can mimic PE
- Thrombolysis if collapsed or hypotensive, if no active GI bleeding or
  intracerebral haemorrhage:
  - Alteplase 100 mg over 2 h, given peripherally, or
  - Streptokinase 250,000 U in 30 min, with 100,000 U/h for 24 h
    (plus hydrocortisone to prevent further circulatory instability), or
  - Urokinase 4,400 IU/kg in 10 min and 4,400 IU/kg/h for 12 h
  - Stop the heparin during thrombolysis, and restart afterwards
  - In cardiac arrest due to suspected massive PE, 50 mg IV alteplase
    immediately may be lifesaving
- Consider liaising with cardiothoracic centre to consider embolectomy,
  particularly if thrombolysis is contraindicated or has failed.

Inferior vena cava (IVC) filter placement

There is little evidence to show improved survival or reduction in recurrent PE rate with IVC filters, and changing to LMWH may be as effective. They are potentially pro-thrombotic and should be removed as soon as possible once no longer required. IVC filters may be indicated in:

• Acute VTE in patients with an absolute contraindication to anticoagulation
• Patients with recent massive PE who survive (a second PE may be fatal)
• Recurrent VTE despite adequate anticoagulation
• Post-pulmonary thromboendarterectomy in PHT.

PE response teams (PERTs)

Are of benefit and provide expertise in complex scenarios where the risk/benefit of thrombolysis and the diagnosis is difficult.

Follow up

All patients need follow up, usually 3 months post diagnosis. Several areas need discussion.

The patient is often keen to ensure their clot has resolved; some centres will use a Q scan or CTPA, while others go on clinical assessment and symptoms

Length of anticoagulation needs to be discussed

• Cancer screening: NICE guidance recommends assessment for the possibility of underlying cancer in those with unprovoked PE aged >40 y, with clinical examination, blood tests, CXR, and CT abdomen/pelvis for all and mammogram for women
• The echo needs to be repeated in those with an initial high PAP or those with ongoing breathlessness
• Consider whether antiphospholipid and hereditary thrombophilia testing is required.

Further information

Howard LSGE et al. British Thoracic Society Guideline for the initial out patient management of PE. *Thorax*. 2018;73: ii1–ii29.

Konstantinides S et al. Heparin plus alteplase compared with heparin alone in patients with submassive pulmonary embolism. *N Engl J Med*. 2002;347: 1143–1150.

Torbicki A et al. European Society of Cardiology acute PE guidelines. *Eur Heart J*. 2008;29: 2276–2315.

NICE Pulmonary embolism guideline (CG144) 2015. ℘ http://www.nice.org.uk

℘ http://www.thrombosisuk.org

℘ https://www.escardio.org/Guidelines/Clinical-Practice-Guidelines/Acute-Pulmonary-Embolism-Diagnosis-and-Management-of

Special circumstances

Pregnancy and thromboembolic disease

PE in pregnancy should be managed as in the non-pregnant patient, although the PESI score is not validated so the decision about outpatient management should be made in consultation with an obstetrician.

- The incidence of DVT ± PE in pregnancy is 1 in 1,000, rising to 2 in 1,000 in the puerperium. The risk of PE in pregnancy is greater with increasing maternal age and with increasing gestational age. More PEs occur during pregnancy than after delivery. There is a 20–30 times increased risk with Caesarean section, compared with normal vaginal delivery. PE is one of the commonest causes of maternal death in pregnancy (1/100,000 pregnancies)
- D-dimers are raised in normal pregnancy and so are unhelpful in the investigation of thromboembolic disease, unless negative
- The CTPA whole body radiation dose is 2–4 mGy, with an absorbed dose to the foetus of 0.01 mSv. This equates to a risk of fatal cancer to age 15 of <1 in 1 million. The absorbed dose to the breast is 10 mSv (higher in pregnancy). CTPA increases the lifetime breast cancer risk in premenopausal women from 10% to 11.4%, with an even higher risk in pregnancy
- The V/Q scan whole body radiation dose is 1.5–2 mGy, with an absorbed dose to the foetus of 0.12 mSv. This equates to a risk of fatal cancer to age 15 of 1 in 280,000. The absorbed dose to the breast is 0.28 mSv. A half-dose perfusion scan reduces radiation dose further
- The overall radiation risk depends on the gestation of the foetus and the metabolic activity of the pregnant breast tissue. There is considerable debate as to which imaging technique is best in pregnancy, in terms of radiation risk to both the mother (including breast tissue) and the foetus. The lowest overall risk favours a Q scan as the first-line investigation, especially as this young healthy population are likely to have normal lungs. Some experts suggest a leg US first (see ⊃ p. 477)
- In those with antenatal thromboembolic disease, LMWH is used. Close to delivery, this is changed to unfractionated heparin, as it is easier to monitor and to reverse its effects. It is unclear whether heparin should be stopped or the dose reduced at the time of delivery. LMWH levels can be monitored with anti-Xa levels
- There are case reports of successful thrombolysis, catheter-directed thrombolysis, and embolectomy in massive PE, but no relevant trials
- Warfarin is teratogenic and is contraindicated in pregnancy, although it is safe in breastfeeding. DOACs are not licensed
- Anticoagulation should be continued for 6 weeks after delivery or 3 months following the initial episode, whichever is longer.

Thromboembolic disease and the OCP/HRT

- Oestrogen-containing OCPs, pregnancy, and HRT increase the risk of PE, but the incidence of fatal PE is low—estimated at 1/100,000 OCP users, with a median age of 29
- Risk of fatal PE is twice as high in those taking third-generation pills
- Previous history of DVT or PE is a contraindication to the OCP
- Meta-analyses show a relative risk of VTE of 2.1 in HRT users, which is highest in the first year of use.

Rare causes

Air embolism

Air within the arterial or venous circulation. Small amounts of air can be tolerated, but large amounts can lodge in the pulmonary vasculature and cause mechanical obstruction and death. This is rare.

Causes

Neck vein cannulation, intrauterine manipulations (such as criminal abortion where a frothy liquid is passed under pressure into the uterus), bronchial trauma, or barotrauma causing air to enter the pulmonary vein and left heart. Air in the LV causes impairment to venous filling and subsequent poor coronary perfusion as air enters the coronary arteries.

Diagnosis

Arterial air emboli may cause dizziness, loss of consciousness, and convulsions. Air may be seen in the retinal arteries or from transected vessels. *Venous* air emboli may cause raised venous pressure, cyanosis, hypotension, tachycardia, syncope, and a 'mill-wheel' murmur over the praecordium.

Treatment

Patients should lie on their right side, with head down and feet up, to allow air to collect and stay at the cardiac apex. From here, it can be aspirated via thoracotomy.

Amniotic fluid embolism

Estimated to occur in 1 in 25,000–80,000 live births. It is the third commonest cause of maternal death, and the most common cause of death in the immediate post-partum period. Usually catastrophic, 80% of women die, 20–50% of these in the first hour. An anaphylactic-type response to amniotic fluid entering the circulation is seen. Amniotic fluid enters the circulation because of torn foetal membranes, which can occur in Caesarean section, uterine or cervical trauma, or uterine rupture. It has a thromboplastic effect, causing disseminated intravascular coagulation (DIC) and thrombi to form in pulmonary vessels. Not all women react in this way to amniotic fluid. It is more common in older multiparous mothers, who have had short tumultuous labour, often involving uterine stimulants.

Clinical presentation

Sudden-onset respiratory distress, hypoxia, bronchospasm, cyanosis, cardiovascular collapse, pulmonary oedema, convulsions, coma, and cardiac arrest. Coagulopathy with intractable uterine bleeding and uterine atony is seen.

Clinical diagnosis

Foetal debris/cells can be identified in blood sampled from the maternal pulmonary artery, but this is not pathognomonic.

Treatment

Supportive, while the thrombi clear from the maternal lungs. Maintain the circulation with fluids and inotropes. Respiratory support with O_2 and ventilation may be needed. Correct coagulopathy with fresh frozen plasma and packed cells. Control placental bleeding.

Fat embolism

Common pathological finding following long bone fractures. Occurs especially with lower limb fractures—pelvis and femur. Commoner in fractures that have not been immobilized. Can also occur after prosthetic joint replacement, cardiac massage, liver trauma, burns, bone marrow transplant, rapid high-altitude decompression, and liposuction. Generally occurs in the young and previously healthy. Presents 24–72 h post-fracture. Marrow fat enters the circulation and lodges in the lungs, causing mechanical obstruction.

Classical presentation

Hypoxia, coagulopathy, with a transient petechial rash on the neck, axillae, and skinfolds, and neurological disturbance such as confusion, disorientation, or sometimes coma. Stable patients may deteriorate with low-grade fever, petechial rash, hypoxia, and confusion. Jaundice and renal dysfunction are possible.

Diagnosis

Usually made clinically in a patient with a lower limb fracture presenting with tachypnoea and hypoxia. Fat globules can be identified in the urine. CXR shows bilateral alveolar infiltrates. Acute respiratory distress syndrome (ARDS) can develop.

Treatment

Early immobilization of fracture, fluid replacement, O_2, and supportive care

Septic, hydatid, and tumour emboli

Also rare causes. Uterine leiomyosarcoma has vascular tropism and can invade the IVC and obstruct the pulmonary arteries. Teratomas can invade the IVC and pulmonary arteries.

Chapter 40

Rare lung diseases

Alveolar microlithiasis 490
Amyloidosis: pathophysiology and classification 492
Amyloidosis: lung involvement 1 494
Amyloidosis: lung involvement 2 496
Hereditary haemorrhagic telangiectasia (HHT) 497
Idiopathic pulmonary hemosiderosis 498
Langerhans cell histiocytosis 500
Lymphangioleiomyomatosis (LAM): clinical features 502
LAM: diagnosis and management 504
Primary ciliary dyskinesia (PCD) 506
Pulmonary alveolar proteinosis (PAP): pathophysiology and clinical features 508
PAP: diagnosis and treatment 510
Pulmonary arteriovenous malformations (PAVMs): aetiology and diagnosis 512
PAVMs: management and complications 514
Recurrent respiratory papillomatosis 515

Alveolar microlithiasis

This is a rare interstitial lung disease (ILD), characterized by the accumulation of numerous and diffuse calcified microliths (round calcium and phosphate hydroxyapatite bodies) in the alveolar space. There is no identifiable abnormality of calcium metabolism. A mutation in the *SLC34A2* gene that encodes a type IIb sodium-phosphate co-transporter in alveolar type II cells, resulting in the accumulation and formation of microliths rich in calcium phosphate (due to impaired clearance), is considered to be the cause of the disease. Microliths are occasionally identified in the sputum. At postmortem, the lungs are heavy and rock hard, often needing a saw to cut them. Fewer than 200 cases are reported.

Clinical features

- Typically presents in young adults, most commonly in the third and fourth decades of life
- May be an incidental chest radiograph (CXR) finding in asymptomatic patients
- Familial tendency—probable autosomal recessive inheritance
- Equal sex distribution in sporadic cases, 2:1 ♀ preponderance in familial cases
- Usually slowly progressive, with progressive breathlessness, hypoxia, respiratory failure, and death
- CXR and chest computed tomography (CT) show fine micronodular lung calcification, predominantly basally or around the hila. It may produce complete radiographic opacification. There is no associated lymph node enlargement. Progressive lung infiltration causes restriction of lung movement and impairs gas exchange, leading to progressive respiratory failure.

Treatment

- There is no effective medical treatment
- Lung transplantation has been successful.

Further information

Francisco F et al. Pulmonary alveolar microlithiasis. State-of-the-art review. *Respir Med.* 2013;107: 1–9.

Amyloidosis: pathophysiology and classification

Definition

Amyloidosis is the extracellular deposition of low molecular weight protein molecules as insoluble fibrils. More than 20 such proteins have been described in different diseases and circumstances. For classification, see Box 40.1.

Box 40.1 Classification of amyloidosis

- 1°/light chain amyloid (AL), from immunoglobulin light chain fragments (λ or κ), usually monoclonal due to a plasma cell dyscrasia (a subtype of lymphoproliferative disorders)
  - 1 in 5,000 deaths due to this type of amyloid
  - Median survival is 6–15 months
  - Frank myeloma is present in 20%, and a subtle monoclonal gammopathy in 70% (MGUS)
  - Systemic form due to circulating monoclonal light chains, widespread organ involvement, particularly heart, liver, and kidneys
  - Localized amyloid production by local clonal B-cells; hence, heterogeneous organ involvement is seen, commonly in the upper respiratory tract and orbit, with urogenital and gastrointestinal (GI) involvement—virtually any organ (except the brain) can be involved
- 2° amyloid (AA)
  - A complication of chronic disease with ongoing/recurring inflammation, e.g. rheumatoid, chronic infections
  - The fibrils are fragments of acute phase reactant, serum amyloid A
  - Commonly renal, hepatic, and lower GI involvement; rarely neurological, lung, and cardiac involvement
  - Median survival 5 y
  - Only a small number of patients with chronic inflammation will develop AA amyloidosis, and the time period for the development of the disease is very variable
- Dialysis-related amyloid (DA), due to fibrils derived from β_2 microglobulin that accumulate in dialysis patients
- Inherited amyloidosis, e.g. due to abnormal pre-albumin (transthyretin, TTR), damaging neural and cardiac tissue
- Organ-specific amyloid such as Alzheimer's disease; plaques of the β protein derived from the larger amyloid precursor protein (APP). Protein presumed to be generated locally.

Pathophysiology

The disease is one of abnormal protein folding and is classified by the origin of the precursor proteins that form the amyloid. For example, AL amyloid forms from the light chains of immunoglobulins. In familial forms, genetic missense mutations produce abnormal folding of the protein.

- Little is known of the specific genetic and environmental factors leading to development of abnormal folding

- Despite different origins, protein molecules fold into alternative forms very similar to each other; in the classic 'β-pleated sheet' structure, fibrils form in an ordered fashion, with uniformity of fibril structure within the sheet
- Substitutions of particular amino acids at specific positions in the light chain variable region lead to destabilization of the light chains, increasing the chance of fibrillogenesis
- In certain models, this abnormal folding can be initiated by the addition of 'amyloid-enhancing factor', rather like the initiation of crystal formation in a supersaturated solution.

Amyloid deposits accumulate in the extracellular space, disrupting normal tissue architecture and leading to organ dysfunction, both directly, and having space occupying effects. The fibrils may be directly cytotoxic (possibly by promoting apoptosis). The subdivisions of amyloid are largely based on the origin of the amyloid protein and shown in Box 40.1.

Epidemiology

The epidemiology is difficult to define accurately, as the disease is often un- or misdiagnosed. The age-adjusted incidence is estimated to be 5–13 per million person years.

Future developments

Anti-amyloid drugs are under investigation, including drugs to stabilize the amyloid precursor proteins in their normal configuration and enhance fibril degradation.

Amyloidosis: lung involvement 1

Clinically significant respiratory tract disease is almost always AL in type, though the presence of a strong family history or chronic inflammatory disease may suggest other types.

Laryngeal amyloidosis

Amyloid causes up to 1% of benign laryngeal disease. May present as discrete nodules or diffuse infiltration and is usually localized, though can be a rare manifestation of systemic (AL) amyloid. Deposits are seen most commonly in the supraglottic larynx (presenting with hoarse voice or stridor). May present with choking and exertional dyspnoea that can be progressive or recurrent.

Tracheobronchial amyloid

Rare (67 worldwide cases reported by the mid-1980s). Macroscopically, is either diffusely infiltrative or 'tumour-like'. It is associated with tracheobronchopathia osteoplastica (a disorder characterized by the deposition of calcified submucosal airway nodules). It presents after the fifth decade with dyspnoea, cough, and rarely haemoptysis. Airway narrowing can lead to atelectasis or recurrent pneumonia; solitary nodules may lead to investigation for presumed lung cancer. Symptomatic disease is usually localized.

Parenchymal amyloid

The most frequently diagnosed amyloid respiratory disease. It is usually divided radiologically into solitary/multiple pulmonary nodules (usually localized AL amyloid) or a diffuse alveolar pattern (usually a manifestation of systemic AL amyloid). Parenchymal amyloid lung nodules are usually peripheral and subpleural, may be bilateral, and are more common in the lower lobes, ranging in diameter 0.4–15 cm. They may cavitate or calcify. Clinical signs are non-diagnostic; pulmonary function tests (PFTs) may show a restrictive defect with reduced transfer factor. The differential diagnosis usually includes fibrosis. Cardiac amyloid may coexist, and distinguishing the contribution to the symptoms of the pulmonary and cardiac disease can be difficult. Median survival with clinically overt lung disease is about 16 months (similar to that of systemic amyloid).

Mediastinal and hilar amyloidosis

Rarely associated with localized pulmonary amyloidosis, and their diagnosis should lead to a search for a systemic cause of amyloid. Amyloid lymphadenopathy can also represent localized AL deposition, in association with B-cell lymphoma.

Pleural effusions

- Occur in up to 2% of those with systemic amyloid
- Seem to be due to pleural infiltration with amyloid deposits
- It can be difficult to distinguish between primary effusions and those due to amyloid related cardiomyopathy
- The sensitivity of pleural biopsy in this situation is unknown
- Pleurodesis has been tried in some cases.

Other

Rare reports of:
- Ventilatory failure due to diaphragm or other respiratory muscle involvement
- Sleep apnoea from macroglossia due to amyloid.

Clinical features

- Dyspnoea and cough
- None—parenchymal disease may be an incidental finding on routine radiography
- Consider the diagnosis particularly in patients with odd upper airway symptoms and parenchymal involvement or those with unexplained congestive cardiac failure (CCF) or nephrotic syndrome.

Diagnosis

Histological confirmation is usually required. Congo red stain producing 'apple green' birefringence in crossed polarized light is the gold standard. Positive histology must lead to immunohistochemistry to determine the fibril type.
- *Histology* transbronchial biopsy (TBB) or occasionally open or video-assisted thoracoscopic surgery (VATS) biopsy (more likely if investigation for solitary pulmonary nodule)
- *123I-labelled scintigraphy* Radiolabelled serum amyloid P (SAP) localizes to amyloid deposits in proportion to the quantity of amyloid present, therefore allowing identification of the distribution and burden of disease. It is most sensitive for solid organ disease, although in lung disease, it can be useful for determining the extent of disease in other organs. It is expensive and carries an infection risk, as the SAP component is currently obtained from blood donors
- *High resolution computed tomography (HRCT)* may show nodules or parenchymal disease
- *Laryngoscopy and bronchoscopy* may be needed to obtain samples for histology, depending on the clinical presentation
- *PFTs* to assess the effect of disease on respiratory function. May show reduced transfer factor and a restrictive pattern. Tracheobronchial involvement may lead to abnormal flow–volume loops due to larger airway obstruction
- Systemic disease:
  - Full blood count (FBC), biochemistry, and urinalysis (?renal involvement)
  - Investigate for underlying blood cell dyscrasia, e.g. myeloma, Waldenström's macroglobulinaemia (bone marrow examination, and search for urine and serum monoclonal protein by immunofixation—the clonal proliferation underlying systemic AL amyloid is usually very subtle, and its identification may be difficult)
  - Echo or cardiac magnetic resonance imaging (MRI) for associated cardiac involvement (when CCF is present; survival is 4–6 months)
  - Thyroid/adrenal function is impaired in up to 10%.

Amyloidosis: lung involvement 2

Treatment

There are limited clinical trials with which to guide management of respiratory tract amyloid. Management decisions are therefore often made empirically. General treatment depends on the cause of the fibril precursor production i.e. treatment for the underlying systemic inflammatory condition in AA amyloidosis, and treatment of the underlying bloods cell dyscrasia in AL amyloid.

- No treatment may be needed
- Local measures may be warranted for endobronchial disease, e.g. symptomatic laryngeal disease—endoscopic excision, CO_2 laser evaporation (useful for small recurrent lesions), stenting. Steroids have no effect on laryngeal amyloid
- Tracheobronchial amyloid—management depends on symptoms, and treatment may involve repeated endoscopic resection, YAG (yttrium–aluminium–garnet) laser therapy, and surgical resection. Repeated endoscopic procedures are thought to be safer than repeated open surgery
- Chemotherapy may be warranted for diffuse parenchymal amyloid if there is objectively measurable disease (prednisolone and melphalan to suppress the underlying blood cell dyscrasia). More intensive chemotherapy has a better clinical response, but there are few trials
- Direct agents targeting amyloidogenic precursors (e.g. transthyretin, TTR) are in early use.

Further information

Blancas-Mejia LM, Ramirez-Alvarado M. Systemic amyloidoses. *Annu Rev Biochem*. 2013;82: 745–774.
Gillmore JD, Hawkins PN. Amyloidosis and the respiratory tract. Rare diseases. *Thorax*. 1999;54: 444–451.
UK National Amyloid Centre is at the Royal Free Hospital, London. ℘ https://www.ucl.ac.uk/amyloidosis/national-amyloidosis-centre

Hereditary haemorrhagic telangiectasia (HHT)

Definition

Also referred to as Osler–Weber–Rendu syndrome, with a prevalence: 1 in 5,000–8,000, it is an autosomal dominant disorder, >80% of all cases of HHT are due to mutations in either *ENG* (HHT1) or *ACVRL1* (HHT2) (endoglin and activin, both TGF-β1 receptors). A total of over 600 different mutations is known. It is characterized by the development of abnormal dilated vessels in the systemic circulation, which may bleed, leading to:

* Recurrent epistaxis
* GI bleeding
* Iron deficiency anaemia
* Other organ involvement, e.g. hepatic (in 30%, commonly asymptomatic), renal, pulmonary, and spinal arteriovenous malformations (AVMs).

Screening

Careful questioning of family members (does anyone in the family have frequent nose bleeds?) and examination for telangiectasia should reveal those in whom screening should occur.

All those with HHT should be screened for pulmonary AVMs (PAVMs; see € p. 514), and all of their offspring post-puberty and pre-pregnancy. There is increasing penetrance with increasing age (62% at age 16, 95% at age 40). Similarly, the detection of PAVMs in a patient should lead to screening for HHT in family members.

There is no consensus regarding the best screening method, but a combination of the following tests may be used:

* CXR
* Supine and erect oximetry
* CT chest
* Shunt quantification techniques, e.g. contrast echo, 100% O_2 rebreathing.

Screening should continue throughout life (every 5–10 y) and during times of enlargement or development of AVMs—post-puberty and pre-pregnancy.

Management

* Usually involves liaison with ENT and gastroenterology colleagues for symptomatic treatment
* Iron replacement, transfusions
* Asymptomatic hepatic AVMs—no treatment usually required
* Cerebral AVMs (in 15% of HHT patients)—some specialists argue these should be treated prophylactically due to the risk of rupture and bleeding (2%/y, often fatal).
* Patients with HHT are increased risk of venous thromboembolism and pulmonary hypertension (PHT), usually due to increased pulmonary flow due to systemic AVMs.

Further information

Shovlin CL, Letarte M. Hereditary haemorrhagic telangiectasia and pulmonary AVMs: issues in clinical management and review of pathogenic mechanisms. *Thorax*. 1999;54: 714–739.

Idiopathic pulmonary hemosiderosis

A rare disease of undetermined aetiology, characterized by recurrent episodes of alveolar haemorrhage and haemoptysis (in the absence of renal disease), usually leading to iron deficiency anaemia.

Pathophysiology

The alveolar space and interstitium contain hemosiderin-laden macrophages, with variable degrees of interstitial fibrosis and degeneration of alveolar, interstitial, and vascular elastic fibres, depending on the chronicity of the condition. Electron microscopy shows damage to the endothelial and basement membranes, but no consistent or diagnostic features have been recognized.

No antibodies have been identified, though serum IgA levels are sometimes raised. With recurrent alveolar haemorrhage, the alveolar blood provokes a fibrotic reaction, with the development of diffuse pulmonary fibrosis.

Iron turnover studies show that the accompanying iron deficiency anaemia is due to loss of iron into the lung through haemorrhage.

Aetiology

Uncertain, but likely to be multifactorial. Possible associations include toxic insecticides (epidemiological studies in rural Greece), premature birth, and fungal toxin exposure. The disease has an equal sex incidence in childhood, with twice as many men affected in adulthood.

Most patients present in childhood, with 85% of cases having onset of symptoms before 16 y. The actual prevalence is unknown, but a cohort study of Swedish children in the 1960s described an incidence of 0.24 per million children. Familial clustering is reported.

Pulmonary hemosiderosis is associated with RA, thyrotoxicosis, coeliac disease, and autoimmune haemolytic anaemia, suggesting a potential autoimmune mechanism.

Clinical features

The clinical course is very variable and ranges from continuous low-level bleeding to massive pulmonary haemorrhage. The latter may be fatal but is fortunately rare.

- Continuous mild pulmonary haemorrhage leads to a chronic non-productive cough with haemoptysis, malaise, lethargy, and failure to thrive in children
- Iron deficiency anaemia is common, as are positive faecal occult blood tests (due to swallowed blood)
- Generalized lymphadenopathy and hepatosplenomegaly are recognized
- With an acute bleed, cough and haemoptysis may worsen, and dyspnoea, chest tightness, and pyrexia may develop
- Chronic bleeding leads to chronic disabling dyspnoea, chronic anaemia, and clubbing (in 25%). Cor pulmonale 2° to pulmonary fibrosis and hypoxaemia may develop.

Examination

May be normal. Clubbing, basal crepitations, and cor pulmonale are all recognized, depending on the severity of the resulting lung disease.

Investigations

The diagnosis is one of exclusion, with no evidence of other organ involvement. The main differential diagnosis is Goodpasture's syndrome, granulomatosis with polyangiitis (Wegener's) (GPA), systemic lupus erythematosus (SLE), and microscopic polyarteritis.

- *Blood tests* Microcytic, hypochromic anaemia, with low iron levels. Antinuclear cytoplasmic antibody (ANCA), double-stranded DNA, and anti-glomerular basement membrane antibodies should be negative
- *CXR* May show transient patchy infiltrates, which worsen during an acute bleed. The apices are usually spared. Progressive disease leads to the development of reticulonodular infiltrates and a ground-glass appearance that is typically perihilar or in the lower zones. Hilar lymphadenopathy may be seen
- *PFTs* kCO is transiently elevated during bleeding episodes (≥130% is abnormal), but this is only useful acutely. A restrictive defect with reduced kCO may develop with chronic disease
- *HRCT chest* The changes seen are fairly non-specific, showing a diffuse bilateral infiltrate, with patchy ground-glass change
- *Bronchoalveolar lavage (BAL)* (if done) contains hemosiderin-laden macrophages.

Management

There is no specific treatment.

- Steroids and immunosuppressive drugs (e.g. cyclophosphamide) may be of benefit during acute bleeding episodes but do not appear to affect the long-term outcome. There are no published data to guide the optimal timing of treatment during the course of disease
- The iron deficiency anaemia responds to replacement therapy, and blood transfusion may be needed in severe bleeds
- Lung transplant has been tried.

At routine clinic appointments
- Check spirometry
- Measure Hb and serum iron levels
- Ask about increases in SOB or haemoptysis.

Prognosis

The prognosis is very variable, with some patients showing spontaneous remission, others progressing to death. The duration of disease in the literature ranges from death within days, following an acute severe illness, to survival with cor pulmonale associated with chronic disease after 20 y.

Langerhans cell histiocytosis

Definition

Pulmonary Langerhans cell histiocytosis (LCH; previously termed pulmonary histiocytosis X or pulmonary eosinophilic granuloma) is a rare condition characterized by infiltration of the lung with histiocytes (Langerhans cells). Pulmonary LCH overlaps with a number of other conditions with similar pathological findings but diverse clinical features. These range from localized infiltration of a single organ (e.g. eosinophilic granuloma of bone) to systemic diseases affecting multiple organs (Letterer–Siwe disease, a multi-organ disease affecting infants and elderly, associated with poor prognosis; also Hand–Schueller–Christian syndrome). Although the isolated pulmonary form most commonly presents to chest physicians, pulmonary manifestations also commonly occur in the systemic forms of the disease.

Epidemiology

Rare. Tends to affect young adults aged 20–40 y. The vast majority of cases occur in current smokers, usually heavy smokers (tobacco and cannabis). May be more common in men, who tend to present at a younger age than women.

Pathogenesis

Langerhans cells are involved in antigen presentation and are characterized by the presence of well-demarcated cytoplasmic organelles called Birbeck granules on electron microscopy. The Langerhans cells seen in LCH appear to be monoclonal, although it is unclear if this represents a true neoplastic process. The antigen stimulus for activating Langerhans cells in the lung is unknown, although cigarette smoke is a possible candidate. Langerhans cells are typically organized into granulomata that are located in bronchiolar walls and subsequently enlarge and invade adjacent structures. This results in the radiological appearance of nodules that, at first, cavitate and then become cystic.

Clinical features

Typically, exertional breathlessness and cough, sometimes with systemic symptoms (e.g. fever, weight loss). Pneumothorax occurs in at least 10% of patients and may be the presenting feature. Rib lesions may also give rise to chest pain. Around 25% of patients are asymptomatic. Examination is usually normal.

Investigations

- *CXR* Typically diffuse reticulonodular shadowing, sometimes with cystic change; upper and middle lobe predominance. May be normal
- *HRCT* Diffuse centrilobular nodules, sometimes with cavitation, and thin- and thick-walled cystic lesions, reflecting lesions of varying age, sometimes bizarrely shaped. These are interspersed with normal lung. Upper and middle lobe predominance; costophrenic angles are typically spared. Purely nodular or purely cystic appearances may occur. Unusual manifestations, such as single nodules or large airways involvement, are also described
- *PFTs* Variable, ranging from normal to obstructive, restrictive, or mixed pattern. Reduced gas transfer and exertional hypoxia are common

- *TBB* may yield diagnostic material although is often unhelpful; risk of pneumothorax is unknown although may be increased. Surgical lung biopsy is often preferable
- *BAL* Increased total cell counts (and high levels of CD-1a positive dendritic cells) and pigmented macrophages, reflecting simply the presence of cigarette smoking. Use of antibodies (e.g. OKT6) to detect Langerhans cells in BAL fluid is limited by poor sensitivity
- *Extrathoracic biopsy* of involved sites (e.g. bone) may be diagnostic.

Diagnosis

Usually based on the combination of clinical and HRCT findings: typically, a young adult smoker with cysts and nodules on HRCT. Confirmation by surgical lung biopsy may be considered in atypical presentations such as the finding of solely nodular or cystic disease on HRCT. The appearance of purely cystic disease on HRCT may be confused with emphysema (where cysts lack walls) or LAM (where cysts are present uniformly in all regions of lung, including the costophrenic angles).

Associations

- Severe PHT—may be seen in the absence of significant parenchymal lung involvement; direct disease involvement of pulmonary vessels has been described
- Manifestations of systemic LCH—particularly diabetes insipidus from pituitary disease, skin involvement, lytic bony lesions, and rarely cardiac or GI disease
- Lymphoma—may precede, complicate, or coexist with pulmonary LCH
- Lung cancer—more common, probably as a result of cigarette smoking.

Management

Treatment, other than smoking cessation, is often not required and may be entirely successful with resolution of radiographic abnormalities. Oral corticosteroids may be tried in symptomatic disease, although there is little evidence to support their use; they are usually administered for at least 6 months. Lung transplantation should be considered in patients with severe respiratory failure or PHT. Pulmonary LCH may recur in transplanted lungs. Experimental treatments, such as the use of IL2 and anti-TNF-α, may be of benefit in the systemic forms of LCH seen in children.

Prognosis

Variable. Spontaneous improvement is common, although later reactivation of disease may occur. A minority of patients deteriorate rapidly, with respiratory failure and death within months. Overall life expectancy is reduced, with median survival 12 y from diagnosis. Death is most commonly due to respiratory failure. Poor prognostic factors include reduced FEV_1, increased RV, and reduced gas transfer.

Further information

Sundar KM et al. Pulmonary Langerhans cell histiocytosis. *Chest*. 2003;123: 1673–1683.
Patient website ♫ http://www.histio.org

Lymphangioleiomyomatosis (LAM): clinical features

Definition and aetiology

A rare disorder characterized by abnormal proliferation of smooth muscle cells, affecting women of childbearing age, usually in their 30s. The disease is hormone-dependent so can occur in post-menopausal women on oestrogen replacement therapy. 'Sporadic LAM' used for disease not associated with tuberous sclerosis.

- Incidence 1 in 1.1 million population
- 40% of adult women with tuberous sclerosis (learning difficulties, subungual fibromas, seizures, facial angiofibromas, autosomal dominant inheritance or spontaneous mutation) develop pulmonary changes identical to those of LAM.

Pathology

Abnormal proliferation of atypical smooth muscle cells (LAM cells) throughout the lung, airways, blood vessels, and lymphatics. There is nodular infiltration, which is initially subtle. Progressive growth causes lymphatic and airway obstruction, leading to cyst formation throughout the lungs. The infiltrating cells stain with antibodies to smooth muscle actin and desmin with HMB-45, an antibody that recognizes an epitope within the protein gp-100 in the melanogenesis pathway. LAM is caused by mutations in the tuberous sclerosis (*TSC*) genes, resulting in activation of the mTOR complex 1 signalling network. Inactivation of both alleles of *TSC2* seems to be necessary.

Clinical features

Common

- 2° pneumothorax (in two-thirds of patients; often a presenting feature; occurs due to lung cystic change; recurrence is common)
- Dyspnoea (in 42%) and cough (in 20%)
- Haemoptysis (in 14%)
- Chylothorax (in 12%, thoracic duct leakage as a result of lymphatic obstruction by LAM cells, may be bilateral).

Less common

- Pleural effusion
- Chest pain
- Pulmonary haemorrhage (due to blocked blood vessels and increased intraluminal pressure).

Other organs affected

Kidney

Angiomyolipoma, a benign tumour, occurs in 50% of LAM patients. Usually diagnosed on CT, these are mostly small and single but can be multiple and larger in tuberous sclerosis. Smaller tumours are usually asymptomatic, but larger ones can cause flank pain and bleeding into the renal tract. Treatment options include tumour resection or embolization. Nephrectomy is not usually required. Screening for these lesions is important, as it allows careful treatment planning should they become symptomatic.

Abdomen

Lymphadenopathy due to lymphatic obstruction. Occurs in one-third of patients and is usually asymptomatic.

Pelvis

Lymphangioleiomyoma—a cystic mass that enlarges during the day and causes fullness and bloating.

Chylous ascites

Can occur in the absence of chylothorax.

Skin

Cutaneous swellings, likely due to localized oedema.

Examination

May be normal. There may be pulmonary crepitations or signs of pleural effusion. Palpable abdominal masses may be present.

Investigations

- *PFTs* may be normal or show a predominantly obstructive pattern. Rarely restrictive. Decreased total lung carbon monoxide transfer factor (TLCO), with a normal or increased total lung capacity
- *CXR* may be normal. Lungs may appear hyperinflated, with reticular shadowing and septal lines due to obstructed lymphatics. There may also be a diffuse interstitial infiltrate
- *HRCT* shows a characteristic appearance, with multiple cysts throughout the lung of varying size, which are usually small (<1cm) and thin-walled. The adjoining lung parenchyma is normal. There may be pleural effusions
- *CT abdomen* to examine for presence of angiomyolipomas and other lymphatic involvement.
- *Positron emission tomography (PET)* scanning is not useful and high FDG update areas should prompt a search for an alternative/additional diagnosis.
- *Vascular endothelial growth factor-D (VEGF-D) levels* if high support the diagnosis, but usually only available in the research setting.

LAM: diagnosis and management

Diagnosis

Consider particularly in young or middle-aged women with:
- Recurrent pneumothoraces, especially those with pre-existing dyspnoea or haemoptysis
- Cystic lung disease, airflow obstruction, or chylous pleural effusions
- Angiomyolipomas or other retroperitoneal tumours
- Tuberous sclerosis and respiratory symptoms.

The disease is easily missed in its early stages. The diagnosis can be made on the characteristic CT appearances or on open lung biopsy. TBBs may not be diagnostic. Large retroperitoneal abdominal lymph nodes can also be biopsied.

Management

The course of LAM is variable. Treatment should be aimed at those who are symptomatic and declining.
- Refer to a specialist centre (Nottingham City Hospital in the UK).
- *Diet* Low-fat diet with medium-chain triglyceride supplementation may prevent chylothorax recurrence; no strong evidence for this, difficult diet to follow
- *Bronchodilators* may improve airflow obstruction
- *Sirolimus* shown to stabilize lung function and improve QoL and is recommended treatment
- *Hormonal manipulation* with progesterone has been tried. It may be beneficial in reducing the decline in FEV_1 and TLCO, particularly in patients with progressive disease, but there are no large studies. Tamoxifen and oophorectomy have also been tried
- *Avoid oestrogens*, i.e. the OCP and HRT
- *Contraception* An increase in symptoms and accelerated disease decline are reported in pregnancy. Use the progesterone-only pill
- *Pleural aspiration* may be required for pleural effusions. For recurrent effusions or chylothoraces, thoracic duct ligation or pleurectomy may be effective. Pleurodesis can be performed, but this is relatively contraindicated if future lung transplant is an option
- *Recurrent pneumothoraces* Advise regarding flying and diving. Thoracic surgery may be necessary
- *Avoid air travel*, if possible, due to risk of pneumothorax
- *Transplant* Single (usually) or double lung, or heart-lung. LAM can recur in the transplanted lung
- *Stop smoking*, as this accelerates the rate of decline
- Influenza vaccine.

Prognosis

Extremely variable. The condition usually slowly progresses to respiratory failure. At 10y, 55% of patients have Medical Research Council (MRC) grade 3 dyspnoea, 23% are on long-term oxygen therapy (LTOT), and 10% are housebound. Survival: 70% of patients are alive at 10 y, 33% are alive at 15 y, and 25% are alive at 20 y.

Further information

Henske EP, McCormack FX. Lymphangioleiomyomatosis—a wolf in sheep's clothing. *J Clin Invest.* 2012;122: 3807–3816.
Patient website ℘ http://www.lamaction.org

Primary ciliary dyskinesia (PCD)

A rare cause of chronic respiratory disease, usually encountered in adult respiratory clinics as a cause of bronchiectasis. Cilia are found in:

- The whole length of the upper respiratory tract
- Brain ventricles
- Fallopian tube/ductus epididymis.

They are made up of dynein arms, with outer and inner connecting rings, and beat at 14 beats/s. Many gene defects have been identified in PCD, causing a number of cilial abnormalities.

Abnormal cilia do not beat normally, leading to reduced mucociliary clearance, microbiological colonization (which further inhibits cilial action), chronic infection, and the development of bronchiectasis.

The main aim following diagnosis in childhood is the prevention of chronic respiratory disease and bronchiectasis.

Clinical features

- Autosomal recessive, >200 phenotypes
- May present with neonatal respiratory distress
- Situs inversus (in about 30%, as cilia determine the side of the organs. Random organ siting occurs with cilial dysfunction, hence the situs inversus of Kartagener's syndrome)
- Nasal blockage/rhinitis/chronic otitis media
- Persistent wet cough in childhood
- Hearing problems/history of glue ear/grommets in childhood
- Clubbing and signs of chest disease are rare in childhood
- Wheeze in 20%
- Infertility due to immotile sperm (sperm tails have same morphological defect as the cilia and do not beat correctly)
- In adults, the disease usually presents with the clinical signs of bronchiectasis: cough productive of purulent sputum, recurrent chest infections, intermittent haemoptysis.

Diagnosis

Saccharin test (nasal mucociliary clearance test, see $\bigodot$ p. 175). Nasal nitric oxide (NO) is very low in PCD (possibly because NO mediates ciliary function); this is the most sensitive and specific screening test. Cilial biopsy via the nasal route. Cilia are examined by high-speed digital video where their beat frequency and pattern can be assessed, confirming the diagnosis. Most cases of PCD are diagnosed in childhood. There is an increased frequency in the children of consanguineous marriages.

Consider the diagnosis in:

- Bronchiectasis
- Situs inversus
- Persistent upper and lower respiratory infection from early childhood
- Infertility—♂ may present in infertility clinics.

Management

In adults, this includes the treatment of 2° bronchiectasis (see ➔ p. 176), with:

- Antibiotics
- Physiotherapy
- Vaccinations
- Management of haemoptysis
- There are four PCD management centres in the UK —London (Royal Brompton), Southampton, Leicester and Leeds/Bradford.

Further information

Bush A, Hogg C. Primary ciliary dyskinesia: recent advances in epidemiology, diagnosis, management and relationship with the expanding spectrum of ciliopathy. *Expert Rev Respir Med.* 2012;6: 663–682.
Patient website ℗ http://www.pcdsupport.org.uk

Pulmonary alveolar proteinosis (PAP): pathophysiology and clinical features

PAP, also referred to as alveolar lipoproteinosis, is a rare alveolar filling defect affecting around 3 per million people. There is a limited published literature: five reported case series of ≥10 cases, and only 410 total cases reported.

Pathophysiology

PAP is due to failure of alveolar macrophages to clear spent surfactant, leading to the filling of alveoli with a phospholipid proteinaceous material. It is thought that the defect has an autoimmune basis and, in the idiopathic form, is due to the presence of antibodies to granulocyte-macrophage colony-stimulating factor (GM-CSF), which cause inhibition of normal alveolar macrophage function, leading to abnormalities of surfactant homeostasis. Defects in GM-CSF signalling have been identified in animal models. Congenital disease is thought to be due to mutations in surfactant gene proteins. Other mechanisms for surfactant accumulation have also been identified:

- *Heavy dust exposure* leads to surfactant hypersecretion, which exceeds the lungs' normal clearance mechanism. Animal models have shown that this condition develops from endogenous lipoid pneumonia, with the accumulation of lipid-laden macrophages, which break down to release surfactant
- *Amphiphilic drugs*, e.g. amiodarone chlorphentermine
- *Lymphoma, leukaemia, and immunosuppression* The mechanism is uncertain, but it is thought that the lipoprotein may be generated from degenerating alveolar cells.

Appearances similar to alveolar lipoproteinosis may also be seen in endogenous lipoid pneumonia resulting from bronchial obstruction and are described in surfactant-secreting alveolar cell carcinoma.

Histology

The alveoli are filled with a granular acellular eosinophilic PAS (periodic acid–Schiff)-positive deposit. Cholesterol clefts and large foamy macrophages may also be seen. The alveolar architecture is usually well preserved. Surfactant protein can be identified using immunohistochemistry. Electron microscopy shows multiple osmiophilic bodies, consistent with denatured surfactant.

Epidemiology

- Presents aged 30–50 y (case reports in children and the elderly)
- ♂:♀ ≈ 4:1
- Increased incidence in smokers
- Rare familial cases reported.

Clinical features

- Typically presents with breathlessness and a non-productive cough. Examination may be normal, or crackles may be heard on auscultation. Clubbing in one-third
- May present with superadded infection, causing an apparent acute onset of symptoms, in association with fever
- Median duration of symptoms before diagnosis is 7 months
- Opportunistic infection is the major complication, most commonly *Nocardia* species, fungi, and mycobacteria. This occurs due to impaired macrophage function and impaired host defence due to surfactant accumulation.

PAP: diagnosis and treatment

Diagnosis

is usually made on the basis of a characteristic CT appearance, although other tests may also be useful.

- Raised serum LDH
- *ABGs* Hypoxia and increased A–a gradient
- *PFTs* Restrictive defect, with reduced lung volumes and transfer factor
- *CXR* Bilateral consolidation with thickened interlobular septa. Usually bilateral. The pattern is very variable and, in up to 50%, may be perihilar (bat-wing appearance)
- *CT* appearance is characteristic, with airspace shadowing in a geographical distribution, alternating with areas of normal lung, the 'crazy paving' pattern. This CT appearance is not specific to alveolar proteinosis, as it is also seen in lipoid pneumonia and bronchoalveolar cell carcinoma
- *BAL* reveals milky washings. Identification of antibodies to GM-CSF in BAL washings is diagnostic. Cytological examination shows a granular extracellular deposit with foamy macrophages and cellular debris
- *Transbronchial/open lung biopsies* when CT is not characteristic.

Treatment of choice

Repeated therapeutic whole lung lavage should be performed at a specialist centre. There are no randomized controlled trials (RCTs) of this treatment, but there is evidence of efficacy in terms of subsequent improvement of symptoms, physiology, and radiology.

- The indication for whole lung lavage is usually breathlessness, limiting activities of daily living
- The procedure is done under general anaesthesia using 100% O_2 and one-lung ventilation using a double-lumen tube. Repeated warm saline lavage using a closed circuit continues until the bronchial washing returns are clear—this may take up to 40 L lavage. One or both lungs may be treated at a time
- The response is variable—some patients need only one treatment; others may need multiple treatments, and about 10% fail to respond
- May be done on bypass if the patient is very hypoxic
- Characteristic milky lavage fluid is obtained
- Inhaled recombinant granulocyte colony-stimulating factor is a novel treatment option (small 2019 RCT), which may prevent progression of disease and improve oxygenation
- There is no benefit from treatment with steroids, and they may exacerbate opportunistic infections.

Prognosis

With whole lung lavage is generally good. Spontaneous remission occurs in one-third; one-third remains stable, and one-third progresses to respiratory failure and death. There are reports of progression to pulmonary fibrosis (which may be a coincidental occurrence).

Further information

Patel SM et al. Pulmonary alveolar proteinosis. *Can Respir J.* 2012;19: 243–245.
Patient website. ℰ http://www.papfoundation.org (USA).

Pulmonary arteriovenous malformations (PAVMs): aetiology and diagnosis

Aetiology

- PAVMs are abnormal blood vessels replacing normal capillaries, making a direct low-resistance connection between the pulmonary arterial and systemic venous circulations. They vary in size, from tiny clusters of vessels (telangiectasia) to larger, more complex aneurysmal-type sacs
- The disorder is rare, affecting 1 in 15,000–24,000
- Several genetic susceptibility loci have been identified on Chr 9 and Chr 12. One identified mutation is in the endoglin gene. This modulates signalling via the TGF-β family of growth factors. This gene is also implicated in the development of primary pulmonary hypertension
- Subjects with significant PAVMs have low pulmonary vascular resistance, a low mean PAP, and a high cardiac output—due to long-standing adaptive mechanisms to the effects of the shunt, in addition to vascular remodelling effects
- Most patients present post-puberty, as AVMs probably develop at this time. They probably grow throughout life, especially during puberty and in pregnancy. They may rarely regress spontaneously. Larger or more numerous AVMs are associated with greater complications and are more likely to present earlier.

Diagnosis

- Most patients present with an abnormal *CXR*, classically showing a smooth, rounded intrapulmonary mass, with draining or feeding vessels
- Mild *hypoxaemia* An AVM is a direct communication between the pulmonary artery and pulmonary vein. Blood therefore bypasses the pulmonary capillary bed, with reduced oxygenation, which poorly corrects with supplementary O_2
- *Orthodeoxia* is desaturation on standing, due to an increase in blood flow in the dependent lung areas. 70% of PAVMs are basal, hence the desaturation seen
- *CT* identifies all AVMs and can determine those suitable for embolization. Contrast is not required, though a computed tomographic pulmonary angiogram is required pre-embolization to better delineate the vascular anatomy
- Patients may present with the complications of a PAVM, particularly bleeding or peripheral abscess formation. The absence of a normal filtering capillary bed means small particles can reach the systemic circulation, leading to sequelae, particularly in the cerebral circulation— strokes and cerebral abscesses. These abnormal vessels are also at risk of rupture.

Shunt quantification

- *100% O_2 rebreathing study*, a non-invasive method of shunt quantification
- *99mTC perfusion scan*, a tracer study; the size of the shunt can be assessed from the proportion of radiolabelled macro-aggregates reaching the systemic circulation, compared with the total number injected. In a normal study, aggregates accumulate in the kidneys

- *Contrast echo* to measure the circulatory transit time of injected echo contrast
- *Angiography* at specialist centre only
- In normal individuals, the anatomical shunt is <2–3.5% of the cardiac output (due to post-pulmonary drainage of bronchial veins into pulmonary vein and drainage into the left atrium).

Clinical features

- Asymptomatic (50%)
- Dyspnoea
- Haemoptysis (10%), probably due to additional bronchial telangiectasia, which can also cause haemorrhage into bronchi or the pleural cavity
- Chest pain (12%); aetiology is uncertain
- Clubbing
- Cyanosis
- Orthodeoxia
- Vascular bruits
- Telangiectasia; 80% of PAVM patients have HHT, and their families should be screened because of the risk of stroke (see ⊅ p. 497)
- May present with acute stroke, with focal neurological signs.

PAVMs: management and complications

Management

- *Embolization* is usually done with coils, which generate local thrombin, leading to cessation of blood flow in AVM feeding vessels. This results in a reduction in the right-to-left shunt and improvement in hypoxaemia and should be done by an expert in a specialist centre only. The small risk of neurological sequelae and angina/arrhythmias is reduced with operator experience.
- 60–70% of patients are left with a small persisting shunt following treatment and retain a small risk of abscess formation. Patients are therefore given prophylactic antibiotics for dental and surgical procedures (ensure the patient has a MedicAlert card).
- *Surgical resection* may be more appropriate than embolization in some cases.
- *Antiplatelet therapy* (rarely) in individual cases, if ongoing transient ischaemic attacks.
- *Transplantation* is not advised, as there is no increased survival benefit over medical treatment.
- *Screening*—the majority of patients with PAVMs have HHT, and so screening of family members is important.
- *Follow-up*—all patients need regular follow-up, with shunt assessment post-surgical resection or embolization, as removal of one shunt may unmask or provoke the development of others.
- ♀ *patients* should be advised to defer pregnancy until completion of formal assessment because of the risks of growth and rupture of PAVMs in pregnancy.

Complications

- PAVM patients never die of respiratory failure in the absence of additional respiratory disease
- All patients are at risk of stroke and cerebral abscesses
- Transient ischaemic attack/stroke (in 25%) due to rupture of abnormal capillaries in aneurysms
- Abscess (in 10%) due to paradoxical emboli, through the right-to-left shunt, and the absence of a filtering capillary bed.

Pregnancy

Associated with an increase in size of AVMs, and new ones may develop, with potentially catastrophic consequences. Careful shunt assessment is therefore needed prior to pregnancy, with contraceptive advice prior to specialist assessment. Close liaison between the specialist centre and obstetric team is paramount. AVMs may need embolization in the third trimester to allow safe delivery.

Further information

Shovlin CL. Hereditary haemorrhagic telangiectasis: pathophysiology, diagnosis and treatment. *Blood Rev.* 2010;24: 203–219.

Recurrent respiratory papillomatosis

These are essentially warts of the upper respiratory tract, caused by the human papillomavirus (HPV 6 or 11). The virus infects epithelial cells and mucous membranes, similar to that seen in cutaneous and anogenital infection. The infection is most commonly acquired during ororespiratory exposure from the mother during vaginal delivery and typically presents in childhood from 6 months onwards, with signs and symptoms of upper respiratory tract infection (URTI). It may also present for the first time in adulthood. It is associated with HLA-DR3 and with sexual transmission in adults. Recurrent respiratory papillomatosis is rare (2 per 100,000), but oral HPV infection is common.

A UK national HPV vaccination programme for all 12–13-year-olds started in 2019, which should ultimately reduce the frequency of this (and other HPV related diseases).

Clinical course

This is variable.

- May remit spontaneously
- Progressive voice loss and airway obstruction
- Most cases are confined to the larynx, although up to 25% of patients subsequently develop extralaryngeal spread to the bronchial tree
- 1% have malignant change to squamous cell carcinomas.

Management

- Surgical excision to maintain airway patency
- Laser therapy—but potential problems of thermal injury, stricture formation, and spread of papillomas
- Photodynamic therapy reduces recurrence rate, using oral or IV photosensitizing recurrent agent, then a laser to destroy photosensitive tissue
- Microdebrider is now used more commonly
- Medical treatment—interferon, aciclovir, ribavirin, isotretinoin, and methotrexate have all been tried
  - *Interferon alfa* as a daily SC injection leads to complete remission in 30–50%, and partial resolution in 30%. One-third recur when treatment is stopped. Adverse reactions are common: flu-like symptoms, deranged liver function tests (LFTs), leucopenia, and alopecia
  - *Cidofovir* is a nucleoside monophosphate analogue and inhibits viral polymerase. It is given as an intralesional injection. Theoretical side effects include nephrotoxicity and neutropenia, but these have not been seen in practice.

Further information

Pian T et al. Safety of intralesional cidofovir in patients with recurrent respiratory papillomatosis. *Eur Arch Otorhinolaryngol.* 2013;270: 1679–1687.

Respiratory infection—bacterial

Community-acquired pneumonia (CAP) 518
CAP: severity assessment 520
CAP: investigations 522
CAP: general management 524
CAP: antibiotics 526
CAP: specific pathogens 528
CAP: antibiotic treatment of pathogens 530
CAP: treatment failure 531
CAP: discharge, follow-up and vaccination 532
Hospital-acquired pneumonia (HAP): clinical features 534
HAP: management 536
Ventilator-associated pneumonia (VAP) 538
Aspiration pneumonia: risk factors 540
Aspiration pneumonia: clinical features 542
Lung abscess: clinical features 544
Lung abscess: management 546
Nocardiosis 548
Actinomycosis 550
Anthrax 552
Tularaemia 554
Melioidosis 555
Leptospirosis 556

Community-acquired pneumonia (CAP)

Respiratory infection is the single largest contributor to the global burden of disease and community-acquired pneumonia (CAP) is the leading cause of death in children worldwide. Even in high-income countries CAP remains common and is associated with significant morbidity and mortality.

Definition

CAP is an infection of lung tissue characterized by symptoms and signs of an acute lower respiratory tract infection in association with chest radiograph (CXR) shadowing not due to any other cause.

Epidemiology

* CAP is the commonest infectious cause of death and the sixth leading cause of death in the UK and USA (with age-adjusted death rates of between 1 and 24/100,000)
* Up to 42% of UK adults with CAP require hospital admission
* Mortality in patients hospitalized with CAP is 5–14%
* In the UK 5–10% of patients with CAP require intensive care unit (ICU) admission
* Mortality is >30% in patients admitted to ICU with CAP
* CAP managed in the community has a mortality of <1%.

Aetiology

Specific pathogens are discussed on ➜ p. 528. A pathogen is identified in only around 40% of hospitalized patients, which may reflect a combination of insensitive testing techniques, a lack of direct respiratory specimens, previous antibiotic treatment, or the presence of currently unidentifiable pathogens. Respiratory viruses appear to be a much more common cause of CAP in adults than traditionally appreciated. Around a third of cases of CAP appear to have infection with more than one pathogen, usually a bacterial-virus combination.

Risk factors for CAP

* *Aspiration* Typically caused by anaerobes and Gram-negative organisms
* *Alcoholism and diabetes* Typically associated with bacteraemic pneumococcal pneumonia; anaerobes and mixed infections are more common in alcoholics
* Oral steroids/immunosuppression—Legionella infection is more common
* *Cigarette smoking* is the strongest independent risk factor for invasive pneumococcal disease in immunocompetent patients
* *Chronic obstructive pulmonary disease (COPD)—Haemophilus influenzae* and *Moraxella catarrhalis* are more common, and COPD is more common in those with bacterial pneumonia
* *Nursing home residents* have an increased frequency of CAP, with aspiration, Gram-negative organisms, and anaerobes more common than in age-matched elderly people.

Clinical features

- Fever
- Cough
- Sputum
- Breathlessness
- Pleuritic chest pain
- Non-specific features in the elderly: may present 'off legs' or with confusion, in the absence of fever.

Examination

- Raised respiratory rate (RR) (may be the only physical sign of CAP in the elderly)
- Tachycardia
- Localizing signs on chest examination: reduced chest expansion on the affected side, with signs consistent with consolidation (reduced air entry, with bronchial breathing, reduced percussion note, increased vocal resonance) and crackles. A normal chest examination makes the diagnosis less likely.

Diagnosis

Diagnosis of CAP is made on the basis of:
- Symptoms and signs of an acute lower respiratory tract infection
- New focal chest signs
- New radiographic shadowing, for which there is no other explanation
- At least one systemic feature (e.g. sweating, fevers, myalgia)
- No other explanation for the illness.

Most helpful in diagnosis
- Fever, pleuritic pain, dyspnoea, and tachypnoea
- Signs on chest examination.

CAP: severity assessment

- Severity assessment enables the most appropriate care to be delivered in the most appropriate clinical setting
- Early identification of patients at high risk of death allows early decisions about hospital admission and need for assisted ventilation and ICU admission to be made
- Assessment of disease severity depends on the experience of the clinician; a number of predictive assessment models have been trialled. Severity models should be regarded as adjuncts to clinical assessment, and the presence and stability of comorbid conditions and patients' wishes and social circumstances should also be taken into account
- Regular reassessment of response to treatment should follow initial severity assessment.

Poor prognostic factors

Those with two or more adverse prognostic factors are at high risk of death and should be managed as for severe CAP (see ⊃ p. 526):

- *Age* ≥65 y
- *Coexisting disease* incl. cardiac disease, diabetes, COPD, stroke
- *RR* ≥30/min—one of the most reliable predictors of disease severity
- *Confusion* Abbreviated mental test score (AMTS) ≤8
- *BP* Systolic ≤90 mmHg and/or diastolic ≤60 mmHg
- *Hypoxaemia* Respiratory failure, with PaO_2 <8 kPa and the need for assisted ventilation, predicts mortality
- *Urea* ≥7 mmol/L
- *Albumin* <35 g/L
- *WCC* >20 or <4 ×109/L are each predictive of poor outcomes
- *Radiology* Bilateral or multilobe involvement. In patients admitted to ICU, progression of CXR changes is a poor prognostic marker
- *Microbiology* Positive blood culture, whatever the pathogen isolated.

Severity scores

The most widely used severity assessment score in the UK is CURB65, which is recommended by the British Thoracic Society (BTS) and by the National Institute for Health and Care Excellence (NICE) to guide both patient assessment and choice of empirical antibiotic treatment (see ⊃ p. 526). CURB65 is validated to predict 30-day mortality in CAP. The CURB65 derivative CRB65 does not rely on laboratory blood tests and may be used in the community to help assess which patients require hospital admission. The Pneumonia Severity Index (PSI) is an alternative, which may be more sensitive, but is more complicated and includes information on comorbid disease and laboratory tests before stratifying patients into five risk classes.

CURB65 score – assign one point for each of:

- *Confusion* New mental confusion defined as AMTS ≤8 (Box 41.1), or new disorientation in person, place or time
- *Urea* >7 mmol/L
- *Respiratory rate* Raised ≥30/min
- *Blood pressure* Systolic BP <90 and/or diastolic BP ≤60 mmHg
- *Age* ≥65 y.

Stratify patients according to CURB65 score as follows:
* *High severity* CAP (CURB65 score of 3–5) is associated with a mortality of 15–40%. These patients require early consultant review and consideration of ICU or high dependency unit (HDU) care
* *Moderate severity* CAP (CURB65 score of 2) is associated with a mortality of 9%. Consider short inpatient admission or hospital-supervised outpatient treatment
* *Low severity* CAP (CURB65 score of 0–1) is associated with a mortality of <3%. Patients with low severity CAP may be suitable for home treatment, depending upon their social circumstances, wishes, and comorbid conditions
* CRB65 may be used by GPs in the community to help assess patients: a score of 0 suggests patients with a low risk of death who may be appropriately treated in the community; scores of ≥1 should be considered for hospital admission.

Remember that pneumonia severity scores aim to contribute to, rather than supersede, clinical judgment; drawbacks of CURB65 scoring include:
* Little evidence to support its use in antibiotic prescribing
* May overestimate severity in the elderly, leading to inappropriate broad-spectrum antibiotic therapy
* May underestimate severity in young patients, potentially leading to suboptimal treatment
* Poor at predicting need for ICU (only 51% of pts requiring ICU admission have CURB65-defined severe disease)
* BTS 'real world' UK audit data demonstrates a surprisingly high mortality at low CURB65 scores
* May be calculated incorrectly (only 4% of trainee doctors are able to correctly name the components of CURB65)
* Many low-risk pts require hospitalization for other reasons, e.g. social circumstances.

Box 41.1 Abbreviated mental test score (AMTS)

(1 point per question, max = 10)
* Age
* Date of birth
* Time (to nearest hour)
* Year
* Hospital name
* Recognition of two people (e.g. nurse, doctor)
* Recall address
* Date of First World War
* Name of monarch
* Count backwards 20 to 1.

CAP: investigations

General investigations

Investigations are aimed at confirming the diagnosis, assessing disease severity, guiding appropriate treatment, assessing the presence of underlying disease, enabling identification of complications, and monitoring progress.

- *Oxygenation assessment* Patients with an O_2 saturation of <92% on admission or with features of severe pneumonia should have arterial blood gases (ABGs) measured, with documentation of inspired O_2 concentration
- *CXR* should be performed promptly in hospitalized patients, with the aim of securing the diagnosis in time for antibiotics to be administered within 4 h of hospital presentation. Classically shows consolidation although other appearances include interstitial infiltrate or cavitation. CXR appearance is not usually helpful in predicting the causative pathogen (➔ p. 528), although multilobar involvement or pleural effusion are more common in bacteraemic pneumococcal disease and cavitation may suggest *Staphylococcus aureus* infection (➔ p. 529)
- *Computed tomography (CT) chest* may be useful if the diagnosis is in doubt or the patient is severely ill and failing to respond to treatment (➔ p. 531) in order to exclude abscess formation, pleural infection, underlying malignancy, or other underlying lung disease
- *Blood tests*
  - Full blood count (FBC)—White cell count (WCC) >15 × 109 suggests bacterial (particularly pneumococcal) infection. Counts of >20 or <4 indicate severe infection
  - Deranged renal and liver function tests can be indicative of severe infection or point to the presence of underlying disease. Liver function tests (LFTs) may be abnormal, particularly with right lower lobe pneumonia. Raised urea is a marker of more severe pneumonia
  - Metabolic acidosis is associated with severe illness
  - C-reactive protein (CRP) is a useful aid to management, with high levels being a more sensitive marker of infection than the WCC or temperature. Serial measures are very useful in assessing response to treatment (➔ p. 531)
  - Procalcitonin may be useful in predicting bacterial infection and shortening antibiotic duration, but the evidence of clinical benefit is limited and it has no routine role currently in CAP management
- *Bronchoscopy* May be helpful, especially after intubation on intensive care unit (ICU), to suction retained secretions, particularly if these are causing lobar collapse, to obtain further samples for culture, and to exclude an endobronchial abnormality.

Microbiological investigations

Microbiological investigations can help to aid selection of optimal antibiotics, hence limiting antibiotic resistance and the possible problems of *Clostridium difficile*-associated diarrhoea. They also inform public health and infection control teams, aiding in the monitoring of pathogen trends causing CAP over time. Despite these investigations the microbiological cause for CAP is not found in 60% of patients.

- *Blood cultures* Recommended for all hospitalized patients with moderate and high severity CAP, ideally before antibiotics are started. About 10% of patients with CAP will have positive blood cultures. The early availability of blood culture results (within 24 h of admission) improves outcome
- *Sputum culture* Useful for those patients who have failed to improve with empirical antibiotic treatment and in those with moderate severity pneumonia admitted to hospital who are expectorating purulent samples and who have not received prior antibiotics, as well as all patients with severe pneumonia. Not routinely recommended for those treated in the community. Sputum examination is recommended for possible tuberculosis (TB) in those with weight loss, a persistent cough, night sweats, and risk factors for TB, e.g. ethnic origin, social deprivation
- *Pleural fluid* (if present) for microscopy, culture, and sensitivity and pH to exclude pleural infection (see ⊃ p. 412)
- *Pneumococcal urinary antigen* testing is recommended for all patients with moderate or high severity CAP: sensitivity is 100% and specificity 60–90% for invasive pneumococcal disease
- *Legionella urinary antigen* testing is recommended for all patients with moderate and high severity CAP, for other patients with specific risk factors (⊃ p. 528), and for all patients with CAP during outbreaks. It is 70–80% sensitive and >95% specific for serotype 1, and rapid results can be obtained early. A positive urinary antigen test correlates with subsequent ICU admission. Samples for Legionella culture (sputum, endotracheal aspirate, BAL, pleural fluid) should be collected, if possible, from antigen-positive patients in order to support epidemiological assessment of outbreaks and identify environmental sources
- *Polymerase chain reaction (PCR) for viral and 'atypical' pathogens* where available is preferable to serological testing. Paired serology samples (from within 7 days of the onset of the illness, repeated 10–14 days later) can be considered in patients with severe CAP who fail to improve but they are unlikely to guide initial treatment
- *PCR of respiratory samples (sputum, BAL) or throat swab* may be diagnostic where mycoplasma pneumonia (⊃ p. 529) is suspected
- *PCR or antigen detection testing of invasive respiratory samples (BAL)* for *Chlamydophila* (⊃ p. 529) should be considered in high severity CAP or where psittacosis is suspected.

CAP: general management

Supportive treatment

- *Oxygen therapy* Hypoxia is due to V/Q mismatching, as blood flows through unventilated lung. Optimal target O_2 saturation for most patients is 94–98%. Patients at risk of hypercapnic respiratory failure may require a lower O_2 saturation target (e.g. 88–92%) and close monitoring of blood gases. A rising CO_2 in a patient without prior respiratory disease may indicate they are tiring and need respiratory support—discuss with ICU urgently
- *Non-invasive ventilatory support* NIV may be initially beneficial in severe CAP although many patients subsequently deteriorate and require intubation. A higher initial RR (>30) is associated with failure of NIV or CPAP. NIV should only be trialled in a high dependency setting, with close monitoring and available expertise for immediate intubation and invasive ventilation if required
- *Fluids* Assessment of volume status by jugular venous pressure (JVP) and BP is essential. Encourage oral fluids. Intravenous (IV) fluids may be needed if volume-depleted and severely unwell. Monitor urine output
- *Analgesia* Paracetamol or non-steroidal anti-inflammatories (NSAIDs) initially, if required. Paracetamol also has an antipyretic role
- *Nutrition* Supplements may be of benefit in prolonged illness
- *Early mobilization* should be encouraged
- *Physiotherapy* Airway clearance techniques may be considered in patients having difficulty expectorating sputum although there is no clear evidence to support routine airway clearance physiotherapy in CAP
- *Venous thromboembolism (VTE) prophylaxis* is recommended for patients who are not fully mobile.

Adjunctive treatment

- *Corticosteroids*
  - Have been proposed as an adjunctive treatment in CAP, with a potentially beneficial anti-inflammatory effect
  - Clinical trials have differed significantly in steroid formulation and dose, inclusion criteria, and end-points
  - The most recent, individual patient-level data meta-analysis (➔ p. 533) showed that low-dose corticosteroids reduce length of hospital stay and time to clinical stability by 1 day in adults hospitalized with CAP, without a significant effect on mortality; on the other hand corticosteroids also increased the risk of CAP-related rehospitalization and hyperglycaemia
  - Current opinion is that steroids are not routinely recommended for the treatment of CAP
- *Granulocyte colony stimulating factor* is not currently recommended for treatment of CAP.

Monitoring

- Temperature, RR, heart rate (HR), blood pressure (BP), mental status, oxygen saturation, and inspired O_2 concentration should be monitored regularly, and patients with high severity CAP require medical review at least 12-hourly
- Consider repeat CRP and repeat CXR in patients who are not improving after 3 days of treatment (→ p. 531).

ICU admission

Those fulfilling criteria for severe CAP on admission or who fail to respond rapidly to treatment should be considered for transfer for close monitoring, either to an HDU or ICU. Persisting hypoxia (PaO_2 8 kPa), acidosis, hypercapnia, hypotension, or depressed conscious level, despite maximal therapy, are indications for assisted ventilation. Continuous positive airway pressure (CPAP) may be of benefit while awaiting the arrival of the ICU team.

When to discuss patient with CAP with ICU

- Always sooner rather than later
- Respiratory failure (PaO_2 <8 kPa) despite high-flow O_2
- Tiring patient, with a rising CO_2
- Worsening metabolic acidosis, despite antibiotics and optimum fluid management
- Hypotension despite adequate fluid resuscitation.

CAP: antibiotics

- Empirical antibiotic treatment is required at diagnosis of CAP in the absence of microbiological information
- Empirical antibiotic choice may be based on site of care (community vs hospital) or on CAP severity; in the UK severity-based antibiotic guidance is recommended, based on CURB65 score
- Typical empirical antibiotic choices for CAP are outlined in Table 41.1, but prescribing of empirical antibiotics should be in line with local protocols: consult hospital prescribing guidelines and liaise with microbiology if needed
- Strongly consider narrowing antibiotic coverage if a specific pathogen is identified (⮊ p. 528).

General points

- Early antibiotic administration is associated with an improved outcome in CAP
- Immediate antibiotic administration in the community is recommended for patients with suspected life-threatening CAP
- Confirmation of CAP with CXR and antibiotic administration should occur within 4 h of hospital admission

Table 41.1 Suggested empirical antibiotics for CAP treatment

	Preferred treatment	Alternative (if intolerant of, or allergic to, preferred treatment)
Community treatment	Amoxicillin 500 mg–1 g tds PO	Doxycycline 100 mg od (after 200 mg loading dose) PO or clarithromycin 500 mg bd PO
Hospital treatment: low severity (CURB-65 = 0–1)	Amoxicillin 500 mg tds PO (or same dose IV if oral treatment not possible)	Doxycycline 100 mg od (after 200 mg loading dose) PO or clarithromycin 500 mg bd PO
Hospital treatment: moderate severity (CURB-65 = 2)	Amoxicillin 500 mg–1 g tds PO and clarithromycin 500 mg bd PO If oral treatment not possible: amoxicillin 500 mg tds IV or benzylpenicillin 1.2 g qds IV and clarithromycin 500 mg bd IV	Doxycycline 100 mg od (after 200 mg loading dose) PO or levofloxacin 500 mg od PO or moxifloxacin 400 mg od PO
Hospital treatment: high severity (CURB-65 = 3–5)	Co-amoxiclav 1.2 g tds IV and clarithromycin 500 mg bd IV (add levofloxacin if legionella strongly suspected)	Benzylpenicillin 1.2 g qds IV and either levofloxacin 500 mg bd IV or ciprofloxacin 400 mg bd IV OR Cefuroxime 1.5 g tds IV or cefotaxime 1 g tds IV or ceftriaxone 2 g od IV and clarithromycin 500 mg bd IV (add levofloxacin if legionella strongly suspected)

- In general, use a single antibiotic as initial empirical therapy in low severity CAP and dual combination antibiotics including a macrolide for moderate and high severity CAP (Table 41.1)
- *IV antibiotics* should be administered immediately to patients with high-severity CAP. IV antibiotics will also be required in patients with non-severe CAP who are unable to safely take oral medications (e.g. unsafe swallow or impaired conscious level)
- *Oral antibiotics* should be used in those with community-managed CAP and those with low or moderate severity hospital-managed pneumonia, with no other contraindications
- Consider adding anaerobic antibiotic cover (e.g. metronidazole) if aspiration pneumonia or lung abscess suspected
- Document indication and planned duration of antibiotic treatment; stop antibiotics if it becomes apparent that they are not indicated
- Review the need for IV antibiotics daily and aim to switch from IV to oral antibiotics as soon as possible, usually when a patient has shown clear response to treatment and has been apyrexial for 24 h
- A switch to oral co-amoxiclav, and *not* an oral cephalosporin, is recommended after treatment with IV cephalosporins
- For those treated with benzylpenicillin plus levofloxacin, a switch to oral levofloxacin ± oral amoxicillin is recommended.

Duration of antibiotic treatment

There is no evidence to inform antibiotic treatment duration, but current guidelines recommend:
- Low severity, uncomplicated CAP = 5 days
- Moderate and high severity CAP = 7–10 days (future NICE guidelines may reduce this to 5 days)
- Extended treatment (14–21 days) may be required, depending upon clinical judgement; consider if CAP due to staphylococcal disease or Gram-negative enteric bacteria.

Combination treatment including a macrolide

This remains controversial. Most observational studies in CAP show a mortality benefit favouring combination therapy with a macrolide (β-lactam monotherapy associated with 1.5–6 fold increase in risk of death). These include studies of bacteraemic pneumococcal disease and so any macrolide-derived benefit is unlikely to reflect treatment of 'atypical' pathogens; instead may be due to macrolide-specific immunomodulatory and anti-inflammatory effects, inhibition of microbial virulence factors, and/or a macrolide antiviral effect (which has been demonstrated *in vitro*). Two non-inferiority RCTs of β-lactam monotherapy vs β-lactam plus macrolide combination (Ⓓ p. 533) have demonstrated conflicting results and the definitive trial is awaited.

CAP: specific pathogens

The aetiological agent cannot be accurately predicted from clinical or imaging features alone, although some features are more statistically likely with one pathogen than another. Key features of specific pathogens are listed below, with typical antibiotic recommendations in Table 41.2.

Streptococcus pneumoniae (pneumococcus)

- Leading bacterial cause of CAP. Asymptomatic nasopharyngeal colonization with the pneumococcus occurs in 50% of children aged 2–3 y and 10% of adults
- Pneumococcal pneumonia classically presents with acute onset of high fever and pleuritic chest pain in young adults, although atypical presentations are common particularly in elderly
- Susceptibility factors for pneumococcal disease: smoking; age (<2 y or >65 y); viral respiratory infection, incl. antecedent influenza; recent acquisition of a new virulent strain; poverty, overcrowding, childhood day care; chronic disease (COPD, asthma, diabetes mellitus; cardiac, renal, or hepatic failure); alcohol excess; asplenia (incl. sickle cell disease); primary or secondary immunodeficiency (HIV, myeloma, chronic lymphocytic leukaemia (CLL); CVID, complement deficiency, Toll-like Receptor-Nuclear Factor-kB signalling defects)
- Bacteraemia may cause metastatic infection: Austrian syndrome (triad of meningitis, pneumonia, and endocarditis due to *S. pneumoniae*) is now very rare but carries a mortality of 60%.

Viral causes of CAP

Surveillance studies with enhanced diagnostic testing demonstrate the presence of respiratory viruses in a significant proportion of patients hospitalized with CAP (see → p. 630). Human rhinovirus appears to be particularly common, although its pathogenic role is unclear; influenza A and B are also commonly isolated.

Legionella spp.

- *Legionella pneumophila* is the most common cause of human disease, divided into >15 serogroups: serogroup 1 is the most prevalent but nearly all serogroups can cause human disease
- Legionnaires' disease (pneumonia caused by *Legionella* spp.) is traditionally considered to cause only high-severity CAP, but it causes low-moderate severity CAP in >50% of cases; it can be acquired sporadically or during outbreaks
- Susceptibility factors for Legionella pneumonia: increasing age; male sex; smoking; alcohol excess; chronic lung disease; lung cancer; end-stage renal disease; diabetes mellitus; immunosuppression (hematologic malignancy, HIV, solid organ transplant, corticosteroids, chemotherapy, anti-TNFα); known outbreak; exposure to contaminated water (hot tubs, air conditioning systems, cooling towers); Summer–Autumn period; travel (Mediterranean)
- No specific clinical features are diagnostic of Legionella infection, although altered mental status, prominent neurological or gastro-intestinal symptoms, abnormal liver enzymes, raised CK, and hyponatremia are commonly reported

- Legionella CAP should be treated with a fluoroquinolone (e.g. Levofloxacin). Macrolide therapy is an alternative for low severity CAP if intolerant of fluoroquinolones. Consider adding a macrolide to fluoroquinolone for initial treatment of high severity Legionella CAP (note risk of QTc prolongation with macrolide–quinolone combination)
- All confirmed cases should be notified to the local Health Protection Unit, who will investigate potential sources
- Pontiac fever is a non-pneumonic, self-limiting form of Legionella infection; antibiotics are not required.

Mycoplasma pneumoniae
- Typically affects younger patients, with prominent extrapulmonary involvement, including haemolysis, cold agglutinins, hepatitis, skin and joint problems
- May cause primarily small airways infection with tree-in-bud nodularity on CT.

Staphylococcus aureus
- Occurs most commonly in winter months, often suggested by recent influenza-like illness; coincident influenza infection is common
- Community-acquired multiple-resistant Staphylococcus aureus (MRSA) (CA-MRSA) pneumonia is increasingly recognized. Risk factors include: hospital admission or antibiotics in previous 90 days; recent influenza-like illness; haemodialysis; previous MRSA colonization; congestive cardiac failure
- Panton–Valentine Leukocidin-producing *Staphylococcus aureus* infection characteristically causes high severity CA-MRSA pneumonia, often in previously healthy young adults. It is typically associated with rapid development of lung necrosis and cavitation with multiorgan failure and carries a high mortality. If strongly suspected, inform ICU, discuss with microbiology and add linezolid 600 mg bd IV, clindamycin 1.2 g qds IV, and rifampicin 600 mg bd IV.

Other pathogens
- *Chlamydophila psittaci* (psittacosis)—infection acquired from birds and animals, with 20% of cases having a history of bird contact; human-to-human spread may occur
- *Coxiella burnetii* (Q fever)—epidemics in relation to animal sources (usually sheep or goats), but occupational exposure only present in minority of cases. Often dry cough, high fever, headache
- *Chlamydophila pneumoniae*—may cause epidemics in the community; unclear if it has a direct pathogenic role
- Zoonotic causes of CAP are outlined later (see ⮞ Box 41.8).

CAP: antibiotic treatment of pathogens

Table 41.2 Recommended antibiotic treatment of specific pathogens

Pathogen	Preferred antibiotic	Alternative antibiotic
Streptococcus pneumoniae	Amoxicillin 500 mg–1 g tds PO *or* benzylpenicillin 1.2 g qds IV	Clarithromycin 500 mg bd PO *or* cefuroxime 0.75–1.5 g tds IV *or* cefotaxime 1–2 g tds IV *or* ceftriaxone 2 g od IV
Mycoplasma pneumoniae and *Chlamydophila pneumoniae*	Clarithromycin 500 mg bd PO/IV	Doxycycline 100 mg od PO (after 200 mg loading dose) *or* fluoroquinolone PO/IV
Chlamydophila psittaci and *Coxiella burnetii*	Doxycycline 100 mg od PO (after 200 mg loading dose)	Clarithromycin 500 mg bd PO/IV
Legionella spp.	Fluoroquinolone PO/IV	Clarithromycin 500 mg bd PO/IV
Haemophilus influenzae	*Non-beta-lactamase-producing* amoxicillin 500 mg tds PO/IV *Beta-lactamase-producing* co-amoxiclav 625 mg tds PO or 1.2 g tds IV	Cefuroxime 750 mg–1.5 g tds IV *or* cefotaxime 1–2 g tds IV *or* ceftriaxone 2 g od IV *or* fluoroquinolone PO/IV
Gram-negative enteric bacilli	Cefuroxime 1.5 g tds *or* cefotaxime 1–2 g tds IV *or* ceftriaxone 1–2 g bd IV	Fluoroquinolone IV *or* imipenem 500 mg qds IV *or* meropenem 0.5–1 g tds IV
Pseudomonas aeruginosa	Ceftazidime 2 g tds IV and gentamicin or tobramycin (dose monitoring)	Ciprofloxacin 400 mg bd IV *or* piperacillin 4 g tds IV and gentamicin *or* tobramycin (dose monitoring)
Staphylococcus aureus	*Non-MRSA* flucloxacillin 1–2 g qds IV ± rifampicin 600 mg od/bd PO/IV	*MRSA* vancomycin 1 g bd (dose monitoring) or linezolid 600 mg bd IV or teicoplanin 400 mg bd IV ± rifampicin 600 mg od/bd PO/IV
Aspiration pneumonia	Co-amoxiclav 1.2 g tds IV	Seek local micro advice

CAP: treatment failure

- Lack of symptomatic response or ongoing fevers should prompt clinical reassessment. Causes of failure to improve are listed in Box 41.2
- Review the history again, perform a full physical examination and have a low threshold for repeat CXR
- Review microbiological test results
- Review antibiotic dose, compliance, and route of administration
- Consider further imaging depending upon CXR findings: pleural ultrasound or CT chest
- Send further microbiological specimens: blood and sputum cultures; sample pleural fluid (→ p. 412)
- Failure of CRP to fall by >50% at 4 days is a useful finding and suggests either treatment failure or the development of a complication such as a lung abscess or pleural infection
- If treatment failure suspected, consider changing empirical antibiotic therapy, e.g. add or switch to macrolide if low-severity CAP on amoxicillin monotherapy; consider adding fluoroquinolone if high-severity CAP and not responding to beta-lactam/macrolide combination.

Box 41.2 Causes of failure to improve in CAP

- Slow clinical response, particularly in the elderly patient
- Incorrect initial diagnosis:
  - Pulmonary thromboembolic disease
  - Pulmonary oedema
  - Lung cancer
  - Other CAP mimics e.g. eosinophilic pneumonia; pulmonary lymphoma; bronchoalveolar cell carcinoma; alveolar haemorrhage; organizing pneumonia; vasculitis; drug-induced lung disease
- Secondary complication:
  - Pulmonary, e.g. parapneumonic effusion or empyema; lung abscess; acute respiratory distress syndrome (ARDS)
  - Extrapulmonary, e.g. septicaemia; metastatic infection (meningitis; endocarditis; pericardial collection; septic arthritis; Lemierre's syndrome); IV cannula site infection; *C. difficile* diarrhoea; cardiovascular complication (cardiac failure, myocardial infarction, arrhythmia)
- Inappropriate antibiotics or unexpected pathogen:
  - Consider infection with less common pathogens, e.g. *Legionella*; *Pseudomonas aeruginosa*; *Mycoplasma*; staphylococcal disease (including MRSA); TB; fungal disease; *Nocardia*; PCP
  - Consider drug-resistant pathogen or mixed infection with more than one pathogen
- Underlying lung disease e.g. bronchiectasis; aspiration; bronchial obstruction (lung cancer, foreign body)
- Impaired immunity e.g. hypogammaglobulinaemia; HIV infection; malnutrition; myeloma.

CAP: discharge, follow-up and vaccination

Discharge

Patients should have medical review within 24 h of planned discharge. Postpone discharge if more than one of the following present (unless they represent usual baseline status for patient): temperature >37.8°C, HR >100/min, RR >24/min, systolic BP <90 mmHg, oxygen saturation <90%, inability to maintain oral intake, and abnormal mental status. Encourage smoking cessation in all current smokers with CAP.

CXR resolution

Radiographic improvement lags behind clinical improvement. There is no need to repeat a CXR before hospital discharge in patients who have made a satisfactory clinical recovery.

• In one study of CAP, complete radiographic resolution occurred after 6 weeks in 73% of patients, but only in 51% at 2 weeks
• Radiographic resolution is slower in the elderly, those with multi-lobe involvement, smokers, and hospital inpatients
• *Legionella* and pneumococcal pneumonia are slower to resolve (may take 12 weeks or more).

Follow-up

Patients should be reviewed in primary or secondary care 6 weeks after an episode of CAP. A repeat CXR to exclude an underlying condition (in particular lung cancer) is recommended 6 weeks after CAP:

• In all patients with persisting symptoms or physical signs
• In all patients considered to be at higher risk of underlying lung malignancy, especially smokers and those over the age of 50 y.

Further investigations, such as CT chest and bronchoscopy, should be considered at this time in patients with persisting symptoms and/or a persistently abnormal CXR.

• One study showed lung cancer is diagnosed on follow-up in 17% of smokers aged over 60 treated for CAP in the community
• Other studies have shown a prevalence of lung cancer of 11% in current and ex-smokers aged over 50 y who are inpatients with CAP and who undergo bronchoscopy prior to discharge.

Cardiovascular risk

• Recent studies have demonstrated that the risk of cardiovascular events (acute coronary syndrome, cardiac arrhythmias, and cardiac failure) is significantly higher after CAP and that this risk is proportional to the severity of infection
• The risk falls with time but interestingly remains above baseline even up to 10 years after an episode of CAP
• Mechanisms currently unclear, but may include inflammation-induced destabilization of atheromatous plaques; prothrombotic state associated with infection; direct cardiac infection
• Ongoing research aims to better understand and reduce the excess cardiovascular mortality after CAP, for example with trials of antiplatelet agents.

Vaccination

Influenza vaccination *reduces hospital deaths from pneumonia and influenza by about 65% and respiratory deaths by 45%.* It also leads to fewer hospital admissions. Influenza vaccination is recommended for 'high-risk' individuals:
• Chronic lung disease
• Cardiac, renal, and liver disease
• Diabetes
• Immunosuppression due to disease or treatment
• Those aged over 65 y
• Long-stay residential or nursing care
• Health care workers

Contraindicated in people with hen egg hypersensitivity (the virus is cultured in chick embryos).

The vaccination contains both A and B subtype viruses and provides partial protection against influenza illnesses. It is modified annually, based on recent viral strains.

Pneumococcal vaccination is recommended for:
• Those aged over 65 y
• Asplenic individuals (incl. coeliac disease and sickle cell disease)
• Chronic renal, cardiac, and liver disease
• Diabetes
• Immunodeficiency or immunosuppression due to disease or treatment

Pneumococcal vaccination after CAP should be given at convalescence. It should not be given during acute infection or in pregnancy.

Further information

Lim et al. British Thoracic Society guidelines for the management of community acquired pneumonia in adults: update 2009. *Thorax* 2009;**64**: iii1–55.
2015 Annotated BTS Guideline for the management of CAP in adults available from: ℰ https:// www.brit-thoracic.org.uk/quality-improvement/guidelines/pneumonia-adults/
Lim et al. British Thoracic Society community acquired pneumonia guideline and the NICE pneumonia guideline: how they fit together. *BMJ Open Respiratory Research* 2015;**2**: e000091.
Garin et al. β-Lactam monotherapy vs β-lactam-macrolide combination treatment in moderately severe community-acquired pneumonia: a randomized noninferiority trial. *JAMA Intern Med* 2014;**174**: 1894–1901.
Postma et al. Antibiotic treatment strategies for community acquired pneumonia in adults. *New Engl J Med* 2015;**372**: 1312–1323.
Lee et al. Antibiotic therapy for adults hospitalized with community-acquired pneumonia: a systematic review. *JAMA* 2016;**315**: 593–602.
Briel et al. Corticosteroids in patients hospitalized with community-acquired pneumonia: systematic review and individual patient data metaanalysis. *Clinical Infectious Diseases* 2018;**66**: 346–354.

Hospital-acquired pneumonia (HAP): clinical features

Definition

New radiographic infiltrate with evidence of infection (e.g. fever, purulent sputum) and onset 48 h or more after hospital admission. Hospital-acquired pneumonia (HAP; also referred to as nosocomial pneumonia) represents around 15% of hospital-acquired infections. Most occur outside the ICU, but those at highest risk are mechanically ventilated patients. HAP requires different antibiotic treatment to CAP and is the leading cause of death from hospital-acquired infection.

Pathophysiology

HAP occurs from aspiration of infected upper airway secretions, from the inhalation of bacteria from contaminated equipment, or haematogenous spread of organisms. Aspiration is thought to be the most important cause. Around 45% of normal people aspirate during sleep, and this is increased in hospital inpatients (who may be frailer) and in those with chronic disease. These patients' upper airways become colonized with Gram-negative bacteria (in up to 75% within 48 h of admission), and this proportion is even higher in those who have received broad-spectrum antibiotics. In addition, the severely ill may have impaired host defences, making them more susceptible to pneumonia. Alteration in the gastric pH with illness and various drugs means that the gastro-intestinal (GI) tract is no longer sterile, thereby providing a potential source of bacterial infection. Risk factors for HAP are listed in Box 41.3; cerebrovascular event and reduced conscious level are the major risk factors for aspiration (Ⓢ p. 540).

Risk factors for specific organisms

- *Streptococcus pneumoniae and Haemophilus influenzae* Increased risk in trauma
- *Staphylococcus aureus* Increased risk in ventilated neurosurgical patients (especially closed head injury), blunt trauma, and coma
- *Pseudomonas aeruginosa* Increased risk with intubation >8 days, COPD, prolonged antibiotics
- *Acinetobacter spp.* Increased risk with prolonged ventilation and previous broad-spectrum antibiotics
- *Anaerobic bacteria* Increased with recent abdominal surgery, aspiration.

Box 41.3 Risk factors for HAP

- Age >70 y
- Chronic lung disease and/or other comorbidity (especially diabetes)
- Reduced conscious level or cerebrovascular accident
- Chest or abdominal surgery
- Mechanical ventilation
- Nasogastric feeding
- Previous antibiotic exposure
- Poor dental hygiene
- Steroid and cytotoxic drug treatment.

Clinical features

HAP typically presents with one or more of:

- Fever
- Productive cough
- Raised inflammatory parameters
- New CXR infiltrate
- Deterioration in gas exchange.

Diagnosis

Diagnosis of HAP is usually clinical, and identification of the infecting agent can be difficult, especially if the patient has already received broad-spectrum antibiotics.

Investigations

- *CXR* usually shows a non-specific infiltrate
- *Blood, sputum, and pleural fluid* should be cultured
- *ABGs* to determine severity
- *Renal and liver function tests* to assess other organ dysfunction
- *Serological tests* are of little use in HAP.

HAP: management

Severity assessment

The CURB-65 pneumonia score (➜ p. 520) for CAP has not been validated in HAP but may be useful in assessing disease severity.

Microbiology

- About 50% of HAP cases are mixed infections; 30% are due to aerobic bacteria alone (most commonly Gram-negative enteric bacilli and *Pseudomonas*); anaerobes alone are found in about 25% of cases
- *Pseudomonas aeruginosa* and *Staphylococcus aureus* are common causes
- *Peptostreptococcus, Fusobacterium*, and *Bacteroides* spp. are commonly isolated, as well as *Enterobacter* spp., *Escherichia coli, Serratia marcescens, Klebsiella*, and *Proteus* spp.
- *Acinetobacter* is an emerging pathogen
- MRSA is increasing in prevalence
- Viruses are recognized as causes.

Management

- Patients developing pneumonia within 48 h of arrival in hospital can be treated with standard CAP antibiotics (➜ p. 526), as the pneumonia is likely to be due to bacteria acquired in the community
- Patients developing pneumonia >48 h after hospital admission need antibiotics to cover different organisms
- Prolonged IV treatment is usually needed, with cover for Gram-negative bacteria. Empirical antibiotics are recommended in hospital guidelines based on knowledge of local microbial resistance patterns, but typical choices include co-amoxiclav, ceftriaxone, piperacillin-tazobactam, or a carbapenem. A single (or ongoing) dose of gentamicin (e.g. 5–7 mg/kg, guided by renal function) may be appropriate for patients with severe sepsis. Addition of an antibiotic with MRSA coverage should be considered, particularly if the patient is known to be recently colonized with MRSA
- Supportive treatment is also required, with O_2, fluids, and ventilation, if necessary
- In penicillin-allergic patients, clindamycin or ciprofloxacin can be used (as long as *Streptococcus pneumoniae* is not thought to be the infecting agent). Levofloxacin has better pneumococcal cover
- Complications of HAP are the same as for CAP (➜ p. 531), including lung abscess and empyema. Drug fever, sepsis with multi-organ failure, and PE with secondary infection are more common in HAP. Pleural US (to look for pleural infection) or CT scanning may demonstrate abscess, underlying tumour, or infection at extrathoracic sites.

Prognosis

HAP is associated with a high mortality, ranging between 20 and 50%.

Prevention

- Meticulous hygiene and hand washing by medical staff, in addition to careful infection control measures, have been shown to reduce rates of HAP
- Early mobilization post-operatively, careful cleaning and maintenance of respiratory equipment, and preoperative smoking cessation also reduce infection rates
- Some ICUs use antibiotics to selectively decontaminate the GI tract of Gram-negative bacilli. This has been shown to reduce infection rates, but there is no proven effect on mortality or length of ICU admission.

Ventilator-associated pneumonia (VAP)

Definition
Pneumonia in a mechanically ventilated patient, developing 48 h or more after endotracheal intubation. Ventilator-associated pneumonia (VAP) is the commonest nosocomial infection in ICU and is an independent predictor of mortality. Up to two-thirds of patients requiring mechanical ventilation for >48 h will develop VAP. It has a mortality of 15–50%, increasing the length of ICU stay by an average of 6.1 days. The major cause is bacterial contamination of the lower respiratory tract from the aspiration of oropharyngeal secretions, which is not prevented by cuffed endotracheal tube or tracheostomy.

Diagnosis
Suggested by:
- New or progressive CXR infiltrate, in association with fever, high inflammatory markers, purulent secretions, and worsening ventilatory parameters (increasing RR, decreasing tidal volumes, increasing O_2 requirements)
- There are many non-infectious causes of fever and CXR infiltrate in ICU patients (Box 41.4), so the diagnosis is not always straightforward. Consider other common sources of fever in ventilated patients: infected IV catheters, urinary infection, *C. difficile* colitis.

Investigations
- *CXR* often shows a non-specific infiltrate, with air bronchograms being the best predictor of the disease
- *Airway sampling for microbiology:*
  - *Bronchoscopic sampling* Protected specimen brush (PSB) samples (with the tip of the bronchoscope placed opposite the orifice of an involved segmental bronchus, and PSB advanced through its protective sheath into the airway) or BAL samples (from a subsegmental bronchus, with the end of the bronchoscope wedged into the airway) are the optimal methods to obtain lower airway samples with minimal contamination. VAP is diagnosed when

> **Box 41.4 Differential diagnosis of fever and CXR infiltrate in ventilated patients**
> - VAP
> - Chemical aspiration without infection
> - Atelectasis
> - ARDS
> - Left ventricular failure
> - Pulmonary embolism with lung infarction
> - Pulmonary haemorrhage
> - Organizing pneumonia
> - Drug-induced lung disease
> - Lung malignancy
> - Pulmonary contusion.

an arbitrary threshold of organisms is grown on a BAL or PSB sample: usual cut-offs are 1,000 colony-forming units/mL (cfu/mL) for PSB samples and 10,000 cfu/mL for BAL samples. Thresholds vary between units, as do thresholds for starting treatment. Meta-analysis of three RCTs showed no significant mortality differences between quantitative and qualitative culture assessments

- *Non-bronchoscopic airway sampling*, e.g. blind bronchial sampling of lower respiratory tract secretions (so-called 'mini-BAL') is cheaper and does not need an expert operator. A catheter is advanced through the endotracheal tube until there is resistance, and saline (20 mL) is infused and then aspirated
- *Serial sampling* is favoured in some units. Regular non-invasive serial airway sampling may aid early diagnosis of VAP. Requires careful interpretation, as the microbiology of the respiratory tract changes over time in critically ill mechanically ventilated patients
- *Tracheal aspiration samples* are easy to obtain but non-specific in diagnosing VAP, as upper airway colonization is common.

Antibiotic treatment

Problems with the emergence of resistant bacteria mean that empirical treatment with antibiotics is used less commonly. Follow local prescribing policy and liaise with microbiology. The most common antibiotic-resistant pathogens are *P. aeruginosa*, MRSA, *Acinetobacter* spp., and *Klebsiella* spp. Risk factors for infection with resistant pathogens are listed in Box 41.5. Delay in commencing antibiotics is associated with a poorer outcome.

Box 41.5 Risk factors for resistant organisms as causes of VAP

- Hospitalization in the previous 90 days
- Nursing home residence
- Current hospital admission >5 days
- Mechanical ventilation >7 days
- Prior broad-spectrum antibiotic use (e.g. third-generation cephalosporin)
- High frequency of local antibiotic resistance.

Empirical antibiotic choice often includes coverage for anaerobes and MRSA, *Legionella* (if long stay), *P. aeruginosa*, and *Acinetobacter*.

Length of treatment depends on the clinical response, with one trial showing that 8-day treatment had similar efficacy to 15-day treatment, although patients with *P. aeruginosa* infection had a greater risk of recurrence following discontinuation of antibiotics at 8 days. Failure to respond should lead to a change of antibiotics and a search for additional infection or another cause for the radiographic infiltrate; further cultures should be sent.

Aspiration pneumonia: risk factors

Definition

Pneumonia that follows the aspiration of exogenous material or endogenous secretions into the lower respiratory tract.

Epidemiology

Aspiration pneumonia is the commonest cause of death in patients with dysphagia due to neurological disorders and is the cause of up to 20% of pneumonias in nursing home residents. It occurs in about 10% of patients admitted to hospital with a drug overdose.

Pathophysiology

Micro-aspiration is common in healthy individuals, but for an aspiration pneumonia to occur there must be compromise of the normal defences protecting the lower airways (glottic closure, cough reflex), with inoculation of the lower respiratory tract with a significant amount of material. Most pneumonias occur as a result of aspiration of micro-organisms from the oral cavity or nasopharynx.

Risk factors for aspiration pneumonia

- *Reduced conscious level* (cough reflex and impaired glottic closure)
  - Alcohol
  - Drug overdose
  - Post-seizure
  - Post-anaesthesia
  - Cerebrovascular accident
- *Dysphagia*
  - Motor neurone disease
  - Cerebrovascular accident (patients with impaired swallow reflex are 7 times more likely to develop a pneumonia than those in whom the gag reflex is unimpaired)
- *Upper GI tract disease*
  - Surgery to the stomach or oesophagus
  - Mechanical impairment of glottic or cardiac sphincter closure, e.g. tracheostomy, nasogastric feeding, bronchoscopy
  - Pharyngeal anaesthesia
- *Increased reflux*
  - Large-volume vomiting
  - Large-volume nasogastric feed
  - Feeding gastrostomy
  - Recumbent position
- *Nursing home residents*
  - Risk of aspiration is lower in those without teeth, who receive aggressive oral hygiene
  - There is a higher incidence of silent aspiration in the otherwise healthy elderly
  - Strong correlation between volume of aspirate and the risk of developing pneumonia.

Aspiration pneumonia: clinical features

Three pulmonary syndromes result from aspiration. The volume and nature of the aspirated material, the site and frequency of the aspiration, and the host response together determine which pulmonary syndrome occurs.

Chemical pneumonitis

Chemical pneumonitis refers to aspiration of substances toxic to the lower airways, in the absence of bacterial infection. This causes a chemical burn of the tracheobronchial tree, causing an intense parenchymal inflammatory reaction with release of inflammatory mediators that may lead to ARDS. Animal studies show that an inoculum with a pH <2.5 of relatively large volume (about 25 mL in adults) is needed to initiate an inflammatory reaction. Animal models show rapid pathological changes within 3 min, with atelectasis, pulmonary haemorrhage, and pulmonary oedema. This was first described by Mendelson, whose syndrome refers to the aspiration of sterile gastric contents and its toxic effects; the original case series was in obstetric anaesthesia.

Clinical features
- Rapid onset of symptoms including breathlessness (within 1–2 h)
- Low-grade fever
- Severe hypoxaemia and diffuse lung infiltrates involving dependent segments
- CXR changes within 2 h.

Treatment
- If aspiration is observed—suction and/or bronchoscopy to clear aspirated secretions or food. This may not prevent chemical injury from acid, which is similar to a flash burn
- Support of cardiac and respiratory function with IV fluids, $O_2\pm$ ventilation
- Steroids are controversial; no benefit has been shown in human studies
- Antibiotics are usually given, even in the absence of evidence of infection, because secondary bacterial infection is common and may be a contributing or primary factor in the aspiration. Acid-damaged lung is more susceptible to the effects of secondary bacterial infection; up to 25% will develop secondary bacterial infection. Activity against Gram-negative and anaerobic organisms is needed, e.g. cefuroxime plus metronidazole, or penicillin plus clindamycin.

Bacterial infection

Aspiration of bacteria normally resident in the upper airways or stomach. The normal bacterial flora are anaerobes, in a host susceptible to aspiration, and less virulent than the bacteria causing CAP.

Clinical features
- Cough, fever, purulent sputum, breathlessness
- The process may evolve over weeks and months, rather than hours
- May be more chronic, with weight loss and anaemia
- Absence of fever or rigors
- Foul-smelling sputum

- Periodontal disease
- Involvement of dependent pulmonary lobes
- Anaerobic bacteria are more difficult to culture so may be present, but not identified in microbiological culture
- May present with later manifestations, e.g. empyema, lung abscess.

Major pathogens are *Peptostreptococcus*, *Fusobacterium nucleatum*, *Prevotella*, and *Bacteroides* spp. Mixed infection is common.

Treatment
- Antibiotics including anaerobic cover, e.g. co-amoxiclav, clindamycin, or a carbapenem
- Swallow assessment/neurological review if no obvious underlying cause found.

Mechanical obstruction

Aspiration of matter that is not directly toxic to the lung may lead to damage by causing airway obstruction or reflex airway closure. Causative agents include:
- Saline
- Barium
- Most ingested fluids, including water
- Gastric contents with a pH >2.5
- Mechanical obstruction, such as occurs in drowning, or those who are unable to clear a potential inoculum, e.g. neurological deficit, impaired cough reflex, reduced conscious level
- Inhalation of an object, with the severity of the obstruction depending on the size and site of the aspirated particle. This is commoner in children but does occur in adults, e.g. teeth, peanuts.

Treatment
- Tracheal suction
- Remove obstructing object if possible
- No further treatment is needed if no CXR infiltrates.

Lung abscess: clinical features

Definition

A localized area of lung suppuration leading to necrosis of the pulmonary parenchyma, with or without cavity formation. Lung abscesses may be single or multiple, acute or chronic (>1 month), primary or secondary. They may occur spontaneously, but, more commonly, an underlying disease exists. Lung abscess is now rare in the developed world but has a high mortality of up to 20–30%.

Pathophysiology

Many are the result of aspiration pneumonia and share the same predisposing factors (➲ p. 540).

- Dental disease
- Impaired consciousness—alcohol, post-anaesthesia, dysphagia
- Diabetes mellitus
- Lung cancer (with bronchial obstruction)
- Secondary to pneumonia (cavitation occurs in 16% of *Staphylococcus aureus* pneumonia)
- Immunocompromise
- Septic embolization (right heart endocarditis due to, e.g. *Staphylococcus aureus* in IV drug users).

The bacterial inoculum reaches the lung parenchyma, often in a dependent lung area. Pneumonitis, followed by necrosis, occurs over 7–14 days. Cavitation occurs when parenchymal necrosis leads to communication with the bronchus, with the entry of air and expectoration of necrotic material leading to the formation of an air-fluid level. Bronchial obstruction leads to atelectasis with stasis and subsequent infection, which can predispose to abscess formation.

Presentation

- Often insidious onset
- Productive cough, haemoptysis
- Breathlessness
- Fevers
- Night sweats
- Non-specific features of chronic infection—anaemia, weight loss, malaise (especially in the elderly)
- Foul sputum or purulent pleural fluid
- Lemierre's syndrome (Box 41.6).

Box 41.6 Lemierre's syndrome (necrobacillosis)

Jugular vein suppurative thrombophlebitis. This is a rare pharyngeal infection in young adults, most commonly due to the anaerobe *Fusobacterium necrophorum*. It presents with a classical history of painful pharyngitis, in the presence of bacteraemia. Infection spreads to the neck and carotid sheath, often leading to thrombosis of the internal jugular vein. This may not be obvious clinically (neck vein US or Doppler may be needed). Septic embolization to the lung, with subsequent cavitation, leads to abscess formation. Can be complicated by empyema and abscesses in the bone, joints, liver, and kidneys.

Microbiology

- Commonly mixed infection, usually including anaerobes
- The most common organisms are those colonizing the oral cavity and gingival crevices—*Peptostreptococcus*, *Prevotella*, *Bacteroides*, and *Fusobacterium* spp.
- Aerobes—*Streptococcus 'milleri'* group, *Staphylococcus aureus*, *Klebsiella* spp., *Streptococcus pyogenes*, *Haemophilus influenzae*, *Nocardia*
- Non-bacterial pathogens are also reported—fungi (*Aspergillus*, *Cryptococcus*, *Histoplasma*, *Blastomyces*) and mycobacteria
- Opportunistic infections in immunocompromised—*Nocardia*, mycobacteria, *Aspergillus*; abscesses due to *Pneumocystis jirovecii*, *Cryptococcus neoformans*, *Rhodococcus* spp., and fungi in HIV-positive patients.

Diagnosis

The diagnosis is usually made from the history, along with the appearance of a cavity with an associated air-fluid level on CXR.

Lung abscess: management

Investigations

- Microbiological culture, ideally before commencing antibiotics
  - *Blood cultures*
  - *Sputum* or bronchoscopic specimen (including for AFBs)
  - Transthoracic percutaneous needle aspiration (CT- or US-guided) may provide samples. Risk of bleeding, pneumothorax, and seeding of infection to pleural space, if abscess not adjacent to the pleura.

In practice, blood cultures and sputum microbiology usually suffice. Samples are usually only obtained by more invasive means if appropriate antibiotics are not leading to an adequate clinical response.

- *Imaging*—exclude aspirated foreign body, underlying neoplasm, or bronchial stenosis and obstruction
  - *CXR* may show consolidation, cavitation (see Box 41.7), air-fluid level (if the patient is unwell, the CXR is likely to be taken in a semi-recumbent position, so an air-fluid level may not be visible). Half of abscesses are in the posterior segment of the right upper lobe or the apical basal segments of either lower lobe
  - *CT* is useful if the diagnosis is in doubt or if the clinical response to treatment is inadequate. It can also help to define the exact position of the abscess (if surgery is being considered)
    - CT also is useful to differentiate an abscess from a pleural collection: a *lung abscess* typically appears as a rounded intrapulmonary mass, with no compression of adjacent lung, with a thickened irregular wall, making an acute angle at its contact with the chest wall; an *empyema* typically has a 'lenticular' shape and compresses adjacent lung, which creates an obtuse angle as it follows the contour of the chest wall
    - CT can determine the presence of obstructing endobronchial disease, due to malignancy or foreign body, and may be useful in defining the extent of disease in a very sick patient who has had significant haemoptysis. Even with CT, differentiating an abscess from a cavitating cancer can be very difficult.

Box 41.7 Differential diagnosis of a cavitating mass on CXR

- Cavitating carcinoma—primary or metastatic
- Cavitary TB
- Granulomatosis with polyangiitis (GPA; Wegener's)
- Infected pulmonary cyst or bulla
- Aspergilloma
- Pulmonary infarct
- Rheumatoid nodule
- Sarcoidosis
- Bronchiectasis.

Antibiotics

- Antibiotic cover is required for both aerobic and anaerobic infection, including β-lactam/β-lactamase inhibitors, e.g. co-amoxiclav and clindamycin. Risk of *Clostridium difficile* diarrhoea
- No data to guide length of antibiotic treatment but consensus that long courses are needed. Common practice is 1–2 weeks IV treatment, with a further 2–6 weeks oral antibiotics, often until outpatient clinic review.

Drainage

- Spontaneous drainage of lung abscesses is common, with the production of purulent sputum. This can be increased with postural drainage and physiotherapy
- No data to support routine use of bronchoscopic drainage, which may carry the risk of endobronchial spread of infection
- Percutaneous drainage with radiologically placed small percutaneous drains for peripheral abscesses may be useful in those failing to respond to antibiotic and supportive treatment, although there is a potential risk of introducing infection into the pleural space.

Surgery

Surgical resection is rarely required if appropriate antibiotic treatment is given. It is usually reserved for complicated infections failing to respond after at least 6 weeks of treatment. Surgery is more likely to be required if:
- Very large abscess (>6 cm diameter)
- Resistant organisms
- Haemorrhage
- Recurrent disease.

Lobectomy or pneumonectomy is occasionally needed if severe infection with an abscess leaves a large volume of damaged lung that is hard to sterilize.

Complications

Haemorrhage (erosion of blood vessels as the abscess extends into the lung parenchyma) can be massive and life-threatening (◆ p. 47) and is an indication for urgent surgery. If clinically slow to respond, consider:
- Underlying malignancy
- Unusual microbiology, e.g. mycobacteria, fungi
- Immunosuppression
- Large cavity (>6 cm) may rarely require drainage
- Non-bacterial cause, e.g. cavitating malignancy, GPA (Wegener's)
- Other cause of persistent fever, e.g. *Clostridium difficile* diarrhoea, antibiotic-associated fever.

Prognosis

Cure rate is 85% in the absence of underlying disease. Mortality is reported as high as 75% in immunocompromised patients. The prognosis is much worse in the presence of underlying lung disease, with increasing age and large abscesses (>6 cm) with *Staphylococcus aureus* infection.

Nocardiosis

Definition

Nocardia are Gram-positive, partially acid-fast, aerobic bacilli that form branching filaments. They are found in soil, decaying organic plant matter, and water and have been isolated from house dust, garden soil, and swimming pools. Infection typically follows inhalation, but percutaneous inoculation also occurs. The *Nocardia asteroides* spp. complex accounts for the majority of clinical infections.

Consider *Nocardia* infection when soft tissue abscesses and/or central nervous system (CNS) manifestations occur in the setting of a pulmonary infection. The combination of respiratory, skin, and/or CNS involvement may lead to a misdiagnosis of vasculitis, and the respiratory manifestations may mimic cancer, TB, or fungal disease.

Epidemiology

Nocardia occurs worldwide, and the frequency of subclinical exposure is unknown. Clinically apparent infection is rare and usually occurs in patients with immunocompromise (haematological malignancy, steroid therapy, organ transplant, diabetes, alcoholism, and HIV infection, especially intravenous drug users) or pre-existing lung disease (particularly pulmonary alveolar proteinosis, TB). Infection also occurs in apparently healthy people (10–25% of cases). Nosocomial infection and disease outbreaks have been reported.

Clinical features

Pulmonary disease

- The lung is the most common site of involvement
- Patients typically present with productive cough, fever, anorexia, weight loss, and malaise; dyspnoea, pleuritic pain, and haemoptysis may occur but are less common
- Empyema occurs in up to a quarter of cases, and direct intrathoracic spread causing pericarditis, mediastinitis, rib osteomyelitis, or superior vena caval obstruction (SVCO) is also reported.

Extrapulmonary disease

- Dissemination from the lungs occurs in 50% of patients
- CNS is the most common site of dissemination, occurring in 25% of pulmonary nocardiosis cases. Single or multiple abscesses occur and may be accompanied by meningitis
- Other sites include the skin and subcutaneous tissues, kidneys, bone, joints and muscle, peritoneum, eyes, pericardium, and heart valves.

Investigations

- Identification by smear and culture is the principal method of diagnosis. *Nocardia* grows on routine media, usually within 2–7 days, although more prolonged culture (2–3 weeks) may be required
- Direct smear of appropriate specimens (e.g. aspirates of abscesses, biopsies) is highly sensitive and typically shows Gram-positive beaded branching filaments, which are usually acid-fast on modified Ziehl–Neelsen (ZN) stain. Examination of BAL fluid may also be diagnostic

- Sensitivity testing of isolates and identification to species level is done by reference laboratories
- Biopsies typically show a mixed cellular infiltrate; granulomata occur rarely and may result in misdiagnosis as TB or histoplasmosis
- CXR and CT may demonstrate parenchymal infiltrates, single or multiple nodules (sometimes with cavitation), or features of pleural infection
- Sputum smear is usually unhelpful. Sputum culture has a greater yield, but *Nocardia* growth may be obscured in mixed cultures. The significance of *Nocardia* growth on sputum culture in asymptomatic patients is unclear; it may represent contamination or colonization in the setting of underlying lung disease
- Blood cultures are almost always negative, although *Nocardia* bacteraemia may occur in the setting of profound immunocompromise
- Consider magnetic resonance imaging (MRI) of the brain to exclude asymptomatic CNS involvement in patients with pulmonary nocardiosis.

Management

- Discuss treatment with an infectious diseases specialist
- Drug treatment choices include sulphonamides/co-trimoxazole, minocycline, imipenem, cefotaxime, ceftriaxone, or amikacin. Sulpha drugs, in particular co-trimoxazole, have traditionally been the mainstay of therapy. Imipenem and amikacin combination therapy has been shown to be active *in vitro* and in animal models and is recommended for pulmonary nocardiosis and for very ill patients. Extended-spectrum cephalosporins, such as ceftriaxone and cefotaxime, have the advantages of good CNS penetration and low toxicity
- Optimal treatment duration is unclear: typically given for 6 months in non-immunocompromised patients, and for 12 months or longer for CNS involvement or immunocompromised patients
- Surgery may be required for abscess drainage.

Prognosis

Clinical outcome is dependent on the site and extent of disease and on underlying host factors. Disease remissions and exacerbations are common. Cure rates are 90% in pleuropulmonary disease and 50% in brain abscess. Mortality of *Nocardia* infection is generally low, although it approaches 50% in cases of bacteraemia.

Actinomycosis

Definition

Actinomycosis is caused by a group of anaerobic Gram-positive bacilli, of which *Actinomyces israelii* is the commonest. These organisms are present in the mouth, GI tract, and vagina. Clinical infection may follow dental procedures or aspiration of infected secretions. Infection is slowly progressive and may disseminate via the bloodstream or invade tissue locally, sometimes resulting in sinus tract formation.

> Consider this diagnosis particularly in patients with pulmonary disease accompanied by soft tissue infection of the head and neck. The diagnosis of actinomycosis is often unsuspected, and the clinical and radiological features may mimic cancer, TB, or fungal disease.

Epidemiology

Actinomycosis is rare. It can occur at any age and is more common in men. Predisposing factors include corticosteroid use, chemotherapy, organ transplant, and HIV infection.

Clinical features

Thoracic disease

Occurs in about 15% of cases. Symptoms of pulmonary involvement are non-specific and include cough, chest pain, haemoptysis, fever, anorexia, and weight loss. Chest wall involvement may occur, with sinus formation or rib infection, and empyema is common. Mediastinal involvement is documented.

Extrathoracic disease

Soft tissue infection of the head and neck, particularly the mandible, is the commonest disease presentation (about 50% of cases). Discharging sinuses may form. Other extrathoracic disease sites include the abdomen (particularly the ileocaecal region), pelvis, liver, bone, and CNS (manifest as single or multiple abscesses).

Investigations

- CXR and CT appearances are variable, including masses (sometimes with cavitation), parenchymal infiltrates, consolidation, mediastinal disease, and/or pleural involvement
- Diagnosis is based on the microscopy and anaerobic culture of infected material. Warn the microbiology laboratory if the diagnosis is suspected, as specific stains and culture conditions are required. Examination of infected material may reveal yellow 'sulphur granules' containing aggregated organisms. Sample sputum, pleural fluid, and pus from sinus tracts; inoculate into anaerobic transport media, and rapidly transport to lab. Endobronchial biopsies have a low sensitivity. Most infections are polymicrobial, with accompanying aerobic or anaerobic bacteria.

Management

- Discuss treatment with an infectious diseases specialist
- Drug treatment choices include penicillin, amoxicillin, clindamycin, or erythromycin. Administration should initially be IV. Optimal treatment duration is unclear (typically given for 6–12 months)
- Surgery may be required for abscess drainage
- Monitor response to treatment with serial CT or MRI scans
- Treat any associated periodontal disease.

Prognosis

Disease relapse is common if prolonged treatment is not administered.

Anthrax

Definition and epidemiology

- *Bacillus anthracis* is an aerobic Gram-positive spore-forming bacterium that causes human disease, principally following either inhalation or cutaneous contact. Spores can survive in soil for many years. Person-to-person transmission does not occur
- Considerable interest has focused on the use of anthrax in bioterrorism; five envelopes containing anthrax spores were sent through the US postal service in 2001, and there were 11 confirmed cases of inhalational anthrax (including five deaths) and seven confirmed cases of cutaneous anthrax. A previous outbreak occurred in Sverdlovsk in the former Soviet Union in 1979, following the release of spores from a biological weapons plant, and resulted in 68 deaths
- Anthrax infection also occurs very rarely in association with occupational exposure to *Bacillus anthracis* in animal wool or hides. The majority of occupational cases result in cutaneous disease, and a diagnosis of inhalational anthrax strongly suggests a bioterrorist attack.

Clinical features

Inhalational anthrax

- Incubation period is variable, although, in the US in 2001, it typically ranged 4–6 days following exposure from opening mail
- Patients typically experience a prodrome of flu-like symptoms such as fever and cough. GI symptoms (vomiting, diarrhoea, abdominal pain), drenching sweats, and altered mental status are often prominent symptoms. Breathlessness, fever, and septic shock develop several days later. Haemorrhagic meningitis is a common complication
- Large haemorrhagic pleural effusions are a characteristic feature.

Cutaneous anthrax

Initial symptoms include itch and development of a papule at the infection site. A necrotic ulcer with a black centre, and often surrounding oedema, subsequently develops. Systemic symptoms, such as fever and sweats, may be present.

Investigations

- *Bacillus anthracis* grows on conventional media and is readily cultured if sampling precedes antibiotic treatment; a definitive diagnosis requires specialized laboratory tests (e.g. PCR, immunohistochemistry of biopsy samples, or serological studies)
- Blood tests typically reveal leucocytosis
- Blood cultures are positive in nearly all cases of inhalational anthrax when taken prior to antibiotic treatment. Staining and culture of pleural fluid may be diagnostic
- CXR in inhalational anthrax classically shows a widened mediastinum (due to necrosis of mediastinal lymph nodes and haemorrhagic mediastinitis); pleural effusions and pulmonary infiltrates may be present. CT may also demonstrate mediastinal and hilar lymphadenopathy
- Gram stain and culture of the ulcer is usually diagnostic in cutaneous anthrax, although biopsy is sometimes required.

Management

- Discuss with infectious diseases and public health specialists if the diagnosis is suspected
- Antibiotic treatment should be administered immediately after taking blood cultures. Recommendations are for initial treatment with either ciprofloxacin or doxycycline IV, in combination with 1–2 additional antibiotics (choices include clindamycin, vancomycin, meropenem, or penicillin). Subsequent treatment should be with either ciprofloxacin or doxycycline orally for 60 days. Oral treatment alone may be sufficient in cases of mild cutaneous disease
- Corticosteroid treatment should be considered in patients with meningitis or severe neck or mediastinal oedema
- Supportive care, including ventilatory support, treatment of shock with IV fluids and/or inotropes, and chest tube drainage of large pleural effusions may be needed.

Prognosis

Inhalational anthrax is associated with a high mortality; five of the recent 11 cases in the USA died. The mortality of previously documented cases has been even higher, perhaps reflecting a delay or lack of antibiotic treatment.

Prophylaxis

US recommendations advise prophylaxis with oral ciprofloxacin or doxycycline for individuals considered to have been exposed to anthrax spores in contaminated areas. A vaccine is available, although its value in post-exposure prophylaxis is unknown.

Tularaemia

Definition and epidemiology

Tularaemia is a rare zoonosis caused by infection with the Gram-negative bacteria *Francisella tularensis*. Two major subspecies are described: subspp. *tularensis* (type A) is highly virulent and found in North America; subspp. *holarctica* (type B) is less virulent and found in North America, Europe, and Asia. Small mammals (particularly rabbits and hares) acquire infection from arthropod bites and act as reservoirs; human infection follows inhalation, direct contact with infected rodents, ingestion of contaminated food, or arthropod bites. Tularaemia is most frequently encountered in rural areas, following activities such as farming and hunting, although laboratory workers are also at risk. There has been considerable interest in the development of *F. tularensis* as a biological weapon, and more recently concerns have arisen as to its possible use in bioterrorism.

Clinical features

Typically abrupt onset of fever, headache, dry cough, and malaise. Development of a tender ulcer and regional lymphadenopathy ('ulceroglandular tularaemia') around an infected arthropod bite is common. Tularaemia pneumonia, following infection with type A, is characterized by cough (productive or dry), breathlessness, and sweating, with often minimal signs on examination; may progress rapidly to respiratory failure and death. Symptoms of pneumonia are milder after infection with type B.

Investigations

* Serology is the principal method of diagnosis, although PCR-based techniques are increasingly used
* *F. tularensis* may be identified in culture of wound specimens, although the laboratory should be warned—type A is sufficiently virulent for some laboratories not to perform culture. Sputum cultures may be diagnostic
* CXR may demonstrate parenchymal infiltrates, often progressing to lobar consolidation. Pleural effusions, hilar lymphadenopathy, and lung abscess may occur.

Management

* Discuss treatment with an infectious diseases specialist
* Drug treatment choices include streptomycin or gentamicin for 10 days. Doxycycline or chloramphenicol are alternatives, although treatment failure rates are higher and a course of 14 days is recommended
* In the setting of a large-scale outbreak (e.g. following use in bioterrorism), doxycycline or ciprofloxacin may be used for treatment or following exposure.

Prognosis

Mortality is 1–2% from type A; type B is benign in humans.

Melioidosis

Definition and epidemiology

Melioidosis is caused by *Burkholderia pseudomallei*, a Gram-negative bacillus that is found in soil and water in South East Asia, northern Australia, China, and India; clinical disease is particularly common in Thailand where it may account for up to one-third of all pneumonia deaths. Infection is thought to follow entry via skin abrasions or inhalation, and pneumonia is the most common clinical presentation. Most cases represent recent infection; re-activation of infection is rare but can occur many years after exposure. Risk factors for melioidosis include diabetes, alcohol excess, renal disease, and chronic lung disease (in particular cystic fibrosis).

Clinical features

- *Acute septicaemic melioidosis* Patients present acutely unwell, with a severe pneumonia and widespread nodular consolidation on CXR; may progress rapidly to death
- *Localized subacute melioidosis* Subacute cavitating lobar (often upper) pneumonia, mimicking TB
- *Chronic suppurative melioidosis* Chronic lung abscess ± empyema; suppurative infection may involve other organs, including skin, brain, joints, bones, liver, spleen, kidney, adrenal, prostate, lymph nodes.

Consider melioidosis in returning travellers from Asia or Australia with CAP or a subacute/chronic 'TB-like' respiratory illness.

Diagnosis

Identification by culture is the principal method of diagnosis. Blood cultures may be diagnostic; alert the laboratory to the possibility of this infection. Enzyme-linked immunosorbent assays (ELISAs) are relatively insensitive.

Management

- *B. pseudomallei* is resistant to multiple antibiotics. Treat with high-dose IV ceftazidime, meropenem, or imipenem for at least 10–14 days (longer if severe pulmonary disease or organ abscesses), followed by oral antibiotic (e.g. co-trimoxazole, alone or in combination with doxycycline) for at least 12 weeks to ensure eradication
- Supportive care, with ICU admission for septic shock or severe pneumonia.

Prognosis

Documented mortality rates range 19–46%.

Leptospirosis

Definition and epidemiology

Leptospirosis is a zoonosis transmitted from water or soil contaminated with urine of infected animals (e.g. rats, dogs, cats, pigs, cattle, hamsters, bats) through skin abrasions or mucosa. Present worldwide, more common in tropical countries, but well described in UK. Individuals most at risk in the UK include farmers, vets, sewage workers, returning travellers from the tropics, military personnel, and canoeists. Incidence peaks in spring/summer. In the tropics, epidemics may occur following storms or floods.

Consider leptospirosis in all patients with diffuse alveolar haemorrhage and in at-risk individuals with pneumonia or ARDS.

Clinical features

Disease manifestations are highly variable, ranging from asymptomatic infection to multi-organ failure, pulmonary haemorrhage, and death. Patients may present solely with pulmonary haemorrhage, without other features of Weil's disease. Manifestations include:

- *Acute (anicteric) leptospirosis* Self-limiting flu-like illness; myalgia, rash, and aseptic meningitis may occur
- *Weil's disease (icterohaemorrhagic fever)* Classic form of leptospirosis. Features include fever, myalgia, conjunctival haemorrhage, rash, jaundice/hepatic failure, renal failure, coagulopathy, and thrombocytopenia, shock, myocarditis/cardiac arrhythmias
- *Pulmonary disease* Occurs in at least a third of hospitalized patients with acute leptospirosis or Weil's disease. Manifestations include mild symptoms/signs (cough, wheeze, and crackles), pneumonia, pulmonary oedema secondary to myocarditis, and ARDS or fulminant alveolar haemorrhage syndrome.

Investigations

- May be isolated in blood cultures
- Serology confirms the diagnosis and is performed in a single Leptospira Reference Unit in the UK. Both ELISA and microscopic agglutination tests may be performed
- CXR and CT typically demonstrate patchy consolidation and ground-glass shadowing, commonly bilateral with lower lobe predominance.

Management

- Discuss treatment with infectious diseases and renal specialists
- Antibiotic choices include penicillin, ceftriaxone, or doxycycline
- Ventilatory support required for alveolar haemorrhage and ARDS
- Ensure adequate hydration; blood products may be required
- High-dose glucocorticoids are occasionally used, although there is no convincing evidence of benefit. Plasma exchange and desmopressin infusions have been tried.

Prognosis

Acute leptospirosis typically resolves spontaneously after about 14 days. Severe pulmonary disease can progress very rapidly (over hours), with reported mortality rates approaching 50%.

Box 41.8 Differential diagnosis of zoonotic microbial causes of CAP (with exposures)
• Avian influenza virus (birds, animals)
• *Bacillus anthracis* (anthrax; animals)
• Brucellosis (animals)
• *Chlamydia caviae* (guinea pigs)
• *Chlamydophila psittaci* (psittacosis; poultry, birds)
• *Coxiella burnetii* (Q fever; parturient cats, cattle, sheep, goats, rabbits)
• *Cryptococcus neoformans* (birds)
• *Francisella tularensis* (tularaemia; rabbits, cats, rodents)
• Hantavirus (rodents, the Americas)
• *Histoplasma capsulatum* (histoplasmosis; birds or bats, the Americas)
• Leptospirosis (water contaminated with infected animal urine)
• *Pasteurella multocida* (pasteurellosis; animals, birds)
• *Ricketsia rickettsii* (Rocky mountain spotted fever; tick bite or exposure to tick-infested habitats, USA)
• *Yersinia pestis* (pneumonic plague; rodents, cats).

Respiratory infection—fungal

Aspergillus lung disease: classification 560
Severe asthma with fungal sensitization 561
Allergic bronchopulmonary aspergillosis 562
Invasive aspergillosis (IA) 564
Chronic pulmonary aspergillosis 566
Summary of *Aspergillus* lung disease 568
Pneumocystis pneumonia (PCP): diagnosis 570
PCP: treatment 572
Cryptococcosis 574
Candidal pneumonia 575
Endemic mycoses: introduction 576
Endemic mycoses: histoplasmosis 578
Endemic mycoses: blastomycosis 580
Endemic mycoses: coccidioidomycosis 582
Endemic mycoses: paracoccidioidomycosis, penicilliosis,
    adiaspiromycosis 583

Aspergillus lung disease: classification

Types of disease

Aspergillus fumigatus and other *Aspergillus* moulds are ubiquitous fungi that can be isolated from the air in most houses, and this increases with increasing indoor humidity. Inhalation of spores (conidia) can produce a range of diseases, some of which are related to each other and some of which are not. While fungi are now thought to be found in healthy lungs, the finding of fungal hyphae (rather than just spores) in the sputum should provoke an assessment.

Classification

Severe asthma with fungal sensitisation (IgE-mediated)

From inhaled *Aspergillus* spores. One of many common antigens provoking airway inflammation and bronchospasm.

Allergic bronchopulmonary aspergillosis-bronchiectasis (APBA-B)

A probable evolution and progression of exuberant IgE and IgG reaction to *Aspergillus* in (usually) asthmatics, with inflammatory damage to the airways and resultant bronchiectasis (but no actual invasion of *Aspergillus* into the airway walls).

Allergic bronchopulmonary aspergillosis-seropositive only (ABPA-S)

Similar to ABPA with mucous plugging and distal consolidation that may flit from area to area, but without resultant bronchiectasis. This is one of the causes of pulmonary eosinophilia.

Invasive *Aspergillus* (IA) pneumonia due to invasion of *Aspergillus*

Typically 2° to immunosuppression, but increasingly recognized in chronic obstructive pulmonary disease (COPD) and critical illness. This can be a multisystem disorder with *Aspergillus* invading almost any part of the body.

Chronic pulmonary aspergillosis (CPA)

Almost exclusively found in those with underlying lung disease leading to air-filled cavity or bulla. Most common risk factors are previous tuberculosis (TB), non-tuberculous mycobacteria (NTM) (can co-exist), COPD. *Aspergillus* IgG is positive with evidence of *aspergillus* in the sputum

Aspergilloma

Asymptomatic *Aspergillus* living and growing as a separate ball of fungus in a pre-existing lung cavity. If symptomatic this is a form of CPA.

Hypersensitivity pneumonitis

Previously known as extrinsic allergic alveolitis; due to an immune inflammatory reaction to inhalation of large numbers of spores (see p. 311).

The presentation and clinical setting of these various *Aspergillus*-related disorders are clearly different and thus are detailed separately.

Severe asthma with fungal sensitization

Approximately 10% of asthmatics are skin prick-positive to *Aspergillus* species, compared with about 70% to house dust mite. It is assumed that this allergy contributes to allergic inflammation in the airways, but, in the few relevant studies, symptoms have not always correlated with exposure. However, in some studies, asthma admissions to hospital correlated better with fungal spore counts than with pollen counts. Fungal spore release may explain an association between thunderstorms and asthma attacks. Particularly high exposure results from working with mouldy vegetable matter, e.g. compost heaps, during late summer/early autumn. A small subset of asthmatic patients with severe asthma may have sensitization without meeting criteria for ABPA (screening test total IgE <1000 IU/mL). There may be a role for anti-fungal therapy in these individuals.

Allergic bronchopulmonary aspergillosis

Definition

This condition is probably an extension of IgE and IgG reaction to *Aspergillus* where the inflammatory response to the *Aspergillus* in the airways leads to damage of the bronchial walls and bronchiectasis. Some authors reserve the use of the term ABPA for when bronchiectasis is present; others subdivide into ABPA-S (seropositive only) in those with positive serology but without bronchiectasis and ABPA-B (bronchiectasis).

The prevalence of ABPA in asthmatic populations has varied considerably between studies and clearly will depend on whether the definition includes bronchiectasis or not. It probably occurs in about 1–2% of asthmatics. A related condition occurs in patients with cystic fibrosis (CF) where it appears about 7% have evidence of colonization and potential ongoing damage.

Pathophysiology

The factors promoting the evolution from atopic asthmatic to ABPA are not known. HLA associations have been shown, with IL-10 promoter alterations are associated with *Aspergillus* colonization. Proteolytic enzymes are released by *Aspergillus* as part of its exophytic feeding strategy, and these enzymes may damage airway mucosa. However, most believe that the damage results from host defence mechanisms. Septated hyphae (rather than just spores) may be visible in the mucus and grown from sputum, but there does not appear to be actual invasion of the bronchial mucosa. This immune inflammatory activity produces mucoid impaction in the airways, eosinophilic pneumonitis, and broncho-centric granuloma formation.

Main criteria for diagnosis

The first four are the most important:
- **Skin prick/IgE +ve to *Aspergillus fumigatus***
- **IgG to *Aspergillus fumigatus***
- **Central (proximal) bronchiectasis**
- **Blood/sputum eosinophilia**
- Total serum IgE >1,000 IU/mL
- Lung infiltrates—flitting.

Other clinical features

- Long-standing asthma, recent deterioration
- Recurrent episodes of mucous plugging
- Fever/malaise
- Expectoration of dark mucous plugs, sometimes as casts of the airways
- Eosinophilia (sputum and blood)
- Occasional haemoptysis.

The major complication is poorly controlled asthma that requires repeated courses of oral steroids.

Investigations

- *Spirometry* Degree of airways obstruction
- *Skin prick sensitivity* to *Aspergillus* (IgE)
- *Sputum Aspergillus* hyphae and eosinophils
- *Blood*
  - IgG to *Aspergillus*
  - IgE RAST to *Aspergillus*
  - Total serum IgE
  - Eosinophil count (suppressed if on steroids)
- *Chest radiograph (CXR)*
  - Flitting infiltrates
  - Bronchiectasis, mucous impaction (gloved finger shadows)
- *Computed tomography (CT)* Central (proximal) bronchiectasis with upper lobe predominance.

Management

The treatment goals are to stop progression to bronchiectasis or fibrosis. The management is essentially that of severe chronic asthma, but with generous use of courses of oral steroids. Several RCTs have shown courses of itraconazole (200 mg bd for 4 months) are well tolerated as an adjunct therapy, reduce steroid requirements, and improve exercise tolerance. There appears to be a sustained effect after the itraconazole is stopped, suggesting at least temporary eradication of the *Aspergillus*. Response and relapse can be monitored with IgG to *Aspergillus*. Itraconazole can cause liver dysfunction, so liver function tests (LFTs) need monitoring. Case reports have shown a reduction in exacerbations of ABPA related to CF but randomized evidence is lacking.

Differential diagnosis

This list revolves mainly around the pulmonary infiltrates and eosinophilia:
- Acute/chronic eosinophilic pneumonia
- Churg–Strauss/EGPA syndrome
- Various parasites (e.g. filariasis, ascaris; Löffler's syndrome)
- Drug-induced eosinophilic pneumonia.

Further information

Schelenz et al. British Society for Medical Mycology best practice recommendations for the diagnosis of serious fungal diseases. *Lancet Infect Dis.* 2015;**15**: 461–474.

Greenberger et al. Allergic bronchopulmonary aspergillosis. *J Allergy Clin Immunol Pract.* 2014 **2**: 703–708.

Invasive aspergillosis (IA)

Definition

The term 'invasive aspergillosis' is reserved for the situation where *Aspergillus* hyphae actually invade tissue (hyalohyphomycosis). This usually occurs with severe immune suppression, but is increasingly recognized outside of this setting (see Risk factors). The port of entry is probably the lungs, but spread can be to almost any area of the body. The species most commonly seen are *Aspergillus fumigatus*, *flavus*, *terreus*, and *niger*. Mortality is very high. The source of *Aspergillus* is unclear but has been found in hospital water supplies.

Pathogenesis

Alveolar macrophages probably normally destroy *Aspergillus* spores. Macrophage failure may allow more spores to germinate, and any subsequent invasion with hyphae seems to be prevented by neutrophils. Inadequate neutrophil function allows invasion across tissue planes and may invade into vessels, with infarction and further spread throughout the body. There is some evidence that cytomegalovirus (CMV) may inactivate macrophages, allowing spores to germinate. The fungal digestive proteases do the damage, rather than the host's limited immunological responses.

Clinical features

Typical setting
Fever, chest pain, cough, haemoptysis, dyspnoea, and pulmonary infiltrate in a neutropenic patient failing to respond to broad-spectrum antibiotics.

Risk factors

- Following chemotherapy, particularly provoking severe neutropenia (<100 cells/microlitre)
- Bone marrow suppression for allogeneic stem cell transplants
- Advanced human immunodeficiency virus (HIV) infection and acquired immune deficiency syndrome (AIDS)
- Immune suppression following transplant
- Infliximab (or other anti-TNF-α) therapy.
- COPD
- Critical illness, such as complicated influenza infection
- Rarely occurs with inhalation of a large number of spores in the apparent absence of underlying disease. This may be the first presentation immunosuppression, classically chronic granulomatous disease.

Spread
Can occur anywhere, with the following well-recognized signs:
- Sinuses (paranasal) and spread into the brain
- Endocarditis
- Eyes
- Skin (papular, ranging to ulcerative, lesions).

Careful examination and particular investigations may be needed to detect spread to these areas.

Investigations

- *Isolate Aspergillus branching septate hyphae* from respiratory tract by:
  - Sputum
  - Expressed sputum (3% saline via nebulizer)
  - Bronchoalveolar lavage (BAL)
  - Transbronchial biopsy (TBB)

(Hyphae may be present when not the 1° cause of the infiltrate.)
- *Biopsies* from other sites (most convincing when acute-angle branching, septated non-pigmented hyphae are seen)
- Circulating levels of *galactomannan*, an exoantigen of *Aspergillus* (70% sensitive in immunosuppressed patients but lower in other populations, false positives due to some antibiotics, e.g. co-amoxiclav and piperacillin-tazobactam). Serial sampling is recommended. Send BAL galactomannan as well
- Presence of β-*glucan* in serum represents fungal invasion but is not *Aspergillus*-specific; false positives due to blood processing and some antibiotics may affect results
- *CXR/CT* CXR changes are usually non-specific. CT may show a halo of low attenuation surrounding a nodular lesion early on. An 'air crescent' sign may develop on CXR, with air appearing at the edge of an area of consolidation. Usually occurs when neutrophil count rising and probably represents gradual containment of the infection into a cavity, not unlike an aspergilloma. IA in the immunocompetent does not typically have angio-invasion so will not usually have the typical halo appearance.

Ultimately, it is the clinical picture that dominates the diagnosis.

Management

Reduction of immunosuppression when possible; consider colony-stimulating factors. Prompt use of antifungals is essential, for a minimum of 6–12 weeks.
- Intravenous (IV) voriconazole is the treatment of choice (may cause visual disturbances, deranged LFTs, skin rash)
- Liposomal amphotericin B is an alternative first-line treatment
- Patients who are intolerant of voriconazole/liposomal amphotericin or who have refractory disease can be treated with lipid-based amphotericin, posaconazole, itraconazole, caspofungin, or micafungin.

Some centres use oral posaconazole as prophylaxis when commencing substantial immune suppression.

Surgical resection of the infected focus should be considered in some (e.g. lung lesions contiguous with the heart or great vessels, chest wall invasion, osteomyelitis, pericardial infection, and endocarditis).

Differential diagnosis

The differential will be the large number of other opportunistic infections seen in immunosuppressed patients. Another invasive mycosis *Candida albicans* is now less common due to its susceptibility to fluconazole.

Chronic pulmonary aspergillosis

Also known as chronic necrotizing aspergillosis, chronic pulmonary aspergillosis, or subacute invasive pulmonary aspergillosis.

Definition

Poorly defined, but it is clear that a low-grade chronic invasion of *Aspergillus* into airway walls and surrounding lung can occur. In the original descriptions, some cause of mild immuno-incompetence was present, e.g. diabetes, steroid therapy, chronic lung disease, poor nutrition.

Aspergilloma

The term aspergilloma is used to describe a ball of fungal hyphae within a cavity in the lung. It is assumed that this is colonization of a prior cavity ('saprophytic infection'), rather than arrested invasion. Aspergillomas can occur in other organs, including the pleural space. Aspergillomas are usually asymptomatic and unless part of CPA and therefore only require treatment in the context of CPA.

Pathogenesis

It is assumed that this form of aspergillosis results from lowered immunity in those with a tendency to make Th2 eosinophilic responses to antigens. There is infiltration of hyphae into lung tissue, ranging from minor patchy consolidation to multiple cavities. There is little, if any, angioinvasion. It is assumed that the fungal digestive proteases gradually do the damage, rather than the host's immunological response.

Clinical features

Suspect semi-IA when:
- Middle-aged
- Reason for mild immunosuppression, e.g. diabetes, alcoholism, and steroid usage (including inhaled)
- A pre-existing chronic lung disease
- Indolent presentation with fever, malaise and weight loss
- Associated with cough, SOB, chest discomfort and occasional haemoptysis
- Patchy indolent CXR changes.

Investigations

- Sputum samples may allow isolation of hyphae
- Varied radiological appearance including lung cavities with or without an aspergilloma, infiltrates, nodules, and various degrees of lung or pleural fibrosis.
- Different forms are recognized with sub-acute or semi-IA (some immunosuppression, more rapid course, nodules, and consolidation predominate on CT), chronic cavitatory pulmonary aspergillosis (constitutional symptoms, thick walled cavities, single or multiple with or without an aspergilloma), and chronic fibrosing pulmonary aspergillosis (characterized by progressive fibrosis)
- Diagnostic test is IgG to *Aspergillus* with associated evidence of *aspergillus* in the sputum (culture or polymerase chain reaction (PCR))

Management

On the assumption that mild immune suppression is the dominant cause, steroids are not usually recommended for fear of further immune suppression. This is in contrast to ABPA where the damage is due to the host's immune defence mechanisms. Oral treatment with itraconazole/voriconazole is usually appropriate, but IV therapy is required for severely ill patients. Alternative treatment options are as for IA.

Haemoptysis

- Tranexamic acid (must be taken during clot formation, as binds to fibrin to prevent action of endogenous fibrinolytics)
- Treat associated bacterial infections
- Consider itraconazole/voriconazole
- Bronchial arteriograms should reveal a leash of vessels supplying part of the cavity wall that can be embolized, even if not actively bleeding. Short-term success rate of embolisation is good; long term, less good
- Surgery can be difficult, as mycetomas may be stuck to the chest wall. Problems of seeding the pleural space are seen less often than in the past, probably due to better antifungal agents
- A few case reports exist of successful reduction of haemoptysis with radiotherapy
- Older approaches involving intracavity injections of amphotericin are rarely used now, although a recent case series of 40 patients seemed promising.

Summary of *Aspergillus* lung disease

The essential differences between the *Aspergillus* lung diseases depends on whether the damage to the lung is mediated by host defence mechanisms (atopic asthma, flitting consolidation, ABPA, possibly aspergilloma) or by the fungus' own digestive proteolytic enzymes (IA, semi-IA, aspergilloma). These two disease states are clearly different, but there probably exists a continuum between each of the subdivisions within each group, and the dominant mechanism in aspergilloma is not entirely clear. Therefore, it is likely that patients with mixed and transitional features will be encountered.

Future developments

- Evaluation of combination antifungal therapies
- Antifungal action of older drugs—flucytosine, rifampicin
- Place of early surgery
- Place of prophylaxis
- Further evaluation of the role of galactomannan and β-glucan levels in blood and BAL fluid for diagnosis.

Further information

Aspergillus/Fungal Research Trust website. ℘ http://www.aspergillus.org.uk.

Kosmidis and Denning. The clinical spectrum of aspergillosis. *Thorax* 2015;**70**: 270–277.

Shah et al. Invasive pulmonary aspergillosis and influenza co-infection in the immunocompetent host: case reports and review of the literature. *Diagn Microbiol Infect Dis* 2018;**91**: 147–152.

Bao et al. Invasive pulmonary aspergillosis in patients with COPD: a case report and literature review. *Oncotarget* 2017;**8**: 38069–38074.

Pneumocystis pneumonia (PCP): diagnosis

Definition

PCP is the clinical syndrome of pneumonia resulting from infection with the fungus *Pneumocystis jirovecii* (previously termed *Pneumocystis carinii*). *Pneumocystis jirovecii* is widespread in the environment, and most people are infected by the age of 2 y; PCP is thought, however, to follow new infection, rather than reactivation of latent infection. Most cases of infection are likely to be person-to-person airborne transmission, rather than environmental.

Causes

Risk factors for PCP include HIV infection (particularly with CD4 count $<200 \times 10^6/L$), treatment with chemotherapy (especially fludarabine), corticosteroids or other immunosuppressive agents, and malnutrition in children. Neutropenia does not appear to be a particular risk factor. PCP occurring in the setting of AIDS is associated with both a greater number of organisms and fewer inflammatory cells in the lungs when compared with infection associated with other causes of immunocompromise. PCP is much less common following the routine use of co-trimoxazole prophylaxis in HIV and post-transplantation, although cases still occur, e.g. in patients presenting with advanced HIV or in those non-compliant with prophylaxis. The threshold steroid dose for predisposition to PCP is unclear, although a dose equivalent to 16 mg prednisolone or greater for 8 weeks appears to significantly increase risk; the risk is likely also to reflect the underlying condition, e.g. PCP may develop in patients with haematological malignancy taking as little as 5 mg prednisolone daily. PCP often appears to present as immunosuppressant drug doses are tapered or increased.

Clinical features

Gradual onset of dry cough and exertional breathlessness, sometimes with retrosternal tightness. Fever and tachypnoea may occur; chest examination is typically normal. May present with pneumothorax. Extrapulmonary disease is very rare.

Investigations

- *CXR* Pattern is classically of bilateral perihilar infiltrates that progress to alveolar shadowing. Less common patterns include small nodular infiltrates or focal consolidation. CXR is normal in about 10%. Pleural effusions are very rare. CT is not routinely required, except in cases of a normal CXR when it may demonstrate a bilateral ground-glass pattern or cystic lesions
- *Hypoxia* is common. Desaturation on exercise may suggest the diagnosis in at-risk individuals with normal saturations at rest
- *White blood count* is usually normal. Serum lactate dehydrogenase (LDH) is typically raised (sensitive but non-specific)
- *β-D-glucan* is a component of the fungal cell wall and can be raised in blood or BAL but is not specific to PCP.

- *Induced sputum* (see ➲ p. 867) has a diagnostic yield of 70–80% in HIV infection but is much less sensitive when performed in the setting of non-HIV immunocompromise where the organism burden is lower. It should not be performed on the open ward or outpatient department
- *Bronchoscopy with BAL* is the diagnostic investigation of choice in non-HIV-infected patients and in patients with HIV in whom induced sputum analysis is non-diagnostic. BAL with silver or immunofluorescent staining has a specificity of nearly 100% and sensitivity of 80–90%. This sensitivity is lower in non-HIV-infected immunocompromised patients, reflecting their lower pathogen loads. PCR is highly sensitive but not specific and cannot tell the difference between infection and colonization. BAL PCR for PCP has good negative predictive value.
- *Transbronchial lung biopsy* has a slightly higher sensitivity (around 95%) but is associated with an increased risk of complications so is reserved for cases where BAL is non-diagnostic. Surgical lung biopsy may be required for diagnosis in a minority of HIV-negative patients.

PCP: treatment

Antimicrobial

- Liaise with infectious diseases or HIV specialist
- High-dose co-trimoxazole (trimethoprim and sulfamethoxazole) remains the drug of choice. Administer 120 mg/kg daily in four divided doses PO or IV (dilute 480 mg ampoules in at least 75 mL 5% glucose; infuse over 60 min). Use IV route initially and then PO during clinical improvement; PO may be used initially in mild cases. Side effects (e.g. rash, nausea, vomiting, blood disorders) are common, particularly in HIV-infected patients. Consider routine use of antiemetics
- Second-line choices, if intolerant or unresponsive to co-trimoxazole, include IV pentamidine, clindamycin and primaquine, dapsone and trimethoprim, atovaquone
- Treatment should be for 21 days
- If PCP is strongly suspected and the patient is unwell, treatment can be started immediately, as the sensitivity of BAL pneumocystis stains only decreases at around 2 weeks. Empirical treatment is also required in the occasional situation where the diagnosis is suspected but bronchoscopy is non-diagnostic or not tolerated
- In cases of HIV presenting with PCP, early introduction of highly active antiretroviral therapy (HAART) has been contentious, with theoretical risks of drug interactions, increasing toxicities, and the potential for immune reconstitution inflammatory syndrome (IRIS). However, a randomized trial and a retrospective analysis both demonstrated a 50% reduction in mortality when HAART was started within 2 weeks of PCP treatment. Suspected IRIS should be treated with corticosteroids ± reintroduction of PCP therapy.

Steroids

High-dose steroids (prednisolone 40 mg bd PO or IV hydrocortisone) are recommended for all patients in respiratory failure. Treat at high dose for 5 days; taper dose over 1–3 weeks (e.g. prednisolone 40 mg daily for days 6–11, then 20 mg daily for days 12–21).

Supportive therapy

Hypoxia is common; administer supplementary high-flow O_2, and consider use of continuous positive airway pressure (CPAP) or high flow nasal oxygen (HFNO). Mechanical ventilation, if considered appropriate, may be required; make this decision prior to initiating CPAP/HFNO.

Outcome

- Mortality 10–20% in the setting of AIDS, but 35–50% in patients with other forms of immunocompromise, probably reflecting the adverse consequences of the greater pulmonary inflammatory response to pneumocystis which is observed in non-HIV immunocompromise. Mortality from PCP requiring mechanical ventilation in HIV-infected patients is about 60% although may be significantly higher in patients with low CD4 counts.

- Relapse rate in AIDS is high (60% in 1 y), so 2° prophylaxis with co-trimoxazole is recommended. 1° prophylaxis is offered to HIV-positive patients with CD4 count <200 × 10^6/L. The indications for prophylaxis in non-HIV patients are less well defined; consider prophylaxis for patients who are likely to receive high doses of prednisolone for prolonged periods.

Further information

Wang et al. Approach to fungal infections in HIV-infected individuals: PCP and beyond. *Clin Chest Med* 2017;**38**: 465–477.

Cryptococcosis

Epidemiology

Cryptococcus neoformans is found worldwide in bird droppings. Following inhalation, yeasts propagate within the alveoli, without usually causing symptoms. *C. neoformans* is dominantly an opportunistic pathogen affecting those with immunocompromise (HIV with CD4 count <100, lymphoma) and disseminated disease with migration to the CNS and meningoencephalitis the most common clinical manifestation of infection

Clinical features

- Clinically evident cryptococcal lung disease is rare, but well described, even in HIV-negative patients. Symptoms are non-specific, including fever and cough, and presentations may be acute or chronic. The CXR may show non-calcified nodules, lymphadenopathy, lobar infiltrates, or pleural involvement
- Pulmonary involvement is associated with meningoencephalitis in those with underlying immunosuppression, and clinical signs of meningism are characteristically absent. CT head (to exclude a space-occupying lesion), followed by lumbar puncture, should therefore be considered in all patients with pulmonary cryptococcal disease who have any condition predisposing to dissemination or neurological signs.

Diagnosis

Diagnostic techniques include:

- India ink stain on cerebrospinal fluid (CSF), or latex agglutination test for capsular antigen in BAL or pleural fluid, blood, or CSF
- Stains and culture of sputum, blood, urine, or BAL fluid. Positive culture from sputum may indicate colonization, rather than active disease, and should be interpreted in the clinical context
- Serum or CSF cryptococcal antigen test is extremely sensitive and specific for the diagnosis. BAL/pulmonary cryptococcal antigen has a lower sensitivity.

Treatment

Cryptococcal infection in the immunocompromised is treated with amphotericin B IV and flucytosine IV for 2–3 weeks, followed by fluconazole. Isolated non-severe pulmonary disease can be treated with oral fluconazole alone. The natural history of disease in immunocompetent patients is poorly understood, and observation alone is often recommended; disseminated disease may occur, however, and some experts advise treatment with fluconazole.

Candidal pneumonia

- *Candida* occurs as part of the normal human flora and is found in the GI tract and on the skin. Invasive disease may occur in the immunocompromised, particularly in neutropenic patients. Prophylaxis with fluconazole is used following bone marrow transplantation
- *Candida* is often isolated from respiratory secretions but very rarely causes respiratory disease. Haematogenous seeding to the lungs causing infiltrates or enlarging nodules may occur with disseminated candidal infection
- Risk factors for candidaemia include immunocompromise, central venous lines, parenteral nutrition, and GI surgery. In lung transplant recipients, a positive donor tracheal culture for *Candida* is a marker for post-transplant candidal infection
- The clinical and radiological features of pulmonary involvement are non-specific. Extrapulmonary manifestations of infection are common, e.g. skin, eye, hepatic, or CNS involvement. Candidaemia is typically associated with a high fever
- Definitive diagnosis of pulmonary disease requires identification of tissue invasion by *Candida* on TBB or surgical lung biopsy
- Treat with an echinocandin (e.g. caspofungin, micafungin), amphotericin B, or fluconazole, and remove any central lines
- Candidaemia carries a mortality of 30–40%.

Further information

Pappas PG et al. Clinical practice guidelines for the management of candidiasis: 2009 update by the Infectious Diseases Society of America. *Clin Infect Dis* 2009;**48**: 503–535.

Endemic mycoses: introduction

Several types of dimorphic fungi, that grow as moulds in the environment but grow as yeasts after inhalation, are known to commonly cause pulmonary disease in endemic regions: *histoplasmosis, blastomycosis, coccidioidomycosis, paracoccidioidomycosis, penicilliosis, and adiaspiromycosis*. Endemic fungi can rarely present in non-endemic areas, and diagnosis is often delayed because of their non-specific and varied clinical features and the failure to obtain a detailed travel history. Fungal infection may mimic other diseases, such as TB and lung cancer, often leading to inappropriate investigations and treatment. Fungal infections can also cause granulomata on lung biopsy, which sometimes results in diagnostic confusion (e.g. with sarcoidosis).

Infection in immunocompetent individuals is usually either asymptomatic or mild and self-limiting, although severe infection may rarely occur in apparently immunocompetent individuals. Outbreaks of disease may occur, as well as sporadic cases. Unlike invasive candidiasis and aspergillosis, where neutrophils are the key host defence mechanism, T-cell-mediated immunity is essential for defence against the endemic mycoses. Patients with impaired T-cell-mediated immunity (e.g. AIDS, lymphoma, steroid use) are therefore at particular risk of developing severe or disseminated infection.

Further information

Wang et al. Approach to fungal infections in HIV-infected individuals: PCP and beyond. *Clin Chest Med* 2017;**38**: 465–477.

Queiroz-Telles et al. Neglected endemic mycoses. *Lancet Infect Dis* 2017;**17**: e367–e377.

England and Hochholzer. Adiaspiromycosis: an unusual fungal infection of the lung. Report of 11 cases. *Am J Surg Pathol* 1993;**17**: 876–886

Endemic mycoses: histoplasmosis

Epidemiology

Histoplasma capsulatum is found in bird- and bat dropping-contaminated soil in the Midwest and south-east USA, particularly the Ohio and Mississippi valleys, as well as in Mexico and parts of South America and Asia. The mycelial form is inhaled and subsequently develops into the yeast form ('dimorphism') within the lung before spread via the lymphatics and the activation of T-cell-mediated immunity with granuloma development.

Clinical features

Manifestations of infection are highly variable.

* *Asymptomatic* infection occurs in the majority of cases. CXR may be normal or demonstrate single or multiple nodules, which may calcify in a characteristic 'target lesion' pattern. Lymphadenopathy may occur with eggshell calcification
* *Acute* symptoms may follow heavy or recurrent exposure (e.g. pigeon fanciers, cavers). Range from a self-limiting flu-like illness of fever, cough, and malaise to fulminant disease with respiratory failure. CXR may be normal or show consolidation, bilateral alveolar shadowing, multiple small nodules, and sometimes lymphadenopathy
* *Chronic* progressive lung disease occurs particularly in patients with underlying COPD; lung cavitation is common, sometimes leading to an incorrect diagnosis of TB or cancer
* *Disseminated* disease mostly affects the immunocompromised (particularly HIV with CD4 <150) and the elderly. Presentation may be acute or chronic, and manifestations include fever, weight loss, and diffuse lung involvement, although almost any organ system may be affected; other features may include hepatosplenomegaly, GI symptoms, headache and meningism, cytopenias, endocarditis, and adrenal failure
* Other unusual manifestations include broncholithiasis, mediastinal fibrosis (with compression of large airways, oesophagus, or superior vena cava (SVC)), or isolated extrapulmonary disease (e.g. arthritis, pericarditis, erythema nodosum, erythema multiforme).

Diagnosis

* Smears or culture of infected material, e.g. sputum or BAL fluid (for chronic pulmonary disease, insensitive for acute disease), blood, urine, or bone marrow (for disseminated disease). May take several weeks
* Serology in acute disease—typically negative at presentation and becomes positive after several weeks. A variety of serological tests are in use, including:
* Complement fixation, designed to detect antibodies to *Histoplasma* mycelial antigen or *Histoplasma* yeast antigen. A positive result (serum titre ≥1:16 for mycelial antigen, ≥1:32 for yeast antigen) for either antigen, in a compatible clinical setting, is considered diagnostic of active disease
  * Immunodiffusion may distinguish active disease from previous exposure but is less sensitive than complement fixation, and a negative result does not exclude the diagnosis

- Serum, urine, or BAL fluid *Histoplasma* polysaccharide antigen test—
  useful for diagnosis of disseminated disease and also pulmonary disease.
  Positive in 85–95% cases in HIV with low CD4 count. Antigenuria is
  seen in 90%, and antigenaemia in <50% of non-HIV patients. Can be
  falsely positive with other endemic mycoses.

Treatment

- Infection in immunocompetent individuals is typically self-limiting, and
  symptoms usually resolve within 2–4 weeks without treatment
- Indications for antifungal treatment are:
  - Persistent symptoms (usually lasting >1 month)
  - Progressive disseminated disease
  - Heavy exposure leading to ARDS
  - Infection in the setting of immunocompromise
- Oral itraconazole is appropriate for persistent symptoms in mild to
  moderate disease and for disseminated disease, including patients
  with HIV who have mild disease. Treat for 6–12 weeks in acute
  histoplasmosis, and for 1–2 y in chronic disease. In the setting of HIV,
  treatment should be lifelong or until CD4 count >200 for at least
  6 months after starting HAART. Check itraconazole drug interactions,
  and monitor liver function (ideally monthly) if taking for >1 month.
  Hypokalaemia may be associated with long-term use
- IV lipid formulations of amphotericin B should be used to treat severe
  infection in the setting of ARDS or immunocompromise.

Endemic mycoses: blastomycosis

Epidemiology

Infection with *Blastomyces dermatitidis* follows the inhalation of spores from contaminated soil, and clinical infection may follow outdoor activities. Blastomycosis is endemic in a distribution similar to that of histoplasmosis in the USA, although extending further north; it is endemic in the south-east USA and the Mississippi, Ohio, and St Lawrence river valleys. Blastomycosis also occurs in Africa, India, and the Middle East. It is significantly less common than histoplasmosis.

Clinical features

Clinical presentation is variable and may mimic other diseases such as bacterial pneumonia, TB, and lung cancer. Clinical manifestations include:
- *Asymptomatic* in at least 50% of those infected
- *Acute* presentation is typically with fever, cough, productive of mucopurulent sputum, and sometimes pleuritic chest pain; misdiagnosis as bacterial pneumonia is common. Acute presentation of fulminant respiratory disease with ARDS may occur. Other acute presentations include a flu-like illness with fever, myalgia, arthralgia, and erythema nodosum
- *Chronic* presentation with fever, productive cough, and weight loss
- *Disseminated* disease occurs in a minority of patients (especially in the immunocompromised) and most commonly involves the lungs, skin, bone, joints, and CNS.

CXR

Airspace infiltrates are the most common finding, but a very wide range of appearances are seen, including nodular pattern, lobar consolidation, diffuse infiltrates, or large peripheral masses (often with air bronchograms). Lymphadenopathy and pleural effusions may rarely occur.

Diagnosis

- Diagnosis is by the staining or culture of infected material. A pyogenic inflammatory response to the fungus is common (unlike in histoplasmosis) and facilitates diagnosis
- Culture of sputum has a high yield and is diagnostic in most cases of acute pulmonary disease. Multiple specimens may be required, however. A drawback of sputum culture is that several weeks may be required before the fungus is identified. Cytological examination of sputum may provide a rapid diagnosis if the examiner is trained appropriately and alerted to the possible diagnosis
- Bronchoscopy has a similar diagnostic yield to sputum culture (92% in one study) and is recommended for patients with negative sputum results; note that lidocaine may inhibit the fungal growth, and minimal concentrations should be used
- More invasive procedures, such as surgical lung biopsy or thoracoscopy, are only rarely needed. Histological specimens require particular stains (e.g. silver stain) to facilitate identification of the fungus
- Currently available serological tests lack sensitivity and are rarely helpful.

Treatment

Usually with itraconazole for at least 6 months. Observation without treatment is not generally recommended, although this is controversial, and symptoms are usually self-limiting in immunocompetent individuals. Lipid formulations of amphotericin B should be used to treat very ill patients. Secondary, but not primary, prophylaxis is recommended for those with HIV and a CD4 count <200.

Endemic mycoses: coccidioidomycosis

Coccidioidomycosis is endemic in semi-arid parts of south-west USA (Arizona, California, Texas, New Mexico, Utah, Nevada), northern Mexico, and Central and South America. Infection follows inhalation of *Coccidioides immitis* or *C. posadasii* spores from soil. Manifestations of infection are variable, including:

- *Asymptomatic* infection, which appears to be common in endemic regions
- *Acute* pulmonary disease. Presents in a similar manner to bacterial pneumonia, with fever, cough, pleuritic chest pain, and often skin rash (e.g. erythema nodosum or erythema multiforme). Eosinophilia may be present. CXR appearance is variable and may show areas of consolidation, lymphadenopathy, and pleural effusion, or be normal. The disease is self-limiting in most cases (Valley Fever); a minority progress to ARDS or chronic disease
- *Chronic* pulmonary disease. Uncommon, may be asymptomatic. CXR typically shows single or multiple nodules that may cavitate; upper lobe infiltrates, similar to those seen in TB, may develop
- *Disseminated* disease. Rare, occurs particularly in the immunocompromised. Presentation may be acute or chronic. Pulmonary disease occurs in association with involvement of the skin, bones, joints, genitourinary system, or CNS.

Diagnosis

With stains or culture of infected tissues. Sputum cultures are often positive in cavitating disease. BAL fluid culture and lung biopsies may also be diagnostic. Serological tests (complement fixation, enzyme-linked immunosorbent assay (ELISA), or immunodiffusion) can support a diagnosis and can be used to monitor treatment response.

Treatment

Not required in the majority of patients who have mild self-limiting disease. Fluconazole is the antifungal of choice, when required in milder disease. In severe or disseminated disease amphotericin B is used followed by fluconazole or itraconazole for up to 12 months. In HIV secondary, but not primary, prophylaxis with itraconazole can be considered in those with CD4 counts <250. In HIV patients with a CD4 count <250, in endemic regions, serological screening is recommended on an annual basis with oral fluconazole treatment for asymptomatic seroconversion.

Endemic mycoses: paracoccidioidomycosis, penicilliosis, adiaspiromycosis

Paracoccidioidomycosis

Endemic in parts of Central and South America and Mexico. It is caused by the dimorphic fungus *Paracoccidioides brasiliensis*. Commonly asymptomatic, only 1–2% of infections are thought to manifest with symptoms. Acute disease is most likely in those less than 30 y, manifesting with fevers, night sweats, weight loss, lymphadenopathy, hepatosplenomegaly, and cytopaenias. The disease progresses over weeks to months. Chronic pulmonary disease occurs through reactivation and has a more insidious onset over months, involving the lungs, skin, lymph nodes, adrenal gland, bones, and CNS. In immunocompromise disseminated disease occurs more quickly.

Diagnosis is made on culture of sputum or BAL fluid, or following staining of lung biopsy samples but it can take time for culture results. Serological antibody tests have a sensitivity of ~90% and can aid more rapid diagnosis. Treatment is with itraconazole, and long courses of 6 to 12 months may be needed. Severe disease is treated with amphotericin B, followed by itraconazole when there is disease response to complete 6 to 12 months of treatment.

Penicilliosis (Talaromycosis)

Endemic in parts of South East Asia and is caused by *Talaromyces marneffei*. Although it can cause disease in the immunocompetent it is dominantly an opportunistic infection. It can cause a wide-range of symptoms with cough, fever, dyspnoea, chest pain, abdominal pain, and diarrhoea. It can involve the lungs, skin, bone, GI tract, and lymph nodes. Diagnosis is with culture of blood, BAL, skin, bone marrow, or biopsy but cytology can be supportive of a diagnosis ahead of culture results. In severe disease treatment is with liposomal amphotericin B in severe disease for two weeks followed by at least 10 weeks of itraconazole.

Adiaspiromycosis

Caused by *Emmonsia* species which are found worldwide and has been reported to rarely cause pulmonary disease. Most cases are reported in those with immunocompromise. Symptoms are non-specific with cough, dyspnoea, fever, and chest pain. Disease severity is related to number of spores inhaled and can present with focal consolidation or reticular nodular shadowing in severe disease. Culture and serological tests are not reliable, and lung biopsy is often required. Diagnosis relies on recognition of giant conidia on cytology or histology. In severe disease treatment is with liposomal amphotericin B with maintenance azole therapy.

Chapter 43

Respiratory infection—mycobacterial

Tuberculosis: epidemiology and pathophysiology 586
TB: pulmonary disease 588
TB: extrapulmonary disease 589
TB: investigations 590
TB: management 1 592
TB: management 2 594
First-line anti-TB drugs 596
TB: adverse drug reactions 598
TB: inpatient admission 600
TB in pregnancy 602
TB chemotherapy with comorbid disease 604
Multidrug-resistant TB (MDR-TB) 606
Latent TB infection 608
TB and anti-TNF-α treatment 610
TB: screening and contact tracing 612
Disseminated BCG infection (BCGosis) 616
Future developments in TB 617
Non-tuberculous mycobacteria (NTM) 618
NTM species and lung disease 620

Tuberculosis: epidemiology and pathophysiology

Tuberculosis (TB) is one of the top ten causes of death and is the leading single infectious cause of death worldwide, despite being a potentially curable disease. It kills around 1.6 million people per year, of whom 300,000 are human immunodeficiency virus (HIV) positive. Rising rates of HIV infection and immigration mean TB remains a large proportion of the workload for respiratory physicians in some parts of the UK. The disease is a great 'mimicker' and should often be considered as part of the differential diagnosis in patients with respiratory disease.

Epidemiology

Globally, the World Health Organization (WHO) estimated that 10 million people developed TB in 2017. Over $2/3^{rds}$ of the global cases of TB are from India, China, SE Asia, Pakistan, Bangladesh, Nigeria, and South Africa. Russia and former Soviet Union countries have rapidly increasing rates, with around 25% multidrug resistance (MDR-TB) in these regions. Worldwide, 50% of MDR-TB cases are from China, India, and Russia. Co-infection with HIV is common, affecting 9% of TB patients, and particularly affects patients in Africa with a HIV co-infection rate in Africa of 72%.

TB rates are now at the lowest recorded level in England, with 5,102 cases of TB in 2017, 9.2 per 100,000. However, while the total number of cases and the total number of deaths from TB are falling, there are significant inequalities that need to be addressed. The majority of cases in the UK are in people born abroad, but 30% of all cases occur in people born in the UK. Particular at-risk groups include the homeless, those with substance misuse, prisoners, and vulnerable migrants. TB is concentrated in the major cities, with 40% of cases in London and some inner-city the incidence of TB exceeds 40 per 100,000.

Pathophysiology

The disease is spread by airborne droplets containing *Mycobacterium tuberculosis* (MTB). Droplets remain airborne for hours after expectoration because of their small size. Infectious droplets are inhaled and become lodged in the distal airways. MTB is taken up by alveolar macrophages, triggering the innate immune system, and spreads via the lymphatics to hilar lymph nodes. Later, a cell-mediated immune process leads to granuloma formation by activated T-lymphocytes and macrophages, which limits further bacterial replication and disease spread. Most (over 90%) immunocompetent individuals successfully contain the infection (either eliminated or contained in a latent state); 10% progress to active 1° disease (1° progressive TB).

Many factors influence whether or not infection leads to active disease, including age, host immunity, and time since infection (risk highest in first few years after infection). The estimated lifetime risk of clinical disease in a child newly infected with MTB is about 10%.

Active disease occurs when the host's immune response is unable to contain MTB replication, with absent or poorly formed granulomas. Active disease occurs most often in the lung parenchyma (due to high O_2 content, in which the bacillus grows well) and hilar lymph nodes. It can occur in any organ from haematogenous spread. This is most common in young children and immunosuppressed adults. Most disease in adults is due to reactivation of childhood disease, so-called 'post-primary disease', from activation of latent TB (the Ghon focus) lying dormant in the lung.

The term *smear-positive TB* refers to the identification of AFB on sputum smear (ZN stain). Patient will require isolation if admitted to hospital.

Culture-positive TB refers to when AFB not seen on smear (smear-negative) but TB is grown on culture (may take up to 9 weeks). Much less infectious than smear-positive disease, although transmission can still occur.

Main risk factors for active TB in the UK
- Place and date of birth:
  - Caucasian population: increasing prevalence with age ($\male > \female$)
  - Afro-Caribbean immigrants: highest prevalence in the young ($\male = \female$)
  - Indian subcontinent: highest prevalence in middle age ($\male = \female$)
- HIV/AIDS
- Poverty, undernutrition, and overcrowding
- Heavy alcohol consumption and smoking
- Medical factors—diabetes, end-stage renal failure, malignant disease, systemic chemotherapy, steroids, and TNF-α antagonists, e.g. infliximab, vitamin D deficiency (vitamin D has pleiotropic effects on the immune system, including macrophage activation).

TB: pulmonary disease

Symptoms

Most cases present with pulmonary disease, classically:
- Productive cough
- Haemoptysis
- Breathlessness
- Systemic symptoms—weight loss, night sweats, and malaise
- Chest pain.

Haemoptysis

More common with cavitatory disease, and up to two-thirds will be smear-positive. Most haemoptysis is small volume. Massive haemoptysis is rare and is most common as a consequence of destruction of a lobe, with consequent bronchiectasis formation (possibly with 2° *Aspergillus* infection or mycetoma in a healed TB cavity). This is seen in those untreated in the pre-chemotherapy era. Most haemoptysis will resolve with antituberculous chemotherapy.

Signs

Often non-specific.
- Examination may be normal
- Lymphadenopathy (particularly cervical)
- Crackles
- Signs of a pleural effusion
- Signs of consolidation (with extensive disease)
- Signs of weight loss/underlying immunocompromise
- Look for evidence of extrapulmonary disease, e.g. skin, joints, CNS, retina, and spinal disease.

Complications

Long-term sequelae of inadequately treated infection include:
- *Bronchiectasis*, bronchial obstruction, and airway stenosis (uncommon) may result from endobronchial disease, though this is much less common in the post-chemotherapy era. It is more common in the presence of extensive parenchymal disease and is associated with lymph node enlargement, with compromise of airway size
- *Pleural disease* (see ➲ p. 420) is due to either 1° progressive disease or reactivation of latent infection. It probably represents an increased immune response—a delayed-type hypersensitivity reaction to mycobacterial antigens, rather than a diminished one, which is the case in other forms of TB infection. Culture is more likely from pleural tissue than fluid (where the organism burden is lower)
- *Pneumothorax* is rare (<1% in the developed world) and results from the rupture of a peripheral cavity. Can lead to the formation of a bronchopleural fistula
- Draining *abscess*
- *Right middle lobe syndrome*—compression of the right middle lobe bronchus by hilar lymph nodes leads to lobar collapse
- Previous treatment with *thoracoplasty* can lead to respiratory failure in later life due to compromised vital capacity (VC).

TB: extrapulmonary disease

Extrapulmonary disease is seen in about 58% of patients with TB in the UK (either with or without pulmonary involvement).

The tuberculin skin test (see ➜ p. 608) is more frequently positive in extrapulmonary disease, as this most commonly represents reactivated disease and less commonly 1° disease. Anergy is more likely in those with poor nutritional status, underlying disease (including HIV), and the elderly.

CNS disease

The most serious manifestation and includes meningeal involvement and space-occupying lesions (tuberculoma) that may lead to cranial nerve lesions. The clinical manifestations are due to the presence of MTB and the host's inflammatory immune response. TB meningitis presents with headache, fever, altered conscious level, and focal neurological signs, including cranial nerve palsies. Fits are common. Cerebrospinal fluid (CSF) contains lymphocytes, high protein, and low glucose. Polymerase chain reaction (PCR) of CSF and adenosine deaminase levels may be useful but are not 100% sensitive.

Pericardial TB

The yield is low from pericardial fluid and biopsy. 85% have a positive tuberculin test. Adenosine deaminase levels may be helpful. A large effusion may lead to cardiac tamponade and may need to be drained.

Spinal disease

Can affect any bone or joint; spine involvement (Pott's disease) is most common in the thoracic spine. Surgery may be needed if there is evidence of cord compression or instability.

Genitourinary disease

From seeding during haematogenous spread. Involvement of the renal and genital tracts is uncommon.
- In men—may cause prostatitis and epididymitis.
- In women—genitourinary TB is a cause of infertility. Sterile pyuria (white and red blood cells in the urine, in the absence of bacterial infection) may indicate TB infection.

Peripheral cold abscess

Can occur at almost any body site.

Disseminated disease

More common in immunosuppressed individuals. Pulmonary disease is typically a miliary (millet seed) pattern, but pulmonary disease is not universal in disseminated disease. This has a higher mortality than localized disease.

TB: investigations

The diagnosis is usually made in one of three ways: *smear or culture* of sputum (or other sample, e.g. pus, CSF, urine, biopsy tissue), or *histology* with the identification of caseating granulomas on biopsy (send biopsy samples for culture in normal saline as well as histology when TB is suspected).

- *Chest radiograph (CXR)* classically shows upper lobe infiltrates with cavitation
  - May be associated with hilar or paratracheal lymphadenopathy
  - May show changes consistent with prior TB infection, with fibrous scar tissue and calcification
  - HIV-infected patients typically have less florid CXR changes and are less likely to have cavitatory disease. Miliary pattern is more common in later stages of AIDS
  - All patients with non-pulmonary TB should have a CXR to exclude or confirm pulmonary disease
- *Sputum ZN stain and culture* is required for definitive diagnosis and is vital for drug resistance testing. ZN is only 50–80% sensitive
  - New sputum processing techniques, along with fluorescence microscopy, have improved smear sensitivity and efficient reading of slides
  - Smear-negative disease accounts for about 20% of disease transmission; smear-positive cases are more infectious
  - Induced sputum is as effective as bronchoalveolar lavage (BAL), especially if the CXR shows changes consistent with active disease (but should not be used for potential MDR-TB, due to the danger to health workers)
  - Conventional culture takes 6 weeks or longer, although use of the mycobacterial growth indicator tube (MGIT) culture system can lead to positive cultures within days
  - Nucleic acid amplification techniques are increasingly used to confirm mycobacteria serotype and drug susceptibility. The Xpert MTB/RIF assay can simultaneously detect MTB and identify rifampicin resistance (which is strongly associated with MDR-TB) within 2h and is recommended to be sent if it will change clinical management (i.e. suspected MDR-TB, coexistent HIV, or critical illness)
- *Tuberculin skin test (Mantoux)* results are described in Box 43.1. If positive assess for active TB and if no features of active TB consider latent TB treatment.
- *Interferon gamma release assays (IGRAs)* (see ➔ p. 608) High sensitivity, but low specificity, of IGRAs mean a negative/low result rules out active or latent TB, but a positive result cannot differentiate between the two
- *Bronchoscopy/endobronchial ultrasound (EBUS)* may be needed to obtain BAL or lymph node samples if there is a high index of clinical suspicion but a non-productive cough or unhelpful sputum culture. In extensive disease, macroscopic bronchoscopic abnormality may be present, with erythematous or ulcerated airways. Granulation tissue or enlarged lymph nodes may be visible. Nodes can perforate or protrude into the bronchial lumen, extruding caseous material into the airway

- *Biopsy from extrapulmonary sites*, e.g. neck lymph nodes, or mediastinoscopy may be warranted. Lymph node biopsy samples, pleural biopsies, and pus aspirated from lymph nodes should be transported to the laboratory in a dry pot (not formalin). Bone marrow or liver biopsy may aid diagnosis in miliary TB. The bone marrow culture yield is higher in pancytopenia
- *Gastric washings* reflect TB swallowed overnight. Rarely performed if bronchoscopy is readily available. Used more commonly in children
- *Urine* Early morning urine (EMU) only if renal or military disease suspected
- *Blood tests* Baseline full blood count (FBC), renal, and liver function tests. Useful to document normal baseline levels before starting antituberculous chemotherapy
- *HIV test* should be offered to all patients
- *CT scan* is more sensitive than CXR, especially for smaller areas of disease. It may show cavitatory disease and signs of airway disease—the 'tree-in-bud' appearance, useful for differentiating between active disease and non-active old disease and guiding area for BAL. May also be needed to assess mediastinal or hilar lymphadenopathy.

A tuberculoma is an encapsulated focus of reactivated TB. These lesions rarely cavitate, and the differential diagnosis is wide, including malignancy (pulmonary nodule, see ➲ p. 372), and vasculitis. Diagnosis may only be possible by percutaneous biopsy, as, in the absence of a main airway component, cultures may be negative.

Box 43.1 Mantoux skin test
- Read at 48 h
- Intradermal. Use 0.1 mL of 1 in 1,000 (= 0.1 mL of 100 TU/mL = 10 TU)
- Graded:
  - <5 mm, negative
  - >5 mm, positive (regardless of BCG history).

TB: management 1

Treatment aims to cure disease without relapse, prevent transmission, and prevent emergence of drug resistance. Long-term treatment with a number of drugs is required, as TB can remain dormant for long periods prior to treatment, making the emergence of naturally resistant mutants possible.

- Send material for bacteriological diagnosis prior to initiating treatment, if possible, to allow for subsequent drug susceptibility testing
- In practice, if there is a high clinical suspicion of TB, treatment should be started before culture and full sensitivities are available
- Never treat with a single drug
- Never add a single drug to a failing regime
- The majority of patients can be treated as outpatients
- Every TB patient should have a named TB case manager
- Smear-positive HIV-negative patients should become smear-negative within 2 weeks of starting treatment (this does not apply to MDR-TB). These patients should be isolated either in hospital (if they are admitted) or at home for this time period
- All patients should be discussed and managed within a TB multidisciplinary team
- From 2007, there are no prescription costs for TB drugs in the UK
- All new cases must be *notified* (including those diagnosed after death) as this initiates contact tracing. In some districts, notification triggers specialist nursing input. The doctor making the diagnosis has a legal responsibility to notify. It also provides epidemiological and surveillance data, enabling treatment and screening services to be planned. A patient can be denotified if the mycobacterium cultured turns out to be an NTM.

Drug treatment

Usually in two phases:

- *Phase 1—initial intensive phase* Designed to kill actively growing bacteria
  - This phase lasts 2 months and shortens the duration of infectivity
  - At least three drugs are needed, e.g. isoniazid, rifampicin, and pyrazinamide, and guidelines recommend four drugs, with ethambutol added because of risks of drug resistance
- Phase 2—continuation phase is usually with two drugs, typically isoniazid and rifampicin for 4 months. Fewer bacteria are present in this phase, and there is therefore a lower chance that drug-resistant mutants will emerge, so drug resistance is less of a problem.

Compliance is of major importance, and all patients should have a risk assessment for treatment adherence. If the clinical response is not satisfactory, check sputum 2 months before the end of the planned treatment period. Compliance can be monitored with urine colour testing (turns red with rifampicin) and tablet counts. If concerns about compliance, consider directly observed treatment (DOT).

DOT

Aims to increase compliance by nurse-supervised and observed daily or weekly tablet swallowing. This has been shown to increase treatment completion, reduce relapses, and reduce development of drug resistance, as the ingestion of each dose is witnessed. This is recommended for patients unlikely to comply, including alcoholics, drug abusers, the homeless, those with serious mental illness (the 'hard to reach'), and those with MDR-TB. Some areas consider other incentives to improve adherence, e.g. providing food and transport costs.

Compulsory detention under Sections 37 and 38 of the Public Health Act (England) is allowed for infectious pulmonary TB, but compulsory treatment is not allowed. This is only used in extreme circumstances to protect public health.

TB: management 2

Standard treatment regimens for drug-sensitive TB

(see ➲ p. 596)

- The standard first-line regimens is for 6 months—four drugs in the initial 2-month phase (rifampicin (R), isoniazid (H), pyrazinamide (Z), and ethambutol (E) (or streptomycin)) and two drugs in the last 4 months (rifampicin and isoniazid) in patients with fully sensitive organisms, with pyridoxine 10–20 mg OD for isoniazid peripheral neuropathy prophylaxis
- Rifampicin should always be given throughout the 6-month course in first-line therapy
- If drug sensitivity is unavailable at 2 months, continue the four-drug regime until it is available
- The fourth drug (usually ethambutol) can be omitted in those at low risk of isoniazid resistance (not previously treated, HIV-negative, UK-born Caucasians, with no drug-resistant contacts). There is a higher risk of isoniazid resistance in ethnic minority groups, immigrants, refugees, those who have had previous treatment, and those who are HIV-positive. This depends on local policy and the ethnic make-up of the local area. If in doubt, treat with four drugs
- Other treatment regimens are also effective (e.g. daily for 2 months, then three times weekly for 4 months with DOT), although these are used less commonly
- Check baseline renal and liver function in all patients. If normal and not at high risk of adverse drug reaction, no need for routine re-checking. Treatment in the setting of liver and renal disease is described on ➲ p. 604 and ➲ p. 605
- Dosages are weight-dependent and may need to be changed for weight loss or gain during the treatment course
- A 6-month treatment course is effective for all other forms of non-CNS extrapulmonary TB (including lymph node and spinal disease), with the same drugs as for respiratory disease. Surgery may be needed, in addition, for spinal disease
- CNS disease needs a 12-month treatment course
- Steroids may be indicated for large pleural effusions, pericardial effusions (60 mg/day for constrictive pericarditis), and CNS disease, especially if associated with neurological impairment. Steroids may also be indicated in ureteric disease and to suppress hypersensitivity reactions to the antituberculous drugs
- Peripheral lymph nodes may enlarge and abscesses may form during treatment; this does not imply failure of treatment but should prompt a compliance check.

Meningitis 12-month course of rifampicin and isoniazid, with pyrazinamide and a fourth drug (e.g. ethambutol) for at least the first 2 months, is effective. If pyrazinamide not used, extend treatment period to 18 months. Steroids may be needed for severe disease, such as prednisolone 20–40 mg od if on rifampicin, otherwise 10–20 mg od. Higher doses of dexamethasone may be used in those with reduced consciousness and/or focal neurological signs. Steroids can usually be tapered after the initial 2–3 weeks of treatment, over a total of 4–8 weeks. Ethambutol should be used with caution in unconscious patients, as visual acuity cannot be tested and there is a small risk of ocular toxicity.

Cerebral tuberculoma without meningitis 12-month regime.

Disseminated TB/miliary TB 6-month regime unless CNS involvement. Exclude CNS disease in miliary TB with CSF examination, whether or not symptoms are present. Start treatment, even if liver function tests (LFTs) are abnormal (this may be due to intrahepatic granulomas). Seek advice if LFTs deteriorate significantly on treatment (see ➲ p. 604; See Box 43.2).

Bone and spinal TB 6-month standard regime. A CT or magnetic resonance imaging (MRI) should be performed in patients with active spinal disease who have neurological symptoms and signs. If there is direct spinal cord involvement (e.g. a spinal cord tuberculoma), treatment should be as for meningeal TB. There is no place for routine spinal surgery (e.g. anterior spinal fusion) in the absence of spinal instability.

Pericardial TB Standard 6-month regime. Steroids, e.g. prednisolone 60 mg od if on rifampicin, tapered after 2–3 weeks of treatment, may be required. Repeat echo may be needed.

Peripheral lymph node TB Standard 6-month regime, which should be used, even if the infected node has been surgically removed. Stop treatment at the end of the 6-month course, regardless of the appearance of new nodes, residual nodes, or draining sinuses.

Patient advice to document on starting TB chemotherapy

- Possibility of nausea and abdominal pain
- Persistent vomiting and/or jaundice—stop drugs *immediately*, and contact doctor
- Red/orange urine with rifampicin
- Red/orange contact lenses with rifampicin
- Contraception advice. If on the oral contraceptive pill (OCP) as efficacy reduced
- Visual acuity (Snellen chart) (ethambutol)
- Visual disturbance (ethambutol)—stop drugs *immediately*, and contact doctor
- Potential drug interactions (see Table 43.2).

First-line anti-TB drugs

- *Isoniazid (H)* Bactericidal. Single daily dose, well tolerated. Major side effect is age-dependent hepatitis. Increased toxicity with alcohol. Peripheral neuropathy is uncommon, although increased risk with diabetes and pregnancy; reduce incidence with 10–20 mg pyridoxine daily
- *Rifampicin (R)* Bactericidal. Single daily dose, well tolerated. Increases hepatic microsomal enzymes; therefore, increases clearance of hepatic metabolized drugs, including prednisolone and the OCP, thus the risks of pregnancy must be highlighted. Red/orange discoloration of urine and contact lenses occurs, and gastro-intestinal (GI) upset
- *Pyrazinamide (Z)* Bactericidal. Single daily dose. GI upset common. Major side effect is hepatic toxicity. Renal excretion leads to hyperuricaemia
- *Ethambutol (E)* has some bactericidal effect, mostly bacteriostatic at usual doses. Single daily dose, well tolerated. Side effect—optic neuritis, uncommon. Document visual acuity (Snellen chart) before starting, and warn patient to stop drugs immediately and contact doctor if any visual disturbance
- *Streptomycin* Bactericidal. Given parenterally. Increased risk of ototoxicity in the foetus and the elderly.

Combined preparations

- *Rifinah® 150* (contains rifampicin 150 mg and isoniazid 100 mg), *Rifinah® 300* (contains rifampicin 300 mg and isoniazid 150 mg)
- *Rifater®* (contains 120 mg rifampicin, 50 mg isoniazid, and 300 mg pyrazinamide).

Table 42.1 shows the recommended doses of the main four drugs.

Table 42.1 Recommended doses of standard anti-TB drugs

Drug		Daily dose	Intermittent dose
Isoniazid (H)		300 mg	15 mg/kg three times weekly
Rifampicin (R)	<50 kg	450 mg	600–900 mg three times weekly
	≥50 kg	600 mg	
Pyrazinamide (Z)	<50 kg	1.5 g	<50 kg—2.0 g
	≥50 kg	2.0 g	≥50 kg—2.5 g three times weekly or 3.5 g twice weekly
Ethambutol (E)		15 mg/kg	30 mg/kg three times weekly or 45 mg/kg twice weekly
Pyridoxine		10–20 mg	

For example, a 75 kg adult commencing quadruple therapy would be given:
- Isoniazid 300 mg od
- Rifampicin 600 mg od
- Pyrazinamide 2.0 g od
- Ethambutol 1.2 g od
- Plus, pyridoxine 10–20 mg od

If using a combined preparation, e.g. Rifater®, with ethambutol:
- 45 kg adult: Rifater® four tablets and ethambutol 700 mg od
- 60 kg adult: Rifater® five tablets and ethambutol 900 mg od
- 80 kg adult: Rifater® six tablets and ethambutol 1.2 g od
- Plus, pyridoxine 10–20 mg od

Drug regimens are often abbreviated to the number of months each phase of treatment lasts, followed by the letters for the drugs being administered during that treatment phase, e.g. 2HRZE/4HR is the standard 6-month re-commended regime; 2HRE/7HR is 2 months of isoniazid, rifampicin, and ethambutol, followed by 7 months of isoniazid and rifampicin.

Examples of potential TB drug interactions are listed in Table 43.2.

Table 43.2 Interactions of TB drugs

Drug	Increases level of	Decreases level of
Rifampicin	(Level decreased by ketoconazole and para-aminosalicylic acid (PAS))	warfarin OCP phenytoin glucocorticoids theophyllines digoxin methadone sulfonylureas ciclosporin
Isoniazid	phenytoin carbamazepine warfarin diazepam	azoles, e.g. ketoconazole
Pyrazinamide	probenecid	

TB: adverse drug reactions

These occur in around 10% of patients, often requiring a change of therapy. Reactions are more common in those on non-standard therapy and in HIV-positive individuals.

Isoniazid peripheral neuropathy

Increased risk in those with diabetes, renal failure, alcoholics, HIV-positive, can be mitigated by pyridoxine 10–20 mg daily.

Rifampicin

May cause shock, acute renal failure, thrombocytopenia. Withdraw, and do not reintroduce the drug. Double maintenance steroid doses at the start of treatment (because of enzyme induction).

Ethambutol

Causes rare optic toxicity; recommend baseline visual acuity assessment with a Snellen chart. Use only in those with adequate visual acuity and those able to report changes in visual acuity or new visual symptoms. Document that the patient has been told to cease the drug immediately at the onset of new visual symptoms. Check baseline renal function before starting ethambutol and avoid in renal failure.

HIV-positive patients

Rifampicin and isoniazid lead to reduced serum concentrations of antifungals. Ketoconazole can inhibit rifampicin absorption. Rifampicin may reduce drug levels of protease inhibitors (as they are metabolized via the cytochrome P450 pathway, which is induced by rifampicin). Rifabutin can cause a severe iritis. Liaise closely with HIV specialist.

Drug resistance

Occurs in <2% of Caucasian cases in the UK, with higher levels in ethnic minority groups.

- Isoniazid resistance is seen in up to 6% in patients of African and Indian subcontinent origin
- Increased drug resistance is seen in HIV-positive patients (fourfold increased risk)
- Second-line drugs are generally more toxic and less effective than first-line drugs, and the treatment of drug resistance can therefore often be complex and difficult—seek specialist advice
- The regime must include at least three drugs to which the organism is known to be susceptible. An injectable drug is often added, as this has shown improved outcomes
- The initial regime will depend on the incidence of drug resistance in the community and should be altered, depending on local drug susceptibility patterns
- In general, always add at least two drugs to which the MTB is susceptible
- Parenteral treatment is usually recommended when there is resistance to two or more drugs.

See Table 43.3.

Table 43.3 Recommended drug regimens for non-MDR drug-resistant TB

Drug resistance		Initial phase	Continuation phase
H	known before treatment	2RZSE	7RE
H	known after treatment	2RZE	10RE
Z		2RHE	7HR
E		2RHZ	4RH
R	(until full sensitivities known)	As MDR-TB	
R	(only if confirmed as isolated resistance)	2HZE	16HE
S	and H	2RZE	10RE

Isoniazid (H), rifampicin (R), pyrazinamide (Z), ethambutol (E) Streptomycin (S)

Rifampicin monoresistance is uncommon but does require regime modification. In most cases, rifampicin resistance is a marker of MDR-TB (see Ɔ p. 606) and should be treated as such, until full sensitivities are known.

TB: inpatient admission

- This is rarely needed, but, if necessary, patients with suspected pulmonary TB should initially be admitted to a side room vented to the outside air (until proven non-infectious)
- Patients with smear-positive non-MDR-TB should be managed as infectious (in a side room, with face mask). This especially applies if they are on a ward with immunosuppressed patients (who may be at higher risk)
- A risk assessment (including an assessment of the immune status of other ward patients) can be made once the infectiousness and likelihood of drug resistance of the patient are known
- Patients with non-pulmonary TB can be nursed on a general ward (but aerosol-generating procedures, e.g. abscess irrigation, may need patient isolation)
- Staff should wear face masks if the patient is potentially infectious
- Inpatients with smear-positive pulmonary TB should be asked to wear a face mask whenever they leave their room, unless they have received 2 weeks' drug treatment
- Barrier nursing is unnecessary for smear-negative non-MDR-TB
- Liaise closely with infection control/microbiology/public health specialists
- If a patient on an open ward is found to have infectious TB, the risk to the other patients is small. Patients whose exposure is considered comparable to that of a household contact should be screened. Only those in the same bay as a coughing infectious case, for at least 8 h, are considered at risk. Exposure should be documented and the patient and the GP contacted
- Non-MDR-TB HIV-negative patients usually become non-infectious after 2 weeks' chemotherapy. Any bacilli seen in smears after that time are likely to be dead
- Patients with HIV and those with TB should not be nursed in close proximity
- All patients with known or suspected MDR-TB should be admitted to a negative pressure ventilated side room. Staff should wear protective face masks (FFP3)
- At discharge, a clear plan must be in place for the administration and supervision of all chemotherapy; this is particularly important for patients with MDR-TB where close liaison with the infection control team and consultant in communicable disease control is paramount.

Treatment failure/disease relapse

- This is usually due to poor compliance
- Consider DOT for treatment failure/disease relapse
- Drug resistance may have developed
- Never add a single drug to a failing regime. Add only two or three, ideally those to which the patient has not been previously exposed
- Assume drug resistance to all, or some, of the drugs in the failed regime
- Repeat cultures and sensitivity testing in this situation. Consider specific molecular tests for rifampicin/isoniazid resistance. If found, then treat as for MDR-TB (see ➜ p. 606)

- UK TB death rates have decreased since 2001, but death is still the most common cause for not completing treatment course. Higher proportions of deaths were found in older patients of white ethnicity who were born in the UK. A higher proportion of deaths were in patients with pulmonary TB than with extrapulmonary. One-quarter of patients who died were diagnosed with TB post-mortem where it was thought to cause or contribute to death in 33%.

TB: treatment follow-up

- CXR is advised at the end of therapy for pulmonary disease
- Relapse is uncommon in those compliant with standard treatment regimes in the UK (0–3%); therefore, long-term follow-up is not recommended
- Follow-up at 12 months after treatment completion is recommended for patients treated for drug-resistant TB
- Relapse after good compliance is usually due to fully sensitive organism; therefore, treatment can be with the same regime again
- Relapse due to poor compliance needs a fully supervised regime.

MDR-TB follow-up

Prolonged follow-up is recommended; lifelong for HIV-positive patients.

TB in pregnancy

There is no increased risk of developing clinical disease in pregnancy. Presentation is the same as in non-pregnant individuals, but the diagnosis may be delayed by the non-specific nature of the symptoms in the early stages of disease, with malaise and fatigue being common in the early stages of pregnancy. A CXR is more likely to be delayed.

The tuberculin skin test result is not affected by pregnancy; this applies to HIV-positive and negative subjects. A negative skin test should not lead to bacille Calmette–Guérin (BCG) vaccination, as live vaccines are contraindicated in pregnancy. In this situation, the skin test should be repeated after delivery and BCG given then after a second negative test.

TB outcome in pregnancy

- If diagnosed in the first trimester, the disease has the same outcome as for non-pregnant women
- If diagnosed in the second or third trimester, studies give more variable outcomes (some studies show a good foetal outcome; some show higher rates of small-for-date babies, pre-eclampsia, and spontaneous abortion), but these effects tend to be related to late diagnosis and incomplete drug treatment. Some studies also show a poorer foetal outcome in extrapulmonary disease
- Late diagnosis of pulmonary TB can lead to a fourfold increased obstetric mortality and ninefold increased risk of pre-term labour in some developing countries.

Treatment in pregnancy

- Isoniazid, rifampicin, and ethambutol are not teratogenic and can be used safely in pregnancy. The 'standard' short-course therapy is recommended (i.e. 6-month treatment)
- Limited pyrazinamide data on the risk of teratogenicity
- Streptomycin may be ototoxic to the foetus
- Active TB must be treated in pregnancy because of the risk of untreated disease to the mother and foetus
- Reserve drugs may be toxic, and the risk/benefit ratio of each case must be assessed individually if second-line drugs are needed
- Babies of sputum-positive mothers, who have had <2 weeks' treatment by delivery, should be treated with isoniazid and have a skin test at 6 weeks. If the skin test is negative, the chemoprophylaxis should be stopped and BCG given 1 week later (as BCG is sensitive to isoniazid)
- Congenital infection is very rare (<300 reported cases). The child can be infected at delivery (this is rare).

Breastfeeding

- Most anti-TB drugs are safe. Isoniazid—monitor infant for possible toxicity, as there is a theoretical risk of convulsions and neuropathy. Give prophylactic pyridoxine to the mother and infant
- Concentrations of drugs reaching breast milk are too low to prevent or treat infection in the infant.

TB chemotherapy with comorbid disease

Liver disease

- Drug-induced hepatitis can be fatal. A raised alanine aminotransferase (ALT) (see Box 43.2) is more common in those who regularly consume alcohol, have viral hepatitis or other chronic liver disease, take concomitant hepatotoxic drugs, are pregnant, or are within 3 months post-partum
- About 20% of those treated with isoniazid alone will have an asymptomatic transient rise in ALT. In the majority, this represents hepatic adaptation. Acetylator status (fast or slow) may influence this
- Isoniazid-induced hepatitis can be symptomatic or asymptomatic and usually occurs within weeks or months of treatment and is age-related
- Isoniazid inhibits several cytochrome P450 enzymes, potentially increasing the plasma concentrations of other hepatotoxic drugs
- Rifampicin can cause subclinical hyperbilirubinaemia without hepatocellular damage. It can also cause direct hepatocellular damage and potentiate the hepatotoxicity of other TB drugs
- Decompensated liver disease—use a drug regime without rifampicin
- Avoid pyrazinamide in patients with known chronic liver disease
- Baseline and regular monitoring of liver function is necessary (weekly LFTs for the first 2 weeks, then at 2-weekly intervals) in patients with chronic liver disease.

Box 43.2 TB drugs and abnormal LFTs

- New drug-induced hepatitis
  - Virological tests to exclude concomitant viral hepatitis
  - Aspartate aminotransferase (AST)/ALT rise 2× upper limit of normal (ULN)—monitor LFTs weekly for 2 weeks, then 2-weekly until normal
  - AST/ALT rise under 2× ULN—repeat LFT at 2 weeks
  - AST/ALT rise 5×ULN or bilirubin rise—cease rifampicin, isoniazid, and pyrazinamide, unless the patient is unwell. If the patient is unwell or sputum still positive, consider admission for parenteral therapy, e.g. streptomycin and ethambutol, with appropriate monitoring
- Drug re-challenge once LFTs less than 2× ULN —reintroduce sequentially, in order:
  - First either Isoniazid at 50 mg/day with sequential increase to 300 mg/day after 2–3 days if no reaction
  - Or Rifampicin at 75mg/day with increase to 300 mg/day after 2–3 days if no reaction, then to maximum dose/kg
  - Pyrazinamide start at 250 mg/day, increase to 1 g/day after 2–3 days, and to maximum dose/kg if no reaction
  - Daily monitoring of LFTs and clinical condition
  - If no further reaction, continue chemotherapy
  - If there is a further reaction, exclude the offending drug, and change to an alternative regime
- If intolerant of pyrazinamide, use rifampicin and isoniazid for 9 months, with ethambutol for 2 months
- If critically unwell and concerned about stopping all chemotherapy can use a 2–3-drug regimen with low likelihood of hepatotoxicity such as ethambutol and streptomycin with or without a fluoroquinolone.

Renal failure

- Isoniazid and rifampicin have biliary excretion so can be given in normal doses in renal disease
- Pyrazinamide metabolites are renally cleared; the dose may need to be less frequent in those with renal insufficiency
- Give pyridoxine, in addition to isoniazid, in those with severe renal disease to prevent isoniazid-induced peripheral neuropathy
- Ethambutol can accumulate, causing optic neuropathy; use only with caution and at a lower dose
- Dialysis patients should receive drugs after dialysis
- Post-renal transplant immunosuppressive drug doses also need alteration.

HIV infection

- Regimes are the same for HIV-positive as HIV-negative patients: standard four-drug regime. Liaise closely with HIV specialists
- Identification of HIV allows additional package of care to be added, including co-trimoxazole prophylaxis and early antiretroviral therapy (ART), which improves mortality—hence the importance of HIV testing in all patients with TB
- In newly diagnosed HIV-positive individuals, the usual practice is to start TB chemotherapy before HIV chemotherapy. ART should be started within the first 8 weeks of TB treatment, and patients with CD4 counts $<50 \times 10^6$/L should start ART within the first 2 weeks; an exception is treatment of tuberculous meningitis when early ART should be avoided
- Protease inhibitors should not be used with rifampicin (they interfere with each other's metabolism)
- Paradoxical worsening of disease (worsening fever, CXR infiltrates, increased lymphadenopathy, or new manifestations of the disease) at the initiation of HIV treatment is common (in ~15%)—so-called TB IRIS. This reflects the restoration of pathogen-specific immune responses. Steroids reduce the morbidity associated with IRIS
- Death during TB chemotherapy is more common in HIV-infected patients, who also have higher relapse rates than non-HIV-infected subjects
- Atypical presentations of TB are common in patients with CD4 counts $<200 \times 10^6$/L and disseminated TB with multi-organ involvement and mycobacteraemia, but sparing the lung may occur with CD4 counts $<75 \times 10^6$/L. Active TB may be asymptomatic in the setting of HIV
- Patients co-infected with TB and HIV should be considered potentially infectious to others at each admission, until proved otherwise, and should be segregated. Review the immune status of other patients and their likely drug resistances and their potential infectivity.

Diabetes

Increased risk of TB and the disease may be more extensive. Note that rifampicin reduces the efficacy of sulfonylureas.

Skin disease

If there is a severe skin reaction to antituberculous therapies consider stopping therapy and re-introducing in a similar fashion to patients with deranged LFTs under close observation.

Multidrug-resistant TB (MDR-TB)

Defined as MTB resistant to two or more first-line agents, usually isoniazid and rifampicin.

• Treatment is complex and time-consuming
• MDR-TB is not more infectious than other forms of TB, but the consequences of acquiring it are more serious
• 3.5% of new TB cases in the world have MDR-TB. The frequency varies between countries. Half of cases in 2017 were in China, India, and Russia
• Specialist advice essential; patients should be managed by experts with experience of managing resistant cases, in a hospital with isolation facilities. The ℅ MDRTBservice@lhch.nhs.uk email address, based in Liverpool, can be used to seek advice from a panel of experts in the management of MDR disease. An MDR-TB UK database is run from the Cardiothoracic Centre in Liverpool
• Rapid molecular tests for rifampicin resistance should be carried out in all patients suspected of having MDR-TB. Liaise closely with the reference laboratory
• Close monitoring (because of increased drug toxicity) is needed
• Compliance is paramount, and all patients should receive DOT (see ➔ p. 593)
• Start treatment with at least four drugs with certain or almost certain effectiveness. Often >4 drugs are started if the susceptibility pattern is unknown (see Table 43.4). Smears and cultures should be performed monthly, even after they become negative. Treatment should be given for a minimum of 18 months after culture conversion, but 24 months may be indicated in chronic disease with extensive pulmonary damage
• If the drug choice is limited by drug resistance and intolerance, consider desensitization and reintroduction of the offending drug. Desensitization must be carried out with concurrent treatment with two other drugs (to minimize emergence of resistant strains)
• Surgery may be indicated
• Successful outcomes reported in 48% of patients worldwide.

Contacts of MDR-TB

Chemoprophylaxis for contacts should include at least two drugs. Base the drug choice on the sensitivities of the index case for a minimum of 6 months (although there are no data to support this treatment period). If there is extensive resistance, no regime may be suitable, and regular follow-up needed instead.

> ### Risk factors for resistant disease
> • Previous anti-TB treatment, prior treatment failure
> • Lack of response to intensive phase of standard short-course therapy/treatment failure
> • HIV infection
> • Contact with patients with drug-resistant disease
> • History of poor adherence, aggravated by social deprivation or substance abuse
> • Residence in regions with high prevalence of drug-resistant disease.

Table 43.4 Second-line TB chemotherapy

Drug	Dose	Potential side effects
Amikacin	15 mg/kg	Tinnitus, ataxia, renal impairment, vertigo
Azithromycin	500 mg od	GI upset, QT prolongation
Capreomycin	15 mg/kg	As for amikacin
Ciprofloxacin	750 mg bd	Abdominal upset, headache, drug interactions, tendinopathy
Clarithromycin	500 mg bd	GI upset, QT prolongation
Ethionamide (or protionamide)	<50 kg: 375 mg bd ≥50 kg: 500 mg bd	GI upset, hepatitis. Avoid in pregnancy
Kanamycin	15 mg/kg	As for amikacin
Ofloxacin	400 mg bd	Abdominal upset, headache
PAS	10. od or 5 g bd	GI upset, fever, rash, hepatitis
Rifabutin	300–450 mg od	As for rifampicin. Uveitis (particularly with HIV infection). Drug interactions, e.g. with macrolides
Streptomycin	15 mg/kg (max dose 1 g od)	As for amikacin
Thioacetazone	150 mg	GI upset, rash, conjunctivitis, vertigo. Avoid if HIV-positive (risk of Stevens–Johnson syndrome)

Extensively drug-resistant TB (XDR-TB)

Defined as MDR-TB with added resistance to all fluoroquinolones and one of three injectable anti-TB drugs (capreomycin, kanamycin, and amikacin); represents 10% of MDR-TB cases. Outcomes are variable, but association with advanced HIV infection in a localized outbreak in South Africa was universally fatal. Some TB strains have also been reported which are resistant to all anti-TB drugs.

Latent TB infection

Definition

A positive skin test or IGRA, showing MTB infection but with no signs, symptoms or CXR changes of active TB. This represents the presence of a small total number of mycobacteria, with the host immune system retaining control over mycobacterial replication. It should be distinguished from active disease, which is usually accompanied by symptoms and CXR signs of active disease (infiltrates or lymphadenopathy).

An estimated 1.7 billion people worldwide have latent TB. Treatment of latent TB with chemoprophylaxis (see further text) reduces the risk of subsequent development of active disease by about 90%, but a proportion of people will be treated who would never have developed active disease.

Tuberculin skin test A positive skin test (Mantoux see box 43.1) results from the development of cell-mediated immunity against TB. Potential problems with skin testing are:

• Low sensitivity in the immunocompromised and cross-reactivity with BCG
• The patient has to return to have the test read after 48–72h
• Criteria for a positive test depend on the population in which it is being used.

IGRA Two blood tests (T-SPOT.TB, Oxford Immunotec Ltd., and QuantiFERON-TB Gold, QIAGEN) are available and are based on the detection of IFN-γ released by T-cells in response to MTB-specific antigens. The T-SPOT.TB test is an ELISpot test, counting individual T-cells producing IFN-γ; the QuantiFERON test is based on a whole blood ELISA and measures the IFN-γ level in the supernatant of the stimulated whole blood sample. Both assays use two proteins (ESAT-6 and CFP10) encoded by a unique genomic sequence of MTB, which is absent from *M. bovis* BCG and the majority of opportunistic mycobacteria. These proteins are the main targets for IFN-γ-secreting T-lymphocytes in individuals infected with MTB. These tests have several advantages over the tuberculin skin test: no return visit for test reading is required, the result is available the next day, and repeated testing does not cause boosting. With both tests, blood must be collected in a heparinized tube and processed within 6–8 h of venepuncture. The blood should be transferred to the laboratory at room temperature. Both tests are more sensitive for the diagnosis of latent TB than the tuberculin skin test, particularly in children and HIV-positive individuals, and, on current available evidence, there is little difference between the two, although the T-SPOT.TB test may be more sensitive in HIV-positive individuals.

HIV infection

The tuberculin skin test may be falsely negative, and radiological changes may be atypical. Current WHO guidelines recommend isoniazid chemoprophylaxis for HIV-infected patients in low-income, high-burden countries, with positive or unknown skin tests in the absence of active disease. Uptake of this recommendation is slow, partly because of the difficulties in distinguishing active from latent disease in the setting of HIV co-infection and concern regarding emergence of resistant strains. Exposure to smear-positive disease should lead to chemoprophylaxis in the absence of active disease. Recommended follow-up is at 3 and 12 months for those not receiving chemoprophylaxis (but who were eligible for it). HIV-positive patients should receive long-term follow-up as part of their ongoing HIV management.

Chemoprophylaxis

Given to contacts or screened immigrants with a positive skin test (≥5mm regardless of BCG status) or positive IGRA, who have no radiological or clinical evidence of active disease. The risk of developing disease after exposure depends on a number of factors, including BCG and HIV/immune status, and whether infection was recent. Younger patients must have had relatively recent infection and have a longer life expectancy from which to gain the benefits of chemoprophylaxis.

Chemoprophylaxis is recommended for:

* Those aged ≤65y (because of the increased risk of drug hepatotoxicity with age)
* Those with recent documented tuberculin conversion
* HIV-infected contacts of smear-positive cases (any age)
* Any age health care worker
* Individuals with HIV, injecting drugs, with haematological malignancy, chronic renal failure, or on dialysis, with silicosis, gastrectomy, solid organ transplant, or receiving anti-TNF-α therapy have a higher risk of developing active TB.

Drug regimes

* Rifampicin and isoniazid daily for 3 months (3RH). Improved compliance but slightly higher side effect profile
* Isoniazid daily for 6 months (6H). Lowest toxicity regime. Has a 60–90% effectiveness in reducing progression of latent infection to clinical disease
* 6H is recommended for people with HIV
* 6R is recommended for contacts of patients with isoniazid-resistant disease
* Individuals who decline chemoprophylaxis should be given 'inform and advise' information, regarding TB risks and symptoms and have a CXR at 3 and 12 months.

TB and anti-TNF-α treatment

Anti-tumour necrosis factor alpha (TNF-α) agents are approved for the treatment of rheumatoid arthritis (RA), Crohn's disease, psoriatic arthropathy, and ankylosing spondylitis. Anti-TNF agents include etanercept, adalimumab, infliximab, golimumab, and certolizumab.

These drugs cause profound immunosuppression, and patients treated with them have an increased risk of infections including TB. Approximately 0.6% of patients started on these agents will develop TB, with no apparent differences between agents. Overall, there is an average 3.5-fold increased risk of developing TB with anti-TNF-α therapy. *All patients due to start anti-TNF-α antibody treatment should be screened for active and latent TB.*

- All patients should have a clinical examination, with history of previous TB treatment and exposure carefully documented. All should have a CXR and tuberculin test or IGRA. The IGRA is less sensitive in those taking concomitant prednisolone and/or disease-modifying drugs, e.g. azathioprine
- Both those with an abnormal CXR consistent with previous TB, or those who have a history of extrapulmonary TB, who have received adequate treatment (as assessed by an expert), can start anti-TNF-α therapy but need monitoring every 3 months with a CXR and symptom assessment. The onset of any new respiratory symptoms, especially within 3 months of starting anti-TNF-α therapy, should be investigated promptly
- Both those with an abnormal CXR consistent with previous TB, or those who have a prior history of extrapulmonary TB, who have NOT had adequate treatment, need to have active TB excluded by appropriate investigations. They should receive chemoprophylaxis before anti-TNF-α therapy commences (assuming active disease is not identified). If there is clinical concern because of the delay in starting anti-TNF-α treatment, a shorter course of chemoprophylaxis can be given, but this may be more toxic
- Any TB diagnosed (pulmonary or extrapulmonary) should be treated with standard chemotherapy
- If active TB is present, patients should receive a minimum of 2 months' anti-TB chemotherapy before starting anti-TNF-α therapy
- If the CXR is normal, the tuberculin test or IGRA may be helpful if the patient is not on immunosuppressants. The skin test must be interpreted knowing the BCG history. A tuberculin skin test is unhelpful if the patient is on immunosuppressants. In this situation, an individual assessment should be made (see Table 43.5); if the risk of drug-induced hepatitis is less than the annual risk of developing TB, chemoprophylaxis should be given. However, if the risk of hepatitis is greater, the patient should be monitored regularly and any suggestive symptoms investigated promptly
- No chemoprophylaxis regime is 100% effective; the protective efficacy is reported at 60% for 6H and 50% for 3HR
- In those without previous BCG, Mantoux 1 in 10,000, 0–5 mm is negative, and Mantoux 1 in 10,000, >6 mm is positive and should lead to a risk assessment

Table 43.5 Sample calculations for aiding TB risk assessment for patients starting anti-TNF-α treatment

Case type	Annual risk of TB disease/ 100,000	TB risk adjusted × 5 for anti-TNF-α effect	Risk of hepatitis following 6H chemo-prophy-laxis/100,000	Risk/benefit conclusion
White, UK born, age 55–74 y	7	35	278	Observation
ISC, in UK >3 y, age >35 y	593	2965	278	Prophylaxis
Black African age 35–54 y	168	840	278	Prophylaxis
Other ethnic group, in UK >5 y, age >35 y	39	195	278	Observation

ISC = Indian subcontinent. The risk of hepatitis with 3RH chemoprophylaxis is 1,766/100,000.

- In those with prior BCG, Mantoux 1 in 10,000, 0–14 mm is negative, and Mantoux 1 in 10,000, >15 mm may represent either latent infection or BCG effect and therefore needs further investigation
- In general, all black African patients aged >15 y and all South Asians born outside the UK should be considered for chemoprophylaxis with 6 months' isoniazid
- If a patient develops TB while on anti-TNF-α therapy, treat with the full standard course of anti-TB chemotherapy. The anti-TNF-α can be continued, if indicated
- Close liaison between the prescriber of the TNF-α antibody treatment and TB specialists is needed.

Further information

Minozzi et al. Risk of infections using anti-TNF agents in rheumatoid arthritis, psoriatic arthritis, and ankylosing spondylitis: a systematic review and meta-analysis. *Exper Opin Drug Saf* 2016;**15(suppl 1)**: 11–34.

BTS recommendations for assessing risk and for managing *Mycobacterium tuberculosis* infection and disease in patients due to start anti-TNF-α treatment. *Thorax* 2005;**60**: 800–805.

TB: screening and contact tracing

Pre-entrant screening

Prior to application for a visa to reside in the UK for >6 months individuals from countries with TB rates of >40/100,000 are required to undergo TB screening at certified centres. This involves a medical history, examination, and CXR. Those with signs of active TB will then undergo sputum testing and treatment. Prior to application for a visa an individual will need a certificate from one of these centres to prove their status as free from TB.

Case finding

Divided into screening of high-risk groups and contact tracing which is covered below in more detail. In addition, to pre-entrant screening, new-entrants to the UK from high-risk TB countries should be offered assessment when they present to health-care services. This should include: assessing risk of HIV, as this will influence decisions for BCG vaccination, and offering screening for HIV as appropriate; offering either a Mantoux or IGRA tests; assessing the risk of active TB. Those with signs of active TB should undergo further assessment, those with a positive IGRA or Mantoux ≥5 mm should be considered for latent TB treatment, and those with a negative IGRA and/or Mantoux should be considered for BCG vaccination. Similarly, case finding should be conducted in groups such as the homeless, substance misusers, prisoners, and other groups. In these groups CXR should also be considered.

Contact tracing

Identifies those with TB and those who are infected but without evidence of disease. It also identifies those suitable for BCG vaccination.

Close contacts are usually those within the same household, sharing kitchen facilities, and frequent household visitors. *Casual contacts* usually include most occupational contacts. Examination is usually only needed if the index case was smear-positive or if the contacts are at high risk. This also applies if >10% of the close contacts have been infected, i.e. the index case is considered highly infectious.

- 10% of TB is diagnosed by contact tracing, with disease occurring in about 1% of contacts
- Smear-negative patients are much less infectious, but contact tracing is still recommended in these patients
- Contacts should be traced for the period the index case has been infectious or for 3 months prior to the first positive sputum or culture, if the time period is uncertain
- Most disease in contacts is found at the first screening visit
- Subjects should be advised to report suspicious symptoms
- Follow-up is recommended at 3 and 12 months for those not receiving chemoprophylaxis
- School index cases—if a pupil is diagnosed with smear-positive TB, the rest of the class and year group who share classes should be assessed as part of routine contact tracing. If a school teacher is diagnosed with

smear-positive TB, the pupils in their class during the previous 3 months should be assessed as part of routine contact tracing. The extension of contact tracing to include non-teaching staff will depend on the infectivity and proximity of the index case and whether the contacts are likely to be especially susceptible to infection.

Airplane transmission rates are low, even on long-haul flights. Contact tracing of passengers and crew is only necessary if the index case was smear-positive and coughing during a flight of at least 8 h. In this situation, screening is only recommended in those at high risk—immunocompromised travellers and children or if the index case was unusually infectious or had MDR-TB.

Extrapulmonary disease Contact screening is not recommended.

Contact examination This usually involves symptom enquiry, BCG vaccination status, Mantoux test and/or IGRA, and CXR.

HIV-infected contacts CXR is indicated, as a negative Mantoux test may be due to anergy and may therefore be a false negative. Mantoux testing is not contraindicated in HIV (PPD is dead). BCG is contraindicated (it is a live vaccine). IGRA usually useful.

BCG vaccination

Remains the only licensed vaccine for TB. The UK national schools' vaccination programme ceased in 2005 and now aims to target vaccination to selected 'at-risk' groups. Vaccination is offered to:

- All neonates who are born in an area with a high incidence (>40/100,000) of TB
- All neonates whose parents or grandparents originate from a country with a TB incidence of 40/100,000 or higher
- All neonates with a family history of TB within the past 5 y
- All Mantoux-negative contacts of patients with respiratory TB if they are previously unvaccinated and aged <35 y. Laboratory and health care workers who are contacts meeting the same criteria should be vaccinated even if they are aged >36 y
- Opportunistically identified children between 4–16 y who are previously unvaccinated and would have been offered vaccination on the currently neonatal scheme
- Mantoux/IGRA negative new entrants from a high-risk country if <16 y, or if originating from sub-Saharan Africa or a country with a TB incidence of ≥500/100,000 and aged 16–35 y
- All Mantoux-negative health care workers, irrespective of age, who are previously unvaccinated and who will be exposed to patients and clinical materials
- Mantoux-negative, previously unvaccinated individuals aged <35 y, if potentially at risk of TB exposure because of their occupation, including veterinary and abattoir workers, prison staff, staff in care homes for the elderly, staff of accommodation for refugees and the homeless, and those going to work in a high-incidence country for >1 month

- BCG has an efficacy of around 70% against TB in children, but difficulties with vaccine supply and regional policies have meant that not all children in the UK have been vaccinated in the past. It is less effective in adults and is not used in America
- Adverse events include pain and suppuration at the injection site and localized lymphadenitis. A course of rifampicin and/or isoniazid for 3–6 months, depending on response, may be needed.

M. bovis

Cattle TB is due to *M. bovis*. Humans are at low risk, as the majority of milk consumed is pasteurized. *M. bovis* is distinguishable from MTB in the laboratory, although initial diagnosis can be difficult (only distinguishable on culture). Around 40 cases are isolated per year in the UK. BCG is live attenuated *M. bovis*.

Disseminated BCG infection (BCGosis)

Live attenuated BCG immunotherapy is the most effective intravesical agent for the treatment and prophylaxis of superficial bladder cancer. BCG leads to a T-cell-mediated immune response, which has anti-tumour activity. After intravesical instillation, live mycobacteria attach to the urothelial lining. BCG organisms are internalized by bladder epithelial cells, leaving bacterial cell surface glycoproteins attached to the epithelial cell membrane. These antigens are thought to mediate the immune response.

- The standard treatment regime is 6-weekly instillations of 100 million to 1 billion cfu of BCG. Some advocate a further 3-week course, 6 weeks after cessation of the first cycle. The dose-response curve is bell-shaped, with excess BCG probably promoting increased tumour activity
- Local side effects are common, with cystitis reported in around 90% of patients; low-grade fever and malaise are frequent. Cystitis persisting >48 h after treatment should be treated with a fluoroquinolone or isoniazid 300 mg od; rifampicin 600 mg od should be added if the symptoms persist at 1 week
- Breaks in the uroepithelium are a risk factor for systemic infection, and, therefore, patients with persistent cystitis or haematuria should have their treatment delayed
- Significant reactions are reported in around 5%, with high fever commonest. A high fever post-treatment (>39°C) may represent the onset of systemic BCG infection or hypersensitivity, and hospital admission is recommended
- BCG sepsis is reported in around 0.4–0.7%, with ten deaths attributed to intravesical BCG to date. The major differential diagnosis is Gram-negative sepsis; thus, patients should be treated with broad-spectrum antibiotics
- Later-onset symptoms (at up to 8–12 weeks, though may occur much earlier), including fever, malaise, arthralgia, and breathlessness, may represent systemic BCG infection, though there is debate as to whether these sorts of systemic symptoms are due to systemic BCG infection or hypersensitivity to BCG. Non-caseating granulomas can be identified on lung and liver biopsy. Culture of organisms is rarely reported, but tissue *M. bovis* can be identified by PCR
- Disseminated infection—treat with rifampicin 600 mg od and isoniazid 300 mg od for 6 months. Some advocate the addition of ethambutol. Prednisolone 40 mg od may be added, and response to corticosteroids is said to support the diagnosis of hypersensitivity. There are no trial data to support these treatment regimens or length of treatment, but *M. bovis* is susceptible to most anti-TB drugs, except pyrazinamide and cycloserine. There is no evidence that isoniazid reduces the anti-tumour effects of BCG
- BCG hypersensitivity pneumonitis is suggested by pulmonary infiltrates; micronodular and miliary appearances are reported with or without eosinophilia
- Granulomatous hepatitis is reported. Standard TB treatment (6 months) is suggested, with prednisolone if symptoms of hypersensitivity predominate
- Systemic BCG infection is reported in HIV-positive infants and infants with severe immune deficiency, undiagnosed at the time of BCG vaccination. Systemic BCG infection is reported after BCG injection into melanoma.

Future developments in TB

- Further research is needed to see if universal use of DNA amplification techniques is more cost-effective than the current risk-based approach
- The best drug regimens for isoniazid resistance are not known despite this being the most prevalent single drug resistance and being associated with treatment failure
- Evidence is needed around drug reintroduction in hepatotoxicity
- All MTB cultures are now undergoing whole genome sequencing which will provide interesting data on clustering of cases in the future.

Further information

NICE Guideline NG33: Tuberculosis 2016. ℘ http://www.nice.org.uk/guidance/ng33.

WHO Global tuberculosis report 2018
   ℘ https://www.who.int/tb/publications/global_report/en/

GOV.UK Tuberculosis in England: annual report 2018
   ℘ https://www.gov.uk/government/publications/tuberculosis-in-england-annual-report

GOV.UK Tuberculosis screening ℘ https://www.gov.uk/guidance/tuberculosis-screening

WHO Consolidated guidelines on drug-resistant tuberculosis treatment ℘ https://www.who.int/
   tb/publications/2019/consolidated-guidelines-drug-resistant-TB-treatment/en/

BNF Tuberculosis ℘ https://bnf.nice.org.uk/treatment-summary/tuberculosis.html

UK's national tuberculosis charity. ℘ http://www.tbalert.org and ℘ http://www.thetruthabouttb.org.

Non-tuberculous mycobacteria (NTM)

NTM (also called atypical, opportunistic, and environmental mycobacteria) are found in the environment, including in soil and water, and may cause disease in susceptible individuals. They are divided into rapid and slowly growing species (for clinically relevant examples see ⊃ pp. 620–621). NTM are less virulent than MTB and—unlike MTB—are unable to adhere to intact, undamaged airway mucosa.

Risk factors for NTM disease

- Chronic lung disease such as cystic fibrosis (CF), bronchiectasis, COPD, cavitary lung disease secondary to prior TB
- Immunodeficiency, e.g. HIV, organ transplantation, anti-TNF-α therapy, rare genetic mutations in IL12/IL23/IFN-γ signalling, autoantibodies against IFN-γ
- GORD, pectus excavatum, and kyphoscoliosis may be risk factors
- NTM disease is well described in otherwise healthy, thin, tall, middle-aged women; the pathogenesis is obscure, although one hypothesis is habitual voluntary cough suppression, leading to failure to clear airway secretions (so-called 'Lady Windermere syndrome').

Clinical features

- Symptoms are non-specific: typically chronic productive cough, fatigue, sometimes with weight loss, dyspnoea, fever, sweats
- Often complicates known underlying lung disease, such as COPD, leading to atypical disease progression
- Colonization of abnormal lung may not cause symptoms but can progress to cause disease later
- Disseminated infection may occur in immunocompromised patients
- Hypersensitivity pneumonitis secondary to NTM may occur following use of hot tubs, indoor swimming pools, or contaminated metalworking fluids; breathlessness tends to be a prominent symptom.

Investigations

- *CXR* can be indistinguishable from that of MTB, with upper zone infiltrate with cavitation. Airway nodularity and associated bronchiectasis are common. CXR may be difficult to interpret in the presence of pre-existing lung disease
- *Sputum samples* Microbiology for AFB stain, culture, and further identification. Following growth of an NTM send two further sputum samples at 7-day intervals for AFB smear and culture
- *Bronchoscopy* with bronchial wash is often required, guided by localization of disease on CT scan
- *HRCT* chest typically shows thin-walled upper lobe cavities, with marked pleural involvement, or small nodules with tree-in-bud pattern and cylindrical bronchiectasis; bilateral diffuse ground-glass infiltrates, nodules, or mosaic pattern may be seen with NTM-associated HP.

Diagnosis

Distinguishing contamination or colonization with NTM from clinical disease ('NTM pulmonary disease') may be challenging. A single positive NTM sputum culture is unlikely to be of significance, although such patients should be followed up with periodic sputum cultures. Treat patients who are deteriorating clinically and who have repeatedly positive cultures or smears for NTM. At least two separate positive sputum cultures or a single positive bronchial lavage or biopsy culture are usually considered sufficient to justify treatment in the appropriate clinical context. Compatible histopathology (granulomatous inflammation), when available, further supports a decision to commence treatment. HRCT may be useful in facilitating treatment decisions and monitoring response.

Management

* The decision to treat is complex and is based on the likelihood of clinical disease, weighed against the side effects and potential toxicity of treatment on an individual patient basis
* No need to notify or contact-trace
* Typical drug regimens for specific NTM species are described on ⊃ pp. 620–621. Prolonged courses of treatment are required, and drug side effects frequently limit therapy. Seek specialist advice
* Avoid macrolide monotherapy, which encourages macrolide resistance
* Be alert to the possibility of drug interactions and toxicity. In the setting of HIV, there are potential drug interactions between rifampicin, macrolides, and protease inhibitors and non-nucleoside reverse transcriptase inhibitors (NNRTIs). Rifampicin induces liver enzymes, and, therefore, the elimination of other drugs (e.g. oral contraceptives, warfarin, phenytoin, prednisolone, ciclosporin) may be increased. Macrolides may cause QT interval prolongation, particularly when taken alongside other QT prolonging drugs
* Curative therapy is not always possible, reflecting antibiotic resistance in the NTM species, drug intolerance due to side effects, and/or significant comorbid disease
* Although rarely employed in the UK, surgical resection of focal disease, in combination with drug therapy, may be curative in patients who are able to tolerate resection—consider in patients with highly resistant isolates who have failed to respond to standard therapy.

Further information

Haworth et al. BTS guidelines for the management of non-tuberculous mycobacterial pulmonary disease. *Thorax* 2017; **72**: ii1–ii64.

NTM species and lung disease

Slowly growing species

Mycobacterium avium complex (MAC)

- MAC (also referred to as *M. avium intracellulare*, MAI) includes the different *M. avium* subspecies as well as *M. intracellulare*
- Classical presentations include upper lobe fibrocavitary disease in elderly male smokers and nodular/bronchiectatic disease in non-smoking females
- Initial treatment should be triple therapy with a macrolide (clarithromycin or azithromycin), rifampicin, and ethambutol. A 3x weekly regimen may be used in less severe disease. Consider adding nebulized/IV amikacin or IV streptomycin in severe (usually cavitary) disease
- Antibiotic susceptibility testing is not predictive of clinical response in MAC with the exception of macrolide susceptibility, and so routine susceptibility testing of MAC isolates is performed for clarithromycin only. Macrolide resistance is associated with a poor prognosis, and its management is complex—seek specialist advice. The major risk factor for macrolide resistance is macrolide monotherapy, and macrolides should *never* be used as monotherapy for active treatment of MAC
- Antibiotic treatment should be continued for at least 12 months of negative sputum cultures while on therapy
- MAC is the leading cause of NTM infection in the setting of HIV and may occur late in the disease when CD4 count <50 or during the first 2 months of ART. Disease is rarely confined to the lungs in this setting, and lymphadenitis and disseminated infection are common.

Mycobacterium kansasii

- Classically presents with progressive upper lobe fibrocavitary disease similar to TB, and isolation of *M. kansasii* is usually associated with disease (rather than reflecting contamination)
- Treatment is usually with rifampicin, ethambutol, and isoniazid for a minimum of 12 months of negative sputum cultures. Clarithromycin and moxifloxacin may be useful agents, e.g. for rifampicin-resistant isolates. Usually good response to treatment: >90% 5 y cure and <10% relapse with full compliance.

Mycobacterium malmoense

- *M. malmoense* typically causes cavitary disease, often in patients with underlying COPD, and isolation of *M. malmoense* is usually associated with disease (rather than contamination)
- Treatment is usually with rifampicin, ethambutol, and a macrolide, for at least 12 months after sputum culture conversion.

Mycobacterium xenopi

- Typically causes upper lobe cavitary disease resembling TB
- Treatment typically comprises rifampicin, ethambutol, and a macrolide, with either isoniazid or a quinolone. Disease may progress, despite treatment, and mortality is relatively high.

Mycobacterium gordonae

- *M. gordonae* is frequently isolated from sputum but is usually a contaminant and only rarely causes progressive lung disease.

Rapidly growing species

Mycobacterium abscessus

- *M. abscessus* comprises three species: *M. abscessus* (*sensu stricto*), *M. massiliense*, and *M. boletii*, which may differ in treatment response (with a better prognosis in *M. massiliense*, compared to *M. abscessus*)
- *M. abscessus* has emerged as a major pathogen in CF where it is the leading mycobacterial cause of progressive lung disease. Transmission of *M. a. massiliense* has been reported between CF patients; segregation in CF centres is increasingly practised
- *M. abscessus* also causes nodular/bronchiectatic disease in patients without CF, classically non-smoking female
- *M. abscessus* is uniformly resistant to standard antituberculous agents, and there is currently no proven curative antibiotic regimen for *M. abscessus* lung disease. Seek advice from a specialist. Regimens based on *in vitro* drug susceptibilities are recommended; a typical treatment protocol comprises induction therapy for at least 4 weeks with IV amikacin, IV tigecycline, IV imipenem, and PO azithromycin, followed by long-term maintenance therapy with nebulized amikacin, PO azithromycin, and another 1–3 PO agents to which the isolate is sensitive (e.g. a quinolone, clofazimine, minocycline, co-trimoxazole, linezolid). IV cefoxitin may be a useful second-line agent for induction
- Although guidelines recommend continuing antibiotic treatment for 12 months once cultures are negative, in practice achieving this level of suppression of *M. abscessus* may be unrealistic. This is a chronic incurable infection for some patients, and intermittent courses of IV agents are typically required to treat exacerbations and control symptoms/minimize progression of lung disease
- Successful treatment of disseminated *M. abscessus* with engineered personalized bacteriophages has been reported in a single patient.

Mycobacterium chelonae

Rarely causes lung disease. Treat with at least two drugs to which the isolate displays *in vitro* susceptibility; often susceptible to macrolides, tobramycin, amikacin, imipenem; resistant to cefoxitin.

Mycobacterium fortuitum

Often does not cause progressive lung disease in the absence of treatment; when therapy is needed, usually susceptible to macrolides, quinolones, imipenem, cefoxitin.

Chapter 44

Respiratory infection—parasitic

Introduction to parasitic respiratory infections 624
Pulmonary hydatid disease 624
Amoebic pulmonary disease 625
Pulmonary ascariasis 625
Strongyloidiasis 625
Toxocariasis 626
Dirofilariasis 626
Schistosomiasis 626
Paragonimiasis 627
Tropical (filarial) pulmonary eosinophilia 627

Introduction to parasitic respiratory infections

A wide variety of parasitic organisms may infect the lungs, although clinical disease is rare in the UK. In general, parasites may cause lung disease by two different mechanisms:

- Hypersensitivity reactions, e.g. Löffler's syndrome and eosinophilic lung disease (Ɔ p. 290), most commonly from helminths such as *ascaris*, *toxocara*, and liver flukes
- Direct infection and invasion, e.g. amoebic disease, pulmonary hydatid disease.

Some of the more important examples are noted in this chapter.

Pulmonary hydatid disease

- Hydatidosis is the commonest parasitic lung disease worldwide
- Human infection follows ingestion of parasite eggs, with the adult worm found in dogs, sheep, goats, horses, camels, and moose; infection is common in sheep-raising regions, particularly Central Europe and the Mediterranean, as well as Alaska and Arctic Canada
- Caused by a cestode (tapeworm). Two main forms:
  - *Echinococcus granulosus*, which causes cystic hydatid disease as the larvae grow in the lungs. Common. Symptoms include cough (sometimes productive of cyst contents, 'hydatidoptysis'), haemoptysis, and chest pain. Chest radiograph (CXR) shows rounded cysts, sometimes with calcified walls, most commonly in lower lobes; computed tomography (CT) may show 'daughter cysts'. Cyst rupture may occur, with wheeze, eosinophilia, and bronchial or pleural spread
  - *Echinococcus multilocularis*, which leads to alveolar hydatid disease following tissue invasion. Rare. Lung masses are less clearly delineated on CT than in cystic disease
- Diagnose from serology or sputum analysis. Serology is insensitive for the diagnosis of pulmonary disease (around 50%). Demonstration of liver cysts supports the diagnosis. Avoid needle aspiration of cysts, which may result in hypersensitivity or dissemination
- Treatment is with surgical excision in most cases. Medical treatment with albendazole if the patient is unfit for surgery or following cyst rupture and dissemination.

Amoebic pulmonary disease

- Caused by the protozoa *Entamoeba histolytica*
- Intestinal and liver infection are common, with lung involvement in a minority
- Lung disease can develop either directly via transdiaphragmatic spread from the liver or via the bloodstream or lymphatics
- Pulmonary manifestations include right lower lobe consolidation, empyema, lung abscess, or hepatobronchial fistulae (resulting in large volumes of brown or 'anchovy' sputum). May be associated pericardial disease
- Diagnose using serology (sensitivity >90%) or following identification of trophozoites in stool, sputum, or pleural fluid
- Treatment is with metronidazole plus diloxanide.

Pulmonary ascariasis

- An intestinal nematode (roundworm) distributed worldwide
- Following oral ingestion of *Ascaris lumbricoides* eggs, larvae haematogenously migrate to lungs where they mature over 1–2 weeks
- Clinically presents as a hypersensitivity reaction, with cough, wheeze, fever, retrosternal discomfort, CXR infiltrates, and peripheral eosinophilia (Löffler's syndrome)
- Examination of gastric aspirates or respiratory secretions for larvae is required to definitively diagnose. Stool for eggs may confirm the diagnosis although often not detectable for ~2 months
- Usually resolves spontaneously after 1–2 weeks. Consider treatment with albendazole/mebendazole for gastro-intestinal (GI) infection once larvae have reached maturity.

Strongyloidiasis

- Caused by the nematode (roundworm) *Strongyloides stercoralis*, found in Central and South America and Africa. Filariform larvae (in faecally contaminated soil) migrate through skin and travel to lungs haematogenously
- Pulmonary involvement may lead to a Löffler-type syndrome, with wheeze, skin rash, eosinophilia, and CXR infiltrate. In the setting of immunocompromise, disseminated autoinfection may occur, leading to the 'hyper-infection syndrome'. Acute respiratory distress syndrome (ARDS) may develop, and 2° bacterial sepsis is common
- Diagnose using serology (sensitivity ~85%; false negatives in immunosuppression) or following microbiological analysis of stool (relatively low sensitivity) or duodenal fluid. In disseminated strongyloidiasis, larvae may be found in sputum, bronchoalveolar lavage (BAL) fluid, and pleural fluid
- Treatment is with ivermectin or albendazole.

Toxocariasis

- Caused by roundworm *Toxocara canis*, distributed worldwide in dogs (*T. cati* from cats also causes disease)
- Ingestion of eggs from contaminated soil/food may result in visceral larva migrans. Migration of larvae through the lungs results in an immune response, with wheeze, cough, and eosinophilia. Heavy ingestion causes fever, anorexia, hepatomegaly, and urticarial rashes
- Diagnosis may be made from serology (sensitivity ~80%)
- Treatment often not required; moderate/severe cases are given albendazole; steroids may be beneficial in severe cases.

Dirofilariasis

- Nematode (roundworm) found in USA, Japan, South America
- Infection is caused by *Dirofilaria immitis* following mosquito transfer from animals, especially dogs. Worms lodge in the pulmonary arteries and elicit an inflammatory response, leading to a necrotic nodule
- Presentation is classically asymptomatic, with a single peripheral nodule on CXR mimicking cancer. Patients may present with cough, chest pain, and haemoptysis, presumably due to pulmonary infarction
- Definitive diagnosis requires lung biopsy. Serology lacks sensitivity and specificity
- Treatment is not usually required.

Schistosomiasis

- Found in the Middle East, South America, South-East Asia, Africa, and the Caribbean
- *Schistosoma* species are trematodes (flukes) carried by snails, and infection follows skin penetration, often during swimming
- Pulmonary involvement may reflect acute tissue migration, causing cough, wheeze, and CXR infiltrates. Chronic infection can lead to interstitial infiltrates or arteriovenous (AV) fistulae. In some, portal hypertension opens up portosystemic collaterals, and eggs then embolize into the pulmonary circulation. A granulomatous pulmonary endarteritis develops, causing pulmonary hypertension (PHT) and cor pulmonale
- Diagnosis from observation of ova in sputum, BAL, urine, or stool, or from lung biopsy. Serology testing is possible, but such tests are not standardized
- Treatment is with praziquantel.

Paragonimiasis

- Caused by *Paragonimus* spp., particularly *P. westermani* (oriental lung fluke), a trematode (fluke) distributed in West Africa, the Far East, India, and Central and South America
- Following ingestion of undercooked seafood, flukes migrate to the lung or pleura and become encapsulated, developing into adults in ~6 weeks
- Clinical features may be acute or chronic and include chest pain, pneumothorax, pleural effusion, Löffler's syndrome, and recurrent haemoptysis. Serum eosinophilia is common
- Diagnose with serology (sensitivity ~90%) or observation of eggs (late phase of infection) in sputum, transbronchial biopsy (TBB), BAL, pleural fluid, or stool
- Treatment is with praziquantel.

Tropical (filarial) pulmonary eosinophilia

- Follows infection with *Wuchereria bancrofti*, *Brugia malayi*, or *Brugia timori* in the tropics
- These roundworms reside in the lymphatics and bloodstream
- Pulmonary involvement is common and represents a hypersensitivity reaction to the organism trapped in the lung, with cough, wheeze, CXR infiltrates, peripheral eosinophilia, and raised serum IgE. See ⊃ p. 293
- Diagnosis is serological (modest sensitivity)
- Treatment is with diethylcarbamazine.

Respiratory infection—viral

Overview of viral pneumonia 630
Influenza: background 632
Influenza: diagnosis 634
Influenza: management 636
Cytomegalovirus pneumonia 638
Adenovirus 640
Measles 640
Human metapneumovirus 641
Parainfluenza 641
Respiratory syncytial virus 642
Varicella pneumonia 643
Hantavirus pulmonary syndrome 644
Coronavirus disease 2019 (COVID-19) 645
Severe acute respiratory syndrome (SARS) 651
Middle East respiratory syndrome (MERS) 654

Overview of viral pneumonia

- Viral upper respiratory tract infections (URTIs) are common, but typically self-limiting, and are usually managed in the community. Viral pneumonia is less common but is more serious and usually requires hospitalization. Older studies suggest that viruses are detectable in 15–30% of patients hospitalized with pneumonia, although more recent research using molecular techniques have identified viral pathogens very commonly in both adults and children with community-acquired pneumonia (CAP); viral and bacterial pathogens may commonly exist. A significant challenge in these studies is distinguishing between asymptomatic viral infection and CAP directly due to a viral agent
- Viruses may cause serious respiratory infection in the immunocompromised (particularly in patients with depressed T-cell function, e.g. following organ transplantation). Cytomegalovirus (CMV) is the commonest serious viral pathogen that affects immunocompromised patients. Influenza, parainfluenza, respiratory syncytial virus (RSV), measles, and adenovirus may also cause pneumonia in the immunocompromised, although diagnosis of these viruses is difficult and infection is commonly undetected
- The clinical and radiological features of viral pneumonia are non-specific. Worsening cough and breathlessness following an URTI suggest the development of pneumonia; wheeze may accompany bronchiolitis. Chest X-ray (CXR) typically shows non-specific diffuse interstitial infiltrates, and hypoxia may occur. 2° bacterial infection may complicate viral pneumonia
- A variety of diagnostic techniques are available, including polymerase chain reaction (PCR), viral culture, antigen testing (e.g. enzyme immunoassay (EIA) and direct fluorescent antibody (DFA) testing), and serology
- Treatment consists of supportive care and, in some cases, antivirals. Infection with certain viruses may require isolation. Treat 2° bacterial infection with antibiotics
- Specific features of the common and/or important viruses are noted in the remainder of the chapter

Influenza: background

- Single-stranded enveloped RNA viruses
- Commonest cause of viral pneumonia in immunocompetent adults. It is transmitted via respiratory secretions and is extremely contagious
- Three pathogenic serotypes: A, B, and C. Type A causes more severe disease and occurs in annual epidemics and intermittent pandemics. Types B and C cause epidemics
- The surface antigens haemagglutinin and neuraminidase determine influenza serotype. Genetic mutations may result in antigenic shifts (major genetic rearrangements between strains, associated with pandemics of influenza A—1918 (H1N1), 1957 (H2N2), 1968 (H3N2), and 2009 (H1N1)) and antigenic drifts (more minor genetic variations associated with epidemics)
- Genetic rearrangement of virus occurs in animal and bird reservoirs, and the virus may then be transferred to humans, e.g. 2009 H1N1 was caused by reassortment of strains: two swine, one human, and one avian
- Seasonal influenza is very well recognized in the UK, particularly during the winter months. It may affect previously well individuals, although it occurs more commonly in the elderly, particularly in the setting of chronic heart or lung disease or immunocompromise
- Although debilitating, influenza is usually self-limiting (uncomplicated) but is associated with increased morbidity and mortality in high risk groups (complicated influenza)
- Pandemic 2009 influenza A/H1N1 was first detected in Mexico and lasted until August 2010, affecting >214 countries and territories and an estimated 201,000 respiratory deaths associated with influenza (18,500 of these were laboratory-confirmed cases). The majority of infection and deaths occurred in those aged 18–64, with lower rates in elderly patients probably due to exposure to similar strains earlier in life. High death rates particularly seen in pregnant patients
- Outbreaks of highly pathogenic H5N1 avian influenza have occurred in many countries, raising fears of the development of sustained human-to-human transmission and a new global pandemic. More than 600 cases have been reported worldwide since 2003, associated with a 60% mortality
- Novel avian influenza A/H7N9 was first reported in March 2013 in eastern China, with likely transmission via secretions/excretions of infected poultry, with no evidence (as yet) of sustained human-to-human transmission. Serological studies have found no evidence of human infection with novel H7N9 prior to November 2012 in Chinese poultry workers. The virus seems to have been created by reassortment of at least four avian influenza viruses (probably obtaining its haemagglutinin gene from H7N3 in domestic ducks, its neuraminidase gene from H7N9 in wild birds, and six remaining genes from multiple related H9N2 viruses in domestic poultry). Early reports suggest that the median patient age is ~60y (in contrast with median H5N1 patient age of ~25y) and is associated with a 27% mortality.

Regularly updated information on seasonal, avian, and pandemic influenza is available from the Health Protection Agency, the World Health

Organization, and the US Centers for Disease Control and Prevention websites:

- ♪ https://www.gov.uk/government/collections/
  seasonal-influenza-guidance-data-and-analysis
- ♪ http://www.who.int/csr/don/en/index.html
- ♪ http://www.cdc.gov/flu/weekly

Additional guidelines are available for the management of suspected influenza in the setting of a pandemic with UK Pandemic Alert Levels 2–4 (cases of pandemic influenza identified in UK): ♪ https://www.england.nhs.uk/ourwork/eprr/pi/

Influenza: diagnosis

Clinical and laboratory features

Incubation period typically 1–4 days; adults contagious for 7 days and children for 21 days from illness onset. The clinical picture following infection is variable and may be influenced, in part, by the influenza subtype. Features include:

- *Asymptomatic* infection
- *'Flu'* (acute onset of fever, cough, headache, coryzal symptoms, myalgia, sore throat)
- Complications include:
  - Bronchitis/bronchiolitis
  - *1° influenza viral pneumonia* (onset typically within 48h of initial fever; cough dry or productive, haemoptysis may occur, bilateral crackles, and/or wheeze; may progress very rapidly to respiratory failure and death; described in many patients infected with avian influenza H5N1 and H7N9 and more likely among pandemic H1N1 than for seasonal influenza; often associated with lymphopenia, thrombocytopenia, abnormal liver function, and multi-organ failure)
  - *2° bacterial pneumonia* (more common than viral pneumonia; onset typically 4–5 days after initial fever, during early convalescence, although may occur earlier; pathogens include *S. pneumoniae, S. aureus*—particularly associated with lung abscess—and *H. influenzae*; mixed bacterial/viral pneumonia may occur). Major contributor to morbidity and mortality in those > 65y
  - Gastro-intestinal (GI) symptoms (e.g. watery diarrhoea; more frequently described during influenza A H1N1 and avian H5N1 than seasonal infection)
  - Otitis media (particularly in children), conjunctivitis; rarely parotitis
  - Myositis (creatine kinase (CK) may be elevated; rarely myoglobinuria with renal failure)
  - Neurological (encephalitis, acute necrotizing encephalopathy, transverse myelitis, Guillain–Barré syndrome—all rare; Reye's syndrome with encephalopathy and fatty liver following aspirin use is well described in children and adolescents)
  - Cardiovascular (ECG abnormalities common, myocarditis or pericarditis rare).

Imaging

CXR typically shows bilateral mid-zone interstitial infiltrates in 1° viral pneumonia, although focal consolidation is also well described. Lobar consolidation occurs in 2° bacterial pneumonia.

Differential diagnosis of 'flu-like' illness

Includes adenovirus, RSV, rhinovirus, parainfluenza, *Chlamydophila pneumoniae, Legionella, Mycoplasma*, and *S. pneumoniae*. A very high fever is said to favour a diagnosis of influenza. Consider Middle East respiratory syndrome (MERS) (see ➲ p. 654) in patients with an appropriate travel history.

Diagnosis

Often suggested by knowledge of a local outbreak. Diagnostic investigations include:

* *Virology* (not routinely required if pandemic established with widespread infection across the UK—Alert Level 4—when diagnosis will be clinical—'influenza-like illness')
  * Presentation <7 days after illness onset: nose and throat swabs in virus transport medium (for direct immunofluorescence, enzyme-linked immunosorbent assay (ELISA), virus culture, and/or reverse transcriptase PCR (RT-PCR))
  * Presentation >7 days after illness onset: 'acute' serum and subsequently 'convalescent' serum after 10–14 days (for influenza serological testing)
  * Rapid (point of care testing (POCT)) may be available, second generation nucleic acid amplication tests have the highest sensitivity and specificity and give results in up to 60 minutes
* *Bacteriology* (in patients with influenza-related pneumonia)
  * Blood culture
  * Pneumococcal and *Legionella* urinary antigen
  * Sputum M, C, & S (if purulent sputum and either no prior antibiotics or failure to respond to empirical antibiotics)
  * 'Acute' serum and subsequently 'convalescent' serum after 10–14 days for influenza/other agents serological testing.

Influenza: management

Severity assessment

- Patients with uncomplicated influenza do not require admission
- For influenza-related pneumonia, a CURB-65 of ≥3 or high PSI score (see ➜ p. 521) indicates severe pneumonia and a high risk of death; low risk patients may be considered for home treatment
- Bilateral CXR infiltrates consistent with 1° viral pneumonia should be considered as severe pneumonia, irrespective of severity score.

Infection control

- Outside the setting of a UK pandemic, most suspected cases of influenza are likely to be seasonal
- Very infectious; large amounts of influenza virus are present in respiratory secretions, easily transmitted by sneezing and coughing. Viral shedding can continue for up to 10 days
- H5N1 avian influenza should be seriously considered in patients with:
  - Fever (≥38°C) and lower respiratory tract symptoms or CXR showing consolidation/ acute respiratory distress syndrome (ARDS) or a severe illness suggestive of an infectious process, *and*
  - Close contact (<1m) within 7 days with *either* live or dead domestic poultry or wild birds in countries affected by H5N1 (or known infected animals, e.g. cats or pigs) *or* close contact with human cases of severe unexplained respiratory illness or unexplained illness resulting in death in patients from countries with H5N1
- H7N9 avian influenza should be suspected in patients with:
  - Fever (≥38°C) and clinical or CXR findings of consolidation/ARDS or a severe illness suggestive of an infectious process, *and*
  - Travel to China within 10 days before symptom onset

In such cases of suspected avian influenza, the patient should be assessed either at their home or in a hospital side room, with both patient and staff wearing surgical masks and staff wearing gown and gloves. Immediately inform local Health Protection Unit as well as hospital infection control and occupational health. If hospitalization is required, patients should be in strict respiratory isolation, preferably in a negative pressure room (although patients should not be transferred for this reason alone), and staff should wear high-filtration mask (FFP3), gown, gloves, and eye protection (consider also cap and plastic apron, depending on situation). Mark all laboratory samples as 'high risk', and inform local laboratory of the sample status.

Treatment

- *Supportive care* O₂, intravenous (IV) fluids, nutritional support. Consider intensive care unit (ICU)/high dependency unit (HDU) admission for patients with one or more of more of: 1° viral pneumonia; CURB-65 score of 4 or 5; PaO₂ <8kPa despite high-flow O₂; progressive hypercapnia; pH <7.26; septic shock. NIV may be used for patients with COPD and decompensated type II respiratory failure, although infection control measures should be in place and protective equipment worn by staff to minimize any spread of infection from respiratory droplets

- *Antiviral* treatment with neuraminidase inhibitors is indicated for patients with an influenza-like illness and fever >38°C within 48h of symptom onset; consider also treating immunocompromised or very elderly patients in the absence of fever, and severely ill or immunocompromised patients if >48h from disease onset. Also treat patients with suspected H5N1 or H7N9, regardless of duration of symptoms. Which antiviral is used depends on relative risk of resistance of the dominant circulating strain. Treat with: oseltamivir 75mg bd for 5 days (30mg od if creatinine clearance <30mL/min); anti-emetics may be needed for nausea. Inhaled zanamivir 10mg bd via inhaler for 5 days (up to 10 days if resistance to oseltamivir) is another option for non-severe disease. Antivirals appear to reduce illness duration (by up to 3 days), hospitalization, and subsequent antibiotic requirements; possible effects on mortality have not been adequately studied. The neuraminidase inhibitor zanamivir may be given intravenously (e.g. for ventilated patients), but its effectiveness in this situation is unproven. Antiviral prophylaxis (oseltamivir 75mg od for 10 days) should be given to exposed contacts of those with uncomplicated influenza, health care workers caring for patients with suspected avian influenza, as well as the patient's household contacts. This may be required irrespective of vaccination status
- Treat influenza-related pneumonia with *antibiotics*, according to severity, e.g. oral co-amoxiclav, a tetracycline (e.g. doxycycline), or a macrolide if non-severe; IV co-amoxiclav or cefuroxime or cefotaxime, together with a macrolide, if severe. Follow local pneumonia antibiotic guidelines.

Outcome

Uncomplicated influenza typically resolves within 7 days, although cough and malaise may persist for several weeks. The reported mortality from 1° influenza viral pneumonia is >40% and up to 24% from 2° bacterial pneumonia. Risks of viral pneumonia are increased in older patients with cardiorespiratory disease or diabetes. Pandemics are associated with a shift in the age distribution—the 2009 pandemic saw high rates of mortality and morbidity among children and young adults.

Vaccination

- The influenza inactivated vaccine is modified annually, based on recent viral strains (and now includes antigen from the 2009 pandemic H1N1), and provides partial protection against influenza illness, hospitalization, and death. Vaccination if age >65, chronic comorbidity, nursing home residents, or health workers. Vaccination will not protect against H5N1 avian influenza but may make simultaneous co-infection with human and avian influenza less likely and so reduce the likelihood of viral genetic reassortment
- Annual vaccination has variable efficacy and was reported to be 15% effective (across all age groups) in the 2017–2018 season. Uptake in at risk groups is still only around 72%
- Live attenuated influenza vaccines are currently under investigation.

Cytomegalovirus pneumonia

Epidemiology

- Enveloped dsDNA virus
- Cytomegalovirus (CMV) is the commonest serious viral pathogen in the immunocompromised and is a particular problem following transplantation; however, rates have fallen after widespread use of prophylaxis
- Individuals are described as 'seropositive' for CMV if they have evidence of IgG antibodies, indicating latent infection following previous exposure; seropositivity increases with age. Infection in transplant recipients results from either transmission from a CMV positive donor to a CMV antibody negative recipient (via the organ or a blood transfusion) or reactivation of latent CMV in a seropositive recipient as a result of immunosuppression
- Infection occurs most frequently during the first 4 months following organ or bone marrow transplantation, corresponding to the period of maximal T-cell suppression. Graft-versus-host disease (GVHD) increases the risk of CMV infection
- Infection may occur in immunocompetent individuals with critical illness, this is more likely to be due to reactivation of latent infection.

Clinical and laboratory features

- 'Flu-like' symptoms in immunocompetent patients
- Symptoms of CMV pneumonia in the immunocompromised are non-specific: fever, dry cough, dyspnoea, and malaise
- Extrapulmonary manifestations of CMV infection (e.g. gastro-oesophagitis; hepatitis) may suggest the diagnosis
- Hypoxia may occur. Leukopenia, thrombocytopenia, and abnormal liver function tests (LFTs) are characteristic.

Imaging

- *CXR* Typically bilateral diffuse interstitial infiltrate, although lobar consolidation and localized haziness also described; can be normal. A nodular infiltrate may suggest co-infection with *Aspergillus*
- *CT* Features include localized or diffuse ground-glass and nodular shadowing that may progress to airspace consolidation.

Diagnosis

Antibody tests are used to estimate risk following transplantation, but diagnosis of active disease requires evidence of either viraemia (by antigen or PCR testing of blood) or tissue invasion (by biopsy). A wide range of diagnostic tests are available, and the choice of tests varies between centres—discuss with your local virologist. The nature of the transplant and immunosuppression also influence the interpretation of test results. Methods include:

- Early antigen fluorescence test on bronchoalveolar lavage (BAL) fluid (high sensitivity, low specificity)

- Qualitative PCR on blood or BAL fluid (highly sensitive but unable to differentiate between latent and replicating CMV; negative result practically excludes the diagnosis; positive result is unhelpful)
- CMV antigenaemia on blood (rapid, differentiates between latent and replicating virus)
- Quantitative PCR on blood or BAL fluid (rapid, differentiates between latent and replicating virus)
- Indirect immunofluorescence with monoclonal antibodies to CMV in BAL fluid (rapid, highly sensitive, and specific)
- Histology of lung tissue from transbronchial or surgical biopsies (demonstrate CMV inclusion bodies—the 'owl's eye' appearance—within infected cells; considered gold standard investigation).

In some cases, a definitive diagnosis is not possible and treatment is empirical.

Treatment

Reduce immunosuppression where possible. Ganciclovir 5 mg/kg IV bd for 2–4 weeks (side effects include neutropenia, anaemia). Consider additional treatment with anti-CMV hyperimmune globulin or prolonged oral valganciclovir in cases of severe or relapsed disease. Foscarnet 60mg/kg tds for 2–3 weeks is an alternative to ganciclovir for resistant cases, but toxicity (nephrotoxicity, metabolic disturbance) can limit treatment.

Complications

- Opportunistic infection (e.g. pneumocystis pneumonia (PCP), aspergillosis) due to further suppression of T-cell function by the CMV infection itself
- Increased risk of organ rejection, as allografts are more susceptible to CMV infection than native organs.

Outcome

The reported mortality from CMV pneumonia varies although may be as high as 85%. Relapse occurs in up to one-third of patients.

Adenovirus

- Non-enveloped dsDNA viruses
- Worldwide distribution, occur throughout the year
- More than 50 serotypes, the relative frequency of which is unclear. Some studies suggest serotypes 1–3 are most common, but studies in the armed services found high frequencies of serotypes 4, 7, and 14 (all of these are associated with upper and lower respiratory tract infections)
- Most common symptoms are those of self-limiting upper airways infection, which frequently mimics group A streptococcal infection, particularly in childhood
- Can cause pneumonia and ARDS in adults
- Occasional complications—myocarditis, hepatitis, nephritis, meningoencephalitis, and disseminated intravascular coagulation (DIC)
- Disseminated disease may occur in the immunocompromised (sometimes due to virus reactivation), most severe in those with poor cell mediated immunity and in the elderly or very young
- Diagnosis is from nasopharyngeal fluid, sputum, or BAL fluid viral culture, antigen testing or PCR, or quantitative PCR on blood (particularly in the immunocompromised). Serology and histology (showing intranuclear inclusions) may also be helpful
- Treatment is usually supportive, but the seriously unwell (particularly the immunocompromised) may be treated with cidofovir (unlicensed; nephrotoxicity; poor evidence) ± IV immunoglobulin. Ganciclovir has limited activity against adenoviruses.

Measles

- Enveloped single-stranded RNA virus
- Very rare in adults, although increasing in prevalence due to low recent uptake of vaccination worldwide. Symptomatic respiratory involvement (e.g. croup, bronchiolitis, and pneumonia) occur most commonly in the very young and those >20y and is a common cause of mortality
- Symptoms of fever and URTI are followed by a diffuse maculopapular rash. Leukopenia is common
- CXR may show reticulonodular infiltrates, hilar lymphadenopathy, and pleural effusions
- 2° bacterial infection is common
- Diagnosis is serological; viral culture is possible but rarely performed
- Treatment is supportive. Treat 2° bacterial infection with antibiotics.

Human metapneumovirus

- Single-stranded enveloped RNA virus
- First isolated in 2001, ubiquitous worldwide
- Seasonal variation—peaks in late winter and early spring
- Most children are infected by 5 yo
- Usually causes mild self-limiting upper airways infection ~5 days after infection but may progress to wheezing and pneumonia or ARDS in some adults (especially the immunocompromised or elderly patients with comorbidities)
- Ongoing airways hyperreactivity may last for several weeks
- PCR/serological evidence of metapneumovirus in ~4% of adults admitted with acute lower respiratory tract infection
- Diagnosis is usually using in full reverse transcriptase PCR (RT-PCR), serology, or viral culture of nasopharyngeal or BAL specimens
- Treatment is supportive. Ribavirin may have activity *in vivo*, but this is still under investigation.

Parainfluenza

- Single-stranded enveloped RNA viruses; serotypes 1–4
- >90% of adults have antibodies to parainfluenza, but these are only partially protective
- Types 1–3 usually cause self-limiting upper respiratory infection but can cause pneumonia, particularly among the elderly or immunocompromised. Type 4 usually causes URTI
- Associated with asthma and COPD exacerbations
- Rarely causes myocarditis, meningitis, and Guillain–Barré syndrome
- Diagnosed using PCR, antigen detection, or viral culture on nasopharyngeal secretions or BAL fluid
- Treatment is supportive (no antivirals have proven efficacy), with reduction of immunosuppression (particularly glucocorticoids) when possible.

Respiratory syncytial virus

- Single-stranded enveloped RNA virus; subtypes A and B. Subtype A is associated with more severe disease
- Very common cause of bronchiolitis and pneumonia in children, causing winter outbreaks. Role in adult respiratory disease is more significant than previously appreciated, and infection often goes unrecognized
- Clinical features in adults are usually of URTI or tracheobronchitis, but this may progress to pneumonia, particularly in the setting of underlying cardiac or respiratory disease, malignancy, or immunosuppression; outbreaks affecting adults in hospitals and nursing homes also occur. RSV may be a relatively common viral cause of pneumonia in patients who have undergone bone marrow transplantation
- Nasopharyngeal secretions and BAL fluid are often diagnostic; detection of RSV antigen in BAL fluid has a sensitivity of nearly 90%. PCR-based diagnostic techniques and serological testing may have a role
- Bacterial superinfection may be a frequent complication
- Treatment is principally supportive. Role of aerosolized ribavirin and steroids in the treatment of severe disease in adults is unclear. Reports of successful outcomes in bone marrow transplant recipients following treatment with ribavirin and immunoglobulin.

Varicella pneumonia

- Caused by varicella-zoster virus (an enveloped dsDNA virus)
- Pneumonia occurs in a small proportion of adults with chickenpox or shingles but accounts for the majority of mortality associated with adult disease. Risk factors for its development include smoking, increased number of skin spots (>100), pregnancy (third trimester), steroid treatment, and immunocompromise
- There is typically a history of recent exposure to a contact infected with chickenpox or shingles. Chest symptoms tend to occur several days after the onset of rash (erythematous macules progressing to papules and then vesicles), although rarely may precede the rash. Cough and breathlessness are common, and pleuritic pain and haemoptysis may occur
- CXR typically shows a diffuse small nodular infiltrate; hilar lymphadenopathy and pleural effusions may uncommonly occur. Nodules may subsequently calcify and persist
- Multi-organ involvement may occur
- Diagnosis is usually suspected on the basis of the history of exposure, presence of rash, and CXR features. Cytological examination of smears from skin lesions, serology, or viral culture or PCR on BAL fluid may confirm the diagnosis
- Treatment of varicella pneumonia is with early administration of aciclovir 10–12.5mg/kg IV tds for 7–10 days. Aciclovir is not licensed for use in pregnancy but does not appear to be associated with increased foetal abnormalities, and the benefits of treatment almost certainly outweigh any risk. Varicella is very infectious until lesions enter the 'crusting' stage; inpatients should be isolated. Extracorporeal membrane oxygenation/life support has been used successfully in individuals with fulminant respiratory failure. Consider early administration of varicella-zoster immune globulin for immunocompromised and pregnant patients exposed to varicella
- Most cases resolve spontaneously, but a minority progresses to respiratory failure and death (10–30%). Mortality may be significantly higher in pregnancy.

Hantavirus pulmonary syndrome

- Also known as hantavirus cardiopulmonary syndrome
- Caused by single-stranded enveloped RNA hantaviruses
- First described following an outbreak in the SW USA in 1993. Several different hantaviruses (e.g. Sin Nombre virus) have been associated with this syndrome. Previously described hantavirus-associated diseases occur more commonly in Scandinavia and north-eastern Asia and tended to cause haemorrhagic fever and renal failure, with relative sparing of the lung
- Very rare, and affected individuals are almost exclusively from America, particularly from the Four Corners Region of USA where Arizona, Colorado, Utah, and New Mexico meet. A 2012 outbreak, affecting ten people who visited Yosemite National Park (California), was thought to be associated with rodent infestation in cabin insulation
- Disease develops following inhalation of aerosolized viruses from rodent faeces, urine, or saliva and typically affects previously well young adults
- Common presenting symptoms are fever, chills, cough, myalgia, and GI symptoms such as vomiting and abdominal pain. Breathlessness occurs later in the disease course and is often quickly followed by respiratory failure and the development of ARDS. Shock may occur and is associated with a poor prognosis
- Laboratory testing classically reveals neutrophilia, thrombocytopenia, elevated lactate dehydrogenase (LDH), and sometimes renal impairment and mildly abnormal LFTs. Leucocytosis and immunoblasts in peripheral blood are associated with severe disease
- CXR typically shows initially bilateral basal infiltrates that progress to involve all regions of the lung; a minority are normal
- Diagnosis may be confirmed using serology, PCR for the virus, or by detection of viral antigen using immunochemistry
- Treatment is supportive within an ICU, including the use of extracorporeal membrane oxygenation when appropriate. It is unclear if person-to-person transmission occurs, and patients should be in respiratory isolation. IV ribavirin may be administered, although this has not been demonstrated to improve outcome
- Mortality 10–50%, with death usually occurring within several days of presentation.

Coronavirus disease 2019 (COVID-19)

Severe acute respiratory syndrome coronavirus 2 (SARS-CoV-2) is a novel coronavirus responsible for the illness coronavirus disease 2019 (COVID-19). The first reported cases of infection with SARS-CoV-2 were in Wuhan, China in December 2019 and have since spread into a global pandemic. SARS-CoV-2 is an RNA virus which is genetically similar to the other betacoronaviruses: SARS-CoV-1 (which causes SARS see ❥ p. 651) and Middle East respiratory syndrome coronavirus (MERS-CoV, the cause of MERS see ❥ p. 654).

Like SARS-CoV-1, SARS-CoV-2 enters human cells through the angiotensin-converting enzyme 2 (ACE2) receptor, which is widely expressed in different tissues, including the lung. Although COVID-19 has a lower mortality than SARS and MERS, SARS-CoV-2 is considerably more infectious and, importantly, individuals can transmit infection in the absence of symptoms. SARS-CoV-2 is spread through respiratory droplets on coughing and sneezing and appears to demonstrate prolonged stability on surfaces; there is suspicion of aerosol transmission, although this has not yet been proven. The rapid spread and high mortality of COVID-19 have led many countries to enforce stringent public health measures such as self-isolation and community 'lock-downs' in an attempt to limit infection.

Risk factors

Risk factors for severe disease are still being defined but seem to include increasing age, male sex, non-white ethnicity, obesity, social deprivation, and underlying diabetes, cardiovascular disease, chronic lung disease, and haematological malignancy. Hypertension appears to increase the risk of disease; there does not currently appear to be a clear association with ACE inhibitor or angiotensin receptor blocker drugs, although this is the subject of ongoing research.

Clinical features

- Incubation period from exposure to symptoms typically 4–5 d
- Effects range from asymptomatic infection (studies suggest ~15%) to pneumonia, ARDS, multiorgan failure, and death
- Most present with cough, fever, malaise, and myalgia; anosmia and GI symptoms such as diarrhoea are common. Delirium is well described in the elderly and in severe disease
- Absence of fever is not uncommon. Some cohort studies in China and US showed only 30% of patients had fever on hospital admission
- Breathlessness is a concerning symptom for worsening disease; typically develops 5–7 d after illness onset. May be relatively mild even in patients with significant hypoxaemia, and such apparent tolerance of hypoxia appears to be a characteristic feature of COVID-19.

Laboratory features

- Lymphopenia and elevated CRP typical but not universal
- Transaminitis common
- Clotting derangement common, with prolonged prothrombin time (PT) and significant elevations of D-dimer and fibrinogen

- Elevated troponin occurs in a subgroup of patients. Poor prognostic factor
- Some develop features of secondary haemophagocytic lymphohistiocytosis (sHLH), with markedly elevated ferritin and triglyceride levels and cytopenias in the context of severe lung disease and fever.

Imaging

CXR

- May be normal
- 'Classic' appearances—multiple bilateral lung opacities (lower zone and peripheral predominance)
- Findings not typical for COVID-19—lobar consolidation, pleural effusion, pneumothorax, peri-hilar consolidation of pulmonary oedema
- 'Indeterminate' findings are those that fit neither the Classic nor non-COVID-19 descriptors.

CT

- Not generally undertaken if CXR classic and clinical course as expected
- May be normal
- 'Classic' appearances—bilateral, basal predominant patchy ground-glass, crazy paving (combination of ground glass and interlobular thickening), peripheral consolidation, peri-lobular pattern, and reverse halo sign.
- Findings not typical for COVID-19—lobar consolidation, cavitation, tree-in-bud opacities, centrilobular nodules, effusions, lymphadenopathy
- 'Indeterminate' findings—non-peripheral and unilateral changes
- Low threshold for computed tomographic pulmonary angiogram (CTPA) if clinically worsening, particularly if suspicion of thromboembolic disease (common with COVID-19).

Differential diagnosis

Includes any respiratory disease that causes significant hypoxia, plus other infectious causes.

- Viral pneumonia (typically seasonal Influenza A and B)
- Bacterial pneumonia
- Pulmonary embolism
- Pulmonary oedema
- New diagnosis of ILD (plus infection)

COVID-19 diagnosis may not be confirmed for 24–48 hours, but the history (including exposure), typical CXR appearance and blood parameters will determine clinical probability while awaiting laboratory confirmation.

Diagnosis is currently made on detection of SARS-CoV-2 RNA by RT-PCR testing of naso-oropharyngeal swab. PCR testing has high specificity (~100%) but lower sensitivity (60–70%), perhaps due to poor specimen quality or testing late in the disease course. Repeat the test if negative yet diagnosis suspected; even multiple negative tests are well described in the setting of classical clinical, imaging, and laboratory features and so do not exclude COVID-19. Testing of saliva is under investigation; PCR testing of sputum or BAL samples may have greater sensitivity. Positive PCR testing does not necessarily indicate viable virus in a recovering patient.

Antibody tests to SARS-CoV-2 antigens (spike protein or nucleocapsid) are currently in development; sensitivity likely to be low early in the disease but increase with time. Antibody testing may be useful in diagnosing patients who present late (≥2 weeks) after symptom onset, as well as in studying community and healthcare spread of infection. Not yet clear whether a positive serological test correlates with clinical immunity and protection against reinfection.

Severity assessment

A number of severity scores have been proposed, awaiting validation, including:

- Epidemiological factors (age, pre-existing medical conditions, use of immunosuppressive drugs)
- Laboratory features (elevated CRP, ferritin, LDH, troponin, D-dimer, CK, reduced lymphocyte count)
- NEWS2 (see ➾ p. 757).

Management

Multiple studies of drug treatments are ongoing (see below). Main treatment is management of hypoxia. This is predominantly type 1 ventilatory failure, thought to be due diffuse alveolar damage with interstitial thickening. Hypoxic vasoconstriction and atelectasis also contribute, with some individuals presenting with significant hypoxia without proportional signs of respiratory distress. Some have described this as an atypical ARDS picture.

Hypoxia

Use oxygen to target $SaO_2 \geq 92\%$ in those with no underlying lung disease. SaO_2 88-92% appropriate for those with risk factors for type 2 respiratory failure.

If hypoxia persists despite high-flow mask oxygen, start non-invasive ventilation (NIV) with continuous positive airway pressure (CPAP) (starting pressure 6–8 cm H_2O with supplemental oxygen). High-flow nasal oxygen is an alternative (though this has been used less frequently in the UK during pandemic because of concerns about lack of efficacy, excessive oxygen use, and nosocomial infection risks). Bi-level ventilation, also an NIV, is indicated for those with hypercapnia.

As with any treatment for respiratory failure, a decision should be made about escalation should these treatments fail. CPAP may be the ceiling of care or may be a bridge to avoid/delay invasive mechanical ventilation or an aid post-extubation. Start CPAP in discussion with ICU team if transfer to ICU is appropriate should CPAP fail. Frailty scores may help decision making in those with significant comorbidity (See ✎ https://www.bgs.org.uk/sites/default/files/content/attachment/2018-07-05/rockwood_cfs.pdf)

Practical considerations

CPAP/NIV is classed as an aerosol-generating procedure (AGP) which poses risks of nosocomial infection. A non-vented mask must be used with a viral filter between the mask and the exhalation port, with entrained oxygen at the patient end.

Occasionally, sedation with either as required anxiolytic (e.g. sublingual lorazepam 0.5 mg/4 h) or a continuous syringe driver (e.g. subcutaneous morphine 5 mg plus midazolam 5 mg/24 h) may aid improve tolerance of CPAP and reduce the frightening sensation of breathlessness.

Awake prone positioning may aid oxygenation. Usually delivered by physiotherapy team.

Once started, review CPAP at 30–60 minutes. Indicators of improvement—improved comfort, reduced respiratory rate (RR), improved saturations. Confirm mask fit, leak, pressures, and entrained oxygen. Alert ICU (if appropriate) if increasing pressures or entrained oxygen requirements.

Infection

Antibiotics are not indicated for uncomplicated non-severe COVID-19 infection.

On admission, ill patients requiring oxygen are normally treated with antibiotics for severe bacterial CAP (follow local protocols, check legionella and pneumococcal antigens) for the first 24–48h, pending SARS-CoV-2 swab result. A low procalcitonin level may aid early de-escalation of antibiotics.

Thromboprophylaxis

Given high rates of venous thromboembolism (VTE), increased doses of low molecular weight heparin (LMWH) thromboprophylaxis may be required—follow local protocols and reassess if rising D-dimer.

Remdesivir

At the time of writing, remdesivir has received a favourable opinion for use by the UK MHRA in an Early Access to Medicines Scheme for patients at increased risk of severe COVID-19. Remdesivir is a nucleotide analogue which has been shown to reduce recovery time in patients with severe COVID-19 in one large RCT. Studies are ongoing, some of which have failed to demonstrate benefit.

Complications

In addition to viral pneumonitis, a number of complications of COVID-19 infection are recognised.

- **VTE** is a common complication due to a prothrombotic state. Case series have shown 20–70% of patients with severe infection have PE. This is associated with a poorer outcome and should be treated with anticoagulation. Enhanced VTE prophylaxis for COVID-19 infection is being studied.
- **Microvascular embolic disease** may be a clinically important entity but is not apparent on CT pulmonary angiography.
- **Cytokine release syndrome (CRS)** describes the release of multiple inflammatory cytokines and may cause organ failure, including ARDS. CRS is thought to represent a virus-induced sHLH. Elevated inflammatory cytokines (particularly interleukin-6) are commonly seen in the blood of patients with severe COVID-19 infection and are associated with a poorer prognosis. Anti-inflammatory therapies targeting various cytokine pathways, such as the anti-IL-6 receptor drug tocilizumab, are being trialled.
- **Neurological complications** include critical care neuropathy, hypoxic encephalopathy, and stroke as well as rarer complications, e.g. Guillain-Barré syndrome.
- **Liver function abnormalities** are common, with up to 75% of patients having some derangement.

- **Acute kidney injury** is seen in around 5% of cases and is more common in elderly patients and those with coexisting renal or cardiovascular disease.
- **Cardiac complications** include acute coronary syndrome, myocarditis, and arrhythmias.
- **Bacterial infection** as a secondary lung insult occurs in around 10% of severe COVID-19 infection.

Outcome

Approximately 80% of cases are mild and recover by around two weeks. The long-term consequences of more severe COVID-19 are not yet known. Overall, the reported mortality is variable but ~1-2%. In hospitalised cases, ICU support is required for ~20%, which is often prolonged. This is expected to lead to post-critical care syndrome, which is likely to necessitate extensive rehabilitation. Fibrotic changes and impaired lung function have been reported. Little is known about the impact of severe COVID-19 disease on long-term mental health, physical function, and lung function.

Trials

COVID-19 is a global research priority with hundreds of active clinical trials. At time of writing, few RCTs have been published. Key interventions being evaluated include antiviral therapies, anticoagulation, respiratory support (CPAP and high flow nasal oxygen (HFNO) vs. intubation), and vaccines. Drug therapies include repurposed drugs, RNA polymerase inhibitors, and adjunctive therapies.

Repurposed drugs with antiviral properties being investigated include chloroquine, hydroxychloroquine, azithromycin, and combination lopinavir/ritonavir (Kaletra). An RCT of high- and low-dose chloroquine was stopped early due to 3.5-fold increased risk of death in the high-dose group. Chloroquine, azithromycin, and to a lesser extent hydroxychloroquine can all prolong the QT interval. Combination lopinavir/ritonavir showed no improvement in time to clinical improvement in a 199 patient RCT, although this was underpowered to detect changes in mortality and randomisation was common after 10 days of illness.

Trials of adjunctive therapies include corticosteroids, immunomodulatory drugs (agents targeted against IL-6, e.g. tocilizumab, and agents targeted against JAK-2, e.g. baricitinib), and convalescent plasma from recovered patients. There are no RCTs yet published reporting the effects of adjunctive therapies in COVID-19. It is not known if the benefit of these therapies will outweigh the harms; corticosteroids have been shown to be harmful in other causes of viral pneumonia. In addition to drug therapies, approximately 20 trials are developing vaccines to prevent COVID-19.

Further info

WHO website for COVID-19
🖰 https://www.who.int/emergencies/diseases/novel-coronavirus-2019
JAMA network COVID-19 page
🖰 https://jamanetwork.com/journals/jama/pages/coronavirus-alert
NEJM COVID-19 page
🖰 https://www.nejm.org/coronavirus
Lancet COVID-19 page
🖰 https://www.thelancet.com/coronavirus
Dashboard for COVID-19 cases worldwide
🖰 https://www.worldometers.info/coronavirus/
Lancet dashboard for COVID-19 trials
🖰 https://www.covid-trials.org/

Severe acute respiratory syndrome (SARS)

Caused by SARS-coronavirus (SARS-CoV; an enveloped RNA virus).

Epidemiology

Rapidly progressive acute respiratory illness, first recognized in November 2002 in the Guangdong province of China. By late February 2003, it had spread internationally, with 792 cases reported. First outbreak mainly affected health care workers and contacts. Spread via Hong Kong to Singapore, Thailand, Vietnam, and Canada via travellers. By July 2003, the worldwide epidemic had ended. There were a few cases in 2004, mostly laboratory-related, and no further cases thereafter.

A total of 8,096 cases were reported to the WHO by August 2003, with 774 deaths, giving a case fatality rate of 9.5%. The fatality rate for those aged ≥60 was 43%. Twenty-nine countries on all five continents were affected; 83% of the worldwide cases were in China and Hong Kong. No deaths occurred in the USA or the UK; 43 deaths (of 251 cases) were in Canada.

Case definition

WHO defined criteria for those presenting with the disease after July 2004 (ℬ http://www.who.int/csr/sars/en):
- Fever >38°C, *plus*
- One or more symptom of lower respiratory tract illness (cough, difficulty breathing, SOB), *plus*
- Radiographic evidence of lung infiltrate, consistent with pneumonia or ARDS, *or* autopsy findings consistent with the pathology of pneumonia *or* ARDS without identifiable cause, *plus*
- No alternative diagnosis to explain the illness.

Laboratory case definition

- A person with symptoms or signs suggestive of SARS, *plus*
- Positive laboratory findings for SARS-CoV, based on one or more of:
  - PCR positive for SARS-CoV for two separate samples
  - Seroconversion by ELISA or immunofluorescence assay
  - Virus isolation.

Pathophysiology

A previously undescribed coronavirus (SARS-CoV) is the causal agent. It is thought that animals, possibly palm civets (similar to cats) or bats, act as the main reservoir. SARS is mostly spread by large droplets and person-to-person contact. There have been no reports of foodborne or waterborne transmission. However, SARS-CoV is shed in large quantities in stool, and profuse watery diarrhoea is a common symptom.

Lung post-mortem studies show diffuse alveolar damage, 2° bacterial pneumonia, and interstitial giant cell and macrophage infiltration. Pathological findings similar to those of bronchiolitis obliterans are recognized. There are no specific diagnostic features.

Incubation period

2–10 days prior to the onset of the first symptom, which is typically fever.

Clinical features

A two-stage illness, commencing with a prodrome of fever (>38°C), with or without rigors, with non-specific systemic symptoms, e.g. malaise, headache, and myalgia.

The respiratory stage of the illness starts 3–7 days after the prodromal phase, with dry cough and breathlessness. Progression to respiratory failure needing ventilation is well recognized. Up to 70% of patients develop large-volume watery diarrhoea.

Destruction of lung tissue is thought to result from an excessive immune response to the virus, rather than from the direct effects of virus replication. Peak viral load is at day 12–14 of infection, with virus shed not only in respiratory secretions, but in faeces and other body fluids.

Retrospectively devised, but non-validated, scoring systems show that the presence of cough, myalgia, diarrhoea, and rhinorrhoea or sore throat are 100% sensitive and 76% specific at identifying a patient with SARS.

Children experience a milder form of the disease, with a low death rate.

Investigations

- Blood tests:
  - White blood count is normal or reduced; low lymphocyte count is common. Leukopenia and thrombocytopenia also recognized
  - Raised CK and alanine aminotransferase (ALT). Raised LDH is associated with a poorer outcome
- CXR—ranges from normal to diffuse bilateral interstitial infiltrate. Areas of focal consolidation, initially peripherally and lower zone in distribution, are also described. Cavitation, hilar lymphadenopathy, and pleural effusion are uncommon at presentation
- CT—interstitial infiltrate, ground-glass opacities, and interlobular septal thickening in those with a normal CXR. Spontaneous pneumothorax, pneumomediastinum, subpleural fibrosis, and/or cystic changes can occur in later stages
- SARS-CoV can be detected by RT-PCR (sensitivity 70%, dependent on specimen type and duration of illness). Useful specimens include nasopharyngeal aspirate, throat swab, urine, and faeces. An initial positive result on PCR must be confirmed by another clinical sample. Serology is sensitive, but seroconversion takes 20 days.

Treatment

There is no specific treatment for SARS, other than general supportive care. Ribavirin has been used but no clear benefit and toxicities common. Lopinavir-ritonavir may have some activity, but evidence of benefit is lacking. Vaccinations are in development.

Hospital admission

Nosocomial transmission of SARS-CoV has been a striking feature in most outbreaks. Infected and suspected cases should be managed in negative pressure side rooms. Full protective clothing, including protective eye wear and face masks, is recommended for all visitors and health care workers. Aerosol-generating procedures (endotracheal intubation, nebulization, bronchoscopy) may amplify transmission.

Prognosis

Older age is associated with a poorer outcome. Diabetes and other comorbid illness are independent risk factors for death.

Middle East respiratory syndrome (MERS)

- Caused by the novel MERS-coronavirus (MERS-CoV), an enveloped zoonotic RNA virus first reported in Saudi Arabia in 2012
- Closely related to bat coronaviruses
- Entered the human population by direct or indirect contact with infected dromedary camels, most commonly in the Arabian Peninsula. Human-to-human spread mostly in healthcare settings
- 2,449 laboratory confirmed cases reported as of July 2019, with 845 deaths, predominantly in Middle East countries (particularly Saudi Arabia) and in travellers returning from the Middle East
- Most patients are severely ill with pneumonia and ARDS, and many have acute kidney injury. Case fatality rate of around 35%
- Diarrhoea, DIC, and pericarditis also seen.

Diagnosis

- Using RT-PCR to detect MERS-CoV in respiratory samples (e.g. nasopharyngeal fluid, sputum, or BAL fluid)
- Testing recommended by WHO for the following:
  - People with acute respiratory infection requiring admission and any of:
    - Disease occurring as part of a cluster occurring within 10 days, unless another aetiology found
    - Disease occurring in a health care worker working in an environment where patients with severe acute respiratory infections are cared for, unless another aetiology found
    - Disease occurring within 10 days of travel to the Middle East, unless another aetiology found
    - Disease follows an unexpectedly severe course despite appropriate treatment
    - People with acute respiratory illness of any severity who had exposure to a probable case of MERS-CoV within 10 days
    - Patients requiring mechanical ventilation in countries where MERS-CoV has been detected.

Treatment

Supportive. Antiviral agents are not currently recommended. Infection control precautions are essential.

Vaccinations and specific anti-viral therapies are under investigation.

Further information

Zumla A et al. Middle East Respiratory Syndrome. Lancet 2015; **386**:995–1007.
WHO website. ℰ http://www.who.int/csr/disease/coronavirus_infections/en/

Chapter 46

Sarcoidosis

Epidemiology, aetiology, and immunopathology 656
Chest disease: clinical features 658
Chest disease: diagnosis and monitoring 660
Management 662
Extrathoracic disease 1 666
Extrathoracic disease 2 668

Epidemiology, aetiology, and immunopathology

Definition

- A multi-system disorder of unknown cause, likely resulting from the interplay of environmental and genetic factors
- Characterized by non-caseating granulomata and CD4+ Th1-biased T-cell response in affected organs
- Commonly involves the respiratory system but can affect nearly all organs
- 50–60% of people have spontaneous remissions; others may develop chronic, and sometimes progressive, disease.

Epidemiology

Incidence varies across population studies, from 5 to 100/100,000, according to geographic distribution. UK incidence is about 5–10/100,000. Commoner in African Americans, West Indians, and the Irish. Commonly presents between ages of 20 and 40. Unusual in children and the elderly. Typically more aggressive disease in black populations than in Caucasians—higher incidence of skin disease, peripheral lymphadenopathy, bone marrow, and liver involvement; higher relapse rates and worse long-term prognosis.

Aetiology

Sarcoidosis is the result of an abnormal immunological response to a benign environmental trigger(s) or antigen(s). The environmental trigger is likely to be a poorly degradable antigen but not a specific antigen or infectious agent. This abnormal immunology occurs in a genetically predisposed host.

Genetics

Familial and ethnic clustering of cases suggest a genetic predisposition. Best evidence of human leucocyte antigen (HLA) association comes from large multicentre ACCESS study, showing HLA-DRB1*1101 is associated with susceptibility to disease in blacks and whites; HLA-DRB1*0301 has been associated with acute and remitting disease. Genome-wide association studies have identified polymorphisms in *BTNL2*, *ANXA11*, and *FAM178A* as susceptibility genes in both familial and sporadic cases.

Immunopathology

- Unknown antigen triggers CD4 (helper) T-cell activation and expansion. This response is exaggerated and Th1-biased, with resultant interferon γ and IL2 production from these T-cells
- Activated T-cells proliferate and release mediators, attracting additional inflammatory cells, with concomitant macrophage activation and aggregation
- This leads to immune granuloma formation, which is enhanced by interferon γ
- Granulomata themselves cause increased local fibroblast stimulation and hence eventual fibrosis
- Metabolic activity of macrophages causes raised angiotensin-converting enzyme (ACE levels in serum, lung tissue, and bronchoalveolar fluid.

Increase in T-cell activity causes B-lymphocyte stimulation, which can cause raised serum immunoglobulins and immune complexes
• In most patients, these immune responses resolve over 2–5 y.

Delayed-type hypersensitivity reactions are depressed
This is thought to be due to the migration of activated lymphocytes to the active compartment (lungs), with resultant peripheral blood lymphopenia. Seen as a decreased response to tuberculin, mumps virus, and *Candida albicans* antigens. This is not thought to be clinically significant.

Sarcoid-like reactions
Reported in association with malignancy (mainly lymphoma, cervical, liver, lung, testes, and uterus). Non-caseating pulmonary granulomas are found, but there are no other symptoms or signs of sarcoidosis.

The main differential diagnoses of granuloma on a lung biopsy are shown in Box 46.1.

> **Box 46.1 Differential diagnosis of granuloma on lung biopsy**
> • Sarcoidosis
> • Tuberculosis
> • Hypersensitivity pneumonitis
> • Granulomatosis with polyangiitis (Wegener's)
> • Drug reactions
> • Non tuberculous mycobacteria infection
> • Fungal infections:
>   • Cryptococcosis
>   • Aspergillosis
>   • Coccidioidomycosis
>   • Blastomycosis
> • Aspiration of foreign material
> • Primary biliary cirrhosis
> • Sarcoid-like reaction to malignancy.

Further information

Iannuzzi MC. Advances in genetics of sarcoidosis. *Proc Am Thorac Soc* 2007;**4**: 457–460.
Schurmann M et al. Familial sarcoidosis is linked to the major histocompatibility complex region. *Am J Respir Crit Care Med* 2000;**162**: 861–864.
Schurmann M et al. HLA-DQB1 and HLA-DPB1 genotypes in familial sarcoidosis. *Respir Med* 1998;**92**: 649–652.

Chest disease: clinical features

More than 90% of patients with sarcoidosis have thoracic involvement, with an abnormal chest radiograph (CXR) (see Box 46.2 and Box 46.3). Pulmonary sarcoidosis can be an incidental CXR finding in ~30% of patients. There is spontaneous remission in two-thirds, and 10–30% have a chronic course.

Clinical features

There are probably at least two distinct clinical courses:
- *Löfgren's syndrome* Acute disease, which is usually self-limiting. Presents with fever, bilateral hilar lymphadenopathy, erythema nodosum, and arthralgia. Occurs particularly in Caucasians. Has a good prognosis and resolves completely and spontaneously in 80% within 1–2 y. A minority may develop lung disease
- *Persistent or progressive* infiltrative lung disease.

Hilar/mediastinal lymphadenopathy

May be asymptomatic or cause cough or chest pain. Usually bilateral and symmetrical, rarely unilateral and asymmetrical (this would suggest alternative diagnosis more likely). Can be associated with systemic symptoms of malaise and arthralgia, which are helped by non-steroidal anti-inflammatories (NSAIDs). Benign course.

Important to exclude other causes of lymphadenopathy such as tuberculosis (TB) and lymphoma (see Box 46.3). May need computed tomography (CT) and lymph node aspirate or biopsy.

Does not require systemic steroid treatment.

Stage I: 85% resolve spontaneously over 2 y; 15% develop lung infiltrates. The average time for bilateral hilar lymphadenopathy resolution is 8 months.

Interstitial lung involvement

May be asymptomatic or cause morbidity and mortality, with dyspnoea, cough, chest ache, or frank pain, malaise, fatigue, and impaired quality of life (QoL). Rarely have crackles or clubbing on examination. Pulmonary infiltrates on CXR. Can return to normal over time or progress to fibrosis and respiratory failure. Lung function tests may be normal or may show a restrictive defect with reduced transfer factor.

Differential diagnosis

Other interstitial lung disease (ILD), malignancy, infection.

Box 46.2 Scadding radiological classification of thoracic sarcoidosis

Stage 0 Normal
Stage I Hilar lymphadenopathy only
Stage II Hilar lymphadenopathy and parenchymal infiltrate
Stage III Parenchymal infiltrate
Stage IV Fibrosis

Seeing a patient with possible sarcoidosis in clinic
- Make diagnosis—clinically, HRCT ± histology
- Assess extent/severity/presence of extrapulmonary involvement—full blood count (FBC), CXR, pulmonary function tests (PFTs), electrocardiogram (ECG), eyes, rash, renal function, serum calcium, liver function, immunoglobulins, and ACE (last two can be raised in active sarcoidosis)
- Stable or progressive? FBC, CXR, PFT (vital capacity (VC) ± kCO), oximetry, ACE, urea (if renal involvement)
- Treatment?

Box 46.3 Differential diagnosis of bilateral hilar lymphadenopathy on CXR

- Sarcoidosis
- Tuberculosis
- Lymphoma
- Lung cancer, especially small cell
- Coccidioidomycosis and histoplasmosis
- Berylliosis
- Mycoplasma
- Hypersensitivity pneumonitis

Chest disease: diagnosis and monitoring

Diagnosis

Based on a characteristic clinical picture, plus:
- Histological evidence of non-caseating granuloma in any tissue
- Characteristic picture on imaging (thoracic high-resolution computed tomography (HRCT) scan or gallium scan)
- Lymphocytosis on bronchoalveolar lavage (BAL).

Other diseases capable of producing similar clinical and histological picture, particularly TB and lymphoma, should be excluded.

Investigations

- *HRCT* Micronodules in a subpleural and bronchovascular distribution. Fissural nodularity and bronchial distortion. Irregular linear opacities, ground-glass shadowing related to bronchovascular bundles, and nodular or ill-defined shadows. Air trapping due to small airway granulomata is common. Endobronchial disease in 55%. Minority have a usual interstitial pneumonia (UIP) pattern, associated with worse prognosis. Hilar and mediastinal lymphadenopathy.
- CT-guided biopsy of nodes seen on CT may be possible and yield a tissue diagnosis
- *Bronchoscopy (transbronchial biopsy (TBB), transbronchial needle aspiration (TBNA), bronchial biopsy, endobronchial ultrasound (EBUS), or BAL)* may not be necessary if no diagnostic doubt. May be important to exclude infectious agents. Positive yield of endobronchial biopsy is 40–60%. Higher if visible abnormal mucosa. Positive yield of TBB is 40–90% (yield still high even if lungs appear normal on HRCT). Initial procedure of choice for suspected pulmonary sarcoidosis. TBNA of mediastinal lymph nodes yields a diagnosis in 60–90% of cases. TBB and TBNA have a higher yield together than either alone. However, presence of non-caseating granulomas on TBB or bronchial biopsy more significant than on lymph node sampling, as granuloma can accompany tumour infiltration of lymph nodes. BAL in sarcoidosis shows a CD4:CD8 ratio of >3.5. A lymphocytosis of $>2 \times 10_5$cells/mL supports the diagnosis but is not diagnostic (also seen in hypersensitivity pneumonitis (HP) and drug-induced alveolitis)
- *Mediastinoscopy* for central or paratracheal nodes or *open lung biopsy*: 90% positive yield. May be necessary to exclude lymphoma, or if diagnosis is uncertain and no result/non-accessible nodes for EBUS and TBNA. Lymph node ± lung (usually via video-assisted thoracoscopic surgery (VATS)) can be biopsied
- *Biopsy other affected areas*, skin, liver, etc., if indicated, as these may be easier to biopsy in order to make a diagnosis
- *Mantoux/Heaf test* is typically grade 0 in sarcoidosis (peripheral cutaneous anergy to tuberculin due to migration of T-cells to active sites of disease). Positive Mantoux or Heaf test make sarcoidosis a less likely diagnosis although does not necessarily make TB more likely. Heaf testing not widely used now.

Monitoring disease

There is no single measurement to assess all the aspects of patients with sarcoidosis. Clinical examination and serial measurements are key.

- *PFT* Pulmonary sarcoidosis gives a restrictive defect with decreased TLC and VC. TLCO provides the most sensitive measurement of change, although many use a properly performed VC as an alternative. Likely to improve with steroids. Airflow obstruction may also occur
- *CXR* may improve with time or treatment
- *HRCT* can help with determining burden of active disease
- *Serum ACE* levels raised in up to 80% of patients with acute sarcoidosis although can be normal in active disease. This may be a surrogate marker of the total granuloma burden. Levels become normal as disease resolves. Can be useful to monitor the clinical course, if activity is uncertain, but levels should not be used in isolation to determine treatment. Levels suppressed by steroids, and, when steroids are stopped, levels usually increase, unrelated to sarcoidosis activity. This is not a specific test. False positives include TB
- *Calcium* may rise with active sarcoidosis or in the summer months. This may cause renal impairment, so urea or creatinine should also be checked. Calcium and vitamin D supplementation are not recommended if bone protection for osteoporosis prevention is being considered
- *BAL* not performed routinely to assess progress of sarcoidosis, but reduction in lymphocytosis would indicate improvement
- *PET* scan may be positive in areas of disease activity. Not reliable for studying brain or heart. Limited studies of serial data.

Management

Most patients with pulmonary sarcoidosis do not require treatment. Asymptomatic CXR infiltrates are usually just monitored. The most recent British Thoracic Society (BTS) guidelines were issued in 2008 (see Box 46.4).

> **Box 46.4 BTS guidelines for the management of sarcoidosis (2008)**
> * Because of the high rate of spontaneous remission, treatment is not indicated for asymptomatic stage I disease
> * Because of high rates of remission, treatment is not indicated in asymptomatic stage II or III disease with mildly abnormal lung function and stable disease
> * Oral corticosteroids are the first line of therapy in patients with progressive disease determined by radiology or on lung function, significant symptoms, or extrapulmonary disease requiring treatment
> * Treatment with prednisolone (or equivalent) 0.5 mg/kg/day for 4 weeks, then reduced to a maintenance dose which will control symptoms and disease progression, should be used for a period of 6–24 months
> * Bisphosphonates should be used to minimize steroid-induced osteoporosis
> * Inhaled corticosteroids, either as initial treatment or maintenance therapy, are not of significant benefit. They may be considered for symptom control (cough) in a subgroup of patients
> * Other immunosuppressive or anti-inflammatory treatments only have a limited role but should be considered in patients when corticosteroids are not controlling the disease or side effects are intolerable. At present, methotrexate is the treatment of choice
> * Lung transplantation should be considered in end-stage pulmonary sarcoidosis.

Starting drug treatment
* When required, treatment is usually with *steroids* initially. Good evidence for short- to medium-term improvement in symptoms, respiratory function, and radiology, but long-term benefits less clear
* Give high doses, such as 30 mg prednisolone/day, to control active disease. Rarely need >40 mg/day. Usually give this high dose for 2–3 weeks, and then reduce if there has been a response
* *Maintenance dose* of around 5–20 mg to control symptoms and prevent progression of disease. Leave on this dose for a few months, and then slowly reduce steroid dose further. Maintain on low dose of prednisolone (5–7.5 mg/day or alternate days) for prolonged period of up to 12 months to consolidate resolution, before considering complete withdrawal. Remember bone protection with a bisphosphonate (avoid routine calcium and vitamin D supplementation)
* Some patients, e.g. with progressive pulmonary sarcoidosis, may require longer treatment (years) of low-dose prednisolone to prevent relapse

- *Inhaled steroids* are of limited efficacy in sarcoidosis but may be useful if there is cough or bronchial hyperreactivity
- *Relapses* often occur when treatment is stopped and may require the reintroduction of steroids or the increase of steroid dose. Duration and dose of steroids is dictated by site and response to treatment
- *If steroid treatment fails* or sarcoidosis life-threatening, other immunosuppressive regimes may be indicated (see Box 46.5), e.g. pulsed high-dose intravenous (IV) methylprednisolone, especially for neurosarcoidosis
- In cases where *prolonged immunosuppression* is required (see Box 46.5), or if steroid side effects cannot be tolerated, other immunosuppressive drugs should be considered. Possibilities include azathioprine and methotrexate. There are limited data for their use in sarcoidosis
- Patients who have troublesome symptoms related to sarcoidosis, such as arthralgia, skin disease, fever, sweats, ocular symptoms, systemic symptoms such as fatigue, may require symptomatic steroid treatment. Lower initial doses, such as 20 mg/day, are likely to be sufficient to gain symptomatic control, and doses can then be reduced.

Box 46.5 Indications for immunosuppressive treatment
- Increasing symptoms, deteriorating PFTs, and worsening CXR infiltrates
- Cardiac sarcoidosis
- Neurosarcoidosis
- Sight-threatening ocular sarcoidosis
- Hypercalcaemia
- Lupus pernio
- Splenic, hepatic, or renal sarcoidosis.

Other drugs used in sarcoidosis

(See → p. 739 for more information regarding immunosuppressive drugs.)
  If there is progressive pulmonary sarcoidosis refractory to steroids, consider:
- *Methotrexate* Given once/week 10–15 mg PO for 6-month trial. Use instead of, or in addition to, low-dose prednisolone. Avoid if hepatic or renal failure. Side effects: gastrointestinal (GI) upset, stomatitis, pneumonitis, myelosuppression. Teratogenic. Monitor FBC and mean corpuscular volume (MCV), aspartate aminotransferase (AST), alanine aminotransferase (ALT) every 2 weeks for 3 months, then monthly. Do not use for >2 y without review. Useful for chronic sarcoidosis and cutaneous disease
- *Azathioprine* Used in neurosarcoidosis and stages II/III pulmonary sarcoidosis with partial/no steroid response. 100–150 mg/day. Use instead of, or in addition to, low-dose prednisolone. Side effects: myelosuppression, GI upset, stomatitis, idiosyncratic reaction—fever, rash. Low oncogenic potential. No gonadal toxicity. Check FBC every 2 weeks for 3 months, then monthly. Thiopurine methyltransferase (TPMT) testing should be performed prior to commencement (see → p. 742)

- *Anti-malarials* Hydroxychloroquine 200 mg od/bd. For skin and particularly hypercalcaemia. Steroid-sparing. Can be given with steroids and other immunosuppressant in severe sarcoidosis. Side effects: rarely ocular toxicity
- *Others* Leflunomide, ciclosporin, thalidomide, TNF-α inhibitors (etanercept, infliximab, adalimumab, golimumab), to be used in conjunction with specialist centres.

Prognosis

There are no prognostic markers in sarcoidosis, apart from:
- *Good prognosis* Löfgren's syndrome has complete resolution in 80% of people. Associated with HLA-DQB1*0201
- *Poorer prognosis with chronic disease* Lupus pernio, nasal mucosa involvement, chronic uveitis, chronic hypercalcaemia, nephrocalcinosis, neural involvement, age >40, and black race
- Prognosis according to CXR appearance:
  - Stage II: 50% cases recover spontaneously in 2 y; 30–40% require systemic steroids; 10–15% require long-term steroids
  - Stage III: worse prognosis. Only 30% show significant improvement with steroids
- Gene expression from mRNA profiling has shown early promise in differentiating progressive from non-progressive disease.

Transplant

Consider if patient has end-stage lung disease, rapidly progressive disease despite treatment, or if they are O_2-dependent. Sarcoidosis is a rare indication for lung transplant. Granulomata recur in transplanted lung but do not cause higher rates of graft failure.

Extrathoracic disease 1

Varies according to ethnic origin and sex of patient.

Systemic symptoms

Common symptoms include fever, sweats, loss of appetite, weight loss, fatigue, malaise, chest pain, dyspnoea, and cough. Polyarthralgia often affects the knees, ankles, wrists, and elbows and can be improved by NSAIDs.

Hypercalcaemia

Granulomata convert vitamin D3 to active 1,25 dihydroxycholecalciferol. This causes enhanced calcium absorption from intestine. Sunlight also increases levels of vitamin D and calcium. High calcium may cause systemic effects and is often associated with renal damage and hypercalciuria. Commoner in Caucasians and in men.

Treatment

If mildly raised, limit dietary calcium intake; avoid sun exposure, and drink plenty of fluids. Otherwise, steroids, often low dose once calcium level controlled (should be within 2 weeks—if not, investigate for other cause for hypercalcaemia). Decrease dose when calcium level satisfactory. Some patients may only need steroids during the summer months. Hydroxychloroquine can also be used.

Skin

25% of patients have skin involvement. More common in women.

Erythema nodosum

Raised papules, nodules, or plaques, usually on shins. Also tender, indurated, or bruised appearance. Firm and often have shiny appearance. Nodular change involving different tattoo colours recognized and is characteristic of sarcoidosis. Sarcoid tissue may arise in old scars or cause scar hypertrophy. Typically seen in Löfgren's syndrome.

Lupus pernio

A bluish tinge that occurs on nose, cheeks, and ears. It is associated with chronic disease.

Diagnosis

Usually easily biopsied.

Treatment

Initially with topical preparations. Lupus pernio should be treated with systemic steroids. Hydroxychloroquine or methotrexate may be necessary. Role of long-term tetracyclines for cutaneous sarcoidosis under investigation.

Eye

Common, occurring in 25% plus of cases, especially women and African-Caribbeans.

Uveitis (acute or chronic), episcleritis, scleritis, glaucoma, conjunctivitis, and retinal involvement can occur. May be asymptomatic or cause painful red eye, with photophobia, lacrimation, and blurred vision. Pupil irregular or constricted. Untreated, can cause visual impairment.

Lacrimal involvement in sarcoidosis gives keratoconjunctivitis sicca—dry eye with diminished tear secretion. Painful red eyes. Treat with artificial tears.

Diagnosis

Assessment by an ophthalmologist with slit lamp examination if any ocular symptoms. Some recommend that all newly diagnosed patients with sarcoidosis have slit lamp examination. Mild asymptomatic eye involvement is common. May need conjunctival biopsy if no evidence of sarcoid elsewhere.

Treatment

Local steroids are commonly used if there is no other indication for systemic steroids. However, if it does not respond, systemic steroids should be used.

Heart

Cardiac sarcoidosis occurs in 5% of patients with pulmonary disease. Postmortem studies show cardiac sarcoidosis is present in 25% so is often undiagnosed. Patients may present with chest pain or, more commonly, are found to have conduction defects on the ECG. These may be benign and asymptomatic, like first-degree heart block, but more significant arrhythmias can occur, the first indication of which may be sudden death. Myocardial granulomata can occur in any part of the heart. Commonly, they occur in the interventricular septum where they can affect nodal and conducting tissue. The left ventricular (LV) wall can be affected, with fibrosis causing reduced compliance and contractile difficulties, leading to cardiac failure. Aneurysms can form, and pericarditis can occur. Valvular dysfunction due to infiltration of the papillary muscles is rare. The clinical course can be uncertain.

Diagnosis

Echo may show signs of cardiomyopathy—usually restrictive. MRI, technetium scan, or gallium scan show non-segmental fixed defects. Biopsy is diagnostic but can be difficult, as sarcoidosis is patchy. Not recommended in general. ECG and 24 h tape may be helpful in identifying potentially fatal arrhythmias and conduction defects.

Treatment

Must be treated with systemic steroids 20–40 mg prednisolone/day, which improves symptoms, ECG, and echo features. These should be slowly reduced, but intractable arrhythmias may need continued high dosage. May need other immunosuppressants. Investigate with 24 h tape and electrophysiological studies if uncertain. Amiodarone, a pacemaker, implantable defibrillator, or heart transplant may be necessary.

In clinic

Perform a screening ECG on all patients with sarcoidosis, perhaps every 6 months.

Extrathoracic disease 2

Kidney

A degree of renal involvement is found in 35% of patients with sarcoidosis. Rarely can present with renal failure (especially following onset of hypercalcaemia), obstructive uropathy, nephrolithiasis, or urinary tract disorder. Nephrocalcinosis is a common cause of chronic renal failure. Often associated hypercalcaemia or other manifestation of sarcoidosis.

Diagnosis
Renal biopsy with granulomata found in interstitium, but this is rarely needed in this context. Search for pulmonary sarcoidosis.

Treatment
Steroids ± hydroxychloroquine for hypercalcaemia.

Central nervous system (CNS)

Involved in 4–18% of patients. Can affect any part of the peripheral or central nervous system. Can present as a peripheral nerve or cranial nerve lesion. Most common is lower motor neurone facial nerve palsy, with optic nerve involvement being next most common. Mononeuritis multiplex recognized. May be less specific, with psychiatric features. Hypothalamic granulomata may cause diabetes insipidus, appetite disturbance, or hypersomnolence.

Diagnosis
Difficult but may be made easier if there is another sign of systemic sarcoidosis, e.g. bilateral hilar lymphadenopathy. Lumbar puncture may show a raised cerebrospinal fluid (CSF) ACE and an increased lymphocyte count. Confirm with biopsy, if possible—cerebral or meningeal tissue if no pulmonary involvement.

Treatment
Must be treated with steroids, but often resistant to treatment. May need to try further immunosuppressants, e.g. TNF-α inhibitors.

Anxiety and depression

Associated with sarcoidosis and may be exacerbated by oral steroid use. Can contribute to fatigue. *Treatment* for anxiety and depression by be required.

Musculoskeletal

Arthralgia is common in sarcoidosis, but arthritis is unusual. Arthralgia commonly affects the ankles and feet in men, but also hands, wrists, and elbows. A subacute proximal myopathy can occur as well as bone cysts, especially of terminal phalanges. The latter show little response to systemic steroids.

Diagnosis
Granuloma seen on muscle biopsy.

Treatment
NSAIDs, steroids may be necessary.

Gastrointestinal

60% of liver biopsies on patients with sarcoidosis show granuloma. Frequently asymptomatic and benign course. Hepatomegaly unusual but can get portal fibrosis and cirrhosis. LFTs suggestive if 3× normal, especially alkaline phosphatase (ALP) and gamma glutamyl transferase (γGT).

Diagnosis
Biopsy.

Treatment
Steroids—may reduce size of liver and improve LFTs.

Haematological

Splenomegaly can occur and may be massive, causing abdominal discomfort. A massive spleen may require splenectomy to avoid rupture. Associated anaemia, neutropenia, and thrombocytopenia. Lymphopenia often seen.

ENT

Nasal or laryngeal granuloma. Sinus invasion. Parotid and other salivary gland enlargement, dry mouth.

Rarely

Breast disease, ovarian or testicular masses.

Further information

Baughman RP et al. A concise review of pulmonary sarcoidosis. *Am J Respir Crit Care Med* 2011;**183**: 573–581.

Dempsey OJ et al. Sarcoidosis. *BMJ* 2009;**339**: 620–625.

American Thoracic Society/European Respiratory Society/World Association of Sarcoidosis and other Granulomatous Disorders statement on sarcoidosis. *Eur Respir J* 1999;**14**: 735–737.

BTS interstitial lung disease guideline 2008. http://www.brit-thoracic.org.uk/portals/0/guidelines/dpldguidelines/thorax%20sept%2008.pdf.

Judson MA et al. Two-year prognosis of sarcoidosis: the ACCESS experience. *Sarcoidosis Vasc Diffuse Lung Dis* 2003;**20**: 204–211.

World Association of Sarcoidosis and other Granulomatous Disorders website. http://www.wasog.org/.

Lockstone HE et al. Gene set analysis of lung samples provides insight into pathogenesis of progressive, fibrotic pulmonary sarcoidosis. *Am J Respir Crit Care Med* 2010;**181**: 1367–1375.

Sickle cell disease and the lung

Overview *672*
Acute chest syndrome *674*

Overview

Background

Sickle cell disease is an autosomal recessive condition resulting in a substitution of a valine for glycine in the β-globin subunit of haemoglobin (Hb), forming HbS. HbS is less soluble under reduced O_2 tensions and leads to deformation of red blood cells (sickling) when deoxygenated (e.g. in atelectatic lung), resulting in chronic haemolysis and vascular occlusion with tissue infarction in individuals homozygous for the β-globin gene mutation (sickle cell anaemia/disease). Hb electrophoresis or high-performance liquid chromatography (HPLC) in sickle cell disease demonstrates HbS ~80–99% and no normal Hb HbA; anaemia Hb 6–9g/dL is usual. Heterozygote carriers of the β-globin gene mutation are referred to as having 'sickle cell trait' and are largely asymptomatic, although sickle crises may occur during extreme hypoxia (e.g. during anaesthesia); HPLC analysis demonstrates HbS ~35–40%, and HbA (normal Hb) ~50%. Sickle Hb solubility testing does not distinguish between trait and homozygous disease.

Pulmonary complications

- *Pneumonia* is more common, particularly from S. pneumoniae, Chlamydia pneumoniae, H. influenzae, Mycoplasma, Legionella, and respiratory viruses; may precipitate acute chest syndrome. Invasive pneumococcal disease is significantly more common. Patients should take lifelong prophylactic penicillin, as functionally asplenic
- *Asthma* appears to be a common comorbidity and may be associated with increased vaso-occlusive crises and episodes of acute chest syndrome
- *Nocturnal oxygen desaturation* and *sleep disordered breathing* are common, pathogenesis unclear—tonsillar hypertrophy is common, and OSA is often a contributing factor
- *Pulmonary thromboembolism* is more common and may precipitate acute chest syndrome
- *Acute chest syndrome* (see ➲ p. 674)
- *Sickle cell chronic lung disease* is a poorly described entity, characterized by progressive breathlessness and abnormal pulmonary function, sometimes with pulmonary hypertension (PHT). Thought to follow recurrent episodes of lung infarction/infection, although there may not be a history of previous acute chest syndrome. Radiologically, characterized by multifocal interstitial infiltrate. Pulmonary function tests (PFTs) typically restrictive, although airways obstruction also described
- *Pulmonary hypertension* is a relatively common complication of sickle cell disease and other forms of haemolytic anaemia. Management is largely as for IPAH in a specialist centre (see ➲ p. 454). Hydroxyurea and transfusions reduce episodes of vaso-occlusive crisis and acute chest syndrome and may be of benefit. Inhaled nitrous oxide (NO) may have a role; studies are ongoing. A minority of these patients have chronic thromboembolic pulmonary hypertension (CTEPH).

Acute chest syndrome

Definition and clinical features

Defined as a new pulmonary infiltrate on chest radiograph (CXR), consistent with consolidation but not atelectasis, associated with symptoms such as fever, cough, chest pain, and breathlessness. A form of acute lung injury, may progress to acute respiratory distress syndrome (ARDS) with associated multiorgan failure; one of the leading causes of death in sickle cell disease. However, mortality has fallen due to use of maintenance hydroxyurea therapy and earlier treatment with transfusion. Risk factors include young age, high steady state leucocyte counts and Hb levels, smoking, and past history of acute chest syndrome. May follow surgery and anaesthesia.

Causes may not be immediately apparent and include one or more of infection (including viruses, atypical bacteria, encapsulated bacteria), pulmonary fat embolism (preceded by bony pain), in situ thrombosis or pulmonary embolus (PE), atelectasis following hypoventilation (from acute painful crisis of chest wall or excessive opiates), and possibly pulmonary oedema due to excessive hydration. Each leads to hypoxia with increased sickling and vascular occlusion, and initially mild disease can escalate rapidly to ARDS and death. All patients with a painful vaso-occlusive crisis should be monitored closely for the development of the acute chest syndrome; routine use of incentive spirometry may help prevent its development in these patients.

Investigations

- *Blood tests* Raised white cell count (WCC), anaemia; check HbS %
- *Hypoxia* is common and may be underestimated using pulse oximetry; A–a gradient predicts clinical severity; consider ICU transfer if worsens
- *Culture* blood and sputum
- *CXR* shows multifocal pulmonary infiltrates, sometimes with pleural effusion
- *Computed tomographic pulmonary angiogram (CTPA)* should be performed if PE suspected
- *Bronchoalveolar lavage (BAL)* may be considered in patients not responding to treatment
- *Echo* reveals evidence of PHT and right heart strain in a significant minority of patients, associated with a higher mortality; such patients may also develop excessive haemolysis and thrombocytopenia and may benefit from a more aggressive exchange transfusion policy.

Management

See Box 47.1.

Box 47.1 Management of sickle cell acute chest syndrome

Supportive care on intensive care unit (ICU) may be required. Liaise with haematology team. Treatment comprises:

- Supplementary O_2 to correct hypoxia; monitor arterial blood gases (ABGs)
- Empirical broad-spectrum *antibiotics* (including a macrolide)
- *Rehydration* (intravenous (IV) fluids are often needed; take care to avoid overhydration)
- *Bronchodilators* are often used; airflow obstruction is common, may contribute to high airway pressures during mechanical ventilation
- Ensure adequate *analgesia* for bony pain (opiates are usually required, consider patient-controlled analgesia)
- *Incentive spirometry* and chest physiotherapy to prevent atelectasis are standard practice. Pain may limit their use, and continuous positive airway pressure (CPAP) may be better tolerated
- *Simple* and *exchange blood transfusion* both effectively reduce the proportion of HbS and improve oxygenation in acute chest syndrome, and early transfusion therapy is recommended. Simple transfusion is indicated if anaemic with Hb <10 g/dL, although Hb should not be raised above 11 g/dL, as the increase in blood viscosity exacerbates sickling. Exchange transfusion should be used in patients with a relatively high Hb, aiming for HbS <20%, and is also recommended in severe or rapidly progressive disease
- *Other treatments* Successful use of inhaled *NO* for the treatment of a handful of refractory cases has been reported, but a clinical trial has failed to demonstrate a reduction in the development of acute chest syndrome following treatment of vaso-occlusive crises with NO. *Corticosteroids* may be of benefit in reducing length of hospital admission, but rebound painful crises are more common, and routine use of corticosteroids is not recommended.

Prognosis

About 13% of patients with acute chest syndrome require mechanical ventilation; overall mortality is 4–9%.

Sleep apnoea and hypoventilation

Obstructive sleep apnoea (OSA) 678
OSA: clinical features 682
OSA: sleep studies, definitions and management 684
OSA: CPAP 688
OSA: driving advice to patients 690
OSA: future developments 692
Central sleep apnoea (CSA) and nocturnal hypoventilation 694
Causes and clinical features of CSA/hypoventilation 696
CSA/hypoventilation: investigations 700
Obesity-related respiratory problems 702

Obstructive sleep apnoea (OSA)

Definition and epidemiology

OSA, or obstructive sleep apnoea/hypopnoea (OSAH) are currently the preferred terms for the problem of dynamic upper airway obstruction during sleep.

- OSA is part of a spectrum, with trivial snoring at one end and repetitive complete obstruction throughout the night (such that the patient cannot sleep and breathe at the same time) at the other
- Along this spectrum is a point at which the degree of obstruction and the attendant arousal fragments sleep sufficiently to cause daytime symptoms
- Distinction should be made between finding OSA episodes (OSA) on a sleep study without symptoms and an abnormal sleep study *plus* the presence of symptoms (i.e. *obstructive sleep apnoea syndrome*, OSAS). Asymptomatic OSA is much more common than symptomatic (OSAS).

Thresholds defining 'abnormality' are arbitrary (e.g. 10 s to define an apnoea). Numerical definitions of OSA, based on counting individual events during a sleep study, are not very helpful. The current definition of the clinical syndrome is:

> Upper airway narrowing, provoked by sleep, causing sufficient sleep fragmentation to result in significant daytime symptoms including; excessive sleepiness, fatigue, tiredness, mood change, poor memory, and a lack of concentration.

- Prevalence depends on the chosen thresholds for defining both an abnormality on the sleep study and significant symptoms
- An estimated 5% of middle-aged men and 2.5% middle-aged women in Western populations have OSAS, sufficient to be candidates for treatment
- Estimated prevalence is rising with increasing obesity
- The prevalence in women is thought to be lower due to their different fat distribution. Upper body obesity (and thus neck obesity) is more a ♂ pattern
- OSAS is the third most common respiratory condition, after asthma and COPD. In some respiratory units, it has now become the commonest reason for specialist referral.

Pathophysiology and associated conditions

Control of the upper airway musculature is complex; upper airway patency depends on dilator muscle activity. All postural muscles relax during sleep (including pharyngeal dilators); some narrowing of the upper airway is normal. Excessive narrowing with the onset of sleep is due to the following factors.

Small pharyngeal size when awake

Such that normal muscle relaxation with sleep is enough to provoke critical narrowing.

- Fatty infiltration of pharyngeal tissues
- External pressure from increased neck fat and/or muscle bulk

- Large tonsils
- Craniofacial shape, e.g. micrognathia or retrognathia
- Extra submucosal tissue, e.g. myxoedema, mucopolysaccharidoses.

Excessive narrowing of the airway occurring with muscle relaxation at sleep onset

- Mass loading from an obese or muscular neck may simply 'overwhelm' residual dilator action as well as reduce the starting size
- Neuromuscular diseases with pharyngeal involvement may lead to greater loss of dilator muscle tone, e.g. stroke, myotonic dystrophy, Duchenne dystrophy, motor neurone disease (MND)
- Muscle relaxants such as sedatives and alcohol
- Increasing age.

Other theories

Non-anatomic traits have been identified that contribute to the risk of OSA by perpetuating unstable ventilation. These include a heightened tendency to arouse before the breathing and the upper airway stabilize, brisk hyperventilation in response to airway obstruction, and low responsiveness of dilator muscles. There may also be years of damage to the mucosa from snoring, which reduce the protective reflex dilation of the pharynx in response to narrowing activated by surface receptors.

Predisposing conditions

OSA is found more commonly in certain conditions, such as acromegaly and hypothyroidism, but the reasons are not well understood. It is unclear whether there need to be any other non-anatomical factors to provoke OSA. Most associated abnormalities that have been described are likely to be 2° to long periods of snoring and OSA, rather than 1° causal factors.

Short-term consequences of OSA

In severe OSA, repetitive collapse of the upper airway, with the arousal required to reactivate the pharyngeal dilators, occurs approximately every minute throughout the sleeping period (60 events/h or over 400/night); they are usually attended by hypoxia (see Fig. 48.2) and hypercapnia that are usually fully corrected during the inter-apnoeic hyperventilatory period. Obstructive events, short of complete obstruction, also provoke arousal, as it is usually the compensatory reflex increase in inspiratory effort, rather than the blood gas deterioration directly, that wakens the brain. In this situation, the drops in O_2 saturation may be very much less and, in younger thinner individuals, almost imperceptible on oximetry tracings (see Fig. 48.6). This is because the compensation afforded by the increased inspiratory effort may be adequate, and the bigger O_2 stores in the lungs of the less obese will buffer an apnoea. Compare to Fig. 48.1 (normal overnight oximetry) and Fig. 48.3 (sleep-onset periodic ventilation).

- Recurrent arousals lead to highly fragmented and unrefreshing sleep
- Excessive daytime sleepiness results
- The correlation between the sleep fragmentation and the resultant degree of sleepiness is not tight, with some patients being sleepy with low levels of fragmentation, and vice versa
- This is thought to result partly from inter-individual differences in sensitivity to the effects of sleep fragmentation

- With every arousal, there is a rise in BP, often over 50 mmHg. It is unclear if these BP rises do any damage to the cardiovascular system. There is also a carry-over of hypertension (average of 3 mmHg) into the waking hours, which falls after treatment of OSA at 1 month
- There is true nocturia, mechanism unclear; there may be raised atrial natriuretic peptide (ANP) levels from increased central blood volume, from the sub-atmospheric intrathoracic pressures during the obstructed breathing; or it may be simply a reflection of highly fragmented sleep, preventing the normal reduction in urine flow associated with sleep.

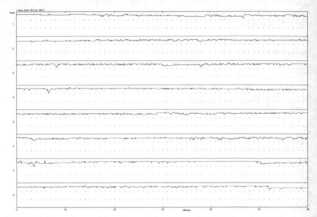

Fig. 48.1 Normal overnight oximetry. Normal baseline and a few dips. Vertical axis, 70–100% SaO_2 for each panel; horizontal axis, 60 min each panel, 8 h total.

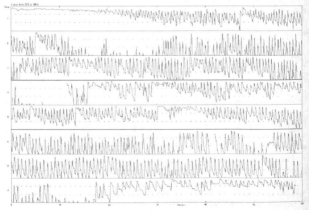

Fig. 48.2 Severe OSA. Large numbers of regular dips, sawtooth-shaped (faster rise in SaO_2 than fall).

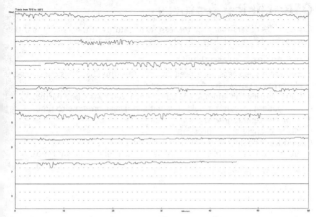

Fig. 48.3 Sleep onset periodic ventilation. Short bursts of dipping, otherwise normal.

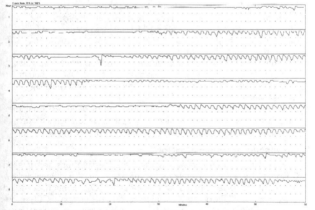

Fig. 48.4 Cheyne-Stokes ventilation. Prolonged periods of dipping, often more sinusoidal, rather than sawtooth.

OSA: clinical features

Chapter 14 covers many of the essential features in the history and discusses the differential diagnosis of excessive daytime sleepiness.

Most patients present with:

- Excessive sleepiness, measured crudely using the ESS; >9 is considered abnormally sleepy (see ➔ p. 103 Fig 14.1)
- Loud snoring and apnoeic episodes recognized by the bed partner
- The patient recognizes waking up with choking from time to time
- Poor concentration and poor memory
- Mood changes and depression
- Unrefreshing sleep and waking unrefreshed
- Nocturia (true nocturia with reversal of the usual day/night ratio).

Less often there will be:

- Insomnia
- Nocturnal sweating
- Reduced libido
- Oesophageal reflux
- Increasingly common are patients arriving with spouses worried by the apnoeic pauses they have observed.

Sleepiness

- Sometimes difficult to assess; failure by the patient to recognize the problem or denial due to concerns over driving and licensing
- The Epworth scale (see ➔ p. 103 Fig 14.1) assesses *tendency to fall asleep*, rather than *perceived sleepiness per se*, as some patients may regard their situation as normal
- It is important to separate the symptom of tiredness from sleepiness (see ➔ p. 100), the latter being much more typical of OSA, although sometimes tiredness is reported (rather than sleepiness) more by women with OSA
- Some centres will used objective measurements of sleepiness (multiple sleep latency tests and maintenance of wakefulness testing), although these are probably more helpful in conditions other than OSA.

Examination and investigations

The examination (often unrewarding) and the investigations are detailed in Chapter 14 (see ➔ p. 102). Look for the presence of additional airflow limitation of the lower airways, with associated CO_2 retention, so-called 'overlap syndrome'. Blood gas is useful to confirm hypercapnia. CO_2 retention in pure OSA is very uncommon (except in the very, very obese). It appears that the additive effect of some airflow limitation of the lower airways (often not enough in its own right to precipitate CO_2 retention) is usually required, which perhaps limits the inter-apnoeic hyperventilation and thus gradually encourages tolerance to raised levels of CO_2. Sleep study is the main diagnostic test and is described on ➔ pp. 684–686.

OSA has a ♂:♀ of 2:1. Patients tend to have a combination of upper body obesity (neck circumference >17 in) and a relatively undersized or set-back mandible. Airway size can be assessed and documented with scoring systems, e.g. see ● p.702 Fig 48.9.

OSA: sleep studies, definitions and management

The sleep study assesses if there is anything likely to be the cause of the patient's symptoms. The considerable grey area between normality and abnormality means that sometimes it is unclear whether the symptoms can be blamed on the sleep study findings. There is also considerable night-to-night variation in sleep study indices that further blurs the distinction between normality and abnormality. In this situation, it may be necessary to undertake a therapeutic trial of CPAP and let the patient decide if the benefits of treatment outweigh the disadvantages. Types of sleep study include:

- Overnight oximetry alone, including heart rate (HR) (see Fig. 48.1–Fig. 48.8)
- More than just oximetry, with other channels, e.g. sound, body movement, oronasal airflow, chest/abdominal movements, leg movements: 'limited' sleep studies or 'respiratory polygraphy (PG)'
- Polysomnography (PSG), with electroencephalogram (EEG), electro-oculogram (EOG), and electromyogram (EMG), to stage sleep electrophysiologically, in addition to the other channels listed above.

There is no evidence that OSA diagnosis needs PSG (with EEG recording of actual sleep); it is very rarely indicated, and its routine use is a waste of resources and is impractical in the COVID-19 era. Oximetry (SaO_2 and pulse rate) identifies most moderate to severe cases, allowing referral for CPAP. Abnormal oximetry, sometimes mimicking OSA, occurs with Cheyne–Stokes breathing (heart failure, post-stroke), in the very obese, and when there is a low baseline SaO_2 (e.g. COPD) (Fig. 48.4; Fig. 48.7); this allows the SaO_2 to oscillate more with small changes in PaO_2, due to the increasing steepness of the Hb dissociation curve at lower SaO_2. False negatives, discussed earlier, can occur with younger and thinner patients.

> With appropriate expertise, a good history, and recognition of its limitations, domiciliary oximetry alone is a valuable tool in the diagnosis and management of OSA. The addition of sound and/or oronasal flow channels reduces the number of equivocal results needing a further study.

Limited sleep studies (respiratory PG) are the usual routine investigation. Different units have expertise in interpreting different sorts of sleep studies. Experience is more important than the particular sleep study equipment used.

Definitions

Definitions of sleep study parameters are arbitrary and treatment decisions should be based on patient symptoms. However, thresholds are used in the Driver and Vehicle Licensing Agency (DVLA) guidelines and in some areas funding of treatments is contingent on these thresholds.

- Apnoea—reduction in airflow by >90% for >10s
- Hypopnoea—variable defined. Latest American Academy of Sleep Medicine guidelines (2012) define hypopnoea as a reduction in airflow >30% in association with either an oxygen desaturation (see below) or an arousal (requires EEG)

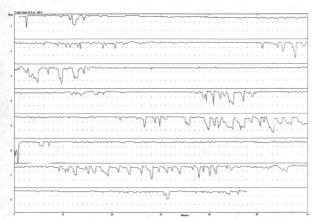

Fig. 48.5 REM sleep hypoventilation in scoliosis. Substantial dips, in bursts, compatible with the occurence of REM periods.

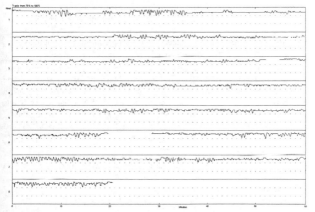

Fig. 48.6 Moderate OSA with many small, <4% dips in SaO$_2$.

- Apnoea hypopnoea index (AHI)—the number of apnoeas and hypopnoeas divided by the total sleep time (or total study length if sleep not measured)
- Oxygen desaturation index (ODI)—the number of dips in SaO$_2$ >3% or 4% from baseline divided by the total sleep time (or the total study length if sleep not measured). This is closely correlated with the AHI as most apnoeas and hypopnoeas will be associated by a fall in SaO$_2$.

Arbitrary AHI thresholds of disease severity (or ODI if AHI not recorded) are:
- AHI <5: normal
- AHI 5–15: mild OSA
- AHI 15–30: moderate OSA
- AHI >30: severe OSA

Management

Not all patients need treatment. There is evidence that treating patients with OSAS improves symptoms, and symptoms rather than the degree of OSA on a sleep study should drive treatment decisions. Treatment decisions require a close dialogue between physician and patient. Patients may underestimate their symptoms so, when in doubt, erring on the side of a CPAP trial is sensible.

Key features in making a treatment choice
- How sleepy is the patient? Does it affect quality of life (QoL)? Is it critical to the patient's livelihood (e.g. heavy goods vehicle (HGV) driving)? Is there motivation for treatment?
- Has the patient underestimated the impact of their sleepiness or misled the doctor because of concerns over driving issues?
- Is there any evidence of the 'overlap' syndrome where additional lower airways obstruction has contributed to hypercapnic respiratory failure? If so, is this a stable state or part of an acute decline with a respiratory acidosis?
- Is obesity the dominant risk factor, or is there a surgically remediable component (e.g. tonsillar hypertrophy)?

There is no randomized controlled trial (RCT) evidence that cardiovascular disease should influence the decision to treat. Many, however, would lower the treatment threshold under these circumstances. OSA is a risk factor for recurrent AF; some evidence exists that treating OSA, when there is left heart failure, improves ejection fraction. Treating OSA can reduce blood pressure and there may be a treatment role for CPAP in treating blood pressure in patients with resistant hypertension.

Simple approaches
- Weight loss. This is difficult; slimming clubs have the best record for non-surgical approaches
- Reduce evening alcohol consumption
- Sleep decubitus, rather than supine, and with the bedhead elevated.

For snorers and mild OSA
- Mandibular advancement devices, assuming adequate dentition
- Pharyngeal surgery as a last resort (limited RCT data, not routinely recommended unless very large tonsils).
- CPAP for selected patients, probably the sleepiest.

For significant OSA
- CPAP therapy
- Bariatric surgery if BMI >35 kg/m^2 (e.g. gastric band or gastric bypass operations)
- Tracheostomy (rarely indicated)
- Mandibular/maxillary advancement surgery in highly selected cases.

Severe OSA with CO_2 retention

- May require a period of non-invasive ventilation (NIV) with positive pressure prior to CPAP, particularly if acidotic
- Stable compensated hypercapnia retention may respond to CPAP alone.

If there are large tonsils, then their removal may be appropriate, but may require treatment with CPAP prior to surgery and is less likely to be successful in treated OSA when BMI > 35 kg/m². Besides tonsillectomy there is little evidence for upper airway surgery. There is usually no role for alerting agents (such as modafinil) in the routine management of sleepiness in OSA. These drugs may possibly reduce the perception of sleepiness more than the sleepiness itself and have mainly been studied in the residual sleepiness sometimes found in patients even when treated successfully with CPAP.

Mandibular advancement devices

- Worn in the mouth at night, holding the lower jaw forward: similar to 'jaw thrust'. Generally used to control snoring and milder OSA, although they can be trialled in patients with more severe OSA who have failed to tolerate CPAP
- Many different designs, but essentially, one half clips to the upper teeth and the other half to the lower, and connected together with the lower jaw held forward by 5–10 mm
- Some give adjustable forward displacement; some are fixed
- The more sophisticated need to be customized to match the patient's dentition, which usually requires the services of a dentist
- Semi-custom fitted devices are probably as effective as dentist fitted devices and are cheaper
- DIY devices exist that are heated and moulded to the teeth directly
- One-size-fits-all devices exist that can work for snoring, but only if they advance the lower jaw
- Side effects include excessive salivation, tooth pain, and jaw ache, which often lessen with time
- Long-term use may be associated with movement of the teeth and alterations to the bite
- The initial cost (usually over £400 for customized versions) is more than that of a CPAP machine (£300), and they may only last about a year
- Although not as effective in reducing the severity of OSA as measured on a sleep study, they can be as effective in reducing symptoms.

Hypoglossal nerve stimulation

There is some evidence that implanted hypoglossal nerve stimulators reduce the severity OSA in patients with moderate to severe OSA. In the UK their use is presently only recommended in research, or special circumstances in select patients.

OSA: CPAP

CPAP consists of a blower/pressure generator that sits by the patient's bed and is connected to a mask by a length of large-bore tubing. Masks are either nasal or cover the nose and mouth (full face mask). The blower raises the pressure at which the patient is breathing (to about 10 cmH$_2$O) and splints open the pharynx, preventing its collapse, sleep fragmentation, and the consequent daytime sleepiness. *CPAP is a highly effective therapy, with resolution of the sleepiness and large gains in QoL.* It is a sufficiently curious and initially uncomfortable therapy to require a *careful set-up programme.* Without this, the take-up and compliance rates are poor. In response to COVID-19, face-to-face CPAP set-up is challenging, due to CPAP delivery being aerosol generating. It remains to be seen if virtual set-up is as effective. Most centres have found that a dedicated CPAP nurse or technician is required. Many centres use special patient education aids, such as video presentations, online resources, and provide helplines. The best method of establishing a patient on CPAP and deriving the required mask pressure is not known, and many different approaches appear to work. This can be done with CPAP machines that automatically hunt for the required pressure, via an inpatient CPAP titration, or via an algorithm calculated pressure (based on neck circumference and number of obstructive events). New mask designs appear at regular intervals, with a slow improvement in their comfort and fit (important to prevent air leaks). Patients require access to long-term support to maintain their CPAP equipment and attend to problems. There are now significant problems supporting the very large numbers of patients on CPAP that accumulate the longer a service has been in operation.

The commonest problems encountered include:

- Mouth leaks lead to increased air through the nose and out of the mouth, with excessive drying of the mucosa, nasal congestion, rhinitis, and sneezing. Usually solved by adding a heated humidifier, a full-face mask, or a chin strip to hold the jaw closed.
- Pain and ulceration of the skin on the nasal bridge. Try different masks or 'interfaces' not resting on the nasal bridge
- Claustrophobia. This usually settles but can be reduced by selecting the right mask
- Temporary nasal congestion, usually during a cold. Try nasal decongestants for these short periods (3–4 days) such as xylometazoline.

Alternative diagnoses

Most patients who snore are sleepy and have an abnormal sleep study, will have OSA, and respond to CPAP. Sometimes, differentiating OSA from central sleep apnoea (see $\bigodot$ pp. 694–701) can be difficult: some patients with Cheyne–Stokes breathing (Fig. 48.4) may have a few obstructed breaths at

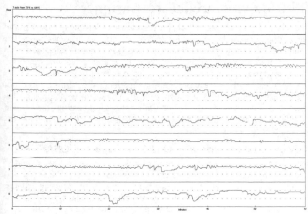

Fig. 48.7 Nocturnal hypoxia in COPD. Low baseline SaO_2, with more dramatic falls (often quite prolonged) during periods compatible with the occurrence of REM.

the end of each apnoeic cycle, even though the problem is primarily central. Poor response to CPAP should at least prompt a reappraisal of the diagnosis. Not all OSA is due to pharyngeal collapse; a very small number of patients have laryngeal closure:

- Multi-system atrophy causing laryngeal closure during sleep, with stridulous obstruction, rather than the usual noise of snoring
- Rheumatoid arthritis can damage the larynx, with resultant OSA
- Arnold–Chiari malformation can compress the brainstem and interfere with the control of the larynx and pharynx, as well as the control of ventilation, with mixed findings on the sleep study
- These forms of obstruction also respond to CPAP. With laryngeal closure there is risk of sudden death normally leading to expedited treatment of these patients.

OSA: driving advice to patients

In UK law, drivers are responsible for their vigilance levels while driving. We know when we are sleepy and should stop driving. Driving while sleepy has been likened to driving while drunk, and a prison sentence can result from sleep-related accidents on the road. No one should drive while they are sleepy, and the same applies to pathological causes of sleepiness.

Regardless of the extent of symptoms patients should be advised not drive while sleepy or tired. If patients are tired or sleepy while driving, they must stop and rest for the day/night. Only if this is not possible, they should be advised to drink a strong caffeine-containing beverage and then nap for 20 min before resuming driving.

Advice to all patients with OSAS or suspected OSAS

- If there is excessive sleepiness having or likely to have an adverse effect on driving, patients must be advised to stop driving.
- In the context of such excessive sleepiness, physicians assessing patients with or suspected of having OSA should advise the following:
  - Suspected OSA; patients must stop driving but need not inform the DVLA unless symptom control (i.e. with CPAP treatment) is not expected to be achieved within 3 months. This applies to both those with Group 1 (car and motorcycle) and Group 2 licenses (bus and lorry)
  - Mild OSA (AHI<15) or another medical condition; patients must stop driving but patients need not inform the DVLA unless symptom control is not expected to be achieved with 3 months. This applies to both Group 1 and 2 drivers. Driving may only resume after satisfactory symptom control
  - Moderate to severe OSA (AHI ≥15); patients must stop driving and must inform the DVLA. Subsequent licensing requires control of their OSA, improvements in sleepiness and treatment adherence. This requires medical confirmation. This applies to both Group 1 and 2 drivers. Drivers must confirm review to undertaken at a minimum of every three years (Group 1) or annually (Group 2)
- When informing the DVLA patients should write to the DVLA to request or download from the DVLA website a SL1 (Group 1) or a SL1V (Group 2). If the patient reports excessive sleepiness then their license is revoked. If already treated and the sleepiness has resolved, then the license is not revoked; hence, rapid treatment is essential. It is the doctor's duty to tell the patient of the diagnosis of OSAS and of the requirement to inform the DVLA if required as outlined above
- In addition, if notifying the DVLA the patient will have to inform their insurer
- In very rare circumstances if there is concern a patient is continuing to drive despite previous advice to the contrary, the clinician is obligated to break confidentiality and inform the DVLA directly because of the risk to public health, as advised by the General Medical Council
- The advice given to the patient should be recorded in the notes.

The DVLA rules change from time to time, and reference to the latest version of their website is recommended.

The latest American Thoracic Guidelines are entirely sensible and useful.* Inappropriate and illogical curbing of driving privileges will push the problem underground, through fear of loss of livelihood, and is the worst of all worlds.

* An official American Thoracic Society Clinical Practice Guideline: sleep apnea, sleepiness, and driving risk in noncommercial drivers. *Am J Respir Crit Care Med.* 2013;**187**: 1259–1266.

OSA: future developments

- OSA is so common that diagnosis will move into general practice. Simpler ways to establish patients on CPAP have evolved. RCTs show that, with appropriate training and supervision, diagnosis and management of OSAS can be carried out in the community.
- There is currently an evidence gap for the use of CPAP in mild OSA which should be addressed by the MERGE study.
- Positional therapy devices that encourage patients not to sleep in the supine position be vibrotactile stimulus are currently being studied.
- Obesity surgery is improving and, in appropriate cases, may become the treatment of choice.
- Pharmacological agents are being developed to prevent the loss of tone in the pharyngeal dilators during sleep, although progress in this area is slow. A phenotyping approach for OSA is gaining popularity in research studies and may lead to targeted therapies.
- New pharyngeal operations are being devised all the time, but none have been very effective when investigated properly; RCTs with objective outcome data are badly needed in this area.
- There is epidemiological evidence that OSA increase the risk of hypertension, cardiovascular disease and worsens glycaemic control. Future studies are needed to determine if these associations are real and to determine the optimal treatment strategies for these comorbidities in OSA.

Further information

Heatley EM et al. Obstructive sleep apnoea in adults: a common chronic condition in need of a comprehensive chronic condition management approach. *Sleep Med Rev* 2013;**17**: 349–355.

Heinzer et al. Prevalence of sleep-disordered breathing in the general population: the HypnoLaus study. *Lancet Respir Med* 2015;**3**: 130–138.

Hu et al. The role of continuous positive airway pressure in blood pressure control for patients with obstructive sleep apnea and hypertension: a meta-analysis of randomized controlled trials. *J Clin Hypertens* 2015; **17**: 215–222.

Chai-Coetzer CL et al. Primary care versus specialist sleep centre management of obstructive sleep apnea and daytime sleepiness and quality of life. *JAMA* 2013;**309**: 997–1004.

McDaid et al. Continuous positive airway pressure devices for the treatment of obstructive sleep apnoea-hypopnoea syndrome: a systematic review and economic analysis. *Health Technol Assess* 2009; **13**: iii–274.

McEvoy et al. CPAP for prevention of cardiovascular events in obstructive sleep apnea. *NEJM* 2016;**375**: 919–931.

DVLA guidance can be found in Chapter 8 (miscellaneous) ⌖ https://www.gov.uk/guidance/assessing-fitness-to-drive-a-guide-for-medical-professionals

Central sleep apnoea (CSA) and nocturnal hypoventilation

Definition and epidemiology

'CSA/hypopnoea', or 'hypoventilation', or 'periodic breathing', are said to occur when there is no evidence of upper airway obstruction as the cause for the episodic reduced ventilation during sleep. Compared with OSA, it is much less common.

- *CSA* tends to be used as a term when there are actual apnoeas; referred to as Cheyne–Stokes breathing when there is regular symmetrical waxing and waning, usually in the context of left ventricular failure
- *Periodic breathing* is an alternative term and can be used to describe regular fluctuations in breathing, with or without actual apnoeas
- The description *nocturnal hypoventilation* tends to be used when the hypoventilation and hypoxaemic dips are not particularly periodic in nature. However, these terms are imprecise and sometimes mixed indiscriminately.

Pathophysiology

CSA, or hypoventilation or periodic breathing, can occur in a number of settings with different aetiologies (see also Chapter 15, ⊃ pp. 105–111). At one end of the spectrum is pure loss of ventilatory drive, while at the other is pure reduction in the ability to expand the chest adequately, with dependence on accessory muscles of respiration. Many clinical presentations are mixtures of these two.

Patients with *reduced ventilatory drive* (e.g. following brainstem damage) can often maintain adequate, or near adequate, ventilation while awake, as there is a non-metabolic 'awake' ventilatory drive equivalent to about 4 or 5 L/min. During non-REM sleep, this awake drive is lost, and ventilation becomes dependent on PaO_2 and $PaCO_2$. During REM sleep, an 'awake-like' drive sometimes returns partially, and ventilation can improve again (seen in congenital forms of absent drive where REM sleep can temporarily restore SaO_2 levels).

In patients with *impaired mechanical ability to ventilate*, accessory muscles of respiration become critically supportive (e.g. in many neuromuscular disorders and obstructive/restrictive respiratory conditions). However, during non-REM sleep, this reflex recruitment of accessory muscles is attenuated and hypoventilation follows. During REM sleep, the physiological paralysis of all postural muscles (REM atonia) can remove all compensatory mechanisms, leaving only the diaphragm working, and may produce profound hypoventilation or apnoea.

Chronic hypoventilation, often 2° to poor respiratory function (as evidenced by CO_2 retention in some patients with COPD or chest wall restrictive disorders), can eventually force resetting of ventilatory control mechanisms. This is an acquired blunting of ventilatory drive and leads to sleep-related changes in ventilation, similar to those described in the previous paragraphs.

Unstable ventilatory control can lead to regular oscillations in ventilation, e.g. as occurs in heart failure and at altitude. During REM sleep, it is normal to have fluctuations in ventilation, sometimes with complete apnoeas.

Sometimes, sleep studies can be misinterpreted, and apnoeas, really of obstructive origin, are mistakenly labelled as central. For example, if inspiratory muscles are very weak, their poor efforts during obstructive apnoeas may be missed on the ribcage and abdominal bands used in sleep studies but may be detectable with oesophageal pressure monitoring.

Causes and clinical features of CSA/hypoventilation

Although there are many different causes, only four relatively common clinical scenarios occur (but with overlap).

Absent or reduced ventilatory drive

Brainstem involvement from strokes, tumours, syringobulbia, surgical damage, post-polio syndrome, congenital (Ondine's curse—usually presents soon after birth, can be later, abnormalities of neural crest development due to increased number of 'alanine repeats' in one of the homeobox genes—*PHOX2B*). Presents clinically with unexplained ventilatory failure, much worse during sleep when the 'awake' drive is lost.

- *May be recognized early*, cyanosis, morning confusion, ankle oedema
- *May be recognized late*, loss of consciousness, and an emergency admission to ICU for ventilation following a chest infection or general anaesthesia.

Lung function is often normal, with no evidence of respiratory muscle weakness, indicating normal innervation from the voluntary motor system. Arnold–Chiari malformation with brainstem compression can present like this, but there is usually involvement of surrounding structures such as the lower cranial motor nuclei supplying the larynx and pharynx (with associated OSA; see ♦ p. 689).

> These patients will have no apparent neuromuscular or respiratory cause for their hypoventilation but may have a previous history of brainstem stroke (or other form of brain damage). The congenital form usually presents shortly after birth when the amount of REM sleep reduces and is replaced by non-REM.

Post-polio syndrome
- Ill-defined syndrome—decline in function, decades after initial illness
- Return of weakness in previously affected areas (mechanism unclear)
- Late development of ventilatory failure is more likely if:
  - Inspiratory muscles were affected in the original illness
  - Additional scoliosis due to paravertebral muscle involvement (in which case vital capacity (VC) will be reduced).

This may be due to premature ageing of the upper and lower motor neurones due to their 'overuse'. This could follow the original destruction of some of the anterior horn cells to the inspiratory muscles and the subsequent reinnervation by surviving neurones which then have to continuously supply more neurones than they were 'designed' for.

Weak or mechanically disadvantaged inspiratory muscles with/without 2° reduction of awake ventilatory drive

Neuromuscular inspiratory muscle weakness
Produces diurnal ventilatory failure in its own right, particularly when the supine VC falls below 20% predicted (~1L), although fall in VC occurs late

with neuromuscular weakness and is not a good predictor of impending ventilator failure.

With increasing inspiratory muscle weakness, other accessory inspiratory muscles are recruited to maintain ventilation. When this is lost during non-REM sleep, and more so during REM sleep, ventilation will fall much more than in normal subjects. While metabolic ventilatory drive is reasonably preserved, this will result in recurrent arousals to 'rescue' the ventilation and consequent marked sleep disturbance.

As ventilatory drive becomes progressively blunted, following the hypoventilation forced on the system by weak muscles, extra sleep hypoventilation (from loss of 'awake' drive) is tolerated, and profound hypoxaemia is observed until there is finally an arousal that recovers the ventilation and SaO_2.

The above patients should have a history of a progressive neuromuscular disorder.

Chest wall restrictive diseases

Scoliosis or post-thoracoplasty patients (Fig. 48.5) can behave in a similar way with gradual onset of ventilatory failure, particularly when VC <1 L. The muscles are not weak but operating at severe mechanical disadvantage.

The same situation occurs in COPD, when muscles are overloaded and accessory muscles provide important support, but this too is reduced with non-REM sleep and lost during REM sleep. Again, any $2°$ reduction in ventilatory drive amplifies the sleep-related falls in SaO_2.

• Chest wall restrictive patients should have an obvious restrictive disorder with reduced VC to 1L or below
• Increasing severity of COPD will produce increasing degrees of sleep hypoventilation (see Fig. 48.7)
• If the awake SaO_2 is already low, the sleep-related falls in ventilation will produce dramatic dips in SaO_2
• COPD and OSA together (overlap syndrome; see ➲ pp. 107–108) provoke profound nocturnal hypoxic dipping (see Fig. 48.8), and probably a more rapid progression to diurnal hypoventilation with CO_2 retention, due to extra blunting of ventilatory drive.

The diaphragm is the only respiratory muscle working during REM sleep, as all other postural muscles are profoundly hypotonic.

• If the diaphragm is paralysed, then REM sleep is a particularly vulnerable time, as there are no muscles of ventilation left working, thus producing particularly profound falls in SaO_2 during REM
• Patients with bilateral diaphragm weakness can present early, with no obvious weakness elsewhere. Diaphragm weakness is best detected with the patient supine. Inspiration, particularly on sniffing, will provoke a paradoxical indrawing of the abdominal wall. The VC will also fall on lying down, increasingly with greater degrees of paralysis (often a >30% fall in VC with complete diaphragm paralysis).

In a progressive neuromuscular disorder, such as MND, the above patterns will be variable between individuals but will gradually worsen. Predominant

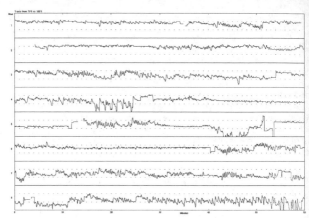

Fig. 48.8 Overlap syndrome-OSA and COPD. Low baseline SaO_2. Some periods with typical sawtooth-dipping; other periods with prolonged falls in SaO_2.

diaphragm weakness, as occurs sometimes in MND, spinal muscular atrophy, and particularly acid maltase deficiency, can lead to ventilatory failure at a time when the patient is still ambulant.

Cheyne–Stokes breathing associated with heart failure

(See Fig. 48.4.)

The raised left atrial pressure in left heart failure increases ventilatory drive through stimulation of J receptors; this in addition to ventilatory stimulation from any hypoxaemia from pulmonary oedema.

- This ventilatory stimulation lowers the awake $PaCO_2$, producing a respiratory alkalosis
- In addition, the use of diuretics may produce a mild metabolic alkalosis, especially if there is hypokalaemia
- J receptor ventilatory stimulation appears to reduce at sleep onset. This, together with the loss of the awake ventilatory drive, allows central hypoventilation or apnoea to occur
- This hypoventilation or apnoea will continue until the $PaCO_2$ builds up driving ventilation again or until the hypoxaemia provokes arousal
- The return of ventilation itself may provoke arousal too. The arousal itself then injects the increased 'wake' ventilatory drive, reducing the $PaCO_2$ again
- Sleep returns, and, once again, the low $PaCO_2$ and alkalosis cause hypoventilation or apnoea.

Thus, a cycle is maintained that involves a fluctuating sleep state with arousals, and usually a fluctuating SaO_2. As with OSA, the patient may be completely unaware of these arousals. The delayed circulatory time of left heart failure may compound this instability by introducing a time delay between any change in $PaCO_2$ in the blood leaving the lungs and its arrival at the carotid body or central chemoreceptors.

Cheyne–Stokes breathing associated with altitude

The acute hypoxia following ascent to altitude provokes increased ventilation. The degree is variable between individuals, and hence the degree of hypocapnia and respiratory alkalosis varies (see ➲ pp. 300–301). With sleep onset, a lessening of the hypoxic drive, and removal of the awake drive, an uncompensated alkalosis will allow hypoventilation, and even apnoea—similar to the situation described previously for Cheyne–Stokes breathing. Again, ventilation will restart, either when the $PaCO_2$ rises to a critical level or the hypoxia provokes arousal. Sleep is fragmented with complaints of insomnia, but the cause of this is rarely recognized by the sufferer.

Skiing in Colorado, altitude 2,400–3,400 m (~10,000 ft), is high enough to provoke significant periodic breathing in about a fifth of individuals. It seems that this fifth are the ones with the highest hypoxic ventilatory response. This gives them the largest respiratory alkalosis and hence the greatest tendency to sleep-onset hypoventilation. In addition, the tendency to arouse with the resultant extra hypoxaemia may be greater too, thus provoking large increases in ventilation on arousal and greater sleep disturbance. As the kidney excretes extra bicarbonate and produces a compensatory metabolic acidosis over a few days, the periodic breathing lessens. See also ➲ p. 300 (altitude sickness).

Two pharmacological approaches have been taken to reduce this sleep-related periodic breathing at altitude.

- Pre-acclimatization with acetazolamide prior to ascent. This produces a mild metabolic acidosis and maintains the ventilatory drive at sleep onset, thus blocking the hypoventilation. RCTs show the efficacy of this approach with doses between 250 and 500 mg/day, 1–3 days prior to ascent
- Hypnotics, such as temazepam, can reduce the degree of periodic breathing by reducing the tendency to arousal with each return of ventilation, and thus damping the system. Randomized trials suggest benefit for the early part of the night, with no impairment of nocturnal hypoxaemia or daytime functioning
- Of course, supplemental O_2 will abolish the problem.

CSA/hypoventilation: investigations

Simple PFTs will characterize weakness of inspiratory muscles. Supine VC is the best predictor of ventilatory failure, as it incorporates diaphragm weakness that is masked during erect testing. Blood gases will reveal diurnal type II ventilatory failure. If the bicarbonate/base excess is raised, with a normal $PaCO_2$ (showing therefore a mild metabolic alkalosis), then this may indicate nocturnal hypoventilation and incipient ventilatory failure. The bicarbonate has been referred to as the 'HbA1c of $PaCO_2$', as it represents an integrated response to the average raised $PaCO_2$ over the last 48 h or so (in the absence of any other reason such as hypokalaemia and some diuretics).

Sleep study

(For examples, see Figs. 48.3, 48.4, 48.5, 48.7 & 48.8.)

Sleep studies in patients with suspected nocturnal hypoventilation or CSA confirm the diagnosis and assess the degree of nocturnal hypoxaemia. Limited sleep studies should reveal falls in SaO_2 in association with hypoventilation, but no evidence of OSA and, in particular, no snoring. Oximetry tracings alone will show a variety of patterns, often resembling OSA. The pattern in neuromuscular weakness will vary from oscillations all the time (due to recurrent arousal) to just REM sleep-related dips in SaO_2. The same will be true for chest wall restrictive disorders and COPD, with REM dips occurring initially and greater hypoxaemia once there is an element of diurnal CO_2 retention and hypoxaemia.

- In OSA, there is a slow fall in SaO_2, as O_2 levels fall in the lung, followed by a rapid rise with the first deep inspiration as the apnoea ends (so-called sawtooth pattern); see Fig. 48.2
- In Cheyne–Stokes of left heart failure, the oscillations in SaO_2 are often more sinusoidal than in OSA, as the pattern of breathing is usually more of a symmetrical waxing and waning of ventilation; see Fig. 48.4. However, if each central apnoea is terminated by an arousal, rather than a smooth return of ventilation, then the pattern will look more like OSA.

In COPD, the degree of hypoxaemia on the sleep study will depend very much on the awake SaO_2. Because of the shape of the Hb dissociation curve, a low awake SaO_2 makes it easier for the SaO_2 to fall further with a given reduction in ventilation. Thus, during non-REM, with removal of awake drive, there will be a fairly stable reduction in SaO_2, but, during REM sleep, there will be further, more dramatic dips. It is important not to diagnose OSA from just an oximetry tracing on the basis of SaO_2 oscillations when there is a low baseline SaO_2 and COPD. In this situation, a fuller sleep study is required to provide evidence of additional upper airway obstruction. The combination of hypoxic COPD and OSA (one of the overlap syndromes) can produce particularly dramatic traces (see Fig. 48.8).

Management

Intervention in CSA, or hypoventilation or periodic breathing, depends on symptoms. *Better control of heart failure* may improve Cheyne–Stokes breathing but often does not. Further treatment will be required for two reasons: either to prevent the cyclical breathing and restore sleep quality, or to globally improve ventilation overnight and reset the respiratory control mechanisms such that the daytime respiratory failure reverses.

In situations where the hypoxia is playing a part in the pathogenesis (e.g. heart failure), then *raising FiO₂* can help (using O₂ via nasal prongs only during sleep). There is limited literature on other forms of treatment for the Cheyne–Stokes of heart failure, although *acetazolamide* and *benzodiazepines* have been tried. The unstable breathing in heart failure has been treated with *CPAP; however, a large RCT has not confirmed long-term benefit.* Treatment with *adaptive servo-ventilation* has been unexpectedly shown to cause a slight increase in mortality in patients with heart failure and reduced left ventricular ejection fraction.

Sedatives are contraindicated with a raised PaCO₂, and extra O₂ may increase the hypercapnia. In these situations, then *overnight NIV*, via either nose or face mask, may be appropriate. In slowly progressive neuromuscular disorders, with either sleep fragmentation or diurnal type II respiratory failure (or both), the symptomatic and physiological response can be dramatic. The use of NIV at night in more rapidly progressive disorders has potential difficulties but is proving very useful in the palliative care of disorders such as MND. Increasing dependence on equipment, not designed to be immediately life-sustaining, is a particular issue. In scoliosis, NIV is commonly used, and again responses are dramatic.

Long-term NIV along with long-term oxygen therapy (LTOT) with persistent compensated hypercapnia following a hospital admission requiring NIV use for acute decompensated hypercapnia improves admission free survival and is now commonly prescribed for such patients.

Future developments

- Introduction of overnight ventilation earlier in the course of a progressive neuromuscular disorder (such as MND) to reduce symptoms and possibly prolong life
- Use of overnight ventilation in patients with stable COPD and hypercapnia, without recent exacerbation. This may reduce exacerbations, hospital admissions, and prolong life. The evidence is inadequate yet to justify its wide use in this patient group.

Further information

Oldenburg O. Cheyne-Stokes respiration in chronic heart failure. Treatment with adaptive servoventilation therapy. *Circ J* 2012;**76**: 2305–2307.

Naughton MT. Cheyne-Stokes respiration: friend or foe? *Thorax*;**67**: 357–360.

Cowie et al. Adaptive servo-ventilation for central sleep apnea in systolic heart failure *NEJM*;**373**: 1095–1105.

Murphy et al. Effect of home noninvasive ventilation with oxygen therapy vs oxygen therapy alone on hospital readmission or death after an acute COPD exacerbation: a randomized clinical trial. *JAMA* 2017;**317**: 2177–2186.

Lanfranchi PA, Somers VK. Sleep-disordered breathing in heart failure: characteristics and implications. *Respir Physiol Neurobiol* 2003;**136**: 153–165.

Berry-Kravis EM et al. Congenital central hypoventilation syndrome. *Am J Respir Crit Care Med* 2006;**174**: 1139–1144.

Gray A et al. Noninvasive ventilation in acute cardiogenic pulmonary edema. *N Engl J Med* 2008;**359**: 142–151.

Obesity-related respiratory problems

Levels of obesity (BMI >30 kg/m^2) are rising. Between 1993 and 2017 levels of obesity increased from 15% to 29% of the adult population in the UK. This has also had many impacts on health care outside of respiratory medicine, particularly the components of the metabolic syndrome.

Obesity, particularly in conjunction with OSA and COPD, provokes ventilatory failure and cor pulmonale (see ➲ p. 232). A common clinical scenario is the obese smoker, with a history of snoring and sleepiness, arriving in the A&E with hypercapnia. Why only some obese patients develop hypercapnia is not clear, but abdominal obesity seems the most hazardous. This may be because of greater lung volume compression, thus breathing occurs nearer residual volume where airway resistance is much higher and total compliance lower, thus increasing the work of breathing considerably.

The term 'obesity hypoventilation syndrome' is used when an obese individual (BMI >30 kg/m^2) has a raised PaCO$_2$ (>6 kPa) with no other apparent explanation, usually in conjunction with worsening sleep-related hypoventilation, and often additional obstructive sleep apnoea.

Obese patients can often have mildly raised PaCO$_2$ and bicarbonate levels for long periods, without apparent problems. Once there is acute decompensation with acidosis, management is more difficult. NIV is usually effective but may require very high inspiratory and expiratory pressures that can be difficult to deliver adequately without pressure damage/ulceration of the nasal bridge. Weight loss is very effective but, as usual, is hard to achieve without bariatric surgery, which will be hazardous if NIV has not lifted the patient out of ventilatory failure.

The main indications for NIV in OHS are decompensated acidotic hypercapnia (PaCO$_2$ >6.5 kPa), hypercapnia with excessive somnolence or hypercapnia and cor pulmonale. Some patients with stable compensated hypercapnia can either be started on CPAP or switched to CPAP from NIV at a later date.

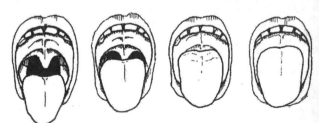

Fig. 48.9 Mallampati index. Simple scoring system for pharyngeal crowding. Affected by craniofacial shape, tongue size, and obesity. Predicts difficulty of intubation and correlates with OSA severity.

Reproduced from Allman and Wilson, Oxford Handbook of Anaesthesia 4th edition, 2015 with permission from Oxford University Press.

Further information

Masa et al. Obesity hypoventilation syndrome. *Eur Respir Rev* 2019;**28**: pii 180097.
Soghier et al. Noninvasive ventilation versus CPAP as initial treatment of obesity hypoventilation syndrome: a systematic review. *Ann Am Thorac Soc* 2019; E. pub 31 July.

Upper airway and tracheal disease

Acute upper airway obstruction 704
Anaphylaxis 706
Upper respiratory tract infections 1 708
Upper respiratory tract infections 2 710
Laryngeal and tracheal disorders 712

Acute upper airway obstruction

This is a life-threatening medical emergency. Call for help and follow an ABC (airway, breathing, circulation) approach.

Presentation

Sudden respiratory distress, cyanosis, and aphonia. Airway obstruction can occur at any level within the airway. Partial airway obstruction leads to noisy breathing, with stridor, gurgling, or snoring. Complete airway obstruction is associated with distress and marked respiratory effort, with paradoxical chest and abdominal movement ('seesaw breathing') and use of accessory muscles of respiration. This may be followed by collapse with loss of consciousness and progress to cardiorespiratory arrest. Look for chest and abdominal movements and listen and feel for airflow at the nose and mouth.

Causes

- Pharyngeal occlusion by tongue and other upper airway muscles, 2° to loss of muscle tone. This may be 2° to drugs, alcohol, a neurological event, or cardiorespiratory arrest
- Vomit or blood
- Inhaled foreign body, which may also cause laryngeal spasm
- Laryngeal obstruction due to oedema from burns, inflammation, or anaphylaxis
- Excessive bronchial secretions, mucosal oedema, bronchospasm: may cause airway obstruction below the larynx
- Infection such as epiglottitis
- Any cause of chronic airway obstruction, such as an airway tumour or extrinsic compression due to goitre, tumour, or lymphadenopathy, may deteriorate precipitously.

Box 49.1 Management of upper airway obstruction

Call for senior anaesthetic help early

- Open the airway with backwards head tilt, chin lift, and forward jaw thrust. In cases of trauma, do not tilt the head in case of cervical spine injury, but perform a jaw thrust only
- If unsuccessful at restoring normal respiration, visually inspect the mouth for obvious obstruction, and remove it with a finger sweep. Be mindful of not pushing any obstructing matter further into the airway. Leave well-fitting dentures in place
- If there is a witnessed history of choking and the patient is conscious, consider performing five black blows, followed by five abdominal thrusts if unsuccessful
- If the patient is unconscious and no signs of life/no spontaneous respiratory effort, start resuscitation. Insert a laryngeal mask or consider anaesthetic/intensive care unit (ICU) placement of an endotracheal tube and deliver O_2 via self-inflating bag with supplemental O_2 15 L/min and reservoir bag. If not breathing and cannot be ventilated, a cricothyroidotomy may be necessary (see ⊃ p. 861)
- Suction out secretions
- Maintain circulation with cardiac compression, if necessary
- Seek definitive treatment for the cause of airway obstruction

Anaphylaxis

This is a life-threatening medical emergency. Call for help and follow and ABC approach.

Causes

IgE-mediated type I hypersensitivity reaction to allergen. Histamine release causes the clinical syndrome. Typical allergens include bee or wasp sting, peanuts, fish, drugs, foods, latex, contrast media, anaesthetic agents, and drugs. Incidence of anaphylaxis is increasing with 1 in 300 Europeans affected at some point in their lifetime.

Presentation

Typically, a rapid onset of symptoms of varying severity:
- Angio-oedema
- Urticaria
- Dyspnoea
- Wheeze
- Stridor
- Hypotension
- Arrhythmias
- Also rhinitis, abdominal pain, vomiting, diarrhoea, sense of impending doom.

Symptoms typically resolve within minutes to hours. It is not clear what determines severity of anaphylaxis in individuals. Asthma and cardiovascular disease are important comorbidities that carry a worse prognosis in anaphylaxis. Patient may have had previous episodes of severe allergic-type reactions. Usually needs in-hospital observation for 6–12 h, sometimes longer.
- *Biphasic anaphylaxis* is a further episode, typically within 10 h, after the initial anaphylaxis seems to have resolved, without further allergen exposure
- *Protracted anaphylaxis* lasts for hours or days.

Subcutaneous allergen immunotherapy (SCIT)

Aims to desensitize a person to an allergen to which they are sensitive, thus minimizing their allergic reaction. Suitable for people with allergic asthma and/or allergic rhinitis, with specific IgE to the allergen identified as causing symptoms. Useful in those who cannot avoid allergen exposure. Small amounts of single or multiple allergens are injected once or twice weekly, with slowly increasing dose strengths until the maximum dose of the allergen is administered, which can take up to 12 months. Mechanism unknown but probably related to increased IgG binding to the allergen, falling allergen-specific IgE levels, and decreased amount of circulating inflammatory cytokines. Can protect against anaphylaxis for 3–5 y, but 'top-up' doses necessary. Effective for dust, grass, tree, and weed pollen, mould spores, latex, and insect venom, as well as some animal allergens. Side effects of administration: anaphylaxis, bronchoconstriction, local reaction. Some centres may not perform in people with severe or unstable asthma because of the risk of death.

Box 49.2 Management of anaphylaxis
- Remove likely allergen where possible
- Cardiopulmonary resuscitation if necessary
- *Airway and breathing* Administer high-flow O_2 through non-rebreathe mask aiming for saturations of 94–98% in most. If airway compromise, consider early tracheal intubation. Airway swelling may make this difficult, and cricothyroidotomy may need to be performed (see ⮑ p. 861)
- Give adrenaline (epinephrine) intramuscular (IM) 1:1,000 solution 0.5 mL (500 micrograms) as early as possible. Repeat after 5 min if no improvement or deterioration.
- *Circulation* treat shock with a fluid challenge (e.g. 500–1000 mL 0.9% sodium chloride). Those experienced with intravenous (IV) adrenaline (1:10,000) can use 50 mcg boluses for profound shock and immediately life-threatening anaphylaxis.
- Antihistamines (e.g. chlorphenamine 10 mg slow IV or IM) and steroids (200 mg slow IV or IM hydrocortisone) are second-line treatments
- Consider nebulized salbutamol or adrenaline if bronchospasm
- On discharge advise on future episodes, MedicAlert bracelet, and card and consider IM self-administered adrenaline
- Offer allergy service/immunology referral
- Send mast cell tryptase blood tests at onset, 1–2 h after symptoms start and at 24 h after symptoms
- Consider C1 esterase inhibitor deficiency, especially if repeated episodes.

Future developments

A diagnostic test to accurately identify anaphylaxis will be useful, as current tests involving measurement of serum or plasma tryptase are not perfect.

Further study of biphasic reactions is needed, along with work on the ideal duration of observation post-anaphylaxis and the effect of specialist allergy services on health care-related quality of life (QoL).

Further information

Resuscitation Council (UK) *Advanced Life Support*, 7th Edition. 2016.

Upper respiratory tract infections 1

Acute upper respiratory tract infections (URTIs) include rhinitis, pharyngitis, tonsillitis, and sinusitis.

URTIs are the commonest cause of time off work in the UK. The majority are managed by GPs and will not reach a respiratory specialist. They are usually self-limiting and often do not require specific treatment.

Acute rhinitis

Nasal congestion with rhinorrhoea, mild malaise, and sneezing. Most commonly due to viral infection (the common cold). Topical decongestants may be useful. There is no evidence for the use of antibiotics or antihistamines.

Candidiasis

Oral *Candida* infection is common in those who have received antibiotics, are immunosuppressed, or are on oral or inhaled steroids. Seen as white plaque-like lesions on the tongue and pharyngeal mucosa. Treat with oral nystatin or amphotericin lozenges, and with oral hygiene. Severe infection can be debilitating, leading to difficulties with eating, especially in the elderly and may need treatment with fluconazole. Exclude underlying immunocompromise (e.g. human immunodeficiency virus (HIV), leukaemia) in those with persisting infection despite treatment.

Acute epiglottitis (supraglottitis)

Infection mainly localized to the epiglottis and surrounding supraglottic structures. It is commoner in children than adults, but a mortality of up to 7% is reported in adults. This is due to upper airways obstruction from grossly oedematous upper airway tissue and can be life-threatening.
* *Haemophilus influenzae*, streptococci, and staphylococci are causative organisms
* Acute epiglottitis typically presents with a sore throat, fever, drooling, hoarseness. Inspiratory stridor is less common, but it can also present with acute upper airway obstruction and chest radiograph (CXR) infiltrates consistent with pulmonary oedema (due to high negative intrathoracic pressure)
* Diagnosis is made by visualizing epiglottis (direct or indirect laryngoscopy), but this may not be possible
* May need airway protection with an endotracheal tube or tracheostomy: liaise with ENT/anaesthetic colleagues early
* In severe infection, epiglottic swabs may be of diagnostic use, but beware of precipitating airway obstruction. Treatment will depend on local guidelines and culture but consider empirical treatments that cover β-lactam-producing *H. influenzae*.

Rhinosinusitis

The paranasal sinuses communicate with the nose and are therefore susceptible to infection from this route. All the sinuses drain by means of the mucociliary escalator. Blockage of free sinus drainage is a predisposing factor for bacterial infection. Sinusitis is a common cause of persistent cough (see **⊃** pp. 18–19). Dental sepsis may lead to maxillary sinusitis by direct spread.

Acute rhinosinusitis

Complicates 1 in 200 URTIs and usually presents with fever, nasal congestion/purulent discharge, maxillary tooth pain, and sinus pain that is worse on leaning forward. It may be associated with systemic upset. Respiratory viral infection interrupts normal defences of the mucosal lining, producing mucous exudates, with 2° bacterial infection. *S. pneumoniae* and *H. influenzae* are the commonest pathogens. *S. aureus* and *S. pyogenes* are also causes, with Pseudomonas in cystic fibrosis (CF). Mixed infections with anaerobes are seen in 10%. Specific diagnostic tests are not usually needed. Antibiotic treatment may be indicated if symptoms persist longer than 10 days, or severe symptoms of fever, facial pain, and purulent discharge at onset lasting >3 days.

Chronic rhinosinusitis

By definition, if present for >3 months. The ciliated epithelial sinus lining is replaced by thickened stratified squamous lining, with absent cilia, due to repeated infection. Anaerobic infection is more common. Fungal infection is more common in atopic people with nasal polyps. Sinus mycetoma is a rare complication in neutropenic patients, diabetics, and the immunocompromised.

Presentation

Frontal headache (frontal sinusitis), maxillary pain, pain over bridge of nose (ethmoidal sinusitis), retro-orbital headache (sphenoidal sinusitis), with purulent nasal discharge and blockage. GPA (Wegener's) may mimic the symptoms of sinusitis.

Investigations

Not usually warranted. CT may be warranted to plan surgical intervention or if malignant disease suspected.

Treatment

Analgesia, topical decongestants, antibiotics if severe infection.

Surgery

May be warranted if prolonged or repeated infection, anatomical abnormality, or other complications, e.g. if infection has spread to the cranial cavity or orbit. Spreading infection is uncommon if there has been prior antibiotic treatment.

Upper respiratory tract infections 2

Acute pharyngitis and tonsillitis

Viruses cause 80–90%; most commonly adenoviruses, coronaviruses, rhinoviruses, and influenza viruses. Group A streptococci, *Streptococcus pneumoniae*, and *Haemophilus influenzae* may cause 2° infection. *Mycoplasma* and *Chlamydia* are seen less commonly.

- Pharyngitis and tonsillitis present with a sore throat, which is usually self-limiting. May be associated with fever, malaise, lymphadenopathy, conjunctivitis, headache, nausea, and vomiting
- Infectious mononucleosis (EBV) is associated with pharyngitis in 80% of cases. Diagnose with Paul Bunnell test for heterophil antibodies and atypical mononuclear cells in peripheral blood
- Coxsackie A and herpes simplex cause 'herpangina syndrome'— ulcerating vesicles on the tonsils and palate
- Cytomegalovirus (CMV) can also cause pharyngitis associated with lymphadenopathy and splenomegaly
- Lemierre's syndrome (jugular vein suppurative thrombophlebitis) is a rare anaerobic pharyngeal infection (see ➲ p. 544 Box 41.6).

Other causative agents
- *Corynebacterium diphtheriae* in unvaccinated populations. A pharyngeal membrane may form, with systemic symptoms, and 'bull neck' due to cervical lymphadenopathy. Low-grade fever, with a relatively high pulse rate. Treat urgently with diphtheria antitoxin
- Vincent's angina is anaerobic infection in those with poor mouth hygiene. Caused by Gram-negative *Borrelia vincenti* and other anaerobic infections. Treat with penicillin
- Group A *Streptococcus* may cause a more unpleasant illness, with systemic upset and dysphagia, due to pharyngotonsillar oedema.

Treatment
Usually supportive, but anti-streptococcal antibiotics may be warranted if there is severe infection (fever, tonsillar exudates, tender anterior cervical lymphadenopathy). There is no evidence that antibiotics reduce the duration of symptoms, but they may reduce complications (e.g. sinusitis, quinsy, and rheumatic fever, which is rare in the Western world). Oral penicillin is the first-line treatment (or a macrolide if penicillin-allergic). Amoxicillin can cause a rash in infectious mononucleosis and so should be avoided. Throat swabs for group A *Streptococcus* may be helpful in directing treatment.

Complications
Untreated infection complications include peritonsillar abscess (quinsy), retropharyngeal abscess, and cervical abscess. Treat with appropriate antibiotics. Surgical drainage is occasionally required.

Laryngitis

This is usually part of a generalized URTI. Often viral, but *Moraxella catarrhalis*, *Haemophilus influenzae*, and *Streptococcus pneumoniae* are also causative. It may cause a hoarse voice or aphonia.

Other causes include inhaled steroids, occupational exposure to inhaled chemicals, and GORD. If a hoarse voice persists in a smoker, a laryngeal or lung cancer (with recurrent laryngeal nerve involvement) must be excluded. Other causes include tuberculous infection, herpes simplex virus (HSV), CMV, diphtheria, fungal infections, and actinomycoses.

Treatment—usually no specific treatment is required, as the illness is typically self-limiting.

Acute bronchitis, tracheitis, and tracheobronchitis

Inflammation due to infection can occur in any part of the tracheobronchial tree and is termed tracheitis, tracheobronchitis, or bronchitis, depending on the anatomical site. It usually follows viral infection, especially of the common cold type, and is commoner during influenza epidemics. 2° bacterial infection is common, with *H. influenzae* and *S. pneumoniae* commonest. There is increased prevalence in the winter months.

Presentation

Productive cough, small-volume streaky haemoptysis, and fever. Breathlessness and hypoxia are uncommon, unless there is coexistent cardiorespiratory disease or a concomitant pneumonia. Retrosternal chest pain is common in tracheitis. Examination is often normal.

Diagnosis

Usually on the basis of the history. A persisting cough, especially in a smoker, may warrant further investigation.

Treatment

Usually symptomatic, particularly in the previously well. Use antibiotics for persistent cough productive of mucopurulent sputum or if there is coexistent cardiopulmonary disease.

Laryngeal and tracheal disorders

Inducible laryngeal obstruction (ILO)

An inappropriate transient closure of the larynx induced by a trigger. Previously incorrectly termed vocal cord dysfunction, although obstruction can be at any laryngeal level. The exact prevalence of ILO is not known but it is thought to affect ~5% of adolescents and young adults, with a female preponderance. Triggers include exercise, irritants, and emotional stress. ILO can mimic or co-exist with asthma.

If induced by exercise the symptoms are typically at maximal exertion. This contrast with bronchospasm where symptoms can occur up to 30 minutes after exercise.

Typically causes dyspnoea with noisy inspiration.

Objective identification, normally with video laryngoscopy is recommended but exercise testing with flow volume loops can be helpful.

There is no randomized data as to how to treat ILO but typically approaches include speech therapy, specialist respiratory physiotherapist, or psychological approaches. Aim to modify breathing patterns, avoid triggers, and treat co-existent reflux or asthma.

Tracheobronchomalacia (TBM) and excessive dynamic airways collapse (EDAC)

Are both conditions that cause part/all of the central airways (trachea and both main bronchi) to collapse during expiration (>50%). Less than 50% collapse of the central airways is normal during expiration. These conditions when mild are often incidental findings on bronchoscopy or dynamic CT. When severe they can cause dyspnoea, cough, haemoptysis, secretion retention, pneumonia, and respiratory failure.

TBM is caused by a weakness in either the anterior or lateral cartilaginous airways rings, whereas EDAC is due to collapse of the posterior wall of the central airways.

TBM can either be congenital (e.g. Ehler–Danlos syndrome), primary (Mounier–Kuhn syndrome) or secondary (e.g. post-traumatic, post-intubation/tracheostomy). EDAC tends to only complicate chronic airways disease such as COPD due in part to forced expiration increasing propensity to upper airway collapse. Treatment for both conditions includes non-invasive ventilation (NIV)/continuous positive airway pressure (CPAP) both during sleep and intermittently in the day, bronchoscopic stent placement, and surgery (depending on the site, including tracheostomy, tracheal resection, and tracheobronchoplasty). They are probably under-recognized as the cause of symptoms in those with COPD and asthma.

Further reading

Halvorsen et al. Inducible laryngeal obstruction: an official joint European Respiratory Society and European Laryngological Society statement. *Eur Respir J* 2017;**50**: pii 1602221.

Kalra et al. Excessive dynamic airway collapse for the internist: new nomenclature or different entity? *Postgrad Med J* 2011;**87**: 482–486.

Biswas et al. Tracheobronchomalacia. *Dis Mon* 2017;**63**: 287–302.

Chapter 50

Vasculitis and the lung

Classification 714

Granulomatosis with polyangiitis (Wegener's): presentation and diagnosis 716

Granulomatosis with polyangiitis (Wegener's): management 718

Microscopic polyangiitis 720

Anti-GBM disease (Goodpasture's) 721

Eosinophilic granulomatosis with polyangiitis (Churg–Strauss syndrome) 722

Rare pulmonary vasculitides 724

Classification

These are rare conditions but are often seen in the specialist chest clinic (see ● p. 27 for an approach to diffuse alveolar haemorrhage). Clinical features can be non-specific and similar to those seen in other diseases, and diagnosis can therefore be difficult. Vasculitides are great 'mimickers' of other diseases, such as lung cancer or acute respiratory distress syndrome (ARDS), and have a high untreated mortality. There is considerable overlap between the different vasculitides, which can make definitive diagnosis difficult. Suspect a diagnosis of vasculitis if:

- Weight loss
- Low-grade fever
- Raised inflammatory markers
- Chest disease is not improving or responding to treatment as expected:
  - Unexplained dyspnoea
  - Hypoxia
  - Unexplained desaturation on exercise
  - Haemoptysis
  - Sinus or nasal disease
  - Wheeze
  - Chest radiograph (CXR) abnormalities/infiltrates
  - Abnormal kCO
- Associated renal impairment or positive urine dip for blood or protein
- Raised autoantibodies
- No other clear diagnosis.

The 1° pathology in vasculitis is inflammation and necrosis of differing sized blood vessels. The pulmonary vessels are involved as part of a multi-systemic vasculitis process.

Small-vessel vasculitides

The most common to involve the lung. Arterioles, capillaries, and venules located within the lung interstitium are affected. Neutrophil infiltration and subsequent fibrinoid necrosis cause vessel wall destruction. Necrotizing pulmonary capillaritis can also occur, characterized by a marked neutrophilic infiltration of the interstitium. Interstitial capillaries become damaged, allowing red blood cells to enter the alveolus; thus, alveolar haemorrhage is a feature of many of the small-vessel vasculitides.

Nomenclature for the vasculitides was released by the International Chapel Hill Consensus Conference in 2012, revising that of 1994 (see Table 50.1).

Table 50.1 Classification of vasculitis, based on the Revised International Chapel Hill Consensus, 2012

1° vasculitis	Lung involvement	ANCA
Small vessel		
ANCA-associated vasculitis (AAV)		
• Microscopic polyangiitis (MPA)	Frequent	c/p-ANCA
• GPA (Wegener's)	Frequent	c-ANCA in 75%,
• EGPA (Churg–Strauss)	Frequent	p-ANCA in 15%
Goodpasture's disease	Frequent	p-ANCA in 70%
		p-ANCA in 10–20%
Medium-sized vessel		
Polyarteritis nodosa (PAN)	Rare	Negative
Large vessel		
Giant cell arteritis	Rare	Negative
Takayasu's arteritis	Frequent	Negative

Box 50.1 Antineutrophil cytoplasmic antibodies (ANCA)

ANCAs react with cytoplasmic granule enzymes in neutrophils and stain them in one of two ways:
• Diffusely cytoplasmic pattern or c-ANCA
• Perinuclear pattern or p-ANCA.

These autoantibodies may have a direct role in pathogenesis as well as being disease markers.

ANCA have two major specificities:
• Antiproteinase 3 antibodies (anti-PR3)—associated with c-ANCA pattern
• Antimyeloperoxidase antibodies (anti-MPO)—associated with p-ANCA pattern.

c-ANCA (anti-PR3) targets PR3 and may suggest GPA (75% of cases are c-ANCA positive). Levels correlate with disease activity and extent. Also found in patients with MPA (45% of those with clinical disease will be c-ANCA positive).

p-ANCA (anti-MPO) targets MPO and has a wider range of disease associations, including other vasculitides and autoimmune diseases, HIV, lung cancer, pulmonary fibrosis, and PEs.

Further information

2012 revised International Chapel Hill Consensus Conference Nomenclature of Vasculitides. *Arthritis Rheum* 2013;**65**: 1–11.

Bosch X et al. ANCA. *Lancet* 2006;**368**: 404–418.

Schwarz M, Brown K. Small vessel vasculitis of the lung. Rare diseases 10. *Thorax* 2000;**55**: 502–10.

Granulomatosis with polyangiitis (Wegener's): presentation and diagnosis

Definition and epidemiology

Necrotizing vasculitis affecting small and medium-sized vessels, especially in the upper and lower respiratory tract and also the kidneys. Associated granulomata. Renamed in 2011.

- Unknown cause
- ♂ = ♀
- 3/100,000, 80–97% Caucasian
- Any age, but most common 40–55 y.

Clinical features

- *ENT* In 90%, upper airways involvement will be the first presenting sign. Nasal congestion and epistaxis, with inflamed, crusty, ulcerated nasal mucosa. Nasal septum perforation. Late sign is a saddle nose deformity. Sinusitis is common and may be painful. Otitis media. Subglottic stenosis, causing upper airway obstruction, dyspnoea, voice change, and cough. Abnormal flow–volume loops
- *Lung* Affected in 85–90% of patients. Haemoptysis, cough, dyspnoea. Pleuritic chest pain
- *Kidney* Affected in 77% of patients. Haematuria, proteinuria, and red cell casts. Only 10% have renal impairment initially, but 80% will have involvement during their disease course. Characteristic progressive deterioration of renal function
- *Systemic* Fever and weight loss
- *Other organ systems (skin, eyes, joints, central nervous system (CNS))* Vasculitic skin rash, with granulomatous involvement in 46%. Muscle and joint pains. Conjunctivitis, scleritis, proptosis, eye pain, visual loss. Mononeuritis multiplex and CNS disease.

Investigations

Consider:

- *CXR* Flitting cavitating pulmonary nodules, consolidation, or pulmonary infiltrates, alveolar haemorrhage, parenchymal distortion, large and small airway disease, pleural effusion, bronchiectasis. Can look like neoplasms, infection, or fluid overload
- *High-resolution computed tomography (HRCT)* of chest
- *O_2 saturations*
- *Full blood count (FBC), urea and electrolytes (U&E), C-reactive protein (CRP), erythrocyte sedimentation rate (ESR)*
- *Serum antinuclear cytoplasmic antibody (ANCA)*, especially c-ANCA, is sensitive and fairly specific. Present in 90% of patients with extensive GPA and 75% with limited. p-ANCA positive in 5–10% of patients with GPA. Combining indirect immunofluorescence with specific immunoassays for antibodies to PR3 and MPO increases sensitivity and specificity for GPA and MPA to over 90%. Remember ANCA can be negative, especially in disease confined to the respiratory tract. ANCA titres rise prior to a relapse and are higher when disease is active, and this can act as a guide to starting treatment. However, high ANCA

levels in the absence of clinical symptoms or signs may not represent active disease, and, therefore, ANCA levels should not be used in isolation to determine treatment. Also consider CRP ± ESR
- *Urine dipstick and microscopy* Red cell casts
- *Pulmonary function tests (PFTs), including kCO*
- *Image sinuses* Bony destruction makes GPA likely
- *Bronchoscopy* May show inflammation and ulceration of larynx, trachea, and bronchi. Scarring and stenosis may be seen. Bronchoalveolar lavage (BAL) is neutrophilic, also with eosinophils and lymphocytes. Transbronchial biopsy (TBB) is unlikely to be diagnostic
- *Biopsy*
  - *Respiratory tract and nose*—granulomata in association with medium- and small-vessel necrotizing vasculitis and surrounding inflammation. Nasal biopsies are often non-specific and may not be diagnostic
  - *Renal biopsy*—focal segmental or diffuse necrotizing glomerulonephritis. Pauci-immune and granulomata rare. Not specific for GPA
  - *Skin biopsy*—leukocytoclastic vasculitis ± granulomata.

Diagnosis

Biopsy and ANCA are key to diagnosis. Biopsy whichever site is affected. May be nasal, lung (open or thoracoscopic), skin, or renal. If there is evidence on urine dip of renal vasculitis, this may be the best and easiest biopsy site. Disease may be patchy in nature, requiring repeat biopsies if the first is negative. High c-ANCA and anti PR3 is highly suggestive of GPA.

Differential diagnosis of GPA

Malignancy, tuberculosis (TB), sarcoidosis, allergic bronchopulmonary aspergillosis (ABPA), anti-GBM disease with pulmonary haemorrhage and nephritis, systemic lupus erythematosus (SLE), MPA, connective tissue disease.

Granulomatosis with polyangiitis (Wegener's): management

Involve the rheumatology and renal team, and share care of the patient. See Chapter 53 for immunosuppressive drug details.

- Standard regimen for *generalized or organ-threatening disease* (e.g. active/progressive pulmonary or renal disease or CNS disease):
  - Induce remission with oral prednisolone (1 mg/kg/day, tapering weekly to a dose of 15 mg or less daily by 3 months) and cyclophosphamide, orally (2 mg/kg/day, up to 200 mg/day) or IV (pulses at 2- or 3-week intervals, 15 mg/kg), for 3–6 months. Reduce cyclophosphamide dose in elderly (e.g. reduce oral dose by 25% if >60 y and by 50% if >75 y) and in setting of renal impairment. Taper cyclophosphamide dose to maintain WCC >4 × 10⁹/L and neutrophils >2 × 10⁹, to reduce infection risk (see ➲ p. 744 for more detail)
  - Rituximab may be used in place of cyclophosphamide (see ➲ p. 746)
  - The aim is to prevent irreversible tissue necrosis. There is evidence that this regime induces remission in 80% of patients at 3 months and 90% at 6 months
  - After induction of remission (at 3–6 months), consider switch from cyclophosphamide and prednisolone to maintenance therapy with prednisolone and either azathioprine (2 mg/kg/day for 12 months, then reduce to 1.5 mg/kg/day; check thiopurine methyltransferase (TPMT) levels; see ➲ p. 742) or methotrexate (15 mg once/week, increase to maximum of 20–25 mg once/week by week 12; see ➲ p. 742). This avoids the morbidity associated with long-term cyclophosphamide use. Both azathioprine and methotrexate have been demonstrated to maintain remission, although the evidence favours use of azathioprine
  - Restart the regime if the patient relapses—this may occur in 50%
- For *severe life-threatening disease* (e.g. rapidly progressive renal failure or massive pulmonary haemorrhage):
  - Plasma exchange/plasmapheresis (7 × 4 L exchanges over 2 weeks) has been shown to be more effective than methylprednisolone in the treatment of GPA. In patients with severe pulmonary haemorrhage, it is also effective and can be given along with fresh frozen plasma
  - In addition, treat with pulsed methylprednisolone (500–1,000 mg/day, depending on body weight for 3 days) and IV cyclophosphamide (15 mg/kg, reduce if elderly or renal impairment)
  - Rituximab may be used in place of cyclophosphamide (see ➲ p. 746).
  - Dialysis for renal failure
  - After induction of remission (over 3–6 months), switch from cyclophosphamide to azathioprine or methotrexate with prednisolone as maintenance therapy

- For *localized disease or early systemic disease* (without threatened organ involvement):
  - Prednisolone with either methotrexate or oral/pulsed cyclophosphamide
  - Use of methotrexate avoids cyclophosphamide-related toxicity but may be associated with a higher relapse rate
  - Localized disease may still be serious (e.g. retro-orbital involvement), and, in these situations, cyclophosphamide should be considered
- *Duration of treatment* Maintenance therapy is recommended to continue for at least 24 months after initial disease remission, as relapses are common. Some recommend continuing treatment for up to 5 y, particularly if the ANCA remains positive
- PCP prophylaxis with co-trimoxazole is recommended (960 mg 3×/week) in patients receiving cyclophosphamide and prednisolone. There is some evidence that co-trimoxazole alone may be effective in the treatment of especially limited GPA, although the reasons for this are not clear—it may be due to suppression of nasal *Staphylococcus aureus* carriage, the presence of which is associated with an increased risk of relapse
- Osteoporosis prophylaxis should be considered
- *Follow-up* monthly for 3 months, then 3–6-monthly. Monitor FBC, U&E, CRP, liver function test (LFT), ANCA, CXR, and kCO. Rising ANCA titres are a poor predictor of relapse; in the absence of other features of a relapse, follow up more closely, but do not increase immunosuppression solely on this basis. Withdrawal of immunosuppression in the setting of a persistently positive ANCA is associated with relapse, however
- *Relapses* Treat minor relapses with an increase in the prednisolone dose. Treat major relapses with cyclophosphamide and increasing prednisolone; consider IV methylprednisolone, plasma exchange
- *Refractory disease* Liaise with specialist; consider alternative therapies such as infliximab, high-dose IV immunoglobulin, rituximab, anti-thymocyte globulin, or CAMPATH 1H (alemtuzumab, anti-CD52). Mycophenolate or leflunomide are alternatives to azathioprine or methotrexate. Exclude underlying infection, malignancy, and non-compliance.

Prognosis

Limited disease with pulmonary, but no renal, involvement and an often-negative c-ANCA test has a better prognosis. However, this can progress over time to *extensive disease*, with classical destructive sinusitis, nephritis, and vasculitis and strong c-ANCA positivity, and is associated with higher mortality. Untreated, 80% of people with extensive GPA will die in 1 y. Overall, 75–90% of patients can be brought into remission with treatment, although 50% relapse in 5 y, and long-term follow-up is required.

Microscopic polyangiitis

At least as common as GPA and may be hard to distinguish. Managed in the same way.

- *Incidence* ♂=♀, mean age 50, mainly Caucasians
- *Kidneys* Main organ affected by a small-vessel necrotizing vasculitis, causing proteinuria and haematuria. Renal biopsy shows focal segmental glomerulonephritis with fibrinoid necrosis and sparse immune deposits
- *Pulmonary involvement* occurs in 30–50% of patients, with pleurisy, asthma, haemoptysis, and pulmonary haemorrhage. CXR may be suggestive of pulmonary haemorrhage
- *p-ANCA* positive, often c-ANCA also.

Treatment

Immunosuppression: steroids and cyclophosphamide first line. Rituximab may be used in place of cyclophosphamide if cyclophosphamide is contra-indicated or not tolerated. (see ⊃ p. 746).

Further information

Ntatsaki E et al. British Society of Rheumatology and British Heath Professionals in Rheumatology guidelines for the management of adults with ANCA associated vasculitis. *Rheumatology* 2014; **53**: 2306–2309.

Langford C, Hoffman G. Wegener's granulomatosis. Rare diseases 3. *Thorax* 1999;**54**: 629–663.

Frankel SK et al. Update in the diagnosis and management of pulmonary vasculitis. *Chest* 2006;**129**: 452–465.

Anti-GBM disease (Goodpasture's)

Definition and epidemiology

Linear deposition of IgG on the basement membranes of alveoli and glomeruli, which damages collagen and in the lungs allows leakage of blood.

- Anti-GBM antibodies are detectable in blood
- Alveolar haemorrhage and glomerulonephritis
- Important differential diagnosis of pulmonary-renal syndrome
- Annual incidence of 1 case per million
- ♂:♀ = 4:1
- Commonest age 20–30 y
- Second peak when women in their late 60s are affected by glomerulonephritis alone
- Cause unknown. Often a preceding viral infection. Smokers at greater risk of pulmonary haemorrhage, but not of anti-GBM disease
- HLA-DR2 association in 60–70%.

Clinical features

- Haemoptysis in 80–90%—more common in smokers
- Cough, dyspnoea, fatigue, and weakness
- Examination: inspiratory crackles common.

Investigations

- *Serum electrolytes* show impaired renal function and often renal failure
- *FBC* Iron deficiency anaemia
- *Urine dip and microscopy* Haematuria, proteinuria, granular, and typically red blood cell casts. Occasionally macroscopic haematuria
- *Anti-GBM* and autoantibody screen
- *CXR± CT* Diffuse bilateral patchy airspace shadowing in mid- and lower zones. May see air bronchograms
- *PFTs* Restrictive defect with raised kCO if alveolar haemorrhage present.

Diagnosis

Renal biopsy usually shows diffuse crescentic glomerulonephritis. Linear IgG deposition detected by immunofluorescence or immuno-peroxidase. Lung biopsy shows active intra-alveolar haemorrhage, with collections of hemosiderin-laden macrophages. These are not specific changes but may also show linear immunofluorescence staining of IgG.

Differential diagnosis

GPA, other pulmonary renal syndromes.

Management

- Involve the renal team, and share care of the patient
- Plasma exchange improves the speed of response to immunosuppression
- High-dose steroids and cyclophosphamide
- May need dialysis. Renal function may not improve, and renal transplant is only an option later if anti-GBM antibody levels become low
- Recurrence is uncommon once disease is controlled. It usually responds to further immunosuppression. Residual defects in PFTs frequent.

Prognosis

Rapidly progressive pulmonary haemorrhage and renal failure. Usually fatal if not treated.

Eosinophilic granulomatosis with polyangiitis (Churg–Strauss syndrome)

Definition and epidemiology

Asthma, blood eosinophilia, and an eosinophilic granulomatous inflammation of the respiratory tract, with necrotizing vasculitis affecting small and medium-sized vessels.

- Rare; 2.4 per million population, but 64 per million of an asthmatic population (who may have been misdiagnosed with asthma)
- Middle-aged adults
- $\male : \female \approx 2:1$
- Unknown cause. Montelukast was postulated as a possible cause, but this is now thought unlikely. Development of eosiophilic granulomatosis with polyangiitis (EGPA) in people on montelukast probably related to their decreased steroid dose 'unmasking' EGPA, or as part of an increasing treatment regime in those with uncontrolled asthma, later diagnosed as EGPA.

Clinical features

A diagnosis of EGPA can be made if four of the following six criteria are present (American College of Rheumatology criteria, 1990):

- Asthma—may have had for years, often maturity onset, difficult to control, associated with rhinitis and nasal polyps
- Blood eosinophilia >10%
- Vasculitic neuropathy such as mononeuritis multiplex (occurs in 75%)
- Pulmonary infiltrates
- Sinus disease
- Extravascular eosinophils on biopsy findings.
- Also may have:
  - Myositis and cardiac failure, cardiomyopathy, coronary artery inflammation, pericardial effusion
  - Eosinophilic infiltration of mesenteric vessels, causing gastrointestinal (GI) disturbance
  - Alveolar haemorrhage
  - Rarely, proteinuria caused by renal disease with focal segmental glomerulonephritis. Renal failure is rare
  - Skin nodules and purpura
  - Myalgia and arthralgia
  - Fever and weight loss.

Typical pattern of disease has three phases: beginning with asthma, then developing blood and tissue eosinophilia, then going on to systemic vasculitis. The asthma precedes the vasculitis, often by years (mean 8 y).

Investigations

- *CXR* Fleeting peripheral pulmonary infiltrates and bilateral multifocal consolidation
- *HRCT* Ground-glass inflammation, pulmonary nodules, bronchial wall thickening, or alveolar haemorrhage
- *Bronchoscopy* BAL - marked eosinophilia

- *Pathology* Extravascular tissue eosinophilia, necrotizing angiitis, granulomata
- *Serum markers* Peripheral blood eosinophilia. p-ANCA and anti-MPO positive in two-thirds. ANCA levels may not correlate with disease activity, but blood eosinophilia is a good guide.

Diagnosis

Predominantly a clinical diagnosis. Pathological confirmation of eosinophilic tissue infiltration or vasculitis desirable. Biopsy easiest site affected, such as skin, kidney, or open or thoracoscopic lung biopsy.

Differential diagnosis

ABPA, sarcoidosis, drug and parasitic causes of eosinophilic pneumonias, HP, hypereosinophilic syndrome.

Management

Depends on severity of disease at presentation.
- *If isolated pulmonary disease*, oral prednisolone 1 mg/kg (max 60 mg/ day) for 1 month or until no evidence of disease, then slowly decrease over 1 y, with increases if symptoms recur
- *If unwell or with alveolar haemorrhage*, pulsed methylprednisolone IV for 3 days, followed by high-dose oral steroids, with or without cyclophosphamide (see ➲ p. 744)
- *In cardiac or GI disease, relapse, or life threatening situations*, such as requiring organ support, cyclophosphamide should be added (see ➲ p. 744)
- Plasma exchange is of no benefit
- Treatment is aimed at reversing organ damage and reducing relapse rate
- *To maintain remission*, prednisolone and one other immunosuppressant drug are usually required. Cyclophosphamide is often changed to azathioprine after 4–6 months
- Prophylactic co-trimoxazole should be given (960mg 3×/week), and consider bone protection for steroids
- *Follow up* regularly, with checks on FBC and eosinophil count, CXR.
- *Mepolizumab*, an anti-IL-5 monoclonal antibody therapy licensed in eosinophilic asthma, has shown some efficacy in an early study for EGPA (*NEJM* 2017). Further studies are underway.

Prognosis

Good prognosis if isolated pulmonary disease. Good response to steroids. May continue to have asthma, despite control of vasculitis, which can be severe and difficult to control. Poor prognosis associated with cardiac disease and severe GI disease, causing bleeding, perforation, or necrosis. Untreated, 5 y survival rate is 25%. Also associated with worse prognosis: proteinuria >1 g/24 h, renal insufficiency, CNS involvement. Cardiac disease is the main cause of death.

Further information

Noth I et al. Churg–Strauss syndrome. *Lancet* 2003;**361**: 587–594.
 http://www.vasculitis.org.uk
Weschler M et al. Mepolizumab or placebo for eosinophilic granulomatosis with polyangiitis. *N Engl J Med* 2017;**376**: 1921–1932.

Rare pulmonary vasculitides

Polyarteritis nodosa

- Similar to MPA but affects medium-sized vessels
- May exist as an 'overlap' disorder with GPA or EGPA
- Lung involvement is rare
- Sometimes associated with previous hepatitis B or rarely hepatitis C infection.

Takayasu's arteritis

- Predominantly young ♀, often Asian
- Vasculitis affecting the aorta and its major branches. Large and medium-sized pulmonary vessels affected, but involvement is usually silent. Pulmonary artery stenosis and occlusion common, occasionally with mild pulmonary hypertension (PHT)
- *Presents* with fevers and weight loss. Absent or weak upper limb peripheral pulses, particularly on left (as left axillary artery comes off aortic arch), and arterial bruits
- *Diagnosis* made by angiography
- *Treatment* Steroids may reduce symptoms but do not affect mortality. Angioplasty and surgical procedures may reduce the complications. Spontaneous remissions may occur.

Giant cell arteritis

- Commonest form of systemic vasculitis affecting large and medium-sized vessels
- 24 cases per 100,000. Predominantly elderly ♀
- *Presents* with non-specific symptoms of fever and weight loss; also headache, scalp tenderness, and jaw pain. Amaurosis fugax and visual loss due to optic neuritis
- *Pulmonary complications* occur in 9–25% of cases. They are relatively minor, with cough, sore throat, and hoarseness. PFTs and CXR normal
- *Diagnosis* High ESR, temporal artery biopsy showing pan-arteritis and giant cell formation
- *Treatment* Good response to oral steroids. Continue for 1–2 y.

Part III

Supportive care

51 Ethical considerations 727

52 Financial entitlements 733

53 Immunosuppressive drugs 739

54 Inhalers and nebulizers 747

55 Intensive care unit (ICU) referral 755

56 Lung transplantation 759

57 Non-invasive ventilation (NIV) 771

58 Oxygen therapy 787

59 Palliative care 799

60 Pulmonary rehabilitation 811

61 Smoking cessation 817

Ethical considerations

Background and capacity 728
Chronic obstructive pulmonary disease (COPD) 730
Lung cancer and neurological disease 732

Background and capacity

Respiratory physicians are often involved in making difficult decisions about the appropriateness of treatment and the prolongation of life in patients with chronic underlying lung disease. Sometimes, artificial ventilation may prolong the dying process; life has a natural end, and the potential to prolong life in the intensive care unit (ICU) can cause dilemmas. In other cases, these interventions are valuable at prolonging life with a reversible complication.

The General Medical Council (GMC), underpinned by longstanding ethical principles, states that doctors have an obligation to respect human life, protect the health of their patients, and put their patients' best interests first, always treating patients with respect and dignity. This means offering treatments where the benefits outweigh any risks and avoiding treatments that carry no net gain to the patient. Following established ethical and legal (including human rights) principles, decisions concerning potentially life-prolonging treatment must start from a presumption in favour of prolonging life. If a patient wishes to have a treatment that, in the doctor's considered view, is not indicated, the doctor and medical team are under no ethical or legal obligation to provide it, but the patient's right to a second opinion must be respected.

Discussions about resuscitation and invasive ventilation are rarely easy but should ideally be held with the patient, their next of kin, and nursing staff, in advance of an emergency situation. Clearly, this is not always possible. Ideally, all decisions regarding resuscitation and the ceiling of treatment (particularly relating to ventilation) should be documented in advance and handed over to on-call teams. Most possible outcomes can be anticipated. In difficult situations the hospital Ethics Committee may need to be involved.

Capacity must be assumed, a legal proxy may be appointed to make decisions on behalf of the patient, or an Independent Mental Capacity Advocate (IMCA) may be required. UK laws aiding decision making for patients who lack capacity include the Adults with Incapacity (Scotland) Act 2000, the Mental Capacity Act 2005; and the requirements of the Human Rights Act 1998. Doctors must seek up-to-date advice when there is uncertainty about how a particular decision might be viewed in law. See Box 51.1 on how to assess capacity.

Where it has been decided that a treatment is not in the best interests of the patient, there is no ethical distinction between stopping the treatment or not starting it in the first place (though the former may be more difficult to do), and this should not be used as an argument for failing to initiate the treatment in the first place.

Lasting power of attorney (LPA)

Allows an appointed attorney to make decisions about health and welfare and/or property and financial affairs, including giving or refusing consent to treatment, if the patient loses their capacity as defined by the Mental Capacity Act 2005. Neither the next of kin nor those with LPA have the legal right to determine any treatment; the responsibility remains with the doctor and multidisciplinary team (MDT), occasionally involving the courts of law.

Advance decisions

Also known as living wills and advance decision to refuse treatment (ADRT). These are statements documenting what treatment the individual would want in the future or would want to refuse in specific circumstances, should they lack capacity. They are legally binding in England and Wales, and doctors giving treatment against the patient's wishes expressed in a directive could be prosecuted. In Scotland and Northern Ireland, advance decisions are governed by common law, rather than legislation. The validity of any document must be validated. Advance decisions do not have to be written down, signed, and witnessed, unless they include decisions about resuscitation and other potential life-prolonging treatments. They must comply with the mental capacity act.

Advance statements

Written by the patient about their preferences, wishes, beliefs, and values, but are not legally binding. They provide a guide for others to make decisions in the patient's best interests if they lose capacity in the future.

Box 51.1 How to assess capacity

Capacity is decision specific. The patient must be able to:
- Understand the information relevant to the decision
- Retain the information long enough to make the decision
- Weigh up the information as part of the decision-making process
- Communicate back their decision.

Chronic obstructive pulmonary disease (COPD)

COPD is the cause of around 30,000 UK deaths per year (2012 data), and most patients die of respiratory failure during an exacerbation. A commonly encountered clinical situation is where a patient with COPD is admitted with an exacerbation and is in type 2 ventilatory failure. Standard treatment does not improve the respiratory acidosis, so non-invasive ventilation (NIV) is commenced. Before starting NIV, a decision must be clearly documented as to whether or not NIV is the ceiling of treatment. It may be, especially if the patient has severe or end-stage COPD.

Invasive ventilation in the ICU may be appropriate in certain specific situations, for example:
- In a relatively young patient (i.e. <65y)
- A patient with a relatively new diagnosis of COPD, in whom the episode is the first or second admission
- In the patient in whom there is a very obviously potentially reversible cause for the exacerbation, e.g. pneumonia.

Sometimes, in this situation, a defined time period for intensive care input may be decided, e.g. ventilation for 48 h (to allow treatments to work and to allow time to assess for any improvement), with extubation after that time period if no improvement has been made.

Decisions about intubation/ventilation and intensive care admission can only be made knowing the patient's usual level of functioning and previous quality of life (QoL). The difficulty is that QoL is a very subjective measure. Objective measures of usual functioning, e.g. measures of daily activity, usual exercise tolerance, and whether home care or assistance with activities of daily living is required, are often more useful in guiding the appropriateness of escalating therapy. With reference to the patient with COPD, the number of hospital admissions and exacerbations and the need for home O_2 or nebulizers will also be useful. Where limited information is available about the patient and therefore uncertainty exists about the appropriateness of ventilation, it should be started until a clearer assessment can be made. This may be relevant for a patient attending the emergency department where little information is available. The point concerning the withdrawal of therapy, should it subsequently be found to be inappropriate, also holds.

There are downsides to invasive ventilation: the risk of pneumothorax is increased in those with end-stage emphysema, and the risk of ventilator-associated pneumonia (VAP) increases with time ventilated (see → p. 538). Knowledge of the risk of these adverse events can help the medical team to balance the argument and make a decision about whether the risks of ventilation are likely to outweigh its benefits. The issue of limited resources should not influence a decision about formal ventilation or ICU admission.

The average length of intubation of patients with COPD admitted to ICU is 3.2 days. These patients have a 20–25% in-hospital mortality, with 50% of patients surviving 1 y post-ICU discharge. About 50% will be living independently 1 y post-hospital discharge. Clearly, only a very selected sub-group of patients is admitted to ICU, but concerns about prolonged periods of ventilation in this group of patients seem to be unfounded. Patients in whom a clear cause for the exacerbation can be identified (e.g. pneumonia) tend to do better, as there is a treatable, reversible cause for the exacerbation, and not just progression of the underlying disease.

Lung cancer and neurological disease

Advanced lung cancer

The use of antibiotic treatment for pneumonia in a patient with advanced lung malignancy may not be in their best interests in some circumstances. The patient's wishes and QoL, stage and extent of disease, and response to other treatments (e.g. chemotherapy) all need consideration. This is another situation in which it might be appropriate to define at the outset the treatments that are appropriate, e.g. 10 days total of IV and oral antibiotics. Note that treatments, such as antibiotics, can lead to improvement in symptoms (e.g. by reducing fever), without necessarily prolonging life, and it may be compassionate to continue antibiotics in this situation.

Progressive neurological disease

The decision about NIV in a patient with a progressive neuromuscular disease can be difficult. There is now strong randomized controlled trial (RCT) evidence that NIV in patients with some neuromuscular diseases (Duchenne muscular dystrophy, motor neurone disease (MND), neuromuscular and chest wall disease), improves QoL and survival. Decisions about the requirement for, and timing of, NIV need to be made by specialists in neuromuscular disease, in conjunction with home ventilation teams. Clinical deterioration can usually be anticipated, with serial measurements of spirometry and overnight O_2 or CO_2. Discussions should take place early on (unless the patient presents in respiratory failure, e.g. due to pneumonia, and subsequent ventilator weaning is difficult). Clinicians, patients, and their relatives may differ in their approaches to NIV in the face of progressive neuromuscular disability, but, of all the palliative options available, NIV can be particularly useful. Further decisions about withdrawal of treatment with progression of the underlying neurological disease of course will still be needed. These can be difficult and require multidisciplinary input. Actual practical NIV withdrawal can also be hard, requiring specialist assistance, but it can usually be done gradually with sedation cover to reduce distress.

Further information

General Medical Council 2010. Treatment and care towards the end of life: good practice in decision making.

Wildman M et al. Survival and quality of life for patients with COPD or asthma admitted to intensive care in a UK multicentre cohort: the COPD and Asthma Outcome Study (CAOS). Thorax. 2009;**64**(2): 128–132.

Chapter 52

Financial entitlements

General points 734
Available financial support 736

General points

Patients with chronic lung disease and their carers may be eligible for financial support. There are a large number of potential benefits that can be claimed, and the process is often time-consuming and complicated. The best sources of information are:
- Benefits Enquiry Line (Dept for Work & Pensions) ☏ 0800 0556688
- Websites:
  - ✍ http://www.gov.uk/financial-help-disabled/overview (useful guide)
  - ✍ http://www.gov.uk/browse/benefits (various online tools)
  - The Citizens Advice Bureau ✍ http://www.citizensadvice.org.uk
- The ward social worker is usually a good source of information.

Available financial support

Patients who are unable to work may be eligible for various types of financial support.

Statutory sick pay (SSP)

A doctor's certificate ('fit note', the statement of fitness for work (form Med3)) ℘ https://www.gov.uk/government/collections/fit-note is usually required for >1 week's SSP. Paid for up to 28 weeks by the employer. Completing the fit note is the responsibility of the hospital consultant under whom the patient was admitted, and it should be completed on discharge to cover the advised period off work. This also applies to patients needing time off work but not admitted to hospital. Nursing staff usually complete the forms for the period during which the patient was in hospital.

Employment and Support Allowance (ESA)

Replaces Incapacity Benefit and Severe Disablement Allowance. Has two phases:
- Assessment phase, in which patients must get Med 3s for first 13 weeks of claim and complete a medical questionnaire (ESA50)
- Work capability assessment phase, during which patients attend a face-to-face assessment to determine ongoing need and set a date for further assessment

For patients who are terminally ill (<6 months' life expectancy), doctors complete a DS1500 form, and such patients normally avoid requirement for face-to-face assessment. There are different types dependent on National Insurance contributions.

Personal Independence Payment (PIP)

For those <65 (replacing Disability Living Allowance) or *Attendance Allowance (AA)* for those >65. These are benefits for the extra costs of disability and are designed for help with personal care or mobility. For PIP, patients have to satisfy a 3-month qualifying period and have a prospective estimate of disability lasting at least 9 months. 'Special rules' allow terminally ill people (<6 months' life expectancy) to claim PIP/AA quickly, using a DS1500 form completed by doctors.

NHS Continuing Healthcare is free social care arranged and funded by the NHS, available for some adults with long term complex healthcare needs. Eligibility depends on assessed need and not on any particular diagnosis. The assessment process is complex and ℘ https://www.beaconchc.co.uk/ gives independent advice.

Direct payments

These are payments from Social Services to allow patients to buy care services for themselves.

Carer's Allowance

Those who care for someone receiving allowances, including PIP/AA, for at least 35 h/week are eligible.

Income Support ± Disability Premiums

For those on a low income, with extra support for disability.

Working Tax Credit (with extra credit for disability)

This is not a benefit as such, but a tax credit from the HMRC (paid in addition to benefits).

Disabled Students' Allowance (DSA)

Available for higher education students in England with disability or long-term health conditions.

Access to Work Grant

Financial support to help disabled people to undertake their job, giving money for, e.g. specialist equipment, travel when unable to use public transport.

Disabled Facilities Grant

Available from local councils to allow essential household modifications (e.g. widen doors, stairlifts).

Other transport assistance

For example, Blue Badge, exemption from paying vehicle tax, disabled person's bus pass/railcard.

Industrial Injuries Disablement Benefit (IIDB)

See Chapter 36 on pneumoconioses, ➔ p. 425, and Chapter 17 on Asbestos and the lung, ➔ p. 123. This is a benefit for illness acquired due to work place exposure or accident. The level of disability determines the level of benefit and is assessed by a medical advisor on a scale of 1–100%. Complete form BI100PD. Patients can additionally claim Constant Attendance Allowance if require daily care and attention because of a disability.

Reduced earning allowance

For those suffering from disability caused by a work-related accident or disease that started before 1 October 1990.

Further information

There are a number of charities who give grants/aid towards the cost of buying equipment.
🔗 https://www.disability-grants.org/
🔗 https://grants-search.turn2us.org.uk/

Immunosuppressive drugs

Patient advice and monitoring 740
Corticosteroids and azathioprine 742
Methotrexate and cyclophosphamide 744

Patient advice and monitoring

Immunosuppressive drugs are used mainly in the management of pulmonary vasculitis, but also in asthma, sarcoidosis, and interstitial lung disease (ILD). Centres differ in their use of these drugs, and local guidelines are often available. A summary of tests to perform before and during immunosuppressive drug treatment is shown in Table 53.1 and general advice for immunosuppression in Box 53.1.

> **Box 53.1 General advice for patients on immunosuppressive drugs**
> - Increased risk of infections and increased likelihood of severe infections. Check FBC if develop febrile illness
> - May have atypical presentation of infections and atypical pathogens
> - Avoid live vaccines such as measles, mumps, rubella, BCG, yellow fever, oral typhoid, oral polio
> - If never had varicella-zoster:
>   - Avoid contacts with chickenpox or shingles, consider passive immunization, immunoglobulin therapy if exposed
>   - Hospital treatment, with close monitoring, if develop chickenpox
> - Avoid measles exposure. Prophylaxis with immunoglobulins if exposed.

Table 53.1 Summary of tests to perform before and during immunosuppressive drug treatment of respiratory disease

Drug	Check before starting	Follow-up
Corticosteroids	Blood pressure (BP), glucose Consider bones/osteoporosis	BP, glucose if symptoms of diabetes
Azathioprine	Full blood count (FBC), liver function tests (LFTs), thiopurine methyltransferase (TPMT) test (see text)	FBC every 2 weeks for 3 months, then monthly LFT monthly
Methotrexate	FBC, urea and electrolytes (U&E), LFT, chest radiograph (CXR) Folic acid	Bloods every 2 weeks for 3 months, then monthly
Cyclophosphamide	FBC, U&E, LFT Urine dip Semen store	Check all every week for 1 month, then every 2 months
Rituximab	FBC, U&E, LFT, hepatitis B&C, electrocardiogram (ECG_, CXR	FBC, U&E, LFT 1 week after each infusion then monthly

Corticosteroids and azathioprine

Corticosteroids

- First-line treatment for suppressing inflammation. At high doses, also cause immunosuppression. Ineffective as sole therapy for induction of remission in systemic vasculitis
- IV methylprednisolone (500–1,000 mg/day) for 3–5 days can be used for aggressive induction of remission, e.g. GPA, followed by maintenance oral steroids (prednisolone 30–40 mg/day)
- Usually taken in the morning, as they may disturb sleep
- Dose should be slowly reduced when control of the disease is achieved. Gastric and bone protection may be necessary, as the patient will be on high doses for some months. Also ensure BP and glucose are controlled
- Ensure patients have steroid treatment card

Side effects include skin and hair thinning, obesity, cataracts, diabetes, and aseptic bone necrosis. Inform patient of these, and document. Pneumocystis pneumonia (PCP) infection can occur 2° to steroid treatment, particularly with high doses for prolonged periods. Some centres use PCP prophylaxis.

Steroids and osteoporosis

Current guidelines suggest patients being started on long-term steroids, with one other osteoporosis risk factor (such as being over 65 or having had a previous osteoporotic fracture), should also start on a bisphosphonate.

In other patients who will be on 7.5 mg/day or more for >3 months, consider checking bone mineral density via DEXA scan of hip and spine, and offer lifestyle advice and bisphosphonates if this is reduced (T score– 1.5 or lower).

(See Royal College of Physicians guidelines, available at ℛ http:// www.rcplondon.ac.uk, and National Osteoporosis Society at ℛ http:// www.nos.org.uk.)

Validated, quantitative fracture risk scores, such as FRAX® and QFracture® are available for use to guide osteoporosis risk and management.

Azathioprine

- Mainly used as a steroid-sparing agent or when vasculitis is under control to enable cyclophosphamide to be stopped. Is a pro-drug for 6-mercaptopurine. Takes ~4 weeks to work
- Cytotoxic drug, less effective than cyclophosphamide. May be reasonable alternative if side effects of cyclophosphamide are unacceptable
- Maximal effect on disease may not be evident for 6–9 months but can be used long term
- TPMT should be performed prior to commencement. TPMT breaks down azathioprine to an inactive product. 90% of the population have normal TPMT levels and 10% have intermediate activity, so azathioprine should be given with caution; 0.3% have no TPMT activity, and azathioprine should be avoided

- For vasculitis, start with 2 mg/kg/day after cyclophosphamide. Maximum dose usually around 150–200 mg/day
- As steroid-sparing regime: could start 50 mg od for 2 weeks, increasing to 100 mg od for 2 weeks if FBC satisfactory, and increasing to 150 mg od (or 75 mg bd) after further 2 weeks if FBC satisfactory. Reduce prednisolone by 5 mg every 4 weeks
- *Check FBC* every 2 weeks for 6 weeks, then at 2 and 4 weeks after each dose increase, and thereafter monthly. *Check LFTs monthly*. Stop treatment if white cell count (WCC) <3, platelets <100, or ALP and transaminases 3× normal. Restart when they recover.

Side effects include sore mouth, ulcers, nausea and vomiting, diarrhoea, skin rash, alopecia (rare). Most respond to stopping the drug and restarting at a lower dose. If taken for a number of years, then increased risk of some types of cancers, including skin. Patients are advised to contact doctor if any concerns about new skin problems. Interacts with allopurinol and leads to increased toxicity.

Methotrexate and cyclophosphamide

Methotrexate

- Can be used as a second-line treatment
- Dose: 7.5–25 mg once/week. Usual starting dose is 10 mg. Can increase after 6 weeks to 15 mg, in increments of 2.5 mg weekly
- Baseline CXR. Monitor FBC, U&E, and LFTs every 2 weeks for 3 months, then monthly. Give folic acid 5 mg 3–4 days after dose to reduce toxicity.

Side effects include mouth ulcers, skin rashes, nausea, macrocytosis, myelosuppression, pneumonitis (dyspnoea and dry cough). Avoid if significant renal or hepatic impairment, or if pleural effusions or ascites, as it can accumulate in these fluids. Stop if WCC <3, platelets <100, transaminases 3× normal, pneumonitis.

Cyclophosphamide

- The 1° cytotoxic drug used for treating systemic vasculitis
- Causes immunosuppression without anti-inflammatory effects
- Used particularly if there are life- or organ-threatening features, e.g. ventilation for lung vasculitis, systemic features, renal involvement
- Takes 12–14 days to work; hence is combined with high-dose steroids at the beginning of treatment. When combined with steroids, it induces remission of vasculitis in 90% of patients
- Perform a baseline urine dip for blood prior to treatment (although note microscopic haematuria is common with active vasculitis). Check routinely for macroscopic haematuria in patients receiving IV cyclophosphamide, and, if it is present, stop drug and arrange cystoscopy (rare if mesna is used and rare with oral cyclophosphamide regimes)
- PCP prophylaxis with co-trimoxazole is recommended (960 mg 3×/week) in patients receiving cyclophosphamide and prednisolone
- Semen storage for men prior to starting treatment.

Usual treatment duration of cyclophosphamide is 3–6 months. Courses longer than 6 months should generally be avoided; they are no more effective and carry the risk of side effects from the cumulative dose. Induce remission with cyclophosphamide and prednisolone, and maintain remission with prednisolone and another immunosuppressant (azathioprine or methotrexate) for at least 2 y.

Side effects Haemorrhagic cystitis is a potentially serious side effect of cyclophosphamide therapy. Risk of bladder cancer is increased (and is greater with increasing cumulative dose), and indefinite monitoring of urinalysis 3–6-monthly after treatment with cyclophosphamide is recommended. Other side effects include nausea, vomiting, infection (including PCP), hair thinning or alopecia (reversible), bone marrow suppression (2%), leukopenia, infertility, lymphoma (0.7%) and leukaemia, pulmonary and bladder fibrosis. Risk of cervical cancer may be higher—recommend annual cervical smear for 3 y and thereafter, as per population screening programme. Should not be taken in pregnancy or if breastfeeding. Both ♂ and ♀ should avoid starting a family during, and for 6 months following, treatment with cyclophosphamide.

Cyclophosphamide regimes
Oral cyclophosphamide is used, if possible, in active vasculitis at a dose of 2 mg/kg (up to 200 mg/day). Reduce dose in elderly (by 25% if >60 y and by 50% if >7 5y) and in setting of renal impairment.

   Monitoring Check FBC and renal function weekly for the first month, 2-weekly for 2nd and 3rd months, and monthly thereafter.
- If WCC <4 × 10⁹/L, neutrophils <2 × 10⁹/L, stop oral cyclophosphamide, and restart with dose reduced by at least 25 mg when WCC recovered, and then monitor weekly for 4 weeks
- If prolonged (WCC <4 × 10⁹/L, neutrophils <2 × 10⁹/L for >2 weeks) or severe (WCC <1 × 10⁹/L, neutrophils <0.5 × 10⁹/L) leukopenia/neutropenia, stop cyclophosphamide, and restart at 50 mg daily when WCC recovered; then increase to target dose weekly, WCC permitting
- If WCC is falling (<6 × 10⁹/L and fall of >2 × 10⁹/L since previous count), reduce dose by 25%.

Pulsed IV cyclophosphamide is given if patients cannot take oral preparations, using doses of 15 mg/kg (reduced for age and renal function, maximum dose 1,500 mg) every 2 weeks for the first three pulses, and then at 3-weekly intervals. The lowest WCC occurs 10 days after a pulse. A randomized study has shown that pulsed doses give a lower cumulative dose than oral regimes, but there is no difference in remission rates between the two. The infection rate is higher with oral regimes (European Vasculitis Study Group).

   If giving IV cyclophosphamide, patients should be well hydrated before (1 L normal saline) and after (3 L/day oral fluids for 3 days) and given mesna, which chelates with the urotoxic cyclophosphamide metabolite acrolein. Dose varies according to the cyclophosphamide dose and is available on product literature. Give during cyclophosphamide infusion and also 4 h and 8 h after. Prescribe anti-emetics.

   Monitoring Check FBC and renal function on day of pulse or previous day.
- If WCC <4 × 10⁹/L, neutrophils <2 × 10⁹/L, postpone pulse until WCC >4 × 10⁹/L, neutrophils >2 × 10⁹/L, while checking FBC weekly, and reduce dose by 25%
- After first pulse, check FBC between days 10 and day of next pulse: reduce dose of next pulse by 40% of previous dose if WCC nadir 1–2 × 10⁹/L or neutrophil nadir 0.5–1.0 × 10⁹/L
- Reduce dose of next pulse by 20% of previous dose if WCC nadir 2–3 × 10⁹/L or neutrophil nadir 1–1.5 × 10⁹/L
- Thereafter, check FBC on day of pulse or previous day, unless dose adjustment when checked additionally at day 10.

Rituximab as an alternative to cyclophosphamide

Rituximab has been shown to be as effective as cyclophosphamide in inducing remission in ANCA-positive vasculitides and may be used in place of cyclophosphamide where there has been progression despite cyclophosphamide, cyclophosphamide is contraindicated, or there are concerns regarding fertility. Treatment needs to be started either by a specialist centre or in collaboration with one via networked care arrangements.

Further information

Ntatsaki E et al. British Society of Rheumatology and British Heath Professionals in Rheumatology guidelines for the management of adults with ANCA associated vasculitis. *Rheumatology* 2014;53(12): 2306–2309.
FRAX® https://www.sheffield.ac.uk/FRAX/
QFracture® https://qfracture.org/index.php

Chapter 54

Inhalers and nebulizers

Background *748*
Examples of different inhaler types *750*

Background

Inhalers

- There are many different inhaler devices that deliver drugs directly to the airways, but essentially two basic types: metered dose inhalers (MDIs) and dry powder inhalers (DPIs). New devices are being introduced all the time, with one, two, or three drugs delivered simultaneously. Check what is available through your local formulary (see Table 54.1 for examples)
- Ideally patients should try a range of devices to choose the most appropriate for them
- Inspiratory flow rates can be measured (e.g. with the In-Check DIAL® device) to help identify the most appropriate inhaler device. Patients should receive advice and a demonstration on inhaler technique and use (see Table 54.2). Technique should be checked regularly, and, if patients cannot manage a particular device, they should be switched to another
- Many pharmacists have been trained to assess inhaler technique
- The percentage of a drug delivered to the airway varies for each device (15–60%, according to the manufacturers) and depends on good technique
- Spacer devices improve the delivery with MDIs and are particularly useful for the elderly, children, and those who find it difficult to coordinate inhaler administration with breathing. They reduce unwanted oropharyngeal deposition of steroids
- Try to use the same type of inhaler device for all the drug classes used by a patient
- Advise the patient how to recognize when a device is empty: some have dose counters; others are shaken to hear if they still have contents
- Titrate inhaler doses with clinical response, using the minimum possible. Inhaled steroids do have side effects, and the dose should be kept to a minimum.

Examples of different inhaler types

Table 54.1 Different medications available for inhalers (not exhaustive; new inhalers come on the market regularly; check with your local formulary)

Class of drug	Examples	Notes
Short-acting β2 agonist (SABA)	Salbutamol (Ventolin®, Asmasal®, Pulvinal®, Salbutamol, Salamol®, Salbutamol Cyclocaps®, Airomir®, Asmasal Clickhaler®, Salamol Easi-Breathe®) Terbutaline (Bricanyl®)	Rapid onset, effects last 4–6 h
Long-acting β2 agonist (LABA)	Salmeterol (Serevent®) Formoterol (Foradil®, Oxis®) Indacaterol maleate (Onbrez Breezhaler®) Olodaterol (Striverdi®)	Duration 12 h for Salmeterol and formoterol—given bd. Duration 24 h for indacaterol and olodaterol—given od
Short-acting muscarinic antagonist (SAMA)	Ipratropium bromide (Atrovent®)	
Long-acting muscarinic antagonist (LAMA)	Tiotropium (Spiriva®) Aclidinium bromide (Eklira®) Glycopyrronium bromide (Seebri®) Umeclidinium (Incruse®)	od dosing other than aclidinium which is bd
Inhaled corticosteroid (ICS)	Beclometasone dipropionate (Clenil®) Beclometasone dipropionate extra-fine (Qvar®) Budesonide (Pulmicort®) Fluticasone propionate (Flixotide®) Mometasone furoate (Asmanex®) Ciclesonide (Alvesco®)	
ICS/LABA combination	Fluticasone/salmeterol (Seretide®) Budesonide/formoterol (Symbicort®) Beclometasone/formoterol (Fostair®) Fluticasone/formoterol (Flutiform®) Fluticasone/vilanterol (Revlar®)	

LAMA/LABA combination	Umeclidinium/vilanterol (Anoro®)	
	Glycopyrronium/indacaterol (Ultibro®)	
	Aclidinium/formoterol (DuaKlir®)	
	Tiotropium/olodaterol (Spiolto®)	
ICS/LAMA/LABA combination	Fluticasone/umeclidinium/ vilanterol (Trelegy®)	Licensed in COPD
	Beclometasone/ glycopyrronium/formoterol (Trimbow®)	

Table 54.2 Instructions for use of different inhaler types

Type of device	Instructions for use
Pressurized aerosol MDI (e.g. aerosol Evohaler®)	Remove the mouthpiece and shake the inhaler well. Hold the inhaler upright, with the thumb on the base below the mouthpiece and the first finger on the metal canister. Breathe out as far as is comfortable, then place the mouthpiece between the teeth, and close lips around it. Do not bite it. As you start to breathe in through the mouth, press on the top of the inhaler to release the medication while still breathing in steadily and deeply. Hold your breath; take the inhaler from your mouth, and continue holding your breath for up to 10 s, if possible. Wait 30 s prior to taking 2nd puff. Use with spacer device to improve drug delivery. CFC-free inhalers need washing every 2–3 weeks, as they can block.
Spacer (e.g. Volumatic® Aero Chamber®)	Ensure spacer is compatible with patient's inhaler. Remove cap of inhaler and shake it. Insert it into end of spacer device. Place the other end of the spacer in the mouth. Press the inhaler canister once to release one dose of the drug. Take one long, slow breath in and hold, or take 3–4 steady breaths in and out. Repeat as indicated. In some, the valve should click. Clean the spacer once a month with mild detergent; rinse, and air dry. Replace after 6–12 months. Some spacer devices will whistle or sound if you breathe in too fast.
Breath-actuated devices (e.g. Autohaler® Easi-Breathe®)	If an Autohaler®, remove the cap and lift the red lever. Insert device into mouth. Inhale slowly and deeply. Continue inhaling when the device 'clicks'. Hold breath for up to 10 s, if possible. Slowly breathe out. To take a 2nd inhaled dose, lower the red lever and lift again. If an Easi-Breathe®, open the hinged cap. Insert device into mouth. Inhale slowly and deeply. Continue inhaling when the device 'clicks'. Hold breath for up to 10 s, if possible. Slowly breathe out. Close the cap, and reopen for further doses. If Easi-Breathe® spacer used, it will need to be removed between each inhalation so that cap can be opened and closed.

Dry powder devices (e.g. Accuhaler® Breezhaler® Turbohaler® Genuair® Handihaler® Ellipta®)	Prime the device. Turbohaler®: hold upright; remove the cap; twist the base as far as possible until the click is heard, and then twist back again. Accuhaler®: open inhaler cover, mouthpiece facing you, and push lever down to pierce the blister containing dose. Handihaler® and Breezhaler®: open devices; insert capsule into chamber; close mouthpiece section; pierce capsule by firmly pressing side button(s). Ellipta®: slide down cover until click is heard. To use all the devices, hold them level; exhale fully; place the mouthpiece into mouth between teeth, and inhale deeply and forcefully. Hold your breath and remove the inhaler. For a 2nd dose, repeat the above actions.
Respimat® for Spiriva® and Spiolto®	To load cartridge, remove clear base; insert cartridge until flush with device; replace clear base. Hold inhaler upright, with cap closed. Turn the transparent base until it clicks. Open the cap. Breathe out slowly and insert the mouthpiece and seal with lips. Point towards the back of the throat. While taking a deep breath, press the button and continue to breathe in. Hold your breath for 10 s, if possible, and breathe out slowly.

There are many YouTube videos showing how to use most of these inhalers.

Table 54.1 and Table 54.2 include some of the most commonly used inhalers and drug preparations. There are frequent additions of new inhaler devices, drugs and generic formulations; check your local formulary. Some inhalers are only licensed for asthma or for COPD.

Nebulizers

Used when they bring greater relief than inhaled therapy, either during acute respiratory illnesses, because of disease severity, or because they are unable to use inhalers. Patients for possible nebulizer therapy should be referred to a respiratory physician. Nebulized antibiotics need a more powerful pump and special neb-set.

How to use

Open the ampoule containing the drug solution, and squirt the solution into the nebulizer chamber. Salbutamol and ipratropium bromide can be taken together, but nebulized budesonide or antibiotics should be used separately. If ipratropium bromide only is being used, this should be delivered via a mouthpiece, as it can lead to glaucoma if used via a mask (atropine-like constricting effects on the pupil). Re-attach the chamber to the nebulizer mask or mouthpiece. Put the mask over nose and mouth, or position mouthpiece between the lips fully in the mouth. Switch the compressor on. Breathe slowly in and out. Continue until all the solution is gone. Switch off the machine. Rinse the nebulizer chamber with hot water (and very dilute washing-up liquid) after each use. If nebulization takes >10 min, change the neb-set (mask, chamber, tubing last 1–3 months). If no improvement, consider servicing the machine. If the patient is using O2, this can still be used during nebulization, either via nasal prongs under the nebulizer mask or by using O2 tubing attached directly to the nebulizer chamber to drive the nebulization; at home, most cylinders do not provide sufficient flow rates to allow this. Nebulizer machines should be serviced annually.

Chapter 55

Intensive care unit (ICU) referral

General points 756
Revised National Early Warning Score (NEWS2) 757

General points

Ideally, communicate with intensive care unit (ICU) early, as it is much better that they know about a potentially sick patient who may need ICU input than to find your patient (and you!) in difficulty later on, with no ICU bed.

Previously, multiple different scoring systems for the early recognition of sick patients were in use in hospitals, enabling doctors and nursing staff to readily identify and assess a deteriorating patient, including response to treatment. National Health Service (NHS) England now requires all hospitals to use the *revised* National Early Warning Score (NEWS2), published by the Royal College of Physicians in 2017 (Table 55.1). In addition to other changes, NEWS2 includes a modified saturation scale for those at risk of hypercapnia and gives an adverse score for those with new confusion/delirium.

The common situations in which ICU input may be required in relation to respiratory disease are principally those relating to decisions about intubation and ventilation. Most commonly these will be:

- Respiratory failure (either type I or type II)
  - Exacerbation of chronic obstructive pulmonary disease (COPD) (usually type II failure). Patients with COPD admitted to ICU have a hospital mortality of 20–25%. Poor prognostic factors include low baseline FEV_1, long-term O_2 use, low sodium and albumin, low body mass index (BMI), poor functional status, and comorbid disease. Age does not add prognostic information
  - Pneumonia (to maintain an adequate pO_2—usually type I failure). In this situation, ICU input may not necessarily lead to intubation, as adequate oxygenation may be achieved by the proper use of a non-rebreathe mask, humidified high-flow nasal O_2, or continuous positive airway pressure (CPAP), with the additional benefits of one-to-one nursing. Altered mental state and difficulty clearing secretions may make invasive ventilation necessary
- Upper airway emergencies
- ≥1 organ failure (not necessarily with respiratory failure)
- Sepsis requiring organ support, particularly circulatory support requiring vasoactive drugs

Many factors are considered when assessing suitability for ICU admission including: diagnosis, illness severity, coexisting disease, physiological reserve, prognosis, availability of suitable treatment, response to treatment to date, anticipated quality of life (QoL), patient's wishes.

Revised National Early Warning Score (NEWS2)

Table 55.1 NEWS2 scoring system for the early recognition of sick patients

Score	3	2	1	0	1	2	3
HR/min	≤40		41–50	51–90	91–110	111–130	≥131
SBP	≤90	91–100	101–110	111–219			≥220
RR/min	≤8		9–11	12–20		21–24	≥25
Temp/°C	≤35		35.1–36	36.1–38	38.1–39	≥39.1	
SaO_2 If not CO_2 retainer	≤91	92–93	94–95	≥96			
SaO_2 If CO_2 retainer	≤83	84–85	86–87	88–92 ≥93 on air	93–94 on O_2	95–96 on O_2	≥97 on O_2
Supplemental O_2		Yes		No			
Conscious level				A			C, V, P, or U

A = alert; C = new confusion; V = responds to voice; P = responds to pain; U = unresponsive.

HR = heart rate; RR = respiratory rate; SBP = systolic blood pressure

Calculate the NEWS2 total by the addition of the scores in each column.

Total score 0 (low risk): minimum 12 hourly observations.

Total score 1–4 (low risk): Increase observations to 4–6-hourly. Nurse decides whether increased observation frequency needed or escalation of care.

Score 3 in any parameter (low–medium risk): observations hourly. Urgent doctor review.

Total score ≥5 (medium risk): observations hourly. Urgent doctor review.

Total score ≥7 (high risk): continuous monitoring. Immediate senior doctor review, including assessment by ICU.

Respiratory rate is the most sensitive marker of illness severity.

Chapter 56

Lung transplantation

Patient selection 760
Contraindications, investigations, and assessment 762
Surgical approaches, follow-up, outcomes, and future
    developments 764
Complications: early 766
Complications: late 768

Patient selection

Lung transplantation was first performed successfully in the 1980s and offers benefits in both prognosis and quality of life to select patients with end-stage lung disease. The number of candidates for transplantation continues to increase and there is a significant shortage of donor organs, and so an increasing number of patients die on the waiting list. There are five UK adult lung transplant centres: Birmingham, Harefield, Manchester, Newcastle, and Papworth. In the most recent UK data (2017–2018), 214 lung transplants were carried out over a 12-month period. Matching is carried out according to patient size and major blood groups; human leucocyte antigen (HLA) matching is not performed.

Underlying conditions

Most common underlying diagnoses, in order: chronic obstructive pulmonary disease (COPD); idiopathic pulmonary fibrosis (IPF); cystic fibrosis (CF); alpha-1 antitrypsin (α1AT) deficiency; pulmonary arterial hypertension (PAH); other diffuse parenchymal lung disease (e.g. sarcoidosis, lymphangioleiomyomatosis (LAM), Langerhans cell histiocytosis (LCH), collagen vascular disease-related lung disease); bronchiectasis; pulmonary hypertension (PHT) secondary to congenital cardiac disease (Eisenmenger's syndrome).

Indications

Referral for transplant assessment should be considered in patients with progressive and advanced lung disease, who are deteriorating despite maximal therapy, with poor quality of life and/or whose predicted 2 y survival is <50%. Candidates should be functionally disabled but still able to walk, with no significant untreatable cardiac, renal, or hepatic impairment; they should have completed pulmonary rehabilitation. Disease-specific guidelines for referral are as follows:

COPD and other obstructive lung disease
- FEV_1 <20% predicted and either TLCO <20% or homogeneous distribution of emphysema (median survival 3 y with medical therapy)
- History of hospitalization(s) for exacerbation(s) associated with acute hypercapnia ($PaCO_2$ >6.5 kPa) and worsening hypoxia
- Pulmonary hypertension or cor pulmonale
- BODE score >7 (see ⊃ p. 194).

Idiopathic pulmonary fibrosis
Any of: TLCO <40% predicted with clinical deterioration; fall in TLCO ≥15% over 6 months; fall in FVC ≥10% over 6 months; O_2 desaturation <88% on 6minute walk test (6MWT); acute, rapid deterioration preceding diagnosis.

Cystic fibrosis and bronchiectasis
- FEV_1 ≤30% predicted or FEV_1 >30% with rapid progressive deterioration, e.g. increasing exacerbation frequency, rapid fall in FEV_1
- History of intensive care unit (ICU) or high-dependency unit (HDU) admission for pulmonary exacerbation
- O_2-dependent respiratory failure, hypercapnia, or pulmonary hypertension

- Severe haemoptysis despite embolization
- Pneumothorax in association with advanced disease
- Young (<20 y) ♀ patients with rapid deterioration have a poor prognosis and should be considered for early referral.

Pulmonary arterial hypertension

World Health Organization (WHO) functional class III or IV despite parenteral therapy for 3 months; worsening right heart failure with increasing fluid retention despite medical therapy; declining 6MWT to <350 m despite medical therapy; need for continuous intravenous (IV) inotropic support; mean right atrial pressure >15 mmHg, and cardiac index <2 L/min/m² on right heart catheter despite optimal therapy.

Timing of referral

This can be difficult; predicted survival should be <2–3 y, but patients must be fit for the procedure during a waiting time of typically 12–16 months in the UK. Allow time for thorough transplant assessment and patient education—early discussion with the transplant team is preferable. The referral decision should not be based on a single factor; rather, a combination of clinical, laboratory, and functional assessments together with individual patient trajectory should be considered. Patients with IPF and CF have particularly high waiting list mortalities and early referral should be considered; consider referral at diagnosis for suitable IPF patients with rapid symptomatic decline. Patients of shorter stature and with blood group O have longer waits and a higher waiting list mortality in the UK and should be considered for earlier referral.

Urgent and super-urgent lung allocation schemes

These schemes were introduced in the UK in 2017 in an attempt to reduce waiting list mortality. They aim to identify patients who are at high risk of death without a transplant, for prioritization at a national level.

Urgent patients are suitable candidates for transplant with predicted survival <90 days, including patients with high oxygen demand (e.g. >10 L/min), refractory right heart failure, and/or continuous non-invasive ventilation (NIV).

Super-urgent allocation applies only to patients suffering acute deterioration requiring extracorporeal life support (e.g. ECMO) who have already been assessed and accepted onto a lung transplant list prior to their deterioration. Suitable patients with an acute decline and good rehabilitation potential who are already listed may be considered for 'bridging to transplant' with awake (ideally ambulatory) ECMO. Patients with sepsis, extrapulmonary organ failure, or requirement for intermittent positive-pressure ventilation (IPPV) are excluded or delisted. Liaise closely with transplant centre.

Further information

Weill D et al. A consensus document for the selection of lung transplant candidates: 2014. *J Heart Lung Transplant* 2015;**34**: 1–15.

Kourliouros A et al. Patient outcomes from time of listing for lung transplantation in the UK: are there disease-specific differences? *Thorax* 2019;**74**: 60–68.

Contraindications, investigations, and assessment

Contraindications

Absolute (although occasional exceptions may occur)

- Severe, untreatable extrapulmonary organ dysfunction (including renal, hepatic, and cardiac disease)
- Solid organ or haematological malignancy within 5 y of listing (excluding cutaneous squamous or basal cell carcinomas)
- Unstable critical condition (e.g. sepsis, shock)
- Uncontrolled extrapulmonary manifestations of systemic disease
- Severe untreatable psychiatric illness
- BMI >35 kg/m²
- Active or recent (within 6 months) substance addiction (cigarette smoking, alcohol abuse, illicit drug use)
- Significant chest wall/spinal deformity
- Non-adherence with treatment or outpatient follow-up
- Lack of social support sufficient to compromise post-transplant outcomes.

Relative

- Age >60 y (not an absolute exclusion but will be assessed by transplant multidisciplinary team (MDT) in context of other relative contraindications)
- Chronic medical conditions that are poorly controlled or associated with target-organ damage (e.g. hypertension, diabetes, coronary artery disease, chronic renal disease with glomerular filtration rate (GFR) <50 ml/min)
- Severe or symptomatic osteoporosis
- Severe obesity (BMI >30 kg/m²) or malnutrition (BMI <17 kg/m²)
- Poor rehabilitation potential: sarcopenia and frailty
- Mechanical ventilation (excluding NIV)
- Chronic high dose oral prednisolone (>15 mg/day)
- Extensive pleural thickening (e.g. from infection or prior surgery or pleurodesis)
- Colonization with *Burkholderia cenocepacia* or other highly resistant pathogens
- Previous (cleared) infection with *Mycobacterium abscessus* is a relative contraindication; a minority of centres may transplant patients with active *M. abscessus* disease, but post-transplant recurrence of *M. abscessus* is associated with very poor outcomes
- Aspergilloma with extensive cavitation
- Chronic extrapulmonary infection (HIV, hepatitis B and C).

Investigations prior to referral

In the UK, referral is via a standardized national proforma. Important investigations include full pulmonary function tests (PFTs), tests of exercise performance (e.g. 6MWT), sputum microbiology, electrocardiogram (ECG), echo, high-resolution computed tomography (HRCT) chest, blood group, liver function tests (LFTs), viral serology (human immunodeficiency virus (HIV), cytomegalovirus (CMV), hepatitis B and C), 24 h creatinine clearance, and in select cases stress echo and coronary angiography. Include in the referral letter details as to the patient's understanding of disease and prognosis. Information regarding individual patient disease trajectory (e.g. serial lung function measurements; exacerbation frequency and severity over time) is particularly valued by the transplant centre.

Assessment process

Following referral, patients and family members/carers typically attend a pre-assessment outpatient clinic which is followed by a 2–4-day inpatient assessment for potential candidates. Following transplant MDT discussion, a listing decision is then made and discussed with the patient.

Management of patients on waiting list

The referring physician remains responsible for continuing regular medical care of the patient to ensure they remain optimally treated while on a lung transplant waiting list. Patients may rarely improve and no longer require transplantation, or they may develop an important contraindication that requires delisting. Liaise closely with transplant centre and inform them promptly of changes in clinical condition. Pay particular attention to:

- Maintenance of nutrition (may require supplementary feeding)
- Avoidance of obesity
- Maintenance of mobility, continuing exercise, and rehabilitation
- Monitoring comorbid disease: heart, kidney, liver, bones. Optimize treatment of diabetes, systemic hypertension, osteoporosis, peptic ulcer disease, gastro-oesophageal reflux, and sinus disease
- Psychological and social support
- Symptom control: palliative care input is often required and should be considered in parallel with active treatment for patients on a transplant waiting list
- Prompt treatment of exacerbations
- Early NIV, if indicated
- Avoiding intubation, if possible.

Surgical approaches, follow-up, outcomes, and future developments

Surgical approaches for lung transplantation

Single lung
• Technically easier, allows two recipients from one donor
• Generally now only used for ILD
• Overdistension of the compliant native lung in emphysema is uncommon but may be problematic.

Bilateral sequential
• Worldwide >80% of lung transplants are now double
• Sequential right and left single-lung transplants at one time
• Selective lung ventilation may render cardiopulmonary bypass unnecessary.

Heart–lung
• Indicated in Eisenmenger's syndrome, or rarely in advanced lung disease with concurrent left ventricular (LV) dysfunction or coronary disease
• Cor pulmonale is not in itself an indication, as right ventricular hypertrophy (RVH) resolves rapidly following lung transplantation alone.

Living lobar transplantation
• Bilateral grafting of lower lobes from two living adult donors to replace lungs of child or small adult
• Appears to be safe for the donor, with lung volume reductions of about 15%, but potential for 300% overall mortality (two donors and one recipient)
• Not widely performed in the UK.

Follow-up after lung transplantation

Patients are typically discharged from hospital about 1 month after transplant, following post-transplant bronchoscopy with bronchoalveolar lavage (BAL) and biopsy. They will be followed up closely by their transplant centre but may also attend local respiratory clinics intermittently between transplant centre visits. Be alert to possible complications (see ➔ p. 766 and ➔ p. 768) and discuss with transplant centre promptly if these are suspected. Spirometric values are generally very stable from 3 months after transplantation, and sustained falls ≥10–15% warrant further investigation. Remember drug interactions (particularly ciclosporin and tacrolimus) if new medications are added. Check immunosuppressant drug blood levels, and perform routine blood tests, according to the local transplant centre policy.

Routine surgery after lung transplantation

Routine surgery >3 months after transplant can be carried out locally, but inform the transplant centre. The morning dose of calcineurin inhibitor (ciclosporin, tacrolimus) should be omitted, as there is a risk of nephrotoxicity with hypovolaemia.

Outcomes following lung transplantation

Post-registration

Outcomes at 1 y after listing for lung transplantation in the UK: 35% of
patients are alive on list; 17% have died on list; 45% received a transplant;
3% removed from list. At 5 y, 64% of patients transplanted and 25% have
died on list.

Survival
- Survival rates in the UK: 89% at 90 days; 80% 1 y; 57% 5 y.
- Rate of death is highest in first year (infection, primary graft failure)
- Risk factors for early death are pre-existing PHT, ventilator dependence,
  recipient age >50 y, donor age >50 y.

Functional outcomes
- Lung function usually normalizes after bilateral transplant and markedly
  improves following single-lung transplant. In COPD, FEV_1 increases to
  50–60% of predicted value after single-lung transplant
- Arterial oxygenation rapidly normalizes
- 6MWT distance typically doubles; most patients resume active lifestyle,
  although fewer than 40% of patients return to work
- Limited data on QoL: initial improvement suggested, but effects after 1
  y are unclear. 85% of survivors have no functional limitations after 5 y.

Future developments

- Future developments are likely to address both the development
  of more effective treatments for chronic rejection (new
  immunosuppressive drugs, induction of immune tolerance) and
  the shortage of donor organs (e.g. living lobar transplantation,
  xenotransplantation, and further research in lung preservation)
- *Ex vivo* lung perfusion (EVLP) may increase the number of organs
  available for transplant. EVLP involves controlled perfusion and
  ventilation of donor lungs for a number of hours in an attempt to
  improve the quality of donor organs, to make previously unusable
  organs suitable for transplantation
- Bronchiolitis obliterans syndrome (BOS; ➋ p. 768) is the leading
  cause of late mortality after lung transplantation; current research
  aims to increase understanding of its pathogenesis and develop novel
  biomarkers of early disease
- The nature of interactions between recipient and donor lung
  microbiomes is a subject of significant current interest and may be
  relevant to allograft tolerance and development of BOS.

Complications: early

Primary graft dysfunction

- Characterized by lung injury (pulmonary infiltrates, hypoxaemia, diffuse alveolar damage, or OP on biopsy) within first 72 hours after transplant; clinical severity ranges from very mild acute lung injury to acute respiratory distress syndrome (ARDS)
- Presumably related to preservation and ischaemia–reperfusion injury
- Exclude other causes, e.g. volume overload, pneumonia, hyperacute rejection, occlusion of venous anastomosis, aspiration
- Treatment is supportive (mechanical ventilation or ECMO)
- High mortality (40–60%).

Acute cellular rejection

- Acute cellular rejection (ACR) is common and results from alloreactive T-cells reacting to donor HLA and other antigens
- ACR occurs particularly within 3 months of transplant and affects approximately 60% in the first year; it is rare after 12 months if adherence with medication is maintained
- Asymptomatic or may be associated with malaise, fever, dyspnoea, cough, hypoxia. May present similarly to pneumonia or cryptogenic organizing pneumonia (COP)
- *Chest radiograph (CXR)* may be normal or show non-specific infiltrates
- Common finding is fall in *spirometry* >10%, although this does not distinguish from other complications, particularly infection
- Ideally confirm histologically: TBBs are safe and typically show perivascular lymphocytic infiltrates. Routine surveillance TBBs can be used to detect acute rejection prior to falls in lung function
- *Treatment* IV methylprednisolone pulses are given within the first 3 months of transplant; after this, high-dose oral corticosteroids are used. The majority of patients respond quickly to augmented immunosuppression
- Recurrent acute rejection is a risk factor for the development of BOS (➜ p. 768)
- Acute rejection is an uncommon cause of breathlessness after 3 months, and other common causes of SOB should be considered
- Antibody-mediated allograft rejection is increasingly recognized and its optimal management is currently unclear; treatment may be attempted with IV immunoglobulin, plasmapheresis, or rituximab.

Airway complications

- Anastomotic stenosis most common and typically occurs weeks to months after transplant; suggested clinically by localized wheeze, recurrent pneumonia, or suboptimal lung function. Treat with balloon dilatation (sometimes repeated) or stent placement via bronchoscopy
- Complete dehiscence of bronchial anastomosis is now rare and requires immediate surgery or re-transplantation
- Partial dehiscence is managed conservatively: drain pneumothorax, reduce steroid dose.

Infection

Bacteria

- May occur early (first month after transplant) or late (associated with BOS)
- Most commonly due to Gram-negative organisms, particularly *Pseudomonas aeruginosa*
- Recipients with CF are not at greater risk than other patients; an exception is *B. cepacia* colonization, which is associated with a high risk of often fatal post-operative infections.

Cytomegalovirus (CMV)

- CMV-seronegative recipients from seropositive donors are at particular risk of severe infection, including pneumonitis; this is usually treated successfully with valganciclovir
- Increases risk of bacterial or fungal superinfection
- Ganciclovir prophylaxis probably results in later, less severe infection
- CMV infection appears to be a risk factor for development of BOS.

Aspergillus

- *Aspergillus* frequently colonizes the airways after lung transplant, but clinically apparent infection develops in only a minority of patients
- Peak disease incidence is at 2 months after transplant
- Sites of disease include airways (may lead to mucosal oedema, ulceration, and pseudomembranes; usually responds to itraconazole, voriconazole, or amphotericin B), fresh bronchial anastomosis, lung parenchyma, and disseminated aspergillosis (associated with high mortality).

Drug-related complications

Immunosuppressive drugs must be taken lifelong following transplantation. Agents used include ciclosporin or tacrolimus, azathioprine or mycophenolate mofetil (MMF), and prednisolone. They are associated with many drug interactions and side effects, particularly nephrotoxicity and osteoporosis. Pulmonary toxicity is described secondary to sirolimus and everolimus. Ciclosporin, tacrolimus, and sirolimus blood levels require close monitoring.

Non-pulmonary complications

Venous thromboembolism and cardiac arrhythmias are not uncommon following lung transplantation. Hyperammonaemia is a rare but serious early complication. Long-term complications include hypertension, renal impairment, hyperlipidaemia, diabetes, stroke, and potentially ischaemic heart disease. Remember also complications of the underlying disease, e.g. distal intestinal obstruction syndrome (DIOS) in patients with cystic fibrosis.

Complications: late

Chronic lung allograft dysfunction (CLAD)

- CLAD represents chronic rejection and accounts for the relatively poor long-term prognosis following lung transplant
- Two main types are now recognized: bronchiolitis obliterans syndrome (BOS) and restrictive allograft syndrome (RAS)

Bronchiolitis obliterans syndrome (BOS)

- BOS is a form of delayed allograft dysfunction characterized by persistent FEV_1 decline in the absence of other causes. It is manifest histologically as *bronchiolitis obliterans*, a fibroproliferative process affecting small airways, sometimes with associated pulmonary vascular atherosclerosis. Histological confirmation is difficult: TBBs have a relatively low sensitivity, so a clinical diagnosis of BOS is defined in the absence of histological confirmation as an unexplained and sustained (≥3 weeks) fall in FEV_1 to ≤80% of peak value post-transplant
- Uncommon in first 6 months, but prevalence increases steadily, affecting 50% of patients at 5 y
- *Pathogenesis* Incompletely understood; likely involves immune-mediated injury to epithelial and endothelial cells, possibly with an environmental trigger; risk factors for development include previous episodes of recurrent acute rejection, infection (e.g. CMV, *A. fumigatus*, *P. aeruginosa*), presence of anti-HLA antibodies pre-transplant, gastro-oesophageal reflux, and medication non-compliance
- *Clinically* Insidious onset of breathlessness and cough, and progressive airflow obstruction on spirometry
- *CXR* is usually unhelpful; *HRCT* may show expiratory air trapping and peripheral bronchiectasis
- *P. aeruginosa* colonization is common, with recurrent purulent tracheobronchitis
- *Treatment* is challenging and acts only to stabilize or reduce the rate of disease progression:
  - Modified immunosuppression may be helpful: consider switching ciclosporin to tacrolimus, and azathioprine to mycophenolate. Systemic glucocorticoids do not appear to be effective
  - Investigate for infection (consider BAL) and treat aggressively
  - Azithromycin is increasingly used and appears to be helpful in stabilizing (and perhaps preventing) BOS
  - Gastro-oesophageal reflux is diagnosed on impedance monitoring and often treated with early fundoplication surgery
  - Emerging therapies include extracorporeal photopheresis, total lymphoid irradiation, montelukast, and inhaled ciclosporin
  - Re-transplantation is the only definitive treatment and is controversial.
- *Prognosis* is poor: mortality is 40% within 2 y of diagnosis; the rate of decline is very variable between individuals.

Restrictive allograft syndrome (RAS)
- RAS is manifest by restrictive spirometry and allograft upper lobe parenchymal fibrosis; lower lobe involvement or blood eosinophilia are associated with a worse prognosis
- Recurrent acute exacerbations often occur
- Much less common than BOS but associated with a worse prognosis.

Recurrence of primary disease
Reported in sarcoidosis, LAM, diffuse panbronchiolitis, desquamative interstitial pneumonitis (DIP), LCH, pulmonary alveolar proteinosis, pulmonary veno-occlusive disease, and bronchoalveolar cell carcinoma.

Malignancy
- Increased risk of certain malignancies, e.g. lymphoma (and other Epstein–Barr virus (EBV)-related post-transplant lymphoproliferative diseases, PTLD), skin, lip, vulval, and perineal carcinomas, *in situ* cervical cancer, and Kaposi's sarcoma
- Most lymphomas appear within the first year, and the lung allograft is the most common site of involvement, with pulmonary nodule(s) ± mediastinal lymphadenopathy. Lymphocyte aggregates from acute rejection may mimic the appearance of PTLD on small TBB specimens
- Lymphomas presenting after the first year are more commonly disseminated or intra-abdominal (e.g. presenting with tonsillar enlargement, peripheral lymphadenopathy, skin nodules, liver involvement, or bowel complications such as intussusception). Patients should be referred back to the transplant centre for treatment, rather than the local haematology team. Usual treatment is a reduction in immunosuppression, plus antivirals and/or rituximab
- Lung cancer occurs and may progress unusually rapidly, mimicking infection.
- Differential diagnosis of CXR nodules following lung transplantation includes:
  - Post-transplant lymphoproliferative disease
  - Infection (e.g. *Pseudomonas, Nocardia*, Aspergillus disease, mycobacteria)
  - Disease recurrence
  - Lung cancer.

Further information
Meyer KC et al. An international ISHLT/ATS/ERS clinical practice guideline: diagnosis and management of bronchiolitis obliterans syndrome. *Eur Resp J* 2014;**44**: 1479–1503.

Non-invasive ventilation (NIV)

Terminology 772
Indications 774
Contraindications 776
NIV in acute respiratory failure: practical use 778
NIV in chronic respiratory failure 782
NIV end-of-life weaning 786

Terminology

Ventilatory support may be invasive (via endotracheal tube or tracheostomy) or non-invasive (via nasal mask or face mask). Non-invasive ventilation (NIV) may be subdivided into positive or negative pressure ventilation (rarely used now).

Abbreviations

- NIV: non-invasive ventilation, also referred to as non-invasive mechanical ventilation (NIMV)
- NIPPV: non-invasive positive pressure ventilation; confusingly, it is also sometimes interpreted as nasal intermittent positive pressure ventilation and sometimes referred to as 'NIPPY', after the name of a particular type of ventilator
- IPAP: inspiratory positive airways pressure
- EPAP: expiratory positive airways pressure, also referred to as positive end expiratory pressure (PEEP)
- BUR: back up rate is the target number of breaths per minute, if spontaneous ventilation is less than this the ventilator will initiate breaths to maintain ventilation
- BiPAP: bi-level positive airway pressure (IPAP > EPAP), refers to a commercial product but now mistakenly used to refer to similar machines
- CPAP: continuous positive airway pressure (IPAP ≈ EPAP)
- VAPSV: volume-assured pressure support ventilation
- ASV: adaptive servo- (or support) ventilation.

Positive pressure ventilators

Also called NIV, bi-level, BiPAP (trade name), NIPPY (trade name). Deliver volume or pressure support; many different types are available. Bi-level pressure support devices are used extensively and provide ventilation with a higher inspiratory positive airway pressure than expiratory pressure (the difference in pressure between the two is also called pressure support), selected by the prescriber. They function in several modes, but usually patient-triggered inspiratory support, with provision of an underlying back-up rate that will cut in if the patient fails to breathe. Non-invasive positive pressure support may be provided by specialized portable ventilators or by standard critical care ventilators.

New 'intelligent' non-invasive ventilators are becoming available that adjust the ventilation on a breath-to-breath basis. Servo-ventilators (ASV) for central sleep apnoea (CSA) adjust ventilator support to the pattern of breathing, effectively 'ironing out' the oscillations without leading to over-ventilation and hypocapnia. A large trial of ASV in patients with CSA and heart failure with reduced ejection fraction showed no benefit of ASV and an excess of mortality in the ASV arm. VAPSV is where tidal volumes and minute ventilation are monitored and the inspiratory pressure is adjusted to maintain the previous 'learned' ventilation. The role of these new ventilators is still being assessed, and they may only be appropriate for certain clinical situations.

Negative pressure ventilators

Assist inspiration by 'sucking out' the chest wall; expiration occurs through elastic recoil of the lungs and chest wall. Includes devices such as tank ventilators and chest 'cuirass' or 'shell' ventilators. The Hayek oscillator is a high-frequency version of the negative pressure cuirass ventilator. Other devices, such as the rocking bed and 'pneumobelt', displace abdominal contents to aid diaphragmatic contraction. Used extensively in the polio epidemics of the 1950s, they are now only very rarely used to manage chronic respiratory failure.

Continuous positive airway pressure (CPAP)

Supplies constant positive pressure during inspiration and expiration and is therefore not a form of ventilation but is sometimes mistakenly referred to as such. It provides a 'splint' to open the upper airway and collapsed alveoli (thus improving ventilation-perfusion (V/Q) matching). CPAP is used extensively in the community to treat obstructive sleep apnoea (OSA) but also has a role in improving oxygenation in selected patients with acute respiratory failure, e.g. patients with cardiogenic pulmonary oedema, pneumocystis pneumonia (see ● p. 572) and seems to have a role in selected patients with severe COVID-19 infection. CPAP can be used used in obesity hypoventilation syndrome (OHS) when OSA is the dominant pathology and hypercapnia is stable (see ● p. 702).

High-flow nasal oxygen (HFNO)

Supplies high-flow, high FiO_2 oxygen therapy and a small constant positive pressure (up to ~7cmH$_2$O) throughout inspiration and expiration (see ● p. 790). As with CPAP this is not a form of ventilation but is mentioned here as it is sometimes incorrectly referred to as such. The constant positive pressure can assist in opening collapsed alveoli (thus improving V/Q matching). HFNO has a role in improving oxygenation in selected patients with acute respiratory failure without hypercapnia and again may have a role in selected patients with severe COVID-19 infection.

Indications

NIV may be used in an attempt to avoid invasive ventilation and its complications (e.g. upper airway trauma, ventilator-associated pneumonia (VAP)); alternatively, NIV may represent the 'ceiling' of treatment in patients deemed unsuitable for intubation. NIV is *not* an alternative to invasive ventilation in patients who require this definitive treatment, as it is not sufficiently secure.

Acute exacerbation of COPD

- Consider NIV in patients with an acute exacerbation of COPD who have a respiratory acidosis (pH <7.35) and hypercapnia ($PaCO_2$>6.5 kPa) despite initial 1 h optimal medical treatment
- Still often required to rescue patients who have been given too high a concentration of O_2 to breathe, reduced hypoxic drive, and have become hypercapnic and acidotic; response to NIV can be rapid
- Benefits include reduced mortality and need for intubation, more rapid improvement in physiological outcomes (respiratory rate (RR), pH, $PaCO_2$), and symptomatic relief from breathlessness, when compared with standard medical treatment
- NIV only assists ventilation; the pressures used are not enough to take over ventilation due to high airway resistance
- Invasive ventilation, if deemed appropriate, should be considered up front, particularly in patients with a severe respiratory acidosis (pH <7.25), as this is associated with treatment failure and increased mortality with NIV alone
- High expiratory pressures (e.g. 6–8 cmH_2O, PEEP) may help reduce the work of breathing by offsetting intrinsic PEEP but will lessen the IPAP–EPAP difference (thus reducing the ventilation component), unless inspiratory pressures are further increased.

Acute cardiogenic pulmonary oedema

- Use of CPAP via face mask is effective and should be considered in patients who fail to improve with medical management alone
- Bi-level NIV has not been shown to be superior to CPAP, and there is a suggestion of increased myocardial infarction (MI) rates following its use. It may, however, have a role in patients who do not respond to CPAP.

Decompensated OSA and obesity hypoventilation

OSA alone very rarely causes significant daytime hypercapnia. NIV is effective in the treatment of OSA and the overlap syndrome (i.e. raised $PaCO_2$, typically with associated obesity hypoventilation or COPD; see ➲ p. 702) when CPAP alone fails to reverse the CO_2 retention. NIV is generally recommended as the first choice over CPAP when an acute respiratory acidosis is present, but conversion to CPAP later may be possible when the ventilatory failure has been reversed. NIV or CPAP are also indicated in patients with compensated hypercapnia and daytime somnolence.

Respiratory failure from neuromuscular weakness

- NIV is the treatment of choice for ventilatory failure resulting from neuromuscular weakness or chest wall deformity
- The pressures used may be adequate to fully take over ventilation, because the chest and lung compliance are often little impaired.

Immunocompromised patients

- Immunocompromised patients who develop acute respiratory failure have an extremely high mortality following endotracheal intubation and ventilation
- CPAP/HFNO can be useful in the hypoxic non-hypercapnic patient
- In those with additional hypercapnia patient NIV/CPAP/HFNO is not recommended outside of the ICU setting
- In immunocompromised patients with pulmonary infiltrates, fever, and hypoxaemic acute respiratory failure, intermittent NIV results in lower intubation rates and hospital mortality when compared with standard treatment.

Community-acquired pneumonia (CAP)

- CPAP/HFNO can be useful in the hypoxic non-hypercapnic patient
- In patients with additional hypercapnia who would be candidates for intubation, use of NIV/CPAP/HFNO should not inappropriately delay invasive ventilation
- Use of NIV may result in a reduction in need for intubation, compared with standard medical treatment, although no significant differences in hospital mortality or length of hospitalization have been shown
- CPAP/HFNO may have a role in improving oxygenation in severe pneumonia and severe COVID-19 infection.

Other conditions

- There is no evidence to support use of NIV in acute severe asthma, and it should not be used; if ventilation is required, then it should be invasive
- NIV is commonly used in decompensated hypercapnic exacerbations of bronchiectasis or cystic fibrosis (CF)
- NIV/HFNO/CPAP may have a role in improving gas exchange following trauma or surgery
- NIV/HFNO are being increasingly used to aid weaning after invasive ventilation.

Contraindications

Contraindications (some relative) to the use of NIV should be considered in the context of individual patients, e.g. severe hypoxaemia may not be considered a contraindication for NIV in a patient who is unsuitable for invasive ventilation.

Contraindications to NIV

- Cardiac or respiratory arrest
- Impaired consciousness or confusion (relative)
- Severe hypoxaemia, as the FiO_2 delivered by NIV is often unreliable
- Copious respiratory secretions
- Haemodynamic instability (relative)
- Facial surgery, trauma, burns, or deformity
- Upper airway obstruction (except from pharyngeal or laryngeal OSA)
- Undrained pneumothorax
- Inability to cooperate or to protect the airway
- Vomiting, bowel obstruction, recent upper gastro-intestinal (GI) tract surgery, oesophageal injury.

Further information

Plant PK et al. Early use of non-invasive ventilation for acute exacerbations of chronic obstructive pulmonary disease on general respiratory wards. *Lancet* 2000;**355**: 1931–1935.

Bourke et al. Effects of non-invasive ventilation on survival and quality of life in patients with amyotrophic lateral sclerosis: a randomized controlled trial *Lancet Neurol* 2006;**5**: 140–147.

Davidson et al. British Thoracic Society/Intensive Care Society guidelines for the management of acute hypercapnic respiratory failure in adults *Thorax* 2016;**71** (Suppl 2): ii1–ii35.

NIV in acute respiratory failure: practical use

When acute decompensated respiratory failure (pH<7.35 and $PaCO_2$ >6.5 kPa) is identified, initial standard medical treatment is usually recommended for 1 h. Medical treatment includes appropriate supplementary and controlled O_2 therapy, where appropriate, bronchodilators and oral/ IV corticosteroids; ~20% will improve within 1 h and will no longer require ventilation. If at 1 h a repeat blood gas shows persistent decompensated respiratory failure, NIV should be considered. Prior to commencing NIV, a senior doctor should make a decision where possible with the patient and their family regarding suitability for NIV, immediate invasive ventilation, invasive ventilation should NIV fail, palliation should NIV fail, or immediate palliation. This decision should be documented clearly in the medical notes. *If the patient is a candidate for invasive ventilation, care must be taken to avoid inappropriate delays in intubation through the use of NIV or CPAP. Liaise with ICU staff early.* Once a decision is made to trial NIV consideration should be given to safely delivering therapy as it is aerosol generating and, depending on the patient, may increase risk of spread of COVID-19.

Setting up NIV

1. Select an appropriate mask type and size for the patient. Masks may be nasal or oronasal (full face). Nasal masks require clear nasal passages and often allow mouth leaks, particularly in the acutely breathless patient, but may be more comfortable. Full-face masks avoid mouth leakage and are now generally favoured for acute ventilatory failure
2. Allow the patient to hold the mask to their face prior to attaching the head straps—this may increase confidence and compliance. Mask adjustments are often necessary to minimize air leaks, although some leakage may have to be accepted. Avoid excessive strap tension; one or two fingers should be able to fit under the strap
3. Set up the ventilator, mask and circuit (nb. depending on local policies and risk of spread of infection may needed a non-vented mask, viral/bacterial filter and expiratory port). Typical initial pressures for ventilating a patient with hypercapnic respiratory failure due to an exacerbation of COPD would be EPAP 4 cmH_2O and IPAP 12 cmH_2O, with a back-up rate of 15/min and inspiratory:expiratory ratio of 1:3 in spontaneous/timed mode. Increase the IPAP in increments of 2 cmH_2O to an initial target of 20 cmH_2O, as tolerated by the patient. Patients with hypercapnic respiratory failure resulting from neuromuscular weakness are often adequately treated with lower pressures. Increase the EPAP (e.g. to 8 or 10 cmH_2O) in obese patients with an 'overlap' syndrome of COPD and OSA to maintain airway patency during inspiration to allow triggering.

    Pressure support ventilators can also be set to provide CPAP by equalizing the IPAP and EPAP; typical pressures range from 5 to 12.5 cmH_2O. CPAP may improve oxygenation in selected patients with cardiogenic pulmonary oedema or pneumonia.
4. Supplementary O_2 concentration (FiO_2) should be guided by the underlying disease process and by oximetry monitoring. For many

hypercapnic patients, aiming for O_2 saturations between 88% and 92% effectively balances the risks of hypoxia vs hypercapnic respiratory acidosis. By adding O_2, there is a risk of potentially masking gradual ventilatory failure (by deceptively achieving adequate oxygenation) and thus hypercapnia, hence more careful blood gas monitoring will be required. If at all possible, use no, or very little, added O_2

5. Patient monitoring should involve assessment of comfort, RR, synchrony with the ventilator, mask leaks, pulse rate, blood pressure (BP), and O_2 saturations

6. Arterial or capillary blood gas analysis should be performed after no more than 1 h, and again after within an hour if there has been no improvement. Improvement in acidosis and decline in RR after 1 h and 4 h of treatment are associated with a better outcome. Repeat the blood gas analysis if the clinical condition changes

7. Lack of response may be indicated by a worsening acidosis or persistently abnormal arterial blood gases (ABGs), or by a reduced conscious level and clinical deterioration. Consider invasive ventilation, if appropriate. The decision to halt NIV depends on the circumstances of the individual patient and should be made by a senior doctor

8. Subsequent management depends on the patient's response. Optimal duration of NIV is unclear, but it is typically administered for about 3 days in acute respiratory failure. NIV does not need to be continuous; the patient may have breaks for meals and nebulizers. Weaning should follow a weaning plan and be gradual and achieved by increasing the period off NIV, with nocturnal use withdrawn last.

There is no substitute for personally assessing the efficacy of NIV (see Table 57.1). For example, failure to see the lungs inflating can be due to head position (best head position is the so-called 'sniffing the morning air' position; produces least pharyngeal resistance). Leaks can be heard. Adjustments can be made; immediately observe the effect. Sometimes, the presence of intrinsic PEEP means significant inspiratory effort is being made (visible intercostal movement) before the ventilator senses inspiration and triggers, thus increasing work of breathing. This can be seen and the EPAP gradually raised, until there is no delay between patient inspiratory effort and the triggering of the ventilator. In situations when patients have extreme difficulties with tolerating NIV, low doses of oral morphine or lorazepam can be helpful in aiding tolerance without significantly worsening hypercapnia.

Table 57.1 Troubleshooting

Problem	Possible solution
Clinical deterioration or worsening respiratory failure	Ensure optimal medical therapy
	Consider complications, e.g. pneumothorax, aspiration, sputum retention
	Does the patient require intubation, if appropriate?
pCO_2 remains high (persistent respiratory acidosis)	Exclude inappropriately high FiO_2 (producing SaO_2 >92%)
	Check mask and circuit for leaks
	Check for patient–ventilator asynchrony
	Check expiration valve or blow off is patent
	Consider increasing IPAP
pO_2 remains low (<7 kPa), with pCO_2 OK	Consider increasing FiO_2
	Consider increasing EPAP
Irritation or ulceration	Adjust strap tension of nasal bridge
	Try cushion dressing
	Change mask type; masks are available that do not rest on the nasal bridge
Dry nose or mouth	Consider humidifier
	Check for leaks
Dry sore eyes	Check mask fit
Nasal congestion	Decongestants, e.g. xylometazoline
Hypotension	Reduce IPAP (or EPAP if already high)

NIV in chronic respiratory failure

Chest wall deformity and neuromuscular weakness

See ➔ pp. 694–701.

- NIV has a well-established role in the management of chronic respiratory failure due to chest wall deformity or neuromuscular weakness and has been shown to improve symptoms, gas exchange, and mortality
- Common underlying diagnoses include chest wall deformity and scoliosis, post-polio syndrome, motor neurone disease (MND), spinal cord injury, neuropathies, myopathies, and muscular dystrophies. The nature of the underlying disease will influence the appropriateness of initiating ventilation; progressive conditions, such as MND, often result in increasing dependence on the ventilator, and the patient and their caregivers should be made aware of this
- NIV is administered at home overnight, and this improves daytime gas exchange. The mechanism for this is unclear; it probably resets the central respiratory drive, although respiratory muscle rest and improved chest wall and lung compliance may also play a part
- Small portable positive pressure ventilators, with either face (usual) or nasal (less often) masks, are used in the majority of cases; negative pressure or abdominal ventilators rarely have a role now, and their use may be limited by upper airways obstruction
- The decision to introduce overnight NIV can be difficult and is based on both symptoms (morning headaches, hypersomnolence, fatigue, poor sleep quality) and evidence of ventilatory failure (daytime hypercapnia (pCO_2 >6.0 kPa, and/or base excess >3) and/or nocturnal hypoventilation (with prolonged periods with O_2 saturations <88% on overnight oximetry). Daytime ventilatory failure, however, is often a late feature and is typically preceded by hypoventilation during sleep
- Supine inspiratory vital capacity (VC) (more sensitive to any diaphragm weakness than sitting or standing) is a good marker of respiratory reserve; supine inspiratory VC <40% predicted is significantly associated with hypercapnic hypoventilation, and such patients should be considered for treatment with NIV. Supine inspiratory VC <20% is typically associated with daytime respiratory failure. VC tends to decline late in patients with neuromuscular weakness where more invasive measurements such as sniff diaphragmatic pressure are earlier predictors of impending ventilatory failure
- Other factors include signs of cor pulmonale or hospital admission with respiratory failure
- Patients with excessive secretions may not be suitable for NIV, although bulbar weakness should not preclude a trial of NIV
- Consider the use of cough assistance techniques and devices in those with excessive secretions, particularly if cough peak flow <270 L/min (see ➔ p. 111)

- Regular follow-up of patients on overnight ventilation is important. Ask about symptoms and compliance, and repeat arterial or capillary blood gas analysis, if indicated. Download machine and review mask. Lack of improvement in gas exchange may reflect non-compliance, excessive air leakage, inadequate pressure support, upper airway obstruction, or progression of underlying disease; consider repeating nocturnal oximetry monitoring on the NIV. Patients with persisting severe hypoxia may benefit from long-term supplementary O_2, although this may worsen CO_2 retention and usually NIV settings are adjusted before trialling this
- There are significant issues of risk management when prescribing home NIV, particularly rapid access to replacement ventilators, battery back-up facilities, careful reassessment when there is evidence of a deterioration, and appropriate training of both the patient and their carer(s)
- Consideration should be given to providing patients who are ventilator dependent with a machine with a battery back-up and a back-up machine. Consider 24 h nursing/medical support
- Tracheostomy ventilation for patients with neuromuscular disease can be considered. Long-term tracheostomies in this situation are controversial, particularly in MND. If a patient is considering this seek specialist advice and input.

Sleep apnoea

See ⊃ Chapter 14.

Overnight NIV can have a role in patients with central hypoventilation, opiate-induced central apnoea, Cheyne–Stokes respiration, obesity hypoventilation, overlap syndromes of OSA with coexisting COPD or obesity. Servo-ventilation has a limited role in CSA, outside the setting of heart failure with preserved ejection fraction (see ⊃ pp. 700–701). There is the prospect of further developments in 'smart' ventilators, where not only is the pressure support monitored and adjusted, but also the level of EPAP required to hold open the pharynx is adjusted; additional forced oscillation is superimposed on the airflow from the ventilator, and the resultant pressure oscillations enable obstructive episodes (both apnoeas and hypopnoeas) to be distinguished from central events. Thus, appropriate inspiratory and expiratory pressures are automatically selected. It is not clear if these new devices work consistently across all aetiologies.

Cystic fibrosis

See ⊃ Chapter 24.

Overnight NIV may have a useful role as a 'bridge' to transplantation in patients with CF and is the preferred method of ventilation in acute and chronic respiratory failure.

COPD

See ➜ Chapter 21.

Use of NIV in the management of chronic stable COPD is controversial. A recent trial showed a reduction in admission free survival in patients with chronic stable hypercapnic respiratory failure with a $PaCO_2 > 7$ kPa treated with NIV and long-term oxygen therapy (LTOT) two-weeks post discharge with an episode of decompensated hypercapnic respiratory failure, compared to LTOT alone. Where appropriate, such patients should be referred for consideration of NIV following discharge at 2–4 weeks. Pragmatically many patients are started on NIV outside of this setting if they have had recurrent admissions, experience decompensation during weaning, have co-existent sleep disordered breathing, have significant day-time somnolence, or require NIV to allow therapeutic LTOT prescription.

Further information

Davidson et al. British Thoracic Society/Intensive Care Society guidelines for the management of acute hypercapnic respiratory failure in adults. *Thorax* 2016;**71**(Suppl 2): ii1–ii35.

Murphy et al. Effect of home non-invasive ventilation with oxygen therapy versus oxygen therapy alone on hospital readmission or death after an acute COPD exacerbation: a randomized clinical trial. *JAMA* 2017;**317**: 2177–2186.

Cowie et al. Adaptive servo-ventilation for central sleep apnea in systolic heart failure. *NEJM* 2015;**373**: 1095–1105.

Turner et al. Tracheostomy in motor neurone disease. *Pract Neurol* 2019;**19**(6): 467–475.

NIV end-of-life weaning

Many patients who receive long-term NIV will have an underlying terminal diagnosis, for example motor neurone disease. NIV is a treatment choice and as such patient can to decide to stop this therapy. Decisions to stop treatment are often very emotive, but the decision to stop a treatment is ethically distinct from euthanasia. A consistent decision to stop NIV by a patient with capacity should be respected. When there is doubt, capacity needs to be carefully assessed (see ⊃ pp. 728–729). Palliative care teams are often very helpful in this setting, both in managing symptoms and in supporting patients, their families, carers, and medical professionals. Consider the patient's preference of where they would like to receive end-of-life care (home, hospice, hospital) and involve the patient's family as much as possible.

Practical steps to stopping NIV once a decision has been made

- Give STAT doses of pre-emptive medications such as 5–10 mg morphine sulphate SC, 5–10 mg midazolam SC, and 20 mg hyoscine butylbromide SC
- Repeat at 10–15min intervals until the patient is settled
- Either switch off NIV machine and remove mask, change to controlled O_2 such as a 28% venturi, or uncontrolled 1–2 L/min nasally
- Or slowly decrease NIV pressures by 2–4 cmH$_2$O giving boluses of medication until settled before further decreases. Stop NIV only once an IPAP of 8 cmH$_2$O has been achieved. Change to controlled O_2 such as a 28% venturi or uncontrolled 1–2 L/min nasally
- Give further boluses of morphine, midazolam, and hyoscine as required
- Consider continuous infusion of medications via a syringe driver.

Further information

Association for Palliative Medicine of Great Britain and Ireland. Withdrawal of Assisted Ventilation at the Request of a Patient with Motor Neurone Disease. 2015.

⅏ https://apmonline.org/wp-content/uploads/2015/02/APM-Guidance-on-Withdrawal-of-Assisted-Ventilation-Consultation-1st-May-2015.pdf

Oxygen therapy

Emergency oxygen therapy 788
Home oxygen therapy 792
Practical issues with home oxygen 796

Emergency oxygen therapy

Oxygen (O_2) is a treatment for hypoxia and not breathlessness.
O_2 therapy is either 'controlled' or 'uncontrolled':
- *Uncontrolled* and high-flow O_2 thought to be important, e.g. in:
  - Shock, sepsis, major trauma
  - Cardiac arrest and during resuscitation
  - Anaphylaxis
  - CO or cyanide poisoning (oxygen saturations unreliable)
  - Pneumothorax
  - Severe hypoxaemia i.e. SaO_2 <85%
- Deliver 15 L/min oxygen via a non-rebreathe mask initially in these situations
- Moderate hypoxia (i.e. SaO_2 <94% but above 85%) can be treated with either nasal cannulae or face mask oxygen aiming for SaO_2 94–98%. Commonly arises:
  - Pneumonia
  - Asthma
  - Acute heart failure
  - Pulmonary embolus (PE)
- When a reliable saturation can be obtained oxygen can often be weaned to achieve SaO_2 94–98%
- In critical illness and with hypoxaemia an arterial blood gas should be obtained as early as possible. Capillary blood gases underestimate the PaO_2 by 0.5–1 kPa and should not be initially used
- British Thoracic Society (BTS) guidelines advise not to remove oxygen to obtain an arterial blood gas on room air in acute settings
- *Controlled* Use when extra O_2 is required, but ventilation critically depends on hypoxic drive (BTS guidelines recommend targeting SaO_2 88–92%), e.g.:
  - Exacerbations of chronic obstructive pulmonary disease (COPD) (particularly when there has been a chronically raised or previously raised $PaCO_2$, as evidenced by a significant base excess/raised bicarbonate or documented previously high CO_2)
  - Exacerbations of cystic fibrosis (CF)
  - Exacerbations of ventilatory failure due to obesity hypoventilation syndrome, scoliosis, or neuromuscular disease

With stable hypercapnic respiratory failure, ventilation still seems to be dominantly driven by $PaCO_2$/pH, but, in exacerbations (when PaO_2 usually falls), peripheral chemoreceptor drive from low PaO_2 becomes dominant. Thus, O_2 therapy must not raise PaO_2 above 8kPa ($\approx$ 92% SaO_2), as this will 'turn off' ventilatory drive, allowing hypoventilation, hypercapnia, acidosis, and potentially death. There is some evidence that high alveolar PO_2 also 'turns off' hypoxic pulmonary vasoconstriction. This allows an increase in pulmonary blood flow to poorly ventilated areas and reduces CO_2 excretion (accounts for ~20% of the $PaCO_2$ rise following excessive FiO_2 in COPD exacerbations).

There is increasing evidence that indiscriminate use of O_2 in some medical emergencies may actually be *harmful* and should only be used if the patient is hypoxaemic (<94%, and then to achieve no higher than 98%), e.g.:
• Ischaemic heart disease, including myocardial infarction (MI)
• Stroke
• Post-cardiac arrest, once stable
• Sickle cell crisis
• Obstetric emergencies
• Most poisonings (other than carbon monoxide (CO) or cyanide)
• Metabolic or renal acidosis with shortness of breath (SOB).

High O_2 levels can be toxic through release of free radicals, and this may be the mechanism of damage in some of the above situations. Following lung injury, particularly from paraquat poisoning and bleomycin lung injury, high O_2 concentrations are clearly damaging to the lung; thus, a degree of controlled hypoxia may be preferable. BTS guidelines recommend target SaO_2 85–88% if O_2 is required in the context of paraquat or bleomycin.

In addition, when SaO_2 are inappropriately maintained >98% changes in the patient's clinical condition with large falls in PaO_2 do not cause falls in SaO_2 masking this indicator of a deteriorating patient.

Delivering uncontrolled O_2
• Standard O_2 face mask (sometimes called high-flow mask). Set the O_2 regulator to at least 4 L/min, much more if very breathless (to prevent dilution by air drawn into mask by high inspiratory flows via exit holes). Can deliver about 50–60% O_2
• Nasal cannulae/prongs/catheters are *uncontrolled* and deliver unpredictable levels of O_2 (depending on flow rate, minute ventilation, and oral vs nasal breathing). Titrate using an O_2 saturation monitor. In patients with hypercapnia who are reliant on their hypoxic drive to breathe nasal cannulae can deliver too high an FiO_2 and ventilation decreases as a consequence. This leads to a vicious cycle where the proportion of the minute ventilation containing the fixed flow nasal O_2 will rise, increasing the FiO_2 and hence the PaO_2 still further
• Non-rebreathe reservoir masks can deliver FiO_2 values over 60% by means of a soft plastic bag between the end of the tubing and mask, plus one-way valves between the bag and mask and on the mask exit ports. This mechanism ensures that most of the inspired air is pure O_2. The ability of the reservoir to empty on inspiration briefly allows higher inspiratory flows than the actual O_2 regulator setting, and the bag valve prevents inhalation of most exhaled CO_2; the mask exit valves close, preventing air inhalation. The usual problem is kinking of the junction between the mask and bag when the head tilts forward, reducing the effectiveness of the reservoir
• Very high FiO_2 requires a tight seal and is generally delivered with high flow nasal oxygen (HFNO; see below) or continuous positive airway pressure (CPAP) masks (using pressures of about 5–7 cmH_2O). This ensures no air is entrained through blow-off vents or leaks, as well as improving ventilation-perfusion (V/Q) matching by recruiting collapsed alveoli.

High flow nasal oxygen (HFNO)
- Brand names include AIRVO™ and Optiflow™
- Allows delivery of high FiO_2 with high flow rates, typically up to 60 L/min
- High flow rates mean that positive pressure is delivered and this equates to CPAP of up to 7 cmH_2O (~1 cmH_2O/10L/min flow). This will be impacted by mouth leak
- HFNO is therefore often used in patients with hypoxic non-hypercapnic respiratory failure (T1RF) despite high-flow oxygen via a non-rebreathe mask
- Needs careful consideration and senior input before starting HFNO, including consideration of location and personal protective equipment as HFNO is aerosol generating
- Immediate invasive ventilation on intensive care unit (ICU) may be more appropriate dependent on the underlying diagnosis
- Depending on the underlying diagnosis and the likelihood of recovery/irreversibility of the disease, starting HFNO may not be appropriate. This is because weaning off HFNO can be difficult in the palliative setting (i.e. in idiopathic pulmonary fibrosis (IPF)) and careful discussion is needed with the patient before starting.

Delivering controlled O_2 therapy
This requires the ability to reliably control the FiO_2 in order to keep the patient's SaO_2 ≤92% (some prefer ≤90%), but high enough to prevent an-aerobic metabolism. This lower acceptable level is debatable: 88% is generous; 85% is likely to be adequate, and 80% may be acceptable if cardiac output is adequate and patient's usual levels are around this figure.
- FiO_2 is controlled through a Venturi mask—O_2 is directed through a narrow nozzle and exits at speed, lowering the air pressure at this point. This draws in surrounding air, diluting the FiO_2
- A proper Venturi mask mixes O_2 and air in the same proportion, *regardless of the O_2 flow*
- The minimum flow setting of the regulator, written on the nozzle, ensures adequate overall flow to prevent diluting air being drawn through the exit holes during inhalation, e.g. a 28% Ventimask® has a 1:10 entrainment ratio—1 L/min O_2 entrains 10 L/min air (total flow 11 L/min); 2 L/min O_2 entrains 20 L/min air (total flow 22 L/min).
- Controlled O_2 via low flows is also needed sometimes with non-invasive ventilation (NIV) and it should be titrated using the patient's SaO_2. At a high FiO_2 the oxygen delivered by NIV is not always reliable and high FiO_2 requirements should trigger consideration of invasive ventilation. This is variable and oxygen is entrained directly into the NIV machine with some models, which allows more accurate FiO_2 delivery. While on NIV the patient is still required to trigger the machine with their own inspiratory effort, so supplemental O_2 should be kept to a minimum so as not to depress ventilatory drive.

O₂ alert card

Should be given to all patients with a previous episode of hypercapnic respiratory failure (see Fig. 58.1). This alerts ambulance crews and medical staff to the potential risk of hypercapnia with high-flow O_2 and documents usual resting baseline SaO_2. However, some ambulance staff protocols are sufficiently rigid that they may not be allowed to override them. In some areas, letters from the patient's consultant and head of the ambulance service must be with the patient.

Patient details	Carry the card with you at all times
Sticky label	**If you need to call the ambulance service or attend the hospital accident and emergency department, show this card to the GP, paramedics, doctor, or emergency department staff looking after you, as it provides them with essential information regarding your personal oxygen needs.**
Introduction	
If you have a sudden worsening of your lung disease (usually due to a chest infection) it is essential that you do not receive too much or too little oxygen, either can be dangerous. Too much oxygen can cause a rise in the level of carbon dioxide in your blood and this can make you drowsy and slow your breathing. Too little oxygen can also be dangerous.	**Latest blood gas recordings:** **Date:** ___/___/_____ **On:** Air, or % oxygen ____% **pH:** ____ pCO₂____ pO₂____ **Oxygen saturation:** _____ %
Purpose of this card	You should receive enough oxygen to achieve a % O2 saturation of no higher than 92%, but higher than 86%, if possible. This is usually done with either a 24% or 28% Venturi mask.
The purpose of this oxygen alert card is to make sure that the doctors or ambulance staff involved in your care are made aware of your special needs regarding oxygen therapy. The card recommends the appropriate amount of oxygen therapy for you based on your previous blood gas tests.	Signed .... Name......................... Designation..

Fig. 58.1 Example of an O_2 alert card.

Further information

O'Driscoll R et al. British Thoracic Society Guideline for oxygen use in adults in healthcare and emergency settings. *BMJ Open Respir Res* 2017; **4**: e000170.

Gooptu B et al. O_2 alert cards and controlled O_2: preventing emergency admissions at risk. *Emerg Med J* 2006;**23**: 636–638.

Home oxygen therapy

Despite the evidence base for oxygen, 25–40% of prescribed home oxygen is not used as prescribed and 20% of COPD patients who might benefit are not currently prescribed oxygen. Home O_2 therapy is now mainly recommended to be used as long-term oxygen therapy (LTOT) to treat select patients with chronic hypoxia, requiring >15 h/day, with the evidence base from two randomized trials. Outside of this setting there are limited indications for oxygen therapy with ambulatory oxygen therapy (AOT), nocturnal oxygen therapy (NOT), and short-burst oxygen therapy (SBOT) only in the context of cluster headaches.

Long-term oxygen therapy (LTOT)

Background and indications

- Two landmark trials of LTOT in the 1980s—the British MRC Working Party trial and the American Nocturnal O_2 Therapy Trial (NOTT) established the value of LTOT
- The *MRC trial* compared COPD patients receiving O_2 for 15 h/day with controls receiving no O_2
- The *NOTT trial* compared continuous daily O_2 (average 17.7 h/day) with overnight O_2 (average 12 h)
- The patients in the MRC trial were on average hypercapnic (mean $PaCO_2$ 7.3 kPa), whereas those in the NOTT trial were on average normocapnic (mean $PaCO_2$ 5.7 kPa)
- The main outcome in both trials was improved survival in those patients receiving O_2 for at least 15 h/day, though this improved survival was not seen in the MRC trial until after a year of O_2 therapy
- The *NOTT trial* showed a reduced exercise pulmonary artery pressure (PAP) after 6 months of continuous or nocturnal O_2 therapy. The 8-y survival was related to the fall in mean PAP during the first 6 months of continuous O_2 use
- The *MRC trial* failed to show a fall in mean PAP with LTOT, but the mean annual increase in PAP (3 mmHg) in patients in the control arm was not seen in the O_2 treated group
- The reason for the improved survival with LTOT is not clear and is unlikely to relate to the small changes in pulmonary haemodynamics seen.

COPD is the disease for which LTOT is most commonly prescribed and the disease in which the original studies were completed. LTOT usage in diseases other than COPD is largely based on the evidence from its use in COPD. Subsequent O_2 studies have shown improved exercise endurance in COPD patients breathing supplemental O_2, with improved walking distance and ability to perform daily activities. FEV_1 is the strongest predictor of survival in COPD; LTOT does not influence the decline in FEV_1.

Additional benefits of LTOT include:

- Reduction of 2° polycythaemia
- Improved sleep quality by reducing hypoxia-associated brain arousals
- Reduced cardiac arrythmias, and potentially reducing the risk of nocturnal sudden death
- Reduced sympathetic outflow, leading to improved renal function, with increased salt and water excretion, and reduced peripheral oedema.

Indications for LTOT

LTOT is the provision of O_2 therapy to patients with a chronically low PaO_2 (≤7.3 kPa, or ≤55 mmHg, or SaO_2 ≤≈88%) for ≥15 h a day (to include the night, when usually most hypoxic), with the aim of achieving an awake PaO_2 >8 kPa, or >60 mmHg, or SaO_2 >≈91%. $PaCO_2$ levels can be normal or raised.

More recent trials have shown no benefit of LTOT in moderately hypoxaemic patients not meeting these established LTOT criteria.

The indications to which LTOT now covers are:
• COPD
• Severe chronic asthma
• Interstitial lung disease (ILD)
• CF
• Bronchiectasis
• Pulmonary vascular disease
• Pulmonary portohypertension
• Pulmonary malignancy
• Chronic heart failure.

LTOT can also be prescribed if the PaO_2 is 7.3–8 kPa, if associated with 2° polycythaemia or pulmonary hypertension (PHT). PaO_2 values above 8 kPa should not lead to a prescription for LTOT.

In addition, it can be prescribed for nocturnal hypoventilation, usually in conjunction with NIV or CPAP, e.g. in:
• Obesity
• Neuromuscular or other restrictive disorders
• OSA treated with CPAP therapy but with continuing hypoxia.

This is entirely non-evidence-based (with no guidance on thresholds, etc.) and should only happen following assessment in a specialist unit and following optimization of the NIV or CPAP.

There are exceptional uses such as nocturnal O_2 for Cheyne–Stokes breathing in heart failure (despite adequate awake levels) which can improve sleep quality.

Assessment for LTOT

• Should occur when patients are stable and at least 8 weeks have passed since any exacerbation of their condition
• Fully optimized treatment
• Two sets of arterial gases are taken at least 3 weeks apart to ensure that the patient remains sufficiently hypoxic to merit LTOT
• Blood gases are also taken after 30 min on supplemental O_2 to ensure the target PaO_2 has been reached.

Capillary blood gas and oximetry-based assessments are not recommended but could be considered if arterial blood gas assessment is not feasible, accepting that a few patients may be prescribed LTOT who do not need it.

Patients should have a repeat arterial blood gas (ABG) on oxygen to check therapeutic oxygen levels and to check $PaCO_2$ levels. Patients need to be warned about the symptoms of CO_2 retention as this can occur even with reassuring clinic CO_2 levels, particularly during an exacerbation.

Ambulatory oxygen therapy (AOT)

Provision of supplemental O_2 during exercise and activities of daily living. This may be on its own or in addition to LTOT. The evidence for AOT is limited, showing improvements in laboratory-based exercise performance only. AOT has not been shown to have long-term benefits on dyspnoea, exercise capacity, functional capacity, time away from home, or QOL. Ambulatory oxygen should not be routinely offered and should only be considered as part of a structured programme of exercise such as pulmonary rehabilitation. AOT should not be considered for patients who are housebound.

Short burst oxygen therapy (SBOT)

Short-burst O_2 is now rarely justified. It may be required for transient situations, such as during exacerbations, but usually either the patient is sufficiently hypoxic to require LTOT or they are not. If it is considered, then proof of efficacy should be sought, particularly given its expense. SBOT at 12 L/min should be considered for cluster headache.

Practical issues with home oxygen

- Fire safety is an important consideration as 1 in 4 oxygen-related fires lead to death. Local fire service should review all homes of those with newly prescribed O_2
- NICE guidelines recommend that home O_2 should not be supplied to patients who still smoke, due to added fire risk and probable reduced efficacy due to ↑ COHb (BTS guidelines dissuade usage in smokers but smoking with adequate risk assessment is not a complete contraindication in the BTS guidelines)
- All patients should have a risk assessment for home oxygen therapy, including a fire risk assessment; risk factors for fires including smoking (87% of all oxygen-related fires), open fires/flames, candles, oil-based emollients, gas stoves
- LTOT is provided by an O_2 concentrator, typically set at 0.5–5 L/min. Some concentrators can deliver higher flow rates. Concentrators contain a molecular sieve of zeolite, which traps gas molecules (mainly nitrogen), depending on size and polarity. Can produce up to 96% O_2, depending on flow (the argon is also concentrated to 4%)
- Patients are provided with back-up cylinders in case of a power cut
- Some patients have liquid oxygen with (portable) cylinders that can be filled from a static reservoir
- Patients may have a higher flow rate for use during activities
- Patients can use nasal prongs or a fixed concentration mask (uncontrolled or controlled O_2, e.g. 24% and 28%), depending on physiological requirements and their preference. A back-up cylinder should be prescribed in case of power cuts
- O_2 humidification (cold) is possible but rarely necessary or effective. Tube lengths of <1.5 m recommended. Tubing should be kept to the length required and out of the way to reduce the risk of trips
- LTOT should be used for ≥15 h/day in patients with COPD, although survival improves when used for longer; therefore, use should not be restricted to 15 h/day
- Patient education in the use of LTOT is important. Specialist respiratory nurses should be involved
- It is important to consider the weight of AOT equipment as this may be prohibitive to its use in some patients.

How to organize home oxygen

- Commonly oxygen is arranged via local specialist respiratory nurses
- The UK-wide integrated O_2 service (2005) ensured provision of all modalities of domiciliary O_2 from one contractor in each area
- The prescriber completes *and signs* a Home Oxygen Order Form (HOOF), providing the supplier with the patient's details, an exact prescription of the O_2 required, including modality, and details of numbers of each piece of equipment needed (e.g. numbers of O_2 cylinders)—the supplier may be able to help advise
- The HOOF is used for the prescription of all forms of O_2; must include details of the O_2 flow rate, % O_2, and delivery device/mask required
- HOOF part A can be used by non-specialists (e.g. GPs, out-of-hours services, palliative care) to temporarily prescribe static O_2 concentrators or static cylinder, pending specialist assessment

- HOOF part B is completed by specialist respiratory services after formal clinical assessment and provides access to the full range of O_2 services
- The O_2 supplier will invoice the local commissioning group; it is vital that the above information is completed, otherwise the HOOF will be returned unfilled
- A Home Oxygen Consent Form (HOCF) must be signed by the patient, consenting for the disclosure of relevant medical information, address, telephone number to the O_2 supplier and fire brigade
- The HOOF is faxed to the O_2 supplier, with copies to the local commissioners, GP, and clinical lead for home O_2 services
- The standard response time for delivery of O_2 services is 3 days although can be ordered as urgent (4 h) or next day. The 4 h option is more expensive

Follow-up is needed to ensure:
- Compliance; withdraw if not using despite support and explanation. Home visit within 4 weeks by specialist nurse recommended
- Confirm the ongoing requirement for LTOT. Some patients improve and no longer need LTOT. ABG tensions at 3 months and then yearly monitoring (may be performed by specialist nurses)
- Cancellation with the O_2 company as soon as a patient dies
- Inform O_2 company of any changes in flow rates/%O_2
- Inform O_2 company of any changes in patient address, etc.

Further information

Hardinge et al. BTS guidelines for home oxygen use in adults. Thorax 2015;**70**(Suppl 1): i1–i43.
NICE   guideline   NG115   ℘   https://www.nice.org.uk/guidance/ng115/evidence/
  b-oxygen-therapy-in-people-with-stable-copd-pdf-6602768751
Patient information. ℘ http://www.nhs.uk/conditions/home-oxygen/pages/introduction.aspx.

Chapter 59

Palliative care

General points *800*

Lung cancer and mesothelioma—pain and dyspnoea *802*

Lung cancer and mesothelioma—other symptoms *806*

Non-malignant respiratory disease (COPD, CF, fibrotic lung disease) *808*

General points

Palliative care is defined by the World Health Organization (WHO) as an approach that improves the quality of life (QoL) of patients and their families facing the problems associated with life-threatening illness, through the prevention and relief of suffering by means of early identification, impeccable assessment, and treatment of pain and other problems, physical, psychosocial, and spiritual. Palliative care is moving away from being involved just at the end of life, especially in developing countries when curative possibilities are less readily available and palliative treatments may be the only option. In the UK, patients may be under palliative care teams intermittently for symptom control, respite care, etc. and may not see the service again for months or years.

Within chest medicine, palliative care is most commonly considered for patients with lung cancer and mesothelioma; many other patients with progressive end-stage respiratory disease (such as chronic obstructive pulmonary disease (COPD), cystic fibrosis (CF), fibrotic lung disease, and motor neurone disease (MND)) also benefit from specific palliative interventions. These two areas are discussed separately in this chapter, although there is much overlap in the management.

Lung cancer and mesothelioma—pain and dyspnoea

- Involve the specialist palliative care team early
- Treat symptoms promptly
- An open discussion of a patient's fears is often helpful, as is a calm and explicit logical approach to symptom management
- Recognize problems are often mixed, complex, and multiple
- Recognize that delirium, dyspnoea, and decreased mobility often herald the terminal phase of cancer.

Pain

- Aim to determine cause, type, and site
- Start with simple analgesia, and increase according to the WHO analgesic ladder, moving from non-opioid analgesia (paracetamol, non-steroidal anti-inflammatories (NSAIDs) through weak opioids (codeine, tramadol) to strong opioids (morphine, diamorphine, fentanyl, etc.), while also considering adjuvant therapy (e.g. antidepressants, antiepileptics). Reassess repeatedly and regularly
- If moving to morphine from a weak opioid, 40–60 mg morphine daily should be adequate (given either 4-hourly immediate release or 12-hourly modified-release preparations). 60 mg codeine qds is equivalent to 24 mg total daily morphine. If the first dose of morphine is no more effective than previous analgesia, increase next dose by 50%
- Prescribe analgesia as required for breakthrough pain (see Box 59.1)
- Give drugs a chance to work at appropriate doses, particularly if they have not had strong opioids before. Allows assessment of analgesic effect and side effects. Usually increase every 3rd day if required
- Once pain is reasonably controlled, morphine dose can be converted to slow-release morphine by dividing total daily amount by two and giving that dose as modified-release morphine 12-hourly (see Box 59.2). The *additional* breakthrough dose is 1/6 of the total 24 h dose (e.g. if using 15 mg *modified*-release morphine bd, then use an additional 5 mg *immediate*-release morphine sulfate for breakthrough pain)
- Be proactive in preventing and treating drug side effects, e.g. constipation, nausea. Prescribe prophylactic laxatives with morphine. Warn people they may feel drowsier if starting morphine or having dose increase, but this usually settles within a few days
- Patients with renal failure are more likely to develop opioid toxicity (drowsiness, confusion, myoclonus), as they have difficulty excreting morphine metabolites. They may need alternatives to morphine (e.g. oxycodone, methadone, alfentanil) if their pain is not controlled on low-dose morphine
- The addition of an anti-inflammatory drug or steroids can be effective for bone pain and for liver capsule pain if there are hepatic metastases
- Consider radiotherapy for localized pain in the chest related to cancer
- *Pleuritic pain* Consider pulmonary embolus (PE); treat any infection. Consider NSAID ± intercostal nerve block

- *Bone metastases causing local tenderness* Start a strong opioid. If there is no improvement after three dose increases, add an NSAID for a 1-week trial. If single site, consider radiotherapy or intercostal nerve block. If multiple sites, consider bisphosphonates (provided not hypocalcaemic), e.g. 90 mg of pamidronate intravenous (IV) every 4 weeks
- *Neuropathic pain* can be treated with tricyclic antidepressants (e.g. amitriptyline started at 10–25 mg nocte or nortriptyline) or antiepileptics (e.g. pregabalin started at 75 mg bd or gabapentin). In some cases, there may be a role for lidocaine patches or capsaicin cream
- *Pain from chest drain tract metastases* Use analgesia, and refer for radiotherapy
- Consider referral to pain clinic or specialist centre for further intervention such as an intercostal nerve block, transcutaneous electrical nerve stimulation (TENS), cervical cordotomy, or complementary therapies.

Box 59.1 Treatment of breakthrough pain
- *If already on non-opioid analgesic* Give one extra dose of the regular analgesic
- *If already on a regular oral opioid* Give 4-hourly oral dose (= 1/6 of total 24 h dose), e.g. 60 mg/day = 10 mg dose
- *If already on continuous subcutaneous (SC) infusion of morphine/ diamorphine* Give 4-hourly dose, e.g. 30 mg/24 h = 5 mg dose SC.

Consider increasing regular analgesic dose if the breakthrough pain occurs before the next regular dose.

If there is no response to the additional breakthrough pain treatment, repeat after 4 h if non-opioid or 1 h if opioid, with same dose. If still no response, consider changing from non-opioid to weak opioid, or weak opioid to strong opioid.

Box 59.2 Conversions between opioids
Different opioids at equivalent doses do not provide greater anal-gesic efficacy but offer alternative routes for administration to ensure adequate absorption and minimize side effects (usually toxicity and confusion).
- *Oral morphine to SC morphine* Conversion factor is ÷ 2, e.g. 60 mg/24 h oral morphine = 30 mg SC morphine
- *Oral morphine to diamorphine infusion* Conversion factor is ÷ 3, e.g. 60 mg/24 h oral morphine = 20 mg/24 h SC diamorphine
- *Oral morphine to 72 h transdermal fentanyl patch* See *British National Formulary* (BNF).

Dyspnoea

- Consider possible causes (see Box 59.3). Dyspnoea may be due to the underlying lung disease or due to an additional pathology. Lung cancer and pulmonary metastases are associated with the sensation of shortness of breath (SOB), often due to stimulation of receptors by malignant infiltration or lymphangitis carcinomatosis
- Dyspnoea is frightening and made worse by anxiety and panic. Explain to patient that alleviation of dyspnoea is possible for most patients with appropriate treatment
- Optimize treatment of any underlying lung disease with bronchodilators and steroids, if appropriate
- Treat concurrent chest infection
- Give advice on planning and adapting daily activities to conserve energy. Consider modifications to home environment
- Teach breathing techniques—diaphragmatic breathing, pursed-lip breathing may help. Consider exercise training
- Fan blowing cool air onto the face/open window can be helpful
- Consider patient positioning when in bed—upright posture assists diaphragmatic excursion; lying tilted may help with copious secretions
- Treat anxiety/depression
- Opioids (e.g. 2.5–5 mg morphine sulfate solution 4-hourly) relieve the sensation of dyspnoea without affecting respiratory function. Consider pre-emptive use for known triggers of breathlessness
- O_2 cylinders/concentrator for intermittent palliative use may help symptoms but may be associated with psychological dependence, may restrict daily activities, and may dry the upper airways
- Consider the need for external beam radiotherapy, endobronchial tumour debulking, or airway stenting in a patient with lung cancer experiencing dyspnoea due to bronchial obstruction or compression with tumour
- If PE diagnosed, consider treatment with low molecular weight heparin (LMWH), instead of warfarin (superior efficacy and avoids need for repeated blood tests; data limited for use of direct oral anticoagulant (DOACs))
- SC opioid infusion may relieve symptoms as death approaches; use with haloperidol, midazolam, or levomepromazine.

Box 59.3 Causes of breathlessness in patients with lung cancer

- Pneumonia
- Underlying chronic lung disease (e.g. COPD, pulmonary fibrosis) or concomitant cardiac disease
- Lobar collapse
- Pleural effusion
- Pneumothorax
- Superior vena caval obstruction (SVCO)
- Upper airway obstruction
- PEs
- Lymphangitis carcinomatosis
- Chest wall infiltration
- Phrenic nerve paralysis
- Pericardial effusion
- Respiratory muscle weakness due to cachexia, paraneoplastic syndromes, steroid myopathy
- Anaemia
- Depression
- Anxiety and panic.

Lung cancer and mesothelioma—other symptoms

Anxiety and depression

- May be due to fear and uncertainty over prognosis
- Leads to dyspnoea, which, in turn, worsens anxiety
- Reassure patients they will not suffocate; symptoms will pass
- Benzodiazepines (such as short-acting lorazepam 0.5–1 mg sublingually 8–12-hourly) are effective for respiratory panic. Longer-acting diazepam 2–5 mg nocte/bd may be helpful for severe anxiety or at night when dyspnoea and panic disturb sleep
- Acute panic may be helped by midazolam 2.5 mg IV, increased in increments of 1 mg, given in a controlled environment with O_2
- Amitriptyline or citalopram may be effective longer-term treatments
- Cannabinoids, such as nabilone, may be useful for patients who have continuous dyspnoea, anxiety, and who do not tolerate other agents
- Relaxation exercises, diaphragmatic breathing training, and complementary therapies may help some patients.

Cough

- Treat the underlying cause
- Try simple, pholcodine or codeine linctus
- Nebulized saline may help expectoration
- Codeine 30 mg qds (or even morphine sulphate solution) may be of use for intractable cough
- Methadone linctus 1–2 mg nocte or bd may be used but has a long duration of action and may accumulate
- Nebulized local anaesthetic may help, e.g. 5 mL 2% lidocaine 6-hourly or bupivacaine 5 mL 0.25% 8-hourly (avoid in asthmatics, as it causes bronchospasm). Pharyngeal numbness is likely to occur, so avoid fluids for 1–2 h afterwards
- Consider radiotherapy if haemoptysis due to lung cancer. Consider discontinuing antiplatelet drugs or anticoagulants
- If massive haemoptysis, consider tranexamic acid, plus emergency supply of opioids and benzodiazepines to ensure pain control and reduction of fear by decreasing awareness. Nebulized adrenaline may be useful. Use dark towels, sheets, and blankets to reduce visual impact.

Pleural effusion

- Drain if symptomatic, and pleurodese early if recurrent, although not if prognosis is poor (<3 months)
- Alternatively, consider indwelling pleural catheter (IPC) to drain fluid— randomized controlled trial (RCT) evidence suggests reasonable to use for 1° therapy (in place of talc pleurodesis). Patient choice is key (see ⊃ p. 858). Avoids inpatient stay. IPC also used for failed talc pleurodesis or with trapped lung.

Poor appetite

- Common symptom; may be 1°, due to cachexia–anorexia syndrome, or 2° due to mouth problems (such as candidiasis), nausea, hypercalcaemia, drugs, or depression
- May be improved in the short term (about 6 weeks) by a course of oral steroids such as dexamethasone 4 mg bd or prednisolone 20 mg daily
- Cachexia leads to decreased respiratory muscle strength and increased SOB
- Consider nutritional supplements.

Brain metastases

- Steroids relieve the cerebral oedema associated with brain metastases, e.g. dexamethasone 8 mg bd (8 a.m. and 2 p.m.) initially and then decrease
- Avoid steroid dosing in the evening, as sleep is affected
- Role of whole brain radiotherapy is controversial after QUARTZ trial demonstrated no overall survival or QoL benefits, although possible role for younger patients with good performance status (PS).

Recurrent laryngeal nerve palsy

- Affects 10% of patients with lung cancer, causes hoarse voice
- Patients with troublesome hoarseness should be referred to ENT for consideration of medialization of vocal cord to prevent paradoxical movement (achieved using injection laryngoplasty of material lateral to vocal fold or surgical placement of an implant).

Non-malignant respiratory disease (COPD, CF, fibrotic lung disease)

The main problems associated with severe non-malignant respiratory disease are dyspnoea, hypoxia, immobility, and psychosocial problems, including depression. End-stage COPD patients may have very frequent exacerbations for some years before a final terminal event. One study has shown those with end-stage COPD are more likely to have depression ± anxiety than those with terminal cancer, but they are less likely to receive specific treatment for their emotional problems or any targeted palliative care. It may be appropriate therefore to shift the focus in patients with severe end-stage respiratory disease away from management of acute exacerbations towards a more palliative approach to care. Emphasizing palliative care's role in 'supportive care' may ease introduction of the concept to the outpatient clinic.

Dyspnoea

- Follow advice in 'Dyspnoea' section (see p. 804)
- Patients may decrease their mobility to avoid dyspnoea and subsequently become more deconditioned. Pulmonary rehabilitation courses are useful
- Sitting upright reduces airway obstruction and optimizes ventilation. Relaxing and dropping the shoulders can improve ventilation when anxiety has caused patient to 'hunch up'
- Stop smoking
- 2014 RCT demonstrated that an integrated breathlessness support service (palliative care and respiratory medicine) improved breathlessness mastery (a QoL domain). Improved survival in those with COPD and ILD but findings needs replicating
- 2019 meta-analysis of interventions for breathlessness management (incl. breathing techniques, psychological support, and relaxation techniques) showed improvement in breathlessness and depression scores but did not alter QoL.

Hypoxia

- SaO_2 <92%
- Long-term oxygen therapy (LTOT) may be appropriate (see p. 792)
- O_2 cylinders for intermittent or ambulatory use may help symptoms, but little data to support their use
- Non-invasive ventilation (NIV) use appropriate for some causes of ventilatory failure (see p. 771).

Anxiety and depression

- Follow advice in 'Anxiety and depression' section (see p. 806)
- Depression rates are high in patients with COPD. Consider antidepressant treatment and counselling. Amitriptyline or citalopram may be effective at helping anxiety also.

Cough

- Treat the underlying cause
- Refer to physiotherapy to improve cough efficacy, particularly if large-volume secretions. Cough-assist device has a role, particularly in neuromuscular diseases
- Consider mucolytics, steroids, antibiotics
- Try simple or codeine linctus. If very problematic, opiates usually helpful (or gabapentin/pregabalin if opiates contraindicated)
- Nebulized saline may help expectoration
- Oral local anaesthetics, such as benzocaine and lidocaine lozenges, may be useful for laryngeal, pharyngeal, or tracheal irritation, but associated risk of aspiration
- Nebulized local anaesthetic may help, e.g. 5 mL 2% lidocaine 6-hourly or bupivacaine 5 mL 0.25% 6-hourly (avoid in asthmatics, as it causes bronchospasm). Pharyngeal numbness is likely to occur, so avoid fluids for 1–2 h afterwards.

Other problems

- Malnutrition, thirst
- Nausea, vomiting, constipation
- Sleep disturbance
- Chest pain
- Fatigue
- Oral candidiasis
- Impact on carers and family of patient with chronic respiratory disease
- Social/spiritual considerations
- Advanced care planning (ACP). Includes treatment options, prognosis, patient's wishes and the process of dying. Some evidence that multidisciplinary team (MDT) platform (palliative care, psychology, and respiratory medicine) improves ACP.

Further information

British National Formulary—useful information on prescribing in palliative care.

Higginson IJ et al. An integrated palliative and respiratory care service for patients with advanced disease and refractory breathlessness: a randomised controlled trial. *Lancet Respir Med* 2014;**2**(12): 979–987.

Brighton LJ et al. Holistic services for people with advanced disease and chronic breathlessness: a systematic review and meta-analysis. *Thorax* 2019;**74**(3): 270–281.

Pulmonary rehabilitation

Aims and patient selection *812*
Programme *814*

Aims and patient selection

Pulmonary rehabilitation (PR) is a well-established evidence-based multi-disciplinary programme of care for patients with symptomatic chronic respiratory impairment, targeting the extrapulmonary manifestations of the disease. The programme is individually tailored and should contain high-intensity progressive aerobic training, strength training, and self-management education. PR is probably the most cost-effective intervention for chronic obstructive pulmonary disease (COPD). It interrupts the vicious cycle of dyspnoea leading to inactivity, subsequent deconditioning, and further worsening dyspnoea on more minimal exertion.

Aims of rehabilitation

- To reduce disability in people with chronic lung disease
- To improve quality of life (QoL) and restore independence
- To diminish the health care burden of disease.

Early studies demonstrated there were improvements in functional status with PR despite no change in severity of airflow obstruction.

Meta-analysis a Cochrane review of 65 randomized controlled trials (RCTs), where PR included exercise training for at least 4 weeks (although the content was varied), confirmed the benefit of rehabilitation, with statistically and clinically significant improvements in functional or maximal exercise capacity and/or QoL. Symptoms of dyspnoea and fatigue are improved, and patients gain an enhanced sense of control over their condition.

Other benefits of PR

- Patients across the disease severity spectrum of COPD (including those with severe airflow obstruction) can benefit from PR
- Studies show patients who completed a rehabilitation course may have fewer hospital admissions for exacerbations than those who had not had rehabilitation, and hospital stays were shorter (10 days vs 21 days)
- Respiratory muscle training improves dyspnoea, but not exercise capacity or health-related QoL, above aerobic training
- High-intensity lower limb aerobic training is recommended, rather than low-intensity training
- Supplemental strength training improves muscle strength but does not provide additional benefit to exercise capacity or health-related QoL than aerobic training alone
- Early PR is recommended after a COPD exacerbation. It is safe and improves exercise tolerance, health-related QoL, and reduces hospital admissions
- Short-term programmes achieve overall similar outcome benefits across the spectrum of patient disability. A minimum programme length of 6 weeks is recommended
- Decline in exercise tolerance and health status tends to occur between 6 and 12 months after completion of a course. Sustained improvement with ongoing rehabilitation sessions has yet to be evaluated.

Candidates

- Anyone with chronic lung disease causing functional impairment despite receiving optimum medical treatment
- Well-motivated patients seem to benefit most
- Patients with poor lower limb mobility may still benefit from upper limb exercise and the education package
- O_2 therapy is not a contraindication to rehabilitation
- Recent exacerbation of COPD is not a contraindication
- Stable ischaemic heart disease and heart failure are not contraindications
- Depression should be addressed prior to participation in PR, if possible, to increase the likelihood of benefit.

Candidates in whom rehabilitation may not be indicated
- Unstable ischaemic heart disease, severe valvular heart disease, severe cognitive impairment, or locomotor difficulties
- Poorly motivated people, with geographical or transport problems making attendance difficult, tend to do less well. It may be, however, that different locations (community or home-based) and different interfaces (manuals or web-based) may help these challenges of hospital-based programmes.

Further information

McCarthy et al. Pulmonary rehabilitation for chronic obstructive pulmonary disease. *Cochrane Database of Systematic Reviews* 2015,**2**.
BTS guideline on pulmonary rehabilitation in adults. *Thorax* 2013;**68**(Suppl 2): ii1–ii30.

Programme

Programmes are usually run on an outpatient basis but can be done in the community, home, or as an inpatient. They are run by a multiprofessional team—physician, physiotherapist, occupational therapist, dietician, nurse, pharmacist, social worker, and psychologist. A minimum programme length of 6 weeks is recommended. Programmes should be regularly audited by the department.

- *Physical training* The main component of the programme is progressive high-intensity aerobic exercise, such as walking and cycling, for a minimum of 2–3 times per week, with two supervised/class sessions. The prescription is individualized, and the benefits are improved with higher-intensity training. Upper or lower limb strength exercise with weights is often included. O_2 supplementation may be required if significant desaturation occurs during exercise to below 80% and if exercise tolerance improves with O_2
- Performance enhancement has been investigated. Improvements shown with: tiotropium, in addition to PR, vs PR alone, non-invasive ventilation (NIV), partitioned training (single leg cycling), testosterone (improves muscle strength). No improvement with: creatine, O_2. Neutral or subgroups: helium hyperoxia, nutrition
- *Disease education*
- *Psychological and social intervention* with advice on anxiety and depression, smoking cessation, plus physiotherapy, and occupational therapy input
- *Nutritional education* to optimize body weight and muscle mass.

Pre-rehabilitation assessment

- Optimize medical treatment
- O_2 saturation on exercise
- ECG may be warranted, especially if history of cardiac disease.

Outcome assessment measures

- *Exercise performance* Often with shuttle walk test (SWT) or 6-minute walk test (6MWT) to assess ability and progress (see Box 60.1)
- *Health status* Disease-specific questionnaires:
  - Chronic Respiratory Questionnaire (CRQ)
  - St George's Respiratory Questionnaire
  - Generic questionnaires, e.g. the Short Form-36 (SF-36)
  - Hospital Anxiety and Depression scores (HADS) are measured
- *Practical* Pedometers can be used for direct feedback and to improve performance.

Future developments

- Access to PR for all who may benefit
- How to optimally maintain the improvements following a rehabilitation programme
- Using technology to enhance compliance and delivery of PR
- Expanding the potential population who may benefit from PR
- Further understanding the mechanisms of health benefits from improving physical activity
- Targeting exercise training earlier in the disease process.

Box 60.1 Shuttle walk test (SWT)

A 10 m course between two points (cones). Walking speed is determined by external audio tape signals ('beeps'), and the patient should pace their walk to reach the cone by the next beep. The patient is required to incrementally increase their speed as the beeps occur more frequently each minute. Test finishes when the patient is too breathless or tired to maintain the required pace, and the distance achieved is calculated. The minimum clinically important difference following rehabilitation is 48 m (~5 shuttles).

6-minute walk test (6MWT)

A 30 m course between two points on a hard, flat surface. Patients do as many 60 m laps as they can around the two points in 6 min. They determine their pace and intensity of exercise. They are allowed to rest in the time if they need to. Total distance walked in 6 min is counted. Results may vary, according to mood and encouragement. An increase from baseline to post-rehabilitation of 35 m or more is considered significant.

Cardiopulmonary exercise testing (CPET)

(See Ⓢ p. 976)

CPET are rarely used to assess pragmatic PR programmes and have been largely replaced by field testing in the UK. CPET is the gold standard for the assessment of peak O_2 uptake, but they also provide more detailed results on exercise progression and limitations to exercise. Occasionally, they may be performed for safety prior to undertaking PR. CPET is still widely used in a research setting for PR.

Smoking cessation

Aims and nicotine replacement therapy *818*
Non-nicotine replacement therapy *822*

Aims and nicotine replacement therapy

Smoking is the main cause of chronic obstructive pulmonary disease (COPD) and lung cancer. In 2015, tobacco smoking accounted for ~19% of all UK deaths and cost the NHS around £3 billion. The UK government has set targets to reduce the number of smokers, with substantial funding for smoking cessation services (£66.4 million in 2011).

- Smoking prevalence in England is slowly falling. In 2018 15% of adults in England were current smokers compared to 20% in 2011. 17% of men and 13% of women over 18 years currently smoke; 82% of smokers start as teenagers
- The incidence of smoking is increasing, particularly amongst women in developing countries
- Smoking is associated with cardiovascular and cerebrovascular disease and bladder, oesophageal, cervical, and renal cancers. It is also associated with increased post-operative complications
- Nicotine exerts its effects on the CNS and is very addictive
- Reducing number of cigarettes smoked may not give health benefits, as cigarettes smoked 'harder'—more puffs, greater inhalation
- Peak nicotine withdrawal time is 2–3 days
- 0.4% of smokers manage to stop each year
- Stopping smoking is associated with an average weight gain of 2–5kg, and this deters many, especially women, from quitting
- The UK government has legislated to reduce smoking rates and harm:
  - 2007—banned smoking in workplaces and public places and increased the age for sale of tobacco from 16 to 18.
  - 2015—banned smoking in cars with children
  - 2016—changed tobacco packaging guidance so that all cigarette and tobacco packs have to come in standardized packaging with prominent health warnings.

Aims of smoking cessation interventions

Smoking cessation is a cost-effective treatment (£2,000 per quality-adjusted life year (QALY) for patients with COPD). To achieve sustained abstinence, the aims are to reduce short-term nicotine cravings (nicotine and non-nicotine replacement therapy) and to modify behaviour in the long term (counselling, telephone or group support-buddy systems). It is vital that the smoker is motivated to quit, or attempts will fail. Health professionals should address smoking cessation at all opportunities, as they can trigger quit attempts by giving brief advice to smokers (advice from doctors often has the strongest impact). This can lead to 1–3 out of 100 people stopping smoking for 6 months. People may be more receptive to smoking cessation advice during times of concern for their own or their families' health. A guide to approaching the topic is:

- Ask how much a person smokes, and document pack years (number of cigarettes smoked per day ÷ 20 × no of years smoked)
- Ask about non-conventional tobacco smoking, e.g. with cannabis, with a waterpipe (Shisha)
- Advise on risks of continued smoking. Assess commitment to quitting
- Assist by offering behavioural therapy ± pharmacotherapy
- Provide self-help material, and refer to stop smoking services
- Arrange follow-up.

Some hospitals and general practices have smoking cessation counsellors. The best results in terms of quit rates are achieved by combining counselling and nicotine replacement therapy (NRT), bupropion, or varenicline, with regular support and follow-up. These can improve quit rates to around 25%. The National Institute for Health and Care Excellence (NICE) has issued guidance on the use of NRT, bupropion, and varenicline for smoking cessation. It advises that pharmacotherapy should only be for smokers committed to a target stop date. Choice of therapy is based on a patient's likely compliance, availability of counselling, previous experience of therapies, contraindications, and personal preference. Prescribe 2 weeks of NRT or 3–4 weeks of bupropion/varenicline, and only give further prescription if individual shows a continuing attempt to quit. If they fail to quit, a second attempt within 6 months is not usually funded.

NRT

Minimizes short- and medium-term nicotine withdrawal symptoms. Should not be used while still smoking, as potential for nicotine overdose (symptoms: agitation, confusion, restlessness, palpitations, hypertension, dilated pupils, shortness of breath (SOB), abdominal cramps, vomiting). Can be bought over the counter or be prescribed by GP. Cheaper than cigarettes. In 2005, Medicines and Healthcare Regulatory Authority licensed NRT products in pregnancy, breastfeeding mothers, people aged 12–17, and those with cardiovascular disease.

- *Patches* Give small amounts of nicotine via transdermal patch to decrease cravings before they occur. Dose (15, 10, 5mg) depends on amount smoked. Use a higher dose if >10 cigarettes/day smoked. Convenient. Worn continuously throughout day, but removed at night due to vivid dreams. Can get localized irritation at patch site. Patches should be used for 6–8 weeks at the higher dose, then weaned to a lower dose for 2–4 weeks. Available over the counter
- *Chewing gum* Different strengths of gum that release nicotine as they are chewed (Smoke <20/day—chew one 2 mg piece slowly for 30 min when urge to smoke occurs. Smoke >20/day or needing >15 pieces of 2 mg gum daily—use 4 mg strength gum. Max 15 4 mg pieces/day). Relieves cravings as they occur. When mouth tingles and has peppery taste, should stop chewing and 'park' the gum inside the cheek. Nicotine is then absorbed through the lining of the mouth. Should not chew continuously or may develop nausea. Nicotine needs to be absorbed through mouth and not swallowed in saliva. Therefore, do not drink with gum. Physical act of chewing can relieve craving. Can taste unpleasant and may need to use several packs of gum a day. Use for 3 months, then reduce the strength and amount of gum used. Available over the counter in a variety of flavours
- *Sublingual tablets* Used on demand to help with cravings. Discrete form of treatment. 1–2 tablets should be placed under the tongue every hour when needed. Dissolve over 30 min. Licensed for use in pregnancy (one tablet only). Use for 3 months, and then gradually reduce the number of tablets used a day. Available on prescription

- *Lozenges* Suck every 1–2 h if urge to smoke (smoke >30/day = 2 mg lozenge, <30/day = 1 mg lozenge). Available over the counter
- *Inhalator* Cigarette-style appliance giving small amounts of nicotine when used. Useful for people who are habitual or ritualistic in that they have 'restless hands' or want the 'hand to mouth' routine. Nicotine is absorbed through the lining of the mouth, not via the lungs. Use for 2 months, then gradually reduce. Available on prescription
- *Nasal spray* Provides rapid relief of craving. Faster absorption than other forms of NRT. May cause local irritation. Use for 2 months, then reduce. Available on prescription.

Non-nicotine replacement therapy

Drugs

Pharmacotherapy should not be used without behavioural support.

Bupropion is promoted as an aid to smoking cessation, in combination with motivational support. It is an antidepressant found to reduce the desire to smoke, even in the absence of depression. It weakly inhibits dopamine, serotonin, and noradrenaline reuptake in the central nervous system (CNS). It counteracts nicotine withdrawal symptoms by increasing these levels in the brain. It is suitable for individuals who smoke ≥10 cigarettes a day. Liver metabolism and 20 h half-life.

Smokers start taking bupropion 1–2 weeks before their intended 'quit day'. Continue for 7–9 weeks after. Leads to improved abstinence rates, compared with placebo or nicotine patch, if associated with counselling (30% 12-month abstinence rate with bupropion, 16% with nicotine patch, 15% with placebo, 35% with patch and bupropion; *N Engl J Med* 1999;**340**:685–691). Also thought to reduce weight gain associated with stopping smoking. Contraindicated in patients with epilepsy or at risk of fits, those with a CNS tumour, those acutely withdrawing from alcohol or benzodiazepines, pregnancy, those with eating disorders, bipolar disorder, and those on monoamine oxidase inhibitors. Preferentially used in some patient groups, e.g. those with schizophrenia or depression. Reduce dose if elderly or has hepatic or renal impairment. Well tolerated. Recognized adverse effects include dry mouth, hypersensitivity, insomnia, seizures (1:1,000), and death. Prescription only.

Varenicline is a drug also promoted as an aid to smoking cessation, in combination with motivational support.

- Binds to the A4B2 nicotinic acetylcholine receptor and acts as a partial agonist
- Binding alleviates symptoms of craving and withdrawal
- Reduces the rewarding and reinforcing effects of smoking by preventing nicotine binding to the A4B2 receptors.

Smokers start taking varenicline 1–2 weeks before their intended 'quit day' and continue for 12–24 weeks. Starting dose is 500 micrograms od for 3 days, 500 micrograms bd for 4 days, then 1 mg bd for 11 weeks, if tolerated. If smokers are abstinent after 12 weeks, they should continue for another 12 weeks to avoid relapse. Avoid abrupt withdrawal.

Side effects include nausea, vomiting, appetite change, change in taste, headache, difficulty sleeping, abnormal dreams, dry mouth, and tiredness. Use with caution if breastfeeding, in renal impairment, and in those with a history of psychiatric disease. It has been associated with neuropsychiatric disorders (depression, agitation, behavioural changes). Randomized controlled trials (RCTs) have shown significantly higher quit rates with varenicline than with bupropion or placebo. Quit rates are higher with higher doses (e.g. continuous quit rate for any 4 weeks: 48% with 1 mg bd ($p = 0.01$ vs placebo), 37% with 1 mg od ($p = 0.01$), 33% with bupropion ($p = 0.02$, 17% with placebo). Adverse drug effects leading to stopping treatment were lower than with bupropion (*Arch Int Med* 2006;**166**: 1561–1568). Prescription only. Recommended by NICE in 2007.

Hypnosis

Aims to improve willpower in the subconscious state with therapeutic suggestion. Anecdotal success, but Cochrane review of trials showed no greater abstinence rate with hypnosis than with any other treatment or placebo treatment.

Acupuncture/acupressure

No evidence in favour of it over placebo acupuncture. Less effective than NRT.

Electronic cigarettes

E-cigarettes are battery-powered and vaporize nicotine and other chemicals in a liquid solution to an aerosol mist. The nicotine contained is approximately the same amount as in a cigarette. They simulate the act of smoking and are therefore controversial. Since 2016 they have been subject to regulation by the Medicines and Healthcare products Regulatory Agency (MHRA) around device safety and e-liquid nicotine levels but are not a licensed product. There is a lack of high-quality evidence of their use in smoking cessation, although some studies suggest that they help smokers decrease cigarette consumption, even when they do not intend to quit. The long-term effects on pulmonary health are unknown, although e-cigarettes are widely accepted as less harmful than smoking tobacco. The Royal College of Physicians have advocated the use of e-cigarettes as an aide to tobacco harm reduction.

Information of reports of e-cigarette related lung injuries are discussed on ➲ p. 268.

Future developments

- Increasing and improving hospital-based smoking cessation services with links to community-based services
- Effectiveness of long-term smoking cessation interventions and relapse rates
- *Dopamine D3 antagonists*—the dopamine D3 receptor is involved in mechanisms of nicotine dependence. Trials currently underway.

Further information

NICE Stop smoking interventions and services. 2018 ℘ https://www.nice.org.uk/guidance/ng92.
Royal College of Physicians. Nicotine without smoke: Tobacco harm reduction. 2016 ℘ https://www.rcplondon.ac.uk/projects/outputs/nicotine-without-smoke-tobacco-harm-reduction-0
Roy Castle Fag Ends. ℘ http://www.stopsmoking.org.uk.
Smoke Free national helpline ☎ 0300 123 1044

Part IV

Practical procedures

62 Airway management 827
63 Bronchoscopy 833
64 Chest drains 851
65 Cricothyroidotomy 861
66 Miscellaneous diagnostic tests 865
67 Pleural biopsy 869
68 Pleurodesis 875
69 Pneumothorax aspiration 881
70 Safe sedation 885
71 Thoracentesis 891
72 Thoracic ultrasound (TUS) 895
73 Thoracoscopy 907
74 Tracheostomy 913

Airway management

Simple airway adjuncts *828*
Supraglottic airway devices (SGAD) *829*
Intubation *830*

Simple airway adjuncts

Simple airway adjuncts

Used to overcome backward tongue displacement causing upper airway obstruction in an unconscious patient.

> ▶▶ *Call for anaesthetic help early*
> Patients may require support of their airway and ventilation/oxygenation in situations when they are unable to adequately maintain these. Such situations may be related to a Glasgow Coma Scale (GCS) of <8, which can cause difficulties with airway maintenance, or related to respiratory compromise or arrest in the critically ill patient.

Oropharyngeal airway (Guedel)

A curved plastic tube with a flanged end that is inserted into the mouth. Size is estimated by holding it at the side of the patient's face and estimating required length from incisors to angle of the jaw. Ensure the mouth is clear, then insert the airway 'upside down', with the curved side towards the tongue. When it is in as far as the soft palate, turn it around by 180°, and push it in further so the flange is at the patient's mouth. If the patient has a gag reflex, remove the airway. Suction can be performed through the airway and O_2 administered via a mask.

Nasopharyngeal airway

A soft plastic tube, with a bevelled end and a flange at the other end. Better tolerated in the semi-conscious. Avoid use in those with base of skull fractures. Sizes 6–7 mm are suitable for adults. Some tubes allow insertion of a safety pin through the flange (prior to use and not for attachment to the patient!) to prevent insertion beyond nares. Lubricate airway with water-soluble jelly, and insert the bevelled end into right nostril, and gently push back with a twisting action along the floor of the nose. Do not force if obstruction is encountered, but remove and try in the other nostril. Nasal bleeding can be caused if the mucosa is damaged. O_2 can be administered through a mask.

Supraglottic airway devices (SGAD)

Used as an alternative to formal intubation. The laryngeal mask airway (LMA) is the most commonly used SGAD. The LMA is a wide-bore tube with an inflated cuff at one end, which is positioned over the larynx and inflated reducing aspiration of gastric contents and gastric inflation. It is easy to insert (see Fig. 62.1) and is used in anaesthetic practice and also in emergencies. Alternative SGAD come with gel cuffs and that do not require inflation (e.g. i-gel®). SGADs are not suitable for patients with high airway resistance such as pulmonary oedema, bronchospasm, or COPD. To insert an LMA select a size 4 or 5 tube, and, after ensuring the cuff works, deflate it. Put water-soluble lubricating jelly over the cuff. The patient should be lying flat, with head extension, if possible. Hold the tube like a pen, and insert from behind the patient's head, with the point of the cuff positioned to the back of the mouth. Advance along the roof of the mouth, and then press it downwards and backwards until resistance is felt. Sometimes a small amount of 'wiggling' helps the tube pass smoothly. Inflate the cuff, which will cause the tube to lift out of the mouth a little. Confirm adequate airway position by auscultating for breath sounds over the chest bilaterally. Secure the tube. With SGADs like the i-gel® a similar technique is used but without the extra steps to inflate the LMA cuff.

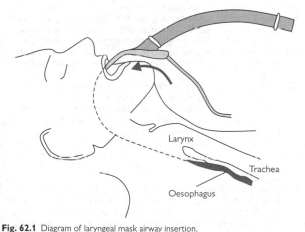

Fig. 62.1 Diagram of laryngeal mask airway insertion.

Reproduced from Wyatt et al. *Oxford Handbook of Emergency Medicine* 3e, 2006, with permission from Oxford University Press.

Intubation

Endotracheal tube

The optimal method of securing a patient's airway and providing airway protection from aspiration of gastric contents. It must be performed by skilled personnel. The tube is bevelled at one end with an inflatable cuff and has a tube connector at the other end.

- Predictors of difficult intubation should be considered, including prior difficult intubation, Mallampati score (see ⊃ p. 702 Fig 48.9), ability to protrude mandible, assessment of neck movements, interincisor distance (<3 cm predicts difficulties), thyromental distance (Patil's test; <7 cm predicts difficulties), and obesity. These all have low sensitivity and specificity for predicting the ease of intubation so careful pre-intubation planning for the possibility of difficulty is required regardless of predicted risk.
- A pre-intubation check list should be used to ensure all equipment is available and that there is a clear plan if difficulty is encountered. Equipment includes a laryngoscope (usually a size 3/4 curved Macintosh blade; check light source), a videolaryngoscope such as McGrath, C-Mac, and Airtraq (now standard equipment on intubation trolleys and should be considered essential), cuffed endotracheal tube (variety of sizes should be to hand; usually use size 7—♀, size 8—♂; check cuff for leak), syringe for cuff inflation, water-soluble lubricating jelly, Magill's forceps, gum elastic bougie, suitable bandage to secure tube in place, capnography and stethoscope (for confirming tube placement), O_2 and suitable breathing circuit (e.g. self-inflating bag or Water's circuit), suction (Yankauer and flexible catheters), and rescue equipment for failed intubation
- Consider appropriate location and personal protective equipment as intubation is aerosol generating (as is extubation)
- Patient lies flat, with neck and head extended (the 'sniffing the morning air' position). A pillow is placed under the head, not the neck, to aid this
- Pre-oxygenate with bag-and-mask ventilation
- Cricoid pressure (30N over the cricoid cartilage—which is equivalent to filling a 20 mL syringe with air, occluding with a bung and then depressing to the 10 mL mark) may reduce gastric inflation and aspiration of gastric contents
- Using the laryngoscope in left hand and standing behind the head, the mouth is opened and the laryngoscope placed over the right side of the tongue and advanced gently around the curve of the tongue
- It may be necessary to apply suction to clear the mouth of secretions
- When the epiglottis is seen, the laryngoscope is advanced into the vallecula, between the root of the epiglottis and the base of the tongue. Upward pressure in the direction of the laryngoscope handle is applied to lift the jaw slightly, and the cords should come into view, taking care not to damage the teeth. Laryngoscopic views are graded (Cormack and Lehane grading): grade 1, entire laryngeal inlet visible; grade 2, arytenoids and posterior vocal cords visible; grade 3, only epiglottis visible; grade 4, epiglottis not seen
- Slide the tube through the glottis so that the cuff is a few cm past the cords, and then withdraw the laryngoscope
- Inflate the cuff

- Confirm adequate tube position by auscultating for breath sounds over the chest bilaterally (also absence of noise over epigastrium) and using end-tidal CO_2 detection (either waveform capnography or using colorimetric litmus-based detectors); five breaths showing CO_2 confirm an adequate tube position
- If the tube is not in position, usually because it has been passed into the oesophagus, deflate the cuff and remove the tube, then re-oxygenate with the bag and mask before trying again. Pull the tube back slightly if the breath sounds are only on the right, as this suggests the tube is in the right main bronchus
- Secure the tube
- Administer O_2 with a self-inflating bag with O_2 and reservoir bag
- Chest radiograph (CXR) to confirm correct tube position, 2–3 cm above the carina
- Suction can be performed through the tube
- Various techniques can be used to assist with difficult tracheal intubation. A gum elastic bougie may be easier to pass through the glottis (allowing endotracheal tube insertion by railroading over the bougie). The BURP technique (external Backward, Upward, and Rightward Pressure on the thyroid cartilage) may improve laryngoscopic view. Videolaryngoscopes are now used increasingly and are often helpful.

Further Information

Resuscitation Council UK. *Advanced Life Support*, 7th Edition. 2016.

Bronchoscopy

Indications and risks *834*
Patient preparation and procedure *836*
Sampling techniques *840*
Central airway obstruction *842*
Advanced bronchoscopy 1 *844*
Advanced bronchoscopy 2 *848*

Indications and risks

Bronchoscopy is the procedure of passing a telescope or camera into the trachea to inspect the large and medium-sized airways. It may be performed with a flexible scope, using local anaesthetic ± sedation (favoured by physicians), or under a general anaesthetic with a rigid scope (used mostly by surgeons). Airways can be visually inspected, samples taken, and therapeutic procedures can be performed. This chapter focuses on flexible bronchoscopy.

Indications for bronchoscopy

- *Suspected lung cancer* Patients who have a central mass <4 cm from the origin of the nearest lobar bronchus, which is likely to be accessible for biopsy at bronchoscopy
- *Suspected pulmonary infection*, such as tuberculosis (TB), in a patient who is unable to produce sputum, or in immunocompromised patients, with fever, cough, hypoxia, or chest radiograph (CXR) changes (induced sputum with hypertonic saline may be an alternative; see ➲ p. 867)
- *Suspected interstitial lung disease (ILD)* if a transbronchial biopsy (TBB) will provide an adequate sample for diagnostic purposes such as in sarcoid. Only indicated in a limited number of ILD, as more adequate biopsies are often obtained through open lung biopsy, which may be preferable
- *Investigation of haemoptysis*
- *Investigation of stridor*
- *Foreign body removal* if this is located proximally
- *Therapeutic indications* include central airway obstruction, sputum plugging, and possibly emphysema (endobronchial lung volume reduction; see ➲ p. 208) and asthma (bronchial thermoplasty; see ➲ p. 156).

Relative contraindications/take care

- If a patient has oxygen saturations below 90% on air at rest or PaO_2<8 kPa, the risk of significant hypoxia during bronchoscopy is increased
- FEV_1 <40% predicted
- Blood clotting abnormalities, particularly platelet level <50 ×10^9/L
- Uraemia, pulmonary hypertension (PHT), superior vena caval obstruction (SVCO), liver disease, and immunosuppression predispose to haemorrhage
- Recent myocardial infarction (MI) may be associated with cardiac ischaemia during bronchoscopy. Wait until 4 weeks after, if possible (otherwise, liaise with cardiology).

Risks associated with bronchoscopy

Flexible bronchoscopy is a safe procedure, with reported mortality rates in large series being 0.01–0.04% and major complications of 0.08–1.1%. Complications include respiratory depression, pneumonia, pneumothorax, airway obstruction, laryngospasm, cardiorespiratory arrest, arrhythmias, pulmonary oedema, vasovagal episodes, fever (especially following bronchoalveolar lavage (BAL)), septicaemia, haemorrhage, nausea, and vomiting.

Bleeding and bronchoscopy

- Significant bleeding occurs in ~0.7% of patients, due to mechanical trauma from the scope, suctioning, brushing, or biopsy, but is more common with TBB (1.6–4.4%). Patients with malignancy, immunocompromise, or uraemia have an increased bleeding tendency
- If bleeding does not stop spontaneously, retract the bronchoscope proximally to maintain vision, and preserve the airway using suction to remove free blood (but do not disturb clot). 1 mL aliquots of 1:10,000 adrenaline solution are administered via the bronchoscope as near to the bleeding point as possible, until it stops. 5–10 mL iced saline may also be useful. If bleeding does not stop, the bronchoscope should be wedged in the segmental bronchus to tamponade the bleeding for 10–15 min
- If massive haemorrhage occurs, the patient should be turned on to the side of the bleeding to protect the other lung. Balloon-tipped vascular catheter may be used to tamponade the bleeding point. If bleeding continues, emergency interventional radiology or thoracic surgery may be indicated. Contact anaesthetics urgently to consider airway protection with double lumen endotracheal tube.

Further information

Du Rand IA et al. British Thoracic Society guideline for diagnostic flexible bronchoscopy in adults. *Thorax* 2013;**68**: i1–i44.

Lee P et al. Therapeutic bronchoscopy in lung cancer. *Clin Chest Med* 2002;**23**: 241–256.

Bungay HK et al. An evaluation of CT as an aid to diagnosing patients undergoing bronchoscopy for suspected bronchial carcinoma. *Clin Radiol* 2000;**55**(7): 554–560.

Laroche C et al. Role of CT scanning of the thorax prior to bronchoscopy in the investigation of suspected lung cancer. *Thorax* 2000;**55**(5): 359–363.

Patient preparation and procedure

Patient preparation

- *Information* Patients should be given written information about the procedure, ideally >24 h prior to the procedure. Provide an information sheet for the patient to take home following the bronchoscopy, with advice about the effects of any sedation and possible complications, as well as telephone numbers in case help is needed
- *Consent* The physician performing the bronchoscopy should obtain written consent, with a description of the procedure and its associated risks
- *Consider stopping anticoagulation* Safe to perform if patient is taking aspirin or prophylactic low molecular weight heparin (LMWH), but omit clopidogrel for 7 days prior (may require cardiology discussion), and, if on warfarin, wait until international normalized ratio (INR) <1.5 (may require full-dose LMWH on days prior to bronchoscopy for high-risk conditions, e.g. mitral prosthetic metal valve, prosthetic valve, and atrial fibrillation (AF), AF and mitral stenosis, <3 months post-venous thromboembolism (VTE), or thrombophilia syndromes)
- *Risks of sedation* Consider factors that may make sedation more hazardous (see ➔ p. 890)
- *Nil by mouth* Patients should have no food for 6 h beforehand and clear fluids only until 2 h beforehand
- *Blood tests* Patients do not need routine pre-procedure blood tests, unless there are specific concerns (active bleeding, uraemia, deranged liver function tests (LFTs), low platelets)
- *Bedside tests* Perform an electrocardiogram (ECG) in patients with a history of cardiac disease. Check blood sugar in patients with diabetes
- *Prophylactic antibiotics* No longer recommended for the prevention of endocarditis, fever, or pneumonia
- *In those with asthma*, a nebulized bronchodilator should be given before the bronchoscopy
- *Those at high risk of infection (TB)* should be last on the list.

Procedure

- Practices vary between centres. Some perform bronchoscopy with the patient sitting up, facing the operator; some from behind, with the patient lying flat
- *IV access* should be present in all patients
- *Pulse oximetry* ± ECG is monitored throughout. *Nasal O_2* should be administered if SaO_2 falls by 4%
- *Sedatives* should be offered to provide conscious sedation (verbal contact possible at all times), anxiolysis, and anterograde amnesia, provided no contraindications (see ➔ p. 890). A benzodiazepine, such as midazolam 1–2 mg, with further 1 mg increments as necessary, may be used with fentanyl/alfentanil. Assess and document sedation depth (see ➔ p. 887). Some patients and operators prefer not to use sedation, due to concerns particularly in elderly patients, those with COPD, or those with cardiac disease. Midazolam can make some patients more agitated. Premedication with anticholinergics is not beneficial during bronchoscopy

- *Lidocaine* Local anaesthetic 2% gel (6 mL = 120 mg) is applied to the nostrils, and the oropharynx is anaesthetized by three actuations of local anaesthetic spray (10% lidocaine, 10 mg/spray) to the back of the throat during inspiration and time allowed to work (~3–5 min).
  - Transcricoid injection may be used to administer 1% lidocaine into the trachea (which will also anaesthetize the vocal cords). Alternatively, vocal cords and trachea may be anaesthetized under direct vision ('spray-as-you-go') through the bronchoscope
  - Further aliquots of 1% lidocaine may be administered to right and left main bronchi via the bronchoscope
  - Maximum dose of lidocaine is unclear, but symptoms of toxicity seen at ≥9.6 mg/kg delivered to the airways. Use the minimal dose required for cough suppression. Toxic effects include central nervous system (CNS) effects (confusion, blurred vision, euphoria, dizziness, myoclonus, seizures) and cardiovascular effects (arrhythmias, cardiac arrest). Risks increased with renal, hepatic, and cardiac dysfunction (see ➔ p. 958)
  - The half-life of lidocaine is 1.5–2 h
- Most access the trachea via the nasal route, as this gives increased stability when taking biopsies and allows the patient to cough and spit out secretions more easily. If this is not possible, a mouth guard is used and access obtained through the mouth
- All sections of the bronchial tree should be visually inspected, including the cords and trachea. See Fig. 63.1 for anatomy. CXR or computed tomography (CT) may help localize the area of concern, so specimen site can then be targeted. This increases the diagnostic yield of bronchoscopy in cases of suspected lung cancer
- Avoid unnecessary suction, as this can increase hypoxia.

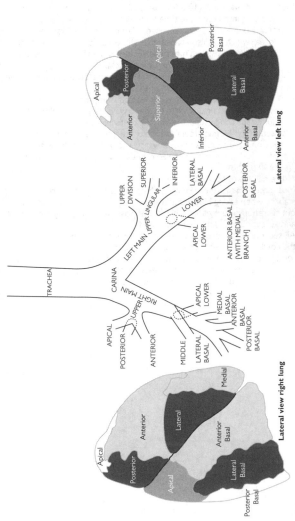

Fig. 63.1 Lung segmental anatomy.

Sampling techniques

Bronchial washings

Taken by instilling ~10 mL of 0.9% saline and then collecting it in a pot/trap using suction through the bronchoscope to obtain superficial airway cells.

Bronchial brushings

Taken by inserting a covered brush into a bronchial segment, uncovering it, rubbing the bronchial wall, covering it, removing it, and either leaving in cell preservation media or wiping it on a slide (which is then sprayed with a cell fixing solution).

Bronchial biopsies

Taken with biopsy forceps; 5–7 should be taken to optimize yield. These may be taken blindly or from a visibly abnormal area, which gives a higher diagnostic yield than blind biopsies. They can be placed in formalin or saline solution, depending on whether they are for histology or microbiology.

Bronchoalveolar lavage (BAL)

Performed by instilling 60–180 mL of saline through the bronchoscope when it is wedged well in a small airway. Ideally, instil fluid during inspiration, and, after allowing the fluid to dwell for 10–30 s, aspirate gently back into the syringe during expiration or collect in a trap. Best performed in the area of abnormality on CXR or CT or non-dependent lobes such as the middle lobe or lingula. Poor return if the patient is coughing excessively or if they have emphysema. Can cause hypoxia proportional to amount of lavage fluid used.

Transbronchial lung biopsy (TBB)

Technique of passing TBB forceps down a terminal bronchus until resistance is first felt and taking a sample of parenchymal tissue. Some perform with radiological screening. One technique is to locate the bronchoscope at segmental bronchus of interest and advance forceps (through working channel) as far as possible. Retract forceps by 1 cm; open forceps while patients inhaling slowly, then advance 5 mm and close forceps while exhaling. Take biopsy (but stop if pain felt, suggesting that forceps have gathered visceral pleura). Repeat 5–6 times.

Associated with a significant risk of bleeding in 9% and pneumothorax in 1–6%, but up to 14% if patient is mechanically ventilated. Half of all pneumothoraces require chest drains. Therefore, perform on one side only, and minimize risk by performing TBB in the lower lobes in dependent segments. Perform CXR after the bronchoscopy if patient symptomatic or clinical suspicion of pneumothorax. Pneumothorax should be managed, according to standard guidelines (see ➋ p. 440). Small pneumothoraces often resolve spontaneously, but the patient may need admission if concerns.

When performing bronchoscopy

• Wear gloves, face mask, and eye shields
• Use FFP3 (duck) masks if there are concerns about TB or human immunodeficiency virus (HIV).

Central airway obstruction

(See also section on acute upper airway obstruction, Chapter 49, ➔ p. 704).

Central airway = trachea and main stem bronchi.

Obstruction can be:
- Extrinsic, e.g. tumour pressing on airway causing obstruction
- Intrinsic, e.g. tumour occluding airway lumen
- Mixed, a combination of extrinsic and intrinsic.

Symptoms and signs
- May be asymptomatic if obstruction is mild
- Productive cough, due to mucosal swelling and mucus production
- Wheeze, unilateral wheeze, positional wheeze (monophonic)
- Stridor
- 2° atelectasis and pneumonia
- Dyspnoea.

Investigations
- Flow–volume loops, FEV_1
- CXR—may be normal
- CT chest + 3D airway reconstruction, if possible
- Bronchoscopy to make tissue diagnosis of underlying disease.

Treatment
- Secure airway
- Consider bronchoscopy—senior physician ± anaesthetist should perform. Bronchoscopy itself can cause obstruction in a compromised airway. Adrenaline administered via bronchoscope may be helpful
- Consider endobronchial treatment—core out tumour; dilate a stenosis, or place a stent (see ➔ p. 849)
- Consider heliox.

Causes of central airway obstruction

- Malignant
  - 1° endoluminal cancer, especially lung cancer or carcinoid
  - Metastatic cancer
  - Laryngeal cancer
  - Oesophageal cancer
  - Mediastinal tumour
  - Lymphadenopathy, lymphoma
- Non-malignant
  - Lymphadenopathy
  - Relapsing polychondritis
  - Tracheomalacia
  - Papilloma
  - Hamartoma
  - Amyloid
  - Web
  - Goitre
  - Foreign body
  - Granulation tissue.

Further information

Ernst A et al. Central airway obstruction. *Am J Respir Crit Care Med* 2004;**169**: 1278–1297.
Janssen JP et al. Series: Interventional pulmonology. *Eur Respir J* 2006;**27**: 1258–1271, **28**: 200–218.
Wood DE et al. Airway stenting for malignant and benign tracheobronchial stenosis. *Ann Thorac Surg* 2003;**76**: 167–174.
Du Rand IA et al. British Thoracic Society guideline for advanced diagnostic and therapeutic flexible bronchoscopy in adults. *Thorax* 2011;**66**: iii1–iii21.

Advanced bronchoscopy 1

Diagnostic procedures

Transbronchial needle aspiration (TBNA) and endobronchial ultrasound (EBUS) allow mediastinal node sampling without the surgical procedure of mediastinoscopy. Some lymph nodes are accessible for sampling in this way, which cannot be accessed via mediastinoscopy.

TBNA

Technique of inserting a biopsy needle (19–25G) through the bronchial wall into an enlarged mediastinal or hilar lymph node or extrabronchial mass and aspirating cells. Usually done with EBUS guidance (see next heading). Used to diagnose (and stage) suspected malignancy, TB, or sarcoidosis. Appropriate lymph nodes should be identified on CT first; stations 2R/L, 3P, 4R/L, 7, 10R/L, and 11R/L are accessible (see Fig. 63.2). Should be performed initially, so the bronchoscope is not contaminated with malignant cells from the airway, and start with the highest-stage lymph nodes first. Push sheath out through end of bronchoscope until the hub is just visible. Flex the bronchoscope so that the sheath tip lies between cartilaginous rings, directed towards the node/mass. Extend the needle so that it passes through the bronchial wall, and then apply suction. A 'to-and-fro' motion of the needle should allow lymph node 'goo' to be aspirated. Subsequently, the suction is stopped; the needle is withdrawn, and the sheath is removed to allow sample preparation. Subcarinal (7) and right lower paratracheal (4R) nodes are the easiest to sample. Aim for 4–6 separate aspirations. Malignancy sensitivity 39–78%. Complications rare (0.3%): pneumomediastinum, pneumothorax, minor bleeding, puncture of adjacent structures.

EBUS

Technique of visualizing the bronchial wall and the immediate surrounding structures via a convex array ultrasound (US) probe incorporated into the tip of the bronchoscope. Airway contact (and therefore US image) can be improved by using a balloon surrounding the probe, which is inflated with water, although many do not use. Useful to assess lymph node involvement in malignancy and for real-time guided TBNA. Possible to sample nodes ≥4 mm in short axis. Mediastinal structures or masses next to the airways can be identified, the depth of bronchial wall tumour invasion assessed, or masses within the lung localized for biopsy. Malignancy sensitivity 88–100%. Oesophageal endoscopic ultrasound (EUS; called EUS-B when using the *bronchoscope* in the oesophagus) is an alternative strategy, which allows examination of the posterior and inferior mediastinum (particularly useful for stations 8 and 9), the liver, the coeliac axis, and the left adrenal gland. It is more accurate at diagnosing mediastinal metastases than CT and positron emission tomography (PET).

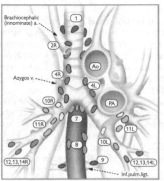

Superior mediastinal nodes

● **1** Highest mediastinal

● **2** Upper paratracheal

● **3** Pre-vascular and retrotracheal

● **4** Lower paratracheal
(including Azygos nodes)

N_2 = single digit, ipsilateral
N_3 = single digit, contralateral, or supraclavicular

Aortic nodes

● **5** Subaortic (A-P window)

● **6** Para-aortic (ascending
aorta or phrenic

Inferior mediastinal nodes

● **7** Subcarinal

● **8** Para-oesophageal
(below carina)

● **9** Pulmonary ligament

N_1 Nodes

○ **10** Hilar

○ **11** Interlobar

● **12** Lobar

● **13** Segmental

● **14** Subsegmental

Labels on figure: Brachiocephalic (innominate) a., 2R, Ao, 4R, 4L, Azygos v., 10R, 11R, PA, 7, 11L, 12,13,14R, 8, 10L, 9, 12,13,14L, Inf.pulm.ligt., 3, Ligamentum arteriosum, Phrenic n., 6, L.pulmonary a., Ao, 5, PA

Fig. 63.2 Mediastinal lymph node stations.

Reproduced from Mountain, Clifton, Regional Lymph Node Classification for Lung Cancer Staging. *Chest* 1997; **111**(6): 1718–1723, with the kind permission of the American College of Chest Physicians.

Radial EBUS
Uses a rotating US probe, inserted down sheath in working channel of bronchoscope, to aid localization of non-visible tumours. Once tumour is found sonographically, the probe is removed, leaving the sheath *in situ*. Subsequently, biopsies and brushings are taken through sheath.

Navigation bronchoscopy
Uses CT imaging to reconstruct airway anatomy and helps operator to precisely locate subsegment of interest for biopsy for non-visible abnormalities. Various systems exist.

Autofluorescence bronchoscopy

Technique to differentiate central malignant areas from normal tissue, including dysplasia and pre-invasive tumours *in situ*. However, the progression of these abnormalities is not known, so the role of autofluorescence bronchoscopy is unclear. Used in conjunction with usual white light bronchoscopy. Uses blue light to induce tissue autofluorescence, which means normal and abnormal tissues appear different colours when viewed through a specialized bronchoscope. Airway trauma, however, can also cause a different mucosal appearance, and the test has low specificity. It is being used in some centres as a surveillance tool following surgical resection of lung cancer, or in patients with head and neck cancer suspected of having a lung 1°, or following positive sputum cytology. Its role is not, however, clear, and advances in standard white light bronchoscopes (such as using narrow band imaging) may be found to be as good at identifying abnormal mucosa.

Rigid bronchoscopy

Visualizes bronchial tree to level of segmental bronchi. Can remove or core out endobronchial tumours, insert a stent, dilate tracheal or bronchial stenosis, and manage massive haemoptysis. Useful to provide information regarding resectability in lung cancer by measuring airway length. Incidence of serious complications <5%: hypoxia, laryngospasm, pneumothorax, bleeding.

Advanced bronchoscopy 2

Therapeutic procedures

Bronchial laser resection, electrocautery, argon–plasma coagulation (APC), and cryotherapy/cryoextraction

These are all procedures that can be used to debulk obstructing endobronchial lesions or coagulate a bleeding point. The use of a laryngeal mask airway (LMA) or uncuffed endotracheal tube is recommended to achieve airway control.

- *Electrocautery* Use of a high-frequency electrical current via a probe/snare/needle knife to heat tissue, causing coagulational vaporization, which enables cutting.
- *Neodymium-doped yttrium aluminum garnet (Nd-YAG)* laser achieves the same effect.
- *APC* A non-contact method of electrocautery, using argon gas which causes desiccation and coagulation. These are all effective immediately. These are used predominantly for obstructing malignant lesions but may be used to remove benign lesions, e.g. papilloma, or to treat benign stenoses, e.g. due to intubation, sarcoidosis, granulomatosis with polyangiitis, trauma, etc. Avoid using FiO_2 >0.4 with laser, electrocautery, and APC to minimize the fire risk. Shave skin on thigh, if necessary, before placing electrode for electrocautery, and avoid placing it over metal prosthetic joints.
- *Cryotherapy/cryoextraction* Technique of repeatedly freezing and then thawing an area with a probe in order to destroy tissue such as an endobronchial obstructing lesion. Standard cryotherapy takes hours to days to have its effects, while cryoextraction allows the bronchoscope and cryoprobe to be removed, complete with attached tumour tissue. It can also be used to remove a foreign body, as freezing attaches foreign body to the end of the probe. The cryoprobe can also be used to take a large transbronchial cryobiopsy in the context of ILD, but significant bleeding risks mean that precautions required (e.g. endotracheal tube and bronchial blocker).

Photodynamic therapy (PDT)

Intravenous (IV) administration of a photosensitizer drug to the patient (selectively concentrated in tumour tissue), followed 48 h later by bronchoscopic exposure of the presensitized tumour to a laser light of specific matching wavelength in order to cause tumour necrosis. Airways cleared of debris immediately after and again a few days later. Skin remains light-sensitive for 8 weeks.

Tracheobronchial stent insertion

Done via the bronchoscope to re-establish airway patency following endobronchial debulking or if there is extrinsic compression. Self-expanding metal airway stents (SEMAS) used in cases of external compression, such as lung cancer, for palliation of breathlessness. Length, diameter, and type of stent need careful selection prior to procedure using CT. Both uncovered stents (for extrabronchial lesions) and covered stents (for tumours with an endobronchial component) are available. These are inserted over a guidewire with flexible bronchoscopic visualization. Repositioning can be tricky after placement. Complications include stent migration or fracture, haemorrhage, mucus impaction, development of granulation tissue, bronchospasm, and even death. Silicone stents are used in mainly benign disease and are inserted via rigid bronchoscopy. They are easily removed and manoeuvred but can migrate and lead to problems with retained secretions.

Brachytherapy

Procedure of endobronchial irradiation using iridium-192 via bronchoscope for endobronchial and intramural tumours. A blind-ending catheter (the applicator) is placed within or alongside a tumour, and the bronchoscope is then removed over a long guidewire, which is then replaced by a radio-opaque graduated metal insert. CXR of the insert is used to plan placement of the radioactive source within the applicator. Treatment occurs over a few minutes. Delayed effect, requires several sessions. Complementary to other bronchoscopic therapies. Can cause radiation bronchitis, stenosis, and haemorrhage.

Chapter 64

Chest drains

Indications, drain types, complications *852*
Insertion technique *854*
Drain management *856*
Indwelling pleural catheters (IPC) *858*

Indications, drain types, complications

Chest drain insertion is associated with significant morbidity and mortality, and careful consideration should be given to the precise indication for drainage. Out-of-hours drain insertion should be avoided, unless an emergency.

Ultrasound guidance should be used for all drains inserted for fluid but is not required for pneumothorax.

Indications

- Tension pneumothorax (following needle decompression)
- Symptomatic pneumothorax with failed aspiration or underlying lung disease or in ventilated patients
- Complicated parapneumonic effusion and empyema
- Malignant pleural effusion for symptomatic relief and/or pleurodesis
- Haemothorax
- Traumatic haemopneumothorax
- Following thoracic surgery
- Rarely, for symptomatic effusions of other aetiology.

Contraindications

- Inexperienced operator
- Lung adherent to chest wall
- Bleeding tendency (a relative contraindication; routine measurement of platelet count and clotting in the absence of risk factors is not required). For anticoagulated patients, do not drain until international normalized ratio (INR) <1.5, unless life-threatening emergency
- Post-pneumonectomy (not an absolute contraindication, but first discuss with cardiothoracic surgical team).

Types of chest drain

Seldinger-style

Inserted by sliding the drain into the pleural cavity over a guidewire. While being the most frequently used, they still require experience and care to be inserted safely and comfortably. Sizes up to 36F are available. *Blunt dissection* drains (e.g. *Portex*® drains) require gentle dissection of subcutaneous tissue and muscles to gain entry to the pleural space. Drains are then inserted, often over a flexible plastic introducer, into the pleural space. Available in sizes up to 36F. Traditional *trocar* drains should no longer be used, being associated with significant potential complications and even death. These drains consist of a flexible plastic tube surrounding a metal rod with a blunt tip.

Small (10–14F) drains are more comfortable and should be the default choice for the majority of situations. Large-bore chest drains (24–36F) are frequently uncomfortable and only rarely required, e.g. 2° pneumothorax with large air leak and/or surgical emphysema, acute haemothorax, and post-operatively.

Complications

- Pain—insertion should not be painful with good local anaesthetic technique. Subsequent pain common, and opiate analgesia may be required. Rarely, significant ongoing pain or intractable cough requires drain to be withdrawn slightly (or completely)
- Inadequate drain position—may require withdrawal or insertion of new drain
- Surgical emphysema (in pneumothorax)—air leaks into subcutaneous tissues. May occur if tube blocked or positioned with holes subcutaneously, or with very large air leaks. See ➲ p. 447 for management
- Infection—iatrogenic pleural infection rate up to 2%, perhaps higher in trauma patients; wound infection
- Organ damage (e.g. lung, liver, spleen, heart, great vessels, stomach). Intrapulmonary placement results in significant continuous bubbling and bleeding; this may occur in up to 6% of all drain insertions. Drainage of gastro-intestinal (GI) contents suggests bowel perforation (or oesophageal rupture as the cause of the effusion)
- Haemorrhage into drain—bloody pleural fluid is a common finding (e.g. in malignant effusions), but unexpected large-volume drainage of frank blood suggests damage to organs or intercostal vessels. Clamp the drain, and leave it in place. Urgent imaging (± interventional radiology to embolize a bleeding vessel) and surgical assessment
- Re-expansion pulmonary oedema (see ➲ p. 448)
- Vasovagal reaction
- Sudden death due to vagus nerve irritation reported.

Further information

Havelock T et al. Pleural procedures and thoracic ultrasound: British Thoracic Society pleural disease guideline 2010. *Thorax* 2010;**65**(suppl. 2): ii61–76.
New England Journal of Medicine. Videos in clinical medicine.
Ⓡ http://www.nejm.org/multimedia/medical-videos

Insertion technique

An assistant is required. Use a dedicated procedure room when possible.
- Discuss procedure with patient, provided written information and obtain written consent (unless emergency situation)
- Insert intravenous (IV) cannula
- Consider giving analgesia. Conscious sedation (e.g. using midazolam) is rarely required and should include O_2 saturation monitoring; be cautious in patients with severe underlying lung disease or respiratory failure; see ➔ p. 888
- Position patient either in lateral decubitus position or lying head elevated at 30°, with insertion side of trunk rotated about 45° upwards and arm on insertion side behind their head. Alternative position is with patient sitting forward, leaning over a table
- Double-check correct side from chest examination and chest radiograph (CXR)
- Choose insertion site: ideally within 'safe triangle' (see Fig. 64.1), which avoids major vessels and muscles (boundaries: anteriorly, anterior axillary line, and border of pectoralis major; posteriorly, posterior axillary line and border of latissimus dorsi; inferiorly, horizontal to level of nipple in man or fifth intercostal space in woman).
- Avoid posterior approaches close to spine, as intercostal artery drops medially to lie in mid-intercostal space. Ultrasound guidance should always be used for fluid—either site marking *immediately* prior to drain insertion or real-time needle visualization using sterile ultrasound sheath and gel.
- Sterile skin preparation. Wear sterile gloves and gown
- Infiltrate skin, intercostal muscle, and parietal pleura with 10–20 mL of 1% lidocaine (maximum 3 mg/kg). Aim just above the upper border of the appropriate rib, avoiding the neurovascular bundle that runs below each rib. The subcutaneous fat lacks pain receptors and does not require anaesthetic. The parietal pleura, however, is extremely sensitive; use the full volume of lidocaine

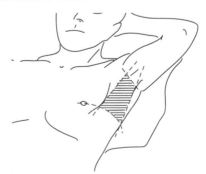

Fig. 64.1 'Safe triangle' for chest drain insertion, bounded anteriorly by pectoralis major, posteriorly by latissimus dorsi, inferiorly by the fifth intercostal space, and superiorly by the axilla.

Reproduced from Havelock et al. Pleural procedures and thoracic ultrasound: British Thoracic Society pleural disease guidelines 2010. *Thorax* 2010;**65**: i61–i76, Figure 2, with permission from BMJ.

- Verify that the site is correct by aspirating pleural fluid or air. Occasionally, a green (21G) needle may be too short in obese patients, and a longer needle is required. If unable to aspirate fluid or air, do not proceed with drain insertion; consider CT-guided drainage
- While waiting for anaesthetic to work, prepare drain and connections. Assistant should prepare underwater seal
- Insert drain:
  - *Seldinger drains* Gently insert the introducer needle, and check that air or fluid can be easily aspirated with a syringe. Remove syringe. Smoothly insert the guidewire through the introducer needle. Remove introducer needle, taking care not to let go of the guidewire at any time. Make a small skin incision ~5 mm. Slide plastic dilator around guidewire to enlarge the entry track. Avoid excessive force; dilator should not be inserted >1 cm into the pleural space. Remove the dilator, and slide the drain into the pleural cavity over the guidewire. Remove the wire when the drain is within the chest
  - *Blunt dissection drains* Small (1 cm) skin incision parallel to rib. Insert horizontal mattress suture across incision to facilitate later closure. Dissect intercostal muscles with blunt forceps (e.g. Spencer–Wells)— the fibres can be teased apart by opening and then removing the forceps; do not close forceps within the chest; this may damage underlying structures. This blunt dissection may take some time. Insert drain (facilitated by introducer) just into the pleural space smoothly and gently—there should not be any significant resistance. *Never apply force when inserting a chest drain.* Once the pleural space has been entered, insert the drain further while removing the introducer. An alternative approach is to remove any introducer and grip the end of the chest tube with blunt forceps, and use these to guide the tube into the chest. Aim towards the apex for a pneumothorax, and the lung base for a pleural effusion. (Note—in emergencies or in patients with extreme obesity or subcutaneous emphysema, it may be appropriate to make a larger initial incision and insert an index finger to assist the drain track)
- Connect the drain to underwater seal bottle via a three-way tap and tubing. If the drain is correctly positioned in the pleural space, it should swing with respiration and drain air or fluid
- Suture and tape the drain in place on the chest wall
- Ensure adequate analgesia
- Warn the patient not to disconnect the tubing or lift the underwater bottle above the level of the insertion site on the chest; supply a 'chest drain information leaflet'
- Obtain CXR to check position. The 'ideal' tube position (apex for pneumothorax, base for effusion) is not necessary for effective drainage, so do not reposition functioning drains on this basis. Computed tomography (CT) may be useful in confirming drain position in certain circumstances. Drains are often positioned in fissures, but, in most cases, this does not affect their functioning
- Small drains may need regular flush to ensure patency; prescribe 20 mL normal saline flush to drain qds
- Provide venous thromboembolism (VTE) prophylaxis with low molecular weight heparin (LMWH) unless contraindicated.

Drain management

General points

- Patients should ideally be managed on a specialist ward by experienced nursing staff. 'Chest drain observations' should be charted regularly, including swinging, bubbling, and volume and appearance of fluid output
- If drain water level does not swing with respiration, the drain is kinked (check underneath dressing as tube enters skin), blocked, clamped, or incorrectly positioned (drainage holes not in pleural space; check CXR). Occluded drains may sometimes be unblocked by a 30 mL saline flush. Non-functioning drains should be removed (risk of introducing infection)
- Suction is sometimes used to encourage drainage, although there is a lack of evidence regarding its use. Consider in cases of pneumothorax with persistent air leak or following chemical pleurodesis. Suction should be high volume/low pressure, typically starting at a level of 5 cmH$_2$O and increasing to 10–20 cmH$_2$O. It may be painful and not tolerated by the patient. Digital suction devices (e.g. Medela Thopaz+™ and Rocket PSU™ portable suction unit), both of which have a battery, enable portable suction while monitoring fluid output and air leak.

To clamp or not to clamp?

Never clamp a bubbling chest drain (risk of tension pneumothorax). Clamping may be considered in two situations:

- To control the rate of drainage of a large pleural effusion. Rapid drainage of large volumes may result in re-expansion pulmonary oedema; clamping, e.g. for 1 h after draining 1.5 L, may prevent this
- To avoid inappropriate drain removal in cases of pneumothorax with a slow air leak, when bubbling appears to have ceased. Clamping a drain for several hours, followed by repeat CXR, in such situations may detect very slow or intermittent air leaks. This is controversial, however, and should only ever be considered on a specialist ward with experienced nursing staff. If the patient becomes breathless, the drain should be immediately unclamped. Digital suction devices, which measure air leak, provide similar information without clamping the drain.

Drain removal

Quickly and smoothly remove the drain, while patient is slowly exhaling (or humming). Tie previously placed mattress suture, if applicable. Apply dressing. CXR to document lung position.

Indwelling pleural catheters (IPC)

Predominantly used for domiciliary drainage of recurrent malignant effusions, with drainage by patients, family members, or district nurses.

Indications

- British Thoracic Society (BTS) guidance for malignant pleural effusions advocates IPC use for completely trapped lung (pleurodesis unlikely to be successful) and for recurrent effusions post-pleurodesis
- Increasing use as 1° therapy. Randomized trials vs talc pleurodesis (TIME2 and AMPLE) demonstrate reduced hospital inpatient time (by 2–3.5 days) and decreased need for further pleural procedures, with similar improvements in dyspnoea and quality of life (QoL). However, increased risk of pleural and soft tissue infection, symptomatic loculation, and catheter blockage.

General points

- IPCs are 15.5/16F fenestrated silicone drains with a tunnelled subcutaneous portion and polyester cuff to prevent accidental removal and bacterial ingress
- Inserted as a day-case. Essential to consider optimum site for insertion, particularly for women (discomfort with bra straps). Using ultrasound, the Seldinger technique is used to insert pleural portion of drain, and blunt dissection is used to insert subcutaneous portion
- Adapter enables connection of IPC valve to conventional drainage bottles when in hospital. If adapter not available and urgent pleural fluid sampling required (e.g. for possible pleural infection), a large-bore IV cannula *without needle* can be used to aspirate fluid aseptically through the valve mechanism
- To drain at home, a pre-vacuumed 500- or 1,000-mL drainage bottle is aseptically connected to the IPC valve, usually 1–3 times/week (dependent on rate of fluid accumulation)
- Spontaneous pleurodesis occurs in 30–70% (dependent on malignancy type and whether lung is trapped). Aggressive daily drainage is associated with a higher rate of spontaneous pleurodesis (47% vs 24% after 12 weeks in ASAP RCT; 37% vs 11% after 60 days in AMPLE-2 RCT). Catheters can be removed if minimal drainage for 3–4 weeks, provided not blocked and minimal fluid remaining on imaging. Approx. 10% risk of catheter fracture on removal leading to retained fragment within thorax (usually asymptomatic)
- IPC-Plus RCT suggested day-case pleurodesis safe and associated with increased rates of pleurodesis
- IPC-related infections can often be treated without catheter removal. Empiric antibiotic therapy should cover *S. aureus* and Gram-negative bacteria
- Use of intrapleural fibrinolytics for symptomatic loculation is not routinely recommended
- Essential for patients to have adequate education and access to support in case of complications. Often provided by district nurses supported by pleural nurses
- Not considered a contraindication to chemotherapy.

Further information

Davies HE et al. Effect of an indwelling pleural catheter vs chest tube and talc pleurodesis for relieving dyspnea in patients with malignant pleural effusion. *JAMA* 2012;**307**(22): 2383–2389.

Fysh ETH et al. Clinical outcomes of indwelling pleural catheter-related pleural infections: an international multicenter study. *Chest*. 2013;**144**(5): 1597–1602.

Thomas R et al. Effect of an indwelling pleural catheter vs talc pleurodesis on hospitalization days in patients with malignant pleural effusion: The AMPLE randomized clinical trial. *JAMA*. 2017;**318**(19): 1903–1912.

Wahidi MM et al. Randomized trial of pleural fluid drainage frequency in patients with malignant pleural effusions. The ASAP trial. *AJRCCM*. 2017;**195**(8): 1050–1057.

Bhatnagar R et al. Outpatient talc administration by indwelling pleural catheter for malignant effusion. *NEJM*. 2018;**378**(14): 1313–1322.

Muruganandan S et al. Aggressive versus symptom-guided drainage of malignant pleural effusion via indwelling pleural catheters (AMPLE-2): an open-label randomised trial. *Lancet Respir Med*. 2018;**6**(9): 671–680.

Chapter 65

Cricothyroidotomy

General points 862
Cricothyroidotomy technique 863

General points

Difficulty in intubating patients often arises unexpectedly, even in those predicted to be low risk. The Difficult Airway Society have produced guidelines to help planning for difficulty and to produce a standardized approach. Cricothyroidotomy or 'emergency front of neck access' is the Plan D on these guidelines. It should be performed in after plans A–C have failed, a situation termed 'can't intubate can't oxygenate' (CICO). Cricothyroidotomy should only be performed by those with appropriate skills and training. The descriptions in this chapter are included to describe the technique and to outline the equipment required.

Scalpel cricothyroidotomy is now the recommended technique. Narrow-bore cannula (<4 mm) techniques had significant limitations and are no longer recommended. Large-bore cannula techniques are available but require more fine motor skill than a scalpel technique. A single standardized approach (scalpel technique) is recommended (see Box 65.1).

Overview of difficult airway management

Before attempting intubation, the steps for management of a difficult airway should be outlined so that the team is clear how to quickly proceed in the eventuality of difficulty

- Plan A: Facemask ventilation and intubation
- If fails proceed to Plan B
- Plan B: Supraglottic airway device
  - If success, stop and think about ongoing plan; wake the patient, intubate the trachea via the supraglottic airway device, proceed without intubation, tracheostomy, or cricothyroidotomy
- If fails proceed to Plan C
- Plan C: Final attempt at face mask ventilation
  - If success, wake the patient if possible
  - If fails (CICO), proceed to Plan D
- Plan D: Cricothyroidotomy (emergency front of neck access).

Cricothyroidotomy technique

Box 65.1 Cricothyroidotomy

Should only be performed by skilled and trained personnel—call for help from ICU/ENT surgery.

- Continue 100% O_2 via the upper-airway
- Ensure neuromuscular blockage
- Extend the head, with the patient lying flat
- Equipment: Scalpel with a number 10 blade, bougie, and tracheal tube (cuffed 6.0)
- Laryngeal handshake to identify the laryngeal anatomy and the cricothyroid membrane (and to stabilize the larynx)
- If palpable cricothyroid membrane, then make a transverse incision through the membrane; then turn the scalpel through 90 degrees with the sharp edge pointing caudally. Then slide the bougie tip along the blade into the trachea. Slide lubricated cuffed size 6.0 tracheal tube along the bougie into the trachea. Ventilate and confirm with capnography. Secure the airway
- If cricothyroid membrane impalpable then make an 8–10 cm incision (caudally to cranially) and then blunt dissect with fingers of both hands to identify the laryngeal structures. Once identified stabilize the larynx and proceed as above.
- Post-procedure, surgery should be postponed unless immediately lifesaving and arrange urgent surgical review.

Further information

Frerk et al. Difficult Airway Society 2015 guidelines for the management of unanticipated difficult intubation in adults. *BJA* 2015; **115**: 827–848.

Miscellaneous diagnostic tests

Skin prick tests *866*
Induced sputum *867*
Bronchial provocation testing *868*

Skin prick tests

These may be useful in identifying specific allergens causing immediate hypersensitivity (IgE-mediated) reactions. Results may influence management and guide allergen avoidance. Can be used to help define the presence of atopy. Triggers for contact urticaria, atopic eczema, and suspected food allergy may also be identified. The results are available almost immediately and correlate well with blood measurements of specific IgE. They should be carried out by staff trained to read the tests and manage adverse reactions.

The allergens tested should be identified from the history and may include common aeroallergens, e.g. pollens (grass, tree, weeds), moulds (*Alternaria alternata*, *Aspergillus fumigatus*, *Cladosporium*, *Penicillium chrysogenum*), house dust mite (*Dermatophagoides pteronyssinus*), and animal dander (dog epithelium, cat pelt).

Practical points

- Testing should be performed off oral antihistamines (7 days) and omalizumab (≥6 months). Tricyclic antidepressants and phenothiazines may also block response. Oral steroids appear not to suppress test results
- Very small risk of anaphylaxis; adrenaline and resuscitation equipment should be available. Particular care is needed with food and latex testing
- Clean the skin with 70% alcohol solution. Put a drop of allergen on the skin (usually the inside forearm). A range of allergens are available commercially. Fresh produce should be used for suspected fruit and vegetable hypersensitivity
- Prick the skin through the allergen drop, using a needle (do not draw blood). This should be with a calibrated lancet (1 mm), held vertically, or a hypodermic needle held at 45° to the skin
- The positive control is usually histamine and the negative control the diluent (usually glycerinated saline)
- Read the histamine control after 10 min and the allergen extracts after 15–20 min. A positive result is an itchy weal, which should be compared with the controls, as some subjects react to the skin prick alone (dermatographism)
- Different test solutions are standardized to give a mean weal diameter of 6 mm across sensitive subjects
- A weal of 3 mm or more is considered positive (indicating sensitization)
- A positive result does not prove that the clinical symptoms are due to bronchial hyperresponsiveness to the tested allergen but do raise clinical suspicion. Positive results can occur in those without symptoms, and false negatives do occur.

Immunoassays

Blood tests can be used to measure antigen-specific IgE. They are more specific, but less sensitive and more expensive than skin prick tests, but give similar information. There is no risk of anaphylaxis, and the patient does not need to stop antihistamines for the test to be performed.

Blood immunoassays are often referred to as RAST (radioallergosorbent tests) tests as historically radioactive tags were added to the antibodies. This technique is now rarely used, with enzyme-linked immunosorbent assay (ELISA) techniques more common, however the term RAST is still used widely to mean specific IgE testing.

Induced sputum

- Used to investigate for infection (e.g. tuberculosis (TB), Pneumocystis pneumonia (PCP)) or airway inflammation
- Patients rinse their mouth to minimize oral contamination. Give inhaled or nebulized salbutamol pre-procedure to minimize bronchospasm due to hypertonic saline. Measure the FEV_1
- Nebulized hypertonic (3–5%) saline is administered via a face mask in increasing concentrations with FEV_1 measurement after each concentration—the procedure is stopped if there is a > 20% fall in FEV_1. Each concentration is nebulized for 5 minutes, after each concentration the patient expectorates sputum into a sterile pot
- If transmission of infection (e.g. TB) is likely, perform the test in a negative pressure room, with appropriate protection of staff and other patients. Do not perform on the open ward or outpatient department
- Send sputum promptly to microbiology for staining and culture and direct immunofluorescent testing for PCP (if indicated). Sputum for differential cell counts needs to be processed immediately by an experienced operator. Sputum is mixed with 0.1% dithiothreitol, diluted with saline, and then filtered and centrifuged. Slides are then prepared with the cells and visualized using a light microscope.

Bronchial provocation testing

Several techniques can be used to assess bronchial hyperreactivity, including pharmacological challenges (non-specific bronchoprovocation testing), exercise challenge (for exercise-induced asthma), food additive challenge, and antigen challenge.

Non-specific bronchoprovocation testing

- Helpful if there is diagnostic doubt regarding the diagnosis of asthma
- Typically use inhaled methacholine or mannitol. Methacholine directly stimulates smooth muscle contraction. Mannitol works indirectly via release of endogenous mediators and is more specific but less sensitive
- Should be performed by experienced personnel, with facilities to deal with acute bronchospasm
- Patients need to omit regular asthma therapy (antihistamines: 3 days; long acting muscarinic antagonist (LAMA): 1 week; long-acting β2 agonist (LABA): 2 days)
- Increasing doses of provocation agent are given sequentially, with the FEV1 measured after each dose
- *Methacholine* Given in a nebulizer using solutions ranging from 0.03 mg/mL to 16 mg/mL. If there is a 20% fall in FEV1 or if the highest dose of methacholine has been given, the test is stopped. The concentration of drug causing a 20% fall is known as the PC20 and may lie between the concentrations of the last two doses. Asthma is indicated by a PC20 ≤8 mg/mL. Normal subjects have a PC20 ≥16 mg/mL. Intermediate responses may be seen in patients with family history of asthma or in those with chronic obstructive pulmonary disease (COPD) or cystic fibrosis (CF) or when recovering from viral infections
- *Mannitol* Proprietary dry powder inhaler (Aridol®) used. Provocation dose causing 15% fall in FEV1 (PD15) is noted. Asthma indicated by PD15 at cumulative dose of ≤635 mg.

Pleural biopsy

General points *870*
Abrams' pleural needle biopsy *872*

General points

Several techniques can be used to obtain a pleural biopsy.

- Using *image guidance* (either computed tomography (CT) or ultrasound (US)), a cutting needle (e.g. 18G Temno® or Cook Quickcore®) takes several 1–2 cm cores along the long axis of any parietal pleural pathology. Positron emission tomography (PET)/CT may have a role guiding pleural biopsy in patients with diffuse pleural abnormality to increase sensitivity. Malignancy sensitivity >85%. US-guided pleural biopsies increase microbiological diagnosis in pleural infection but not routine practice
- Using *thoracoscopic biopsy* (medical thoracoscopy/video-assisted thoracoscopic surgery (VATS)) (see ➲ p. 405). Multiple biopsies are taken of visually abnormal parietal pleura. Malignancy sensitivity >92%
- Using a pleural biopsy needle (e.g. Abrams' or Cope) in a *'blind' percutaneous* fashion to take multiple biopsies. Not advocated for diagnosing malignancy (sensitivity 47%—unsurprising, given patchy nature of pleural malignancy). May have utility in resource-limited settings for diffuse pleural diseases (e.g. tuberculosis (TB) pleuritis), but thoracoscopy still preferred (TB sensitivity ~100% vs ~80%).

Abrams' pleural needle biopsy

Indications

Diagnosis of tuberculous pleural effusion/pleural thickening when access to other biopsy techniques is limited.

Technique

An assistant is required.
- Discuss procedure with patient, and obtain written consent
- Insert intravenous (IV) cannula
- Consider sedation (e.g. midazolam 2–5 mg IV, with O2 saturation monitoring)
- Position patient sitting forward, leaning on a pillow over a table, with their arms folded in front of them or in the lateral decubitus position
- Double-check correct side from chest examination and chest radiograph (CXR)
- Choose biopsy site using pleural US to ensure an adequate volume of pleural fluid under proposed site. Use lateral approach to avoid neurovascular bundle, which lies mid-intercostal space posteriorly
- Sterile skin preparation. Wear sterile gloves and gown
- Infiltrate skin, intercostal muscle, and parietal pleura with 10–20 mL (up to 3 mg/kg) of 1% lidocaine. Aim just above the upper border of the appropriate rib, avoiding the neurovascular bundle that runs below each rib. Anaesthetize area behind rib below the insertion point. Verify that pleural fluid can be aspirated. If unable to aspirate, do not proceed
- While waiting for anaesthetic to work, assemble Abrams' reverse bevel biopsy needle. The needle consists of an outer sheath with a triangular opening (biopsy port) that can be opened or closed by rotating an inner sheath
- Make small (5 mm) skin incision; dissect intercostal muscles with blunt forceps (e.g. Spencer–Wells)
- Insert biopsy needle gently, with biopsy port closed. Do not apply force; the needle should slip into the pleural space without resistance. When in the pleural cavity, fluid can be withdrawn by attaching a syringe to the needle and opening the biopsy port
- To take a biopsy, attach a syringe to the needle. Open the biopsy port and angle it downwards, and then pull the biopsy port firmly against the parietal pleura on the rib beneath the entry point (6 o'clock position relative to entry point). Close the biopsy port, thereby pulling a sample of parietal pleura into the needle
- Remove the biopsy needle; open the biopsy port, and remove biopsy sample
- Repeat procedure 4–6 times in positions 4–8 o'clock; always sampling below the insertion point (to avoid the neurovascular bundle beneath the rib above)
- Send biopsy samples in saline for analysis for TB and in formalin for histological processing
- Apply dressing to biopsy site. May require a single stitch
- CXR to exclude pneumothorax.

Complications

Include pain (up to 15%), pneumothorax (up to 15%), haemothorax (<2%), and empyema. Haemorrhage from trauma to an intercostal artery may necessitate emergency thoracotomy. Fatalities are well documented but rare.

Further information

Maskell NA et al. Standard pleural biopsy versus CT-guided cutting-needle biopsy for diagnosis of malignant disease in pleural effusions: a randomised controlled trial. *Lancet* 2003;**361**: 1326–1331.

Hooper C et al. Investigation of a unilateral pleural effusion in adults: British Thoracic Society pleural disease guideline 2010. *Thorax* 2010;**65**(Suppl. 2): ii4–ii17.

Psallidas I et al. A pilot feasibility study in establishing the role of ultrasound-guided pleural biopsies in pleural infection (The AUDIO study). *Chest.* 2018;**154**(4): 766–772.

Chapter 68

Pleurodesis

General points 876
Chemical pleurodesis 878

General points

Aim of pleurodesis is to seal visceral to parietal pleura with adhesions to prevent pleural fluid or air accumulating. Pleurodesis is dependent upon:
- Lung re-expansion following removal of pleural fluid or air, which allows the apposition of visceral and parietal pleura. This may be encouraged by applying suction to an intercostal drain
- Inflammation of the pleural surfaces and local activation of coagulation, required to produce pleural fibrosis and adhesions. May be induced by chemical sclerosing agent or by mechanical pleural abrasion at video-assisted thoracoscopic surgery (VATS).

Indications
- Recurrent symptomatic pleural effusion (usually malignant, although pleurodesis also rarely used in benign recurrent effusions)
- Recurrent pneumothorax (due to concerns regarding the long-term safety of intrapleural talc, surgical abrasion pleurodesis usually procedure of choice in younger patients; chemical pleurodesis may be used in older patients who are unfit for surgery).

Chemical pleurodesis

Types of sclerosant

Choice of sclerosing agents varies. The most commonly used agents are sterile talc and bleomycin.

- Talc most effective (success rate 60–90%) and usually well tolerated, although risk of acute respiratory distress syndrome (ARDS) (see Complications). Administered either as slurry via chest drain or as poudrage at thoracoscopy, with comparable efficacy
- Bleomycin has success rates of only 60%
- Tetracycline successful in 65% cases, but current lack of drug manufacture.

Other rarely used agents include doxycycline, minocycline, interferon, interleukins, cisplatin, or patient's own blood.

Corticosteroids

May increase failure rate of pleurodesis, by inhibiting inflammatory response and development of adhesions, and should be discontinued.

Technique

Most centres will have written pleurodesis protocol, usually involving pre-medication and intrapleural local anaesthesia. A typical protocol is set out as follows:

- Discuss procedure and risks with patient, provide written information, and obtain written consent
- Insert chest drain (see ➲ p. 854): small bore (10–14F) chest tubes sufficient for fluid drainage and pleurodesis and are more comfortable than larger drains. Flush drain with 20 mL normal saline 6-hourly
- Commence low molecular weight heparin (LMWH) thromboembolism prophylaxis (increased risk following pleurodesis, especially in patients with malignancy)
- Drain fluid in a controlled manner. Small risk of re-expansion pulmonary oedema if large effusions drained too quickly; control output by clamping drain (see ➲ Chapter 64, p. 856)
- Chest radiograph (CXR) when drain output slows (<150 mL/day):
  - Consider pleurodesis if fluid removed and lung fully or partially expanded on CXR (although success rates much lower in the setting of an incompletely expanded lung)
  - Consider trial of suction if lung only partially re-expanded, if pain allows. Aim to increase pressure to –20 cmH$_2$O over 2 h.

For pleurodesis

- Insert intravenous (IV) cannula, and attach pulse oximeter
- Pleurodesis may be extremely painful. Consider premedication with opioid (oramorph 2.5–5 mg or IV opioid) and anti-emetic (e.g. metoclopramide 10 mg). For significant anxiety, consider a benzodiazepine (e.g. midazolam 1–2 mg IV, titrate to conscious level; care in elderly and in patients with respiratory failure). The patient should be comfortable but alert and cooperative
- Administer intrapleural local anaesthetic (e.g. lidocaine 3 mg/kg, max 250 mg, typically 20 ml 1% lidocaine) via chest drain, as intrapleural administration of sclerosants frequently painful. Clamp drain, and wait several minutes

- Prepare talc slurry. Using sterile technique, aspirate 50 mL normal saline into a syringe, and carefully remove plunger while keeping gloved finger over end of syringe. Tip 4–5 g sterile talc into syringe, and replace plunger gently. Shake syringe for 2–3 min to ensure homogeneous slurry. Administer slurry via chest drain over 1–2 min
- Flush drain with 20 mL saline
- Clamp drain for 1 h after administration of sclerosant. Then unclamp, and consider applying suction, increasing to –20 cmH_2O over 2 h. Restart 6-hourly saline flushes
- Further analgesia, if required
- Monitor pulse, blood pressure (BP), temperature, respiratory rate (RR), and O_2 saturations half-hourly for 2 h and then 6-hourly
- Analgesia and antipyretics, as required. Despite previous concerns, the TIME1 randomized controlled trial (RCT) demonstrated that non-steroidal anti-inflammatories (NSAIDs) are not associated with a higher rate of pleurodesis failure than opiates (although are associated with an increased use of rescue analgesia)
- Optimal duration of drainage following pleurodesis unknown; consider drain removal within 24–72 h if adequate drainage of fluid and lung expansion on CXR. Can usually remove tube at 48 h.

Complications

All sclerosants may cause chest pain and fever. Sterile talc may rarely (<1%) result in respiratory failure due to ARDS, manifest as hypoxia and diffuse pulmonary infiltrates within 48 h of pleurodesis. 'Mixed' talc (containing small particles) appears to be associated with greater systemic inflammation and greater deterioration in gas exchange than 'graded' talc (which has small particles removed), so routine use of graded talc is recommended.

Further information

Maskell NA et al. Randomized trials describing lung inflammation after pleurodesis with talc of varying particle size. *Am J Respir Crit Care Med* 2004;**170**: 377–382.

Roberts ME et al. Management of a malignant pleural effusion: British Thoracic Society pleural disease guideline 2010. *Thorax* 2010;**65**(Suppl 2): ii32–ii40.

Rahman NM et al. Effect of opioids vs NSAIDs and larger vs smaller chest tube size on pain control and pleurodesis efficacy among patients with malignant pleural effusion: The TIME1 randomized clinical trial. *JAMA*. 2015;**314**(24): 2641–2653.

Clive AO et al. Interventions for the management of malignant pleural effusions: a network meta-analysis. *Cochrane Database Syst Rev*. 2016;**5**: CD010529.

Pneumothorax aspiration

Indications *882*
Technique *883*

Indications

- 1° *pneumothorax* Consider aspiration if patient breathless, hypoxic, and pneumothorax large
- 2° *pneumothorax* Consider aspiration if evidence of underlying lung disease (or patient with significant smoking history, aged >50 y), with small pneumothorax and breathlessness.

Technique

See Chapter 37 for discussion of pneumothorax management. Carefully re-examine the chest radiograph (CXR) to ensure that the lung is not tethered at any point (may increase procedural risk and require computed tomography (CT)-guided intervention). Use a dedicated procedure room when possible.

- Discuss procedure with patient, and obtain written consent (unless emergency situation)
- Consider inserting an intravenous (IV) cannula
- Position patient sitting upright in bed, supported on pillows
- Double-check correct side from chest examination and CXR
- Choose aspiration site: second intercostal space in mid-clavicular line on side of pneumothorax
- Sterile skin preparation. Wear sterile gloves and gown
- Infiltrate skin, intercostal muscles, and parietal pleura with 10 mL of 1% lidocaine. Aim just above the upper border of the appropriate rib, avoiding the neurovascular bundle that runs below each rib. Parietal pleura is extremely sensitive; use 10–20 mL of 1% lidocaine (maximum 3 mg/kg)
- While waiting for anaesthetic to work, connect 50 mL syringe to three-way tap, with tap turned 'off' to patient
- Confirm presence of pneumothorax by aspirating air with green (21G) needle
- Insert large-bore (e.g. 16G) cannula over upper border of rib. Remove inner needle; quickly connect cannula to three-way tap and 50 mL syringe
- Aspirate 50 mL air with syringe; turn tap, and expel air into atmosphere. Repeat until resistance felt or 2.5 L of air aspirated (aspiration of >2.5 L suggests a large air leak, and aspiration is likely to fail). Halt procedure if painful or patient coughing excessively
- Remove cannula; cover insertion site with dressing
- Repeat CXR
- Aspiration is successful if pneumothorax size has reduced on CXR and patient is symptomatically improved
- If initial aspiration of a 1° pneumothorax fails, a chest drain is likely required. The risks of this procedure need to be outweighed by the clinical necessity (i.e. significant symptoms or adverse physiology).

Further information

Havelock T et al. Pleural procedures and thoracic ultrasound: British Thoracic Society pleural disease guideline 2010. *Thorax* 2010;**65**(suppl. 2): ii61–76.

Safe sedation

Administration of sedation *886*
Drugs used for sedation *888*
Sedation in specific circumstances *890*

Administration of sedation

- Intravenous (IV) sedation commonly used for bronchoscopy and thoracoscopy and, less frequently, for other procedures, e.g. chest drain insertion. Studies show that both patients and physicians usually prefer the use of sedation for bronchoscopy, although some tolerate unsedated bronchoscopy well; consider patient preference and comorbidities
- Follow *Summary of Safe Sedation Practice* (UK Academy of Medical Royal Colleges, 2001) (see Table 70.1). Updated 2013 guidance highlights competency-based sedation training, formation of hospital 'sedation committees', and audit
- Sedation is usually the responsibility of the physician performing a procedure, although some units have anaesthetist-delivered sedation
- Desired depth of sedation is usually *conscious sedation*—patient maintains airway patency and cardiorespiratory function, and verbal contact with the patient is possible at all times. Some procedures (e.g. interventional bronchoscopy) may require deeper sedation provided by anaesthetists, with same level of care and monitoring as for a general anaesthetic
- Significant interpatient variability to IV sedation; therefore, essential to titrate sedatives, using small incremental doses, to avoid oversedation
- Assess (and document) sedation depth. Tools, such as the *Ramsay Scale* (see Table 70.2) and the *Modified Observer's Assessment of Alertness/Sedation (MOAAS)* (see Table 70.3) score, may help documentation
- *NHS Patient Safety Alerts* (NPSA) in 2014 and 2017 emphasize importance of flushing cannulae after administration of sedation to prevent inadvertent injection.

Table 70.1 Summary of Safe Sedation Practice

Domain	Safe practice
Patient assessment	'Checklist' identification of sedation risk factors prior to procedure Provide instructions on activities after procedure
Level of sedation	Sedation provided only to the level of 'conscious' sedation (verbal contact possible)
IV sedation	Secure venous access Antagonist drugs at hand When combination sedation used, give opioids first, and caution to avoid oversedation
Monitoring	Defined professionals have responsibility for monitoring patient safety and making a written record. Pulse oximeter monitoring continued until discharge from unit. Consider monitoring BP and ECG in higher-risk patients
O_2 therapy	Nasal cannula and facial mask O_2 delivery available
Facilities	Trolley can be tipped head-down Resuscitation equipment immediately available

Table 70.2 Ramsay scale

Level	Response
1	Anxious and agitated or restless
2	Cooperative, orientated, and tranquil
3	Responds only to commands
4	Brisk response to light glabellar touch or loud noise
5	Sluggish response to light glabellar touch or loud noise

Ramsay MA et al. Controlled sedation with alphaxalone-alphadolone. *Br Med J* 1974;**2**(5920): 656–659.

Table 70.3 Modified Observer's Assessment of Alertness/Sedation (MOAAS) scale

Level	Response
5	Responds readily to name spoken in normal tone
4	Lethargic response to name spoken in normal tone
3	Responds only after name is called loudly or repeatedly
2	Responds only after mild prodding or shaking
1	Does not respond to mild prodding or shaking

Chernik DA et al. Validity and reliability of the Observer's Assessment of Alertness/Sedation Scale: study with intravenous midazolam. *J Clin Psychopharmacol* 1990;**10**(4): 244–251.

Drugs used for sedation

See → Appendix 5 p. 957 for further details about drug doses, pharmacology, and side effects.

Benzodiazepines

- Benzodiazepines cause sedation, anxiolysis, and anterograde amnesia by binding to, and increasing the activity of, γ-aminobutyric acid (GABA), a brain neuroinhibitory transmitter
- *Midazolam* (used by 78% of bronchoscopists) improves experience of bronchoscopy, reduces procedural discomfort, causes anterograde amnesia, and increases willingness of patients to have further procedures without worsening adverse event profile
- Other benzodiazepines (e.g. diazepam and lorazepam) have also been used, but midazolam has particular suitability with rapid peak effect (over 5–10 mins) and relatively short half-life
- Natural variability in action of cytochrome P450 (CYP) 3A4 and 3A5, responsible for benzodiazepine metabolism, may prolong elimination half-life by up to sixfold
- *Flumazenil* (benzodiazepine antagonist) reverses benzodiazepine oversedation and must be immediately available, although administration should not be routine. Flumazenil has a shorter half-life than midazolam, so potential risk of resedation
- A 2008 NPSA report documented harm and death from excessive midazolam. To prevent inadvertent injection of high-strength midazolam solution (2 or 5 mg/mL), NPSA mandates that only low-strength midazolam solution (1mg/mL) should normally be available in clinical areas
- Following a 2004 NCEPOD report (see Sedation in specific circumstances), no more than 5 mg midazolam should be initially drawn up into any syringe prior to a procedure for patients aged <70 (2 mg midazolam for patients >70), to reduce likelihood of oversedation.

Opioids

- Mechanism of action of *opioids* are not completely understood, but they are known to be μ-opioid receptor agonists, causing analgesia, sedation, and cough suppression
- *Fentanyl* and *alfentanil* both have favourable pharmacological profiles, having a rapid peak effect and a relatively short half-life
- *Naloxone* (competitive antagonist) reverses opioid-induced respiratory depression and oversedation. For oversedated patients who have received both benzodiazepine and opioid, initial reversal with flumazenil (rather than naloxone) recommended, unless the patient has received particularly high dose of opioid
- Addition of an opioid to midazolam for bronchoscopy improves procedural cough, reduces lidocaine usage, and increases patient procedural tolerance. Most frequent combination agents used for bronchoscopy are midazolam and fentanyl/alfentanil. Opioids should be administered (and allowed to reach maximal effect) prior to administration of midazolam. Risk of oversedation may increase when using combination agents, although several studies fail to show an increase in clinically significant adverse events.

Other drugs

* Propofol (and its pro-drug fospropofol) are sedative-hypnotics that exert their actions partly by increasing GABA activity. Together with ketamine, these drugs have a relatively narrow therapeutic window between 'conscious' sedation and general anaesthesia and are *currently recommended for use solely by anaesthetists in the UK.*

Sedation in specific circumstances

- Risks may be increased when using combined sedation for patients in *respiratory failure*, and caution is recommended
- *Elderly patients* are likely to require lower doses of sedatives and may suffer with prolonged after-effects (e.g. amnesia and coordination impairment). A 2004 NCEPOD report for elderly patients undergoing therapeutic gastro-intestinal (GI) endoscopy recommended that no more than 2 mg should be initially drawn up for patients aged >70
- *Other comorbidities* likely to require dose modification include hepatic impairment, heart failure, and renal impairment
- *Concomitant medications* (e.g. antifungals, antiretrovirals, calcium channel blockers (CCBs), and macrolide antibiotics) inhibit cytochrome P450 3A4 (which also metabolizes benzodiazepines and opioids) and may prolong sedation.

Further information

Du Rand IA et al. British Thoracic Society guideline for diagnostic flexible bronchoscopy in adults. *Thorax* 2013;**68**: i1–i44.

Academy of Royal Medical Colleges. Safe Sedation Practice for Healthcare Procedures – Standards and Guidance. Oct 2013.

Thoracentesis

General points *892*
Diagnostic thoracentesis *893*
Therapeutic thoracentesis *894*

General points

Thoracentesis ('pleural tap' or pleural fluid aspiration) may be diagnostic or therapeutic. Site selection using ultrasound (US) guidance (see Chapter 72) gives a higher success rate and a better adverse event profile and should be used routinely. Use a dedicated procedure room when possible. Avoid out-of-hours procedures unless an emergency.

Diagnostic thoracentesis

Indication

Undiagnosed pleural effusion. There are no absolute *contraindications* to pleural aspiration, although, for non-urgent thoracentesis, anticoagulated patients should have their clotting corrected to international normalized ratio (INR) <1.5.

Technique

- Discuss procedure with patient, and obtain written consent.
- Position patient sitting forward, leaning on a pillow over a table, with their arms folded in front of them
- Double-check correct side from chest examination and CXR
- Choose aspiration site using ultrasound, preferably in 'safe triangle' (see ➔ p. 854), unless loculated fluid makes this impossible. Avoid posterior approaches where possible (as the intercostal artery lies in the mid-intercostal space posteriorly)
- Sterile skin preparation and aseptic technique
- Infiltrate skin, intercostal muscle, and parietal pleura with 1% lidocaine. Aim just above the upper border of the appropriate rib, avoiding the neurovascular bundle that runs below each rib. The parietal pleura is extremely sensitive; use 10–20 mL of 1% lidocaine (maximum 3 mg/kg)
- Aspirate pleural fluid with a green (21G) needle and 50 mL syringe
- Following diagnostic tap:
  - Record pleural fluid appearance
  - Send sample to biochemistry for measurement of glucose, protein, and lactate dehydrogenase (LDH)
  - Send a fresh 20 mL sample in sterile pot to cytology for examination for malignant cells and differential cell count
  - Send samples in sterile pot and blood culture bottles to microbiology for Gram stain and microscopy, culture, and acid-fast bacillus (AFB) stain and culture
  - Process non-purulent heparinized samples in arterial blood gas (ABG) analyser for pH (consult biochemistry laboratory for local policy of pH analysis beforehand; never put purulent samples in the arterial blood analyser)
  - Consider measurement of cholesterol, triglycerides, chylomicrons, haematocrit, and amylase, depending on the clinical circumstances
- There is no need for a routine chest radiograph (CXR) following aspiration, unless difficulties were encountered during the procedure
- If unable to obtain fluid, re-ultrasound to confirm depth and conformation of fluid, and consider computed tomography (CT)-guided aspiration.

Complications

Include pain, failure to obtain fluid, pneumothorax (2–4% with US), cough, bleeding, empyema, spleen or liver puncture, and malignant seeding down aspiration site (can be treated with radiotherapy).

Therapeutic thoracentesis

Indication

Symptomatic relief of breathlessness due to a pleural effusion, most commonly due to malignancy.

Technique

- In most cases, can be performed as a day-case procedure. Commercial thoracentesis kits are available, but the following should be readily available
- The initial procedure of local anaesthetic infiltration is identical to that of diagnostic thoracentesis. It is important to verify that the insertion site is optimal using US; *always* ensure that fluid is first obtained with a green (21G) needle
- Carefully advance an intravenous (IV) cannula (with a syringe on the end) along the anaesthetized track
- When fluid is aspirated, remove the inner needle while fully inserting the plastic cannula. Attach the cannula to a three-way tap
- Aspirate fluid from the chest with a 50 mL syringe via the three-way tap, and flush the fluid into a sterile jug through extension tubing (e.g. a blood giving set, cut using sterile scissors). Often, having 'primed' the tubing with pleural fluid, further syringe aspiration is not required, as the fluid siphons down out of the chest itself into the jug. Drain a maximum of 1.5 L of fluid on one occasion (risk of re-expansion pulmonary oedema following sudden removal of large volumes). Stop the procedure if resistance is felt or the patient experiences discomfort or severe coughing
- Some physicians use pleural manometry to measure pleural pressure and derive pleural elastance measurements (change in pressure with removal of given volume of pleural fluid). This may predict non-expandable lung and help determine a maximum amount to drain
- Apply dressing to aspiration site
- CXR post-procedure is helpful in evaluating for non-expandable 'trapped' lung but is discordant with elastance measurements in 1/3.

Further information

Havelock T et al. Pleural procedures and thoracic ultrasound: British Thoracic Society pleural disease guideline 2010. *Thorax* 2010;**65**(suppl. 2): ii61–76.

Thoracic ultrasound (TUS)

Diagnostic and therapeutic utility 896
Training 897
Physics of US 898
Performing a TUS examination 900
TUS appearances 1 902
TUS appearances 2 904

Diagnostic and therapeutic utility

Thoracic ultrasound (TUS) is increasingly used for bedside evaluation of the pleural space and thorax. Given improved safety, National Patient Safety Agency (NPSA) and British Thoracic Society (BTS) guidance 'strongly recommend' TUS for pleural fluid procedure site selection. TUS also gives useful diagnostic information (see Table 72.1) which may alter management (e.g. a patient with a transudative effusion who has pleural nodularity, suggestive of malignancy).

Table 72.1 Diagnostic and therapeutic utility of TUS

Structure	Utility
Pleural fluid	Fluid quantification and characterization. Guided intervention. Obesity and rib crowding cause difficulties
Pleural thickening and nodularity	Detection and guided core biopsy. 'Colour fluid sign' may help differentiate between fluid and thickening
Diaphragm	Assessment of function. Detection of thickening or nodularity (assessment limited by aerated lung)
Pneumothorax	Ruling out post-procedural pneumothorax. Unhelpful for assessing pneumothorax size. Chronic obstructive pulmonary disease (COPD), cystic fibrosis (CF), and prior pleurodesis may mimic pneumothorax
Lung	Detection of atelectasis, consolidation, pulmonary oedema and peripheral lung lesions (abscess/tumour). Guided biopsy. Unable to assess structures deep to aerated lung
Heart	Detection of pericardial fluid, cardiomegaly
Ribs	Rib fracture detection and fine needle aspiration (FNA) of metastases
Liver	Metastases/abscess detection
Lymph nodes	Assessment and guided FNA/core biopsy

Training

- Follow the Royal College of Radiology 'level 1' TUS syllabus
  - ℘ http://www.rcr.ac.uk/publication/ultrasound-training-recommendations-medical-and-surgical-specialties-third-edition
  - ℘ http://www.rcr.ac.uk/publication/focused-ultrasound-training-standards
- Find a suitable mentor (with TUS level 2 or level 1 for ≥2 y)
- Keep a log book, and maintain a record of video clips and still images
- Attend a practical and theoretical TUS course
- Level 1 practical training currently requires ≥1 session/week over ≥3 months (~5 scans/session)
- Maintain level 1 competency by: (1) doing ≥20 scans/y (≤3 months between scans), (2) maintaining contact with a named radiologist 'mentor', (3) auditing practice, (4) remaining current with literature and CPD.

Physics of US

Characteristics of the US wave

- US is a longitudinal wave in which particles move in the same direction as the wave (creating successive compressions and rarefactions)
- Frequencies used typically 2.5–12 MHz (audible sound 20 Hz–20 kHz)
- Key formula (Where c = speed of US in soft tissue (~1,540 m/s)):

$$Frequency\,(f) = constant\,(c)\,/\,wavelength\,(\lambda)$$

- With a typical frequency of 5 MHz, TUS wavelength (which determines resolution) is ~0.3 mm.

Changes to the US wave

- US wave can be transmitted, attenuated, or reflected
- *Transmission* occurs when particles in a tissue move together and have coherent vibration
- *Attenuation* (loss of US energy) occurs due to wave absorption, scatter, and refraction. Absorption occurs when particles do not move together and have chaotic vibration, generating heat. Higher frequencies (i.e. shorter wavelengths) are more likely to be absorbed than transmitted, giving poorer depth penetration but better resolution. Deeper structures lead to greater wave attenuation (travels further through tissue), and US machines compensate for this using *time gain compensation* (TGC), which can be fine-tuned using sliders on machine
- *Reflection* occurs at the interface between tissues with different impedance. High impedance at soft tissue-air interface and soft tissue–bone interface causes near-complete reflection (and explains inability to image aerated lung and the acoustic shadow cast behind ribs). Also, reason why coupling US gel required. Partial reflection is required to generate a return of signal to the US probe (and create an image).

Generation of the US wave

- US probes have piezoelectric crystals responsible for wave generation and detection. Timing and power of the returning wave generates the B/2D-mode image
- *Pulse repetition frequency* (PRF) determines interval between successive US pulses (must avoid collision of successive pulses). Slow PRF when attempting complex imaging (e.g. simultaneous 2D/Doppler imaging) causes jerky images. Reducing size of scan field improves PRF.

US artefacts

- Numerous artefacts occur with TUS, including:
  - *Mirror artefact* Smooth curved surfaces (e.g. diaphragm) reflect liver/spleen so that they seem within the thoracic cavity (appearing as consolidated lung)
  - *Horizontal reverberation artefact ('A' lines)* Tissue interfaces that have significant impedance mismatch (e.g. soft tissue-aerated lung interface) create successive reflections between the interface and the ultrasound probe itself, giving a series of echogenic parallel lines below the pleural stripe

- *Comet tail artefact ('B' lines)* Another reverberation artefact seen at the pleural-aerated lung interface, which creates vertical 'comet tails', particularly at the lung bases. Accentuated in conditions which enlarge/thicken interlobular septae (e.g. pulmonary oedema/interstitial lung disease (ILD))
- *Posterior acoustic shadowing* Poor visualization of structures deep to interfaces with a high reflection coefficient (e.g. ribs, calcified gallstones) due to complete reflection/absorption
- *Posterior acoustic enhancement* Transmission through a medium which causes minimal attenuation (e.g. fluid-filled cyst) causes apparent enhancement of posterior structures.

Probe choice

- *Curvilinear transducers* (2–6 MHz) have a fan-shaped pulse field and give excellent depth penetration and reasonable resolution
- *Linear transducers* (7–14 MHz) have a rectangular pulse field and give excellent near-field resolution but have poor depth penetration.

Performing a TUS examination

Prior to the examination

- Examine any available radiology, particularly computed tomography (CT). Think—are there lesions on the CT which should be visible at TUS (including rib metastases, parenchymal pathology, or liver metastases)?
- Position the patient appropriately. For diagnostic TUS, sat up leaning forward, with arms resting on a table, gives excellent views laterally and posteriorly (where most pleural pathology lies). For pleural procedures, the lateral decubitus position prevents the patient from moving (recommended for real-time US-guided pleural intervention)
- Move the US machine to the patient, taking care not to run over the expensive (~£5,000) probe cables. Think about machine position, particularly if undertaking real-time intervention—the probe and the machine screen should be in a straight line. Clean the US machine and probe with an appropriate wipe.

Operating the US machine

- Confirm and enter patient details on the US machine
- Select 2D/B mode, using 'abdominal' pre-set if 'thoracic' not available (initial depth ~15 cm; ensure that TGC sliders are arranged vertically)
- Use a 5 MHz curvilinear probe for routine TUS (good compromise between depth of penetration and resolution). 10 MHz linear probe better for vascular access and lymph node/rib metastasis FNA (high resolution but poor depth penetration)
- Hold the probe gently, like a pen. Three movements are important to get the most information from narrow intercostal spaces: rotation, angulation, and translation. TUS is a dynamic process; move the probe over both hemithoraces, while continuously optimizing the image, and make sure to first identify the costophrenic angle and liver/spleen to avoid mimics of a pleural effusion (e.g. ascites and loculated intra-abdominal collections).

Optimize machine controls while imaging

- *Depth* should be changed, depending on structure being imaged. Always ensure that you can initially see the full extent of any effusion and structures deep to the fluid
- *Gain* Avoid the temptation to set the gain too high
- *Focal points* Start with one focal point, positioned at the depth of maximal interest. Multiple focal points, while seemingly attractive, reduce the PRF and make the image jerky
- *Frequency* May need to reduce, particularly for larger patients, to increase depth penetration
- *Colour Doppler* Useful for assessing possible vascular structures (including intercostal arteries) and differentiating between pleural thickening and fluid ('colour fluid sign')
- *TGC* May need to increase gain at depth, particularly for larger patients. Conversely, a massive effusion (and accompanying posterior acoustic enhancement) may make deeper structures very bright, necessitating reducing gain at depth

- *Sector width* and *zoom*
- *Freeze and store* Always store at least one still image/video clip per patient. If performing an intervention, store a representative image from your intervention site
- *Measure/callipers* Useful for measuring depth of pleural effusion at site of intervention and the distance from skin to pleural effusion (Consider—will a standard 35 mm 21G needle reach the fluid?)
- Poor image? Restart using the default settings, and ensure that the TGC sliders are vertical and that depth is appropriate. For larger patients, increase the US power to maximum, and consider reducing US frequency (to ~3 MHz). Tissue harmonic imaging may improve tissue boundary differentiation. Some machines have an image 'optimize' button.

TUS appearances 1

Aerated lung

See Fig. 72.1.
- Bright echogenic pleural stripe caused by reflection at the soft tissue-air interface
- Pleural sliding/gliding—a shimmering at the pleural stripe as the visceral pleura slides over the parietal pleura
- Comet tail artefacts (B lines)—fanning out vertically from the pleural stripe, particularly at the lung bases
- Horizontal reverberation artefacts (A lines)—repeating periodic horizontal lines below pleural stripe
- Absent deep detail—high reflection coefficient at pleural stripe means that it is impossible to image aerated lung or structures deep to lung. The only apparent structures are artefacts.

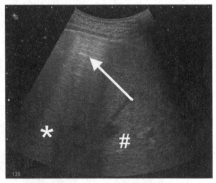

Fig. 72.1 Normal costophrenic angle with aerated lung (left) abutting liver (right, #). Comet tails (*) and horizontal reverberation artefacts (arrow) are seen. Note lack of pleural fluid prevents diaphragm visualization.

Pneumothorax

- TUS may be a useful rule-out test for pneumothorax, but always get a CXR to confirm when pneumothorax suspected
- Absent pleural sliding/gliding
- Absent comet tail artefacts (B lines)
- Horizontal reverberation artefacts (A lines)—may be accentuated in pneumothorax
- Absent deep detail
- A 'lung point' may be seen if the pneumothorax is of a size that some lung is still in contact with the chest wall. One side of the sonographic image looks typical for pneumothorax while the other side shows typical features of aerated lung (including pleural sliding and comet tail artefacts). The 'lung point' is the interface between these parts of the image and represents where the lung starts to contact the chest wall.

Pleural effusion

- See Fig. 72.2
- TUS has a higher sensitivity for pleural fluid detection than CXR
- Fluid is seen deep to parietal pleura as a relatively dark (hypoechoic) structure
- *Anechoic effusions* are black and featureless and may be transudative or exudative
- *Echogenic effusions* are exudative and appear speckled, due to protein/ pus/blood/intrapleural air
- *Septated effusions* are also exudative, and septations can be caused by any pleural inflammation (e.g. pleural infection, malignancy)
- Size—measure maximal effusion depth. A variety of formulae have been proposed to estimate pleural fluid volume, particularly in an ICU setting. Practically, the following is suggested—small (only visible at one intercostal space), moderate (less than half the hemithorax), large (greater than half the hemithorax)
- Possible to image structures deep to fluid.

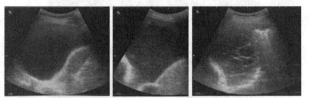

Fig. 72.2 Anechoic (right), echogenic (middle), and septated (right) effusions.

Pleural thickening

Often relatively hypoechoic and may be difficult to distinguish from pleural fluid. Colour Doppler may help—for fluid, there is a wave-like motion of pleural fluid ('colour fluid sign') caused by respiratory/cardiac motion (not seen with thickening).

TUS appearances 2

Diaphragm

- Should be smooth, and it may be possible to discern five alternating hypo- and hyperechoic stripes (see Fig. 72.3; disrupted in pathology)
- Diaphragm poorly visualized without fluid but may be possible by imaging over the liver/spleen and angling probe upwards
- Diaphragm inversion occurs with large effusions and usually associated with significant dyspnoea
- Function may be assessed by watching movement and diaphragmatic thickening with respiration and sniffing (and comparing both sides).

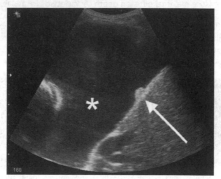

Fig. 72.3 Diaphragmatic nodule (arrow) and echogenic effusion (*).

Abnormal lung

- 'Compressive' atelectasis is commonly seen with pleural fluid. Lung has a concave 'hockey stick' appearance with significant volume loss. Internal structure is visible due to lack of aeration
- Consolidated lung may look similar to liver (or spleen), and parenchymal structure is visible due to lack of aeration (see Fig. 72.4). Minimal volume loss and ill-defined boundaries. Hyperechoic (bright) branching structures and speckles represent air bronchograms. Branching hypoechoic structures are either pulmonary vessels (with demonstrable colour Doppler signal) or fluid bronchograms (without Doppler signal)
- Conditions which cause enlargement/thickening of the interlobular septae, such as heart failure and interstitial lung diseases can cause increased number and prominence of the comet tail artefacts (B lines). These artefacts are thought to occur due to a reverberation of the ultrasound wave at the interface between the interlobular septae and aerated lung.

TUS features in malignancy

Sonographic features with high specificity (95–100%) for malignancy and overall sensitivity 79%:
- Parietal pleural thickening >1 cm
- Nodular pleural thickening
- Visceral pleural thickening
- Diaphragmatic thickening >7 mm
- Disruption of five diaphragmatic layers
- Diaphragmatic nodules.

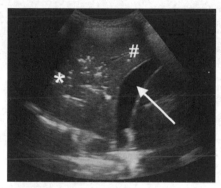

Fig. 72.4 Consolidated lung with visible air bronchograms (*) and pulmonary vessels (#) overlying a subpulmonic effusion (arrow).

TUS features in pleural infection

No sonographic characteristics can rule out pleural infection, and fluid sampling is essential. Septated effusions may drain less well than non-septated effusions (although this should not discourage drain insertion, as many will still drain well). Densely echogenic fluid is likely to be pus or blood.

US-guided intervention

Pleural procedures (aspiration and drainage) can be guided sonographically, either by site marking or using real-time guided intervention. *Site marking* is easier and can be used for most effusions >2–4 cm depth but must be performed immediately prior to intervention without patient repositioning. *Real-time visualization* of the needle in the pleural space requires sterile US gel and sheath and is technically more challenging but is required for smaller or loculated effusions. An in-plane oblique course is taken from the side of the probe, and the entire path of the needle is visible. A similar technique is used for *pleural biopsy* (using a cutting needle such as a Temno® needle) and *lymph node/rib metastasis FNA* (using a linear probe and a 23 or 21G needle).

Cautions

- Avoid risky sampling of small <1 cm effusions (which may not even be apparent on CXR), unless there is a genuine diagnostic need
- Always identify the hemidiaphragm to ensure that the pleural space, rather than the upper abdomen, is being imaged
- Avoid posterior approaches for interventions whenever possible (even though this might be the site of maximal fluid depth), due to the relative exposure of the neurovascular bundle. Provided adequate fluid is present, always use the safe triangle.

Further information

Koh DM et al. Transthoracic US of the chest: clinical uses and applications. *Radiographics* 2002;**22**(1): e1.

Feldman MK et al. US artifacts. *Radiographics* 2009;**29**(4): 1179–1189.

Thoracoscopy

General points 908
Indications and risks 909
Thoracoscopy technique 910

General points

Thoracoscopy is the procedure of examining the parietal pleura, visceral pleura, and diaphragm with a thoracoscope and taking biopsies. Chemical pleurodesis can also be performed. Performed by chest physicians using conscious sedation and local anaesthetic. Occasionally deep sedation is instead delivered by an anaesthetist. Either a rigid or a 'semi-rigid' flexible thoracoscope (similar to a bronchoscope) is used, dependent on local availability. Overlap with video-assisted thoracoscopic surgery (VATS) (equipment similar, but VATS undertaken using general anaesthetic and single lung ventilation).

There needs to be an adequate space into which the thoracoscope is inserted without damaging the underlying lung. Patients suitable for thoracoscopy are therefore usually those who have an underlying pleural effusion or a pneumothorax where the lung is away from the instrument insertion site (although experts may induce a pneumothorax using a Boutin pleural needle, designed to avoid injuring the visceral pleura).

Indications and risks

Indications
- Undiagnosed pleural effusion—usually an exudate (sensitivity for malignancy >92% and tuberculosis (TB) ~100%; similar to VATS)
- Suspected mesothelioma
- Staging of pleural effusion in lung cancer
- Treatment of recurrent pleural effusions with pleurodesis
- Pneumothorax requiring chemical pleurodesis, as an alternative to surgery, e.g. patient unfit for surgical thoracoscopy.

Contraindications/proceed with caution
- Obliterated pleural space
- Mature pleural adhesions
- Bleeding disorder
- Hypoxia <92% on air or hypercapnia
- Unstable cardiovascular disease
- Persistent uncontrollable cough
- Severe obesity (thoracoscopy ports not long enough to reach pleura)
- Obstructing central airway tumour (likely to cause non-expandable lung)

Risks associated with thoracoscopy
Mortality rates low (0% for diagnostic thoracoscopies; 0.69% when talc also used—but studies included ungraded talc). Major complications <2%.
- Haemorrhage—may need diathermy in the pleural space (rare)
- Pulmonary perforations (rare)
- Air or gas embolism during pneumothorax induction (rare <0.1%)
- Local wound infection
- Empyema
- Fever, acute respiratory distress syndrome (ARDS) with talc poudrage (see ➲ p. 879)
- Port site tumour seeding.

Thoracoscopy technique

Preparation of patient and consent

- Patient should have written information >24 h before the procedure. Written consent taken by doctor performing procedure
- Check recent chest radiograph (CXR) and any computed tomography (CT) scans available
- Check full blood count (FBC), urea and electrolytes (U&E)
- Nil by mouth for solids 6 h and liquids 2 h pre-procedure
- IV cannula in arm on the same side as the thoracoscopy to make repeated sedation/analgesia administration during the procedure easy
- Premedication with analgesia, such as single doses of oral paracetamol and ibuprofen, 1 h before. Some centres give a single dose of intravenous (IV) antibiotic as infection prophylaxis (e.g. co-amoxiclav or, if allergic, vancomycin)
- Baseline O_2 saturations, pulse, blood pressure (BP), temperature. Measure oximetry throughout.

Procedure

- The patient is placed in the lateral decubitus position, with the side of the pleural effusion uppermost
- Sedation (IV midazolam) is administered and allowed time to work. O_2 (2–4 L/min) is administered via nasal cannulae
- Pleural ultrasound (US) is used to define pleural anatomy and optimize location for thoracoscope port insertion
- The skin is cleaned and local anaesthetic inserted, in the same way as for a chest drain. Aspiration of fluid or air from the pleural space confirms it is safe to proceed to thoracoscopy
- An incision is made, and a horizontal mattress suture is inserted (for wound closure post-drain removal). Blunt dissection is performed through the parietal pleura, and the port is inserted
- The pleural effusion is drained via a suction tube through the thoracoscope port. Air is simultaneously allowed to enter the pleural space through this port, and effectively a pneumothorax is created
- The thoracoscope, with its light source, can then be inserted through the port and the pleural cavity inspected followed by biopsies being taken. If required, a separate second smaller incision allows forceps or other instruments to be inserted and biopsies taken
- An opioid (e.g. IV fentanyl) is given immediately prior to taking biopsies, as these can be intensely painful
- At the end of the procedure, one port is replaced with a 24F drain, and any further ports are removed and sutures tied
- Thoracoscopic biopsies are usually large and yield good diagnostic results
- If the pleural surfaces have appearances consistent with malignancy, pleurodesis can be performed prior to removing the port, using 4–5 g talc administered using an insufflator (poudrage). Talc poudrage efficacy is at least as good as talc slurry via a chest drain, and insufflation during thoracoscopy reduces the number of procedures required. Alternatively, an indwelling pleural catheter (IPC) can be inserted at the end of the procedure. This may avoid overnight hospital stay while allowing for definitive pleural effusion management.

Post-thoracoscopy care

- Monitor O_2 saturations, pulse, BP, and temperature
- Chest drain on free drainage initially, but suction is started when bubbling stops, incrementing to −20 cmH$_2$O over 2 h, as tolerated
- Analgesia, as required, such as oral morphine 2.5–5 mg PO, codeine 30–60 mg PO, paracetamol 1 g PO
- If talc not used, may be discharged same day provided chest drain stopped bubbling and CXR satisfactory
- If being admitted, venous thromboembolism (VTE) prophylaxis with low molecular weight heparin (LMWH) (increased coagulopathy with talc pleurodesis)
- Mobile CXR the morning after thoracoscopy
- Remove chest drain when the lung is re-inflated on CXR with minimal fluid or air drainage. Trapped lung occurs if the visceral pleura is too thick to allow lung re-inflation (see ➔ p. 409).

Further information

Rahman NM et al. Local anaesthetic thoracoscopy: British Thoracic Society pleural disease guideline 2010. *Thorax* 2010;**65**(Suppl 2): ii54–ii60.

Tracheostomy

Indications and techniques 914
Complications 918

Indications and techniques

Temporary tracheostomy

Usually performed as an adjunct to assisted ventilation. Such patients are now often returned to respiratory wards for 'decannulation', with the potential for complications to occur there.

Indications

There is no uniform agreement for tracheostomy on the intensive care unit (ICU).

- Airway protection following major head and neck surgery
- Prolonged wean from the ventilator due to generalized weakness or pre-existing parenchymal lung disease
- Neurospinal indications; cervical cord injury or pathology, reduced GCS following neurological injury.

Tracheostomy may allow improved patient communication (with cuff deflation/tube fenestration), reduced sedation, possible reduction in laryngeal damage (the evidence for this is limited), facilitation of weaning.

There is no evidence for a reduced incidence of aspiration or pneumonia with tracheostomy vs endotracheal tube.

Timing of tracheostomy is individual. There is now good evidence that there is no benefit from early tracheostomy and so the decision should not be rushed.

Percutaneous vs surgical tracheostomy

Percutaneous tracheostomy (PT) can be performed on the ICU immediately once the decision is made where conventional tracheostomy requires coordination between the ICU, surgeons, and theatres. There are a variety of PT techniques; most institutes now use a single dilator technique. Position should be confirmed endoscopic verification of placement. In the Blue Rhino® system, a curved, cone-shaped dilator is slid over a guidewire and introduced into the tracheal lumen between the second and third tracheal rings until the hole is large enough to accept the required tracheostomy tube. This technique requires controlled force, although posterior tracheal wall injuries are rare. In comparing percutaneous to surgical tracheostomies, the fit of the tracheostomy tube is tighter, with less stomal infection, less post-operative haemorrhage, but the long-term complications of the two techniques are similar. This allows individual ICUs to determine which technique is preferable based on their local availability and each individual patient, as neither technique is superior overall. Humidification of the inspired gas is always required to prevent the build-up of thick viscid mucus, reducing the very serious risk of tracheostomy blockage. Humidification can only be withdrawn in long-term tracheostomy patients after several weeks or months.

Decannulation

Tracheostomy may still be required to administer intermittent ventilation, reduce ventilatory dead space, aid respiratory secretion clearance, limit aspiration (when cuffed), and bypass any upper airway obstruction. This is weighed against the consequences of a tracheostomy: increased tendency to aspirate (because of a reduced ability to swallow), reduced ability to talk, and the increased infection brought about from a foreign body in the trachea as well as bypassing the upper airway. Thus, decannulation should be carried out as soon as:

- Adequate clearance of secretions, i.e. good cough and thin secretions
- Low probability that thick mucus plugs will block off large airways and need urgent suctioning
- No upper airway obstruction
- No significant aspiration (can be checked by drinking methylene blue and then suctioning), although a small amount is not an absolute contraindication
- No need to continue ventilation or simply reduce dead space for maintenance of gas exchange
- Conversion to non-invasive ventilation (NIV), if necessary, is possible and has been demonstrated to work adequately while tracheostomy capped.

Respiratory physiotherapists can often help with these assessments. The ability to cope adequately without the tracheostomy can be repeatedly determined (and for increasing periods) by capping the tube, with the cuff fully deflated and preferably with a fenestrated tube (to maximally reduce airflow resistance). The addition of a speaking valve does not replicate the physiological challenge of decannulation, as there is still relief from a significant amount of dead space ventilation.

Once a tube has been removed, the stoma can close over very quickly, making reinsertion difficult. Introducing a 'guidewire' (over which the old tube is removed and the new can be inserted) is useful, if there is concern that reinsertion is a possibility (a thin suction tube, with the connector cut off, will suffice as a guide 'wire'); alternatively, a mini-tracheostomy can be inserted as an interim measure. The final decision to decannulate is often delayed unnecessarily. Sooner, rather than later, is usually better, as the improved swallowing, reduced aspiration, better coughing, reduced irritation, reduced chance of infection can together outweigh the apparent advantage of easy access to the airway for suction.

Available tube options
- Tracheostomy tubes can be cuffed or uncuffed.
- If ventilation is not necessary and aspiration is not a problem, cuffs are not required.
- Short-term temporary tracheostomy tubes come with a replaceable inner tube.
- Some long-term home tracheostomy tubes may not have them but a replaceable inner tube is needed in the acute setting. A replaceable inner tube allows better cleaning and therefore reduces the chance of the lumen obstructing, but the diameter of the lumen is of course less for a similar-sized external diameter.

Tracheostomy tubes can be fenestrated to allow exhalation via the larynx to aid talking. The fenestration can be closed off with a non-fenestrated inner tube, should intermittent ventilation still be required.

Speaking valves are available that fit on the tracheostomy, allowing inspiration via the tracheostomy but closing and allowing expiration via the larynx (if cuff down and/or fenestration open!). They effectively still reduce dead space, maintain access for suctioning, but allow talking.

In the very obese, tracheostomy tubes are often too short and too curved to cope with the increased distance between skin and trachea; tubes with adjustable flanges that allow customized intra-tracheal lengths are useful here.

Complications

- *Displacement or obstruction* Evidenced by failing gas exchange, unexpected ventilator pressures; patient may be able to talk despite cuff inflated. If available, use capnography to detect oscillating $FiCO_2$ and determine if obstructed or not. Remove inner tube, and check for secretion build-up. Try passing suction catheter. Fibre-optic inspection. Removal and reinsertion, using fibrescope as guide, to ensure correct placement
- *Infection* Early or late. Good stoma care should prevent this
- *Bleeding* Local erosion at entry site, damage from vigorous suctioning; more seriously, erosion by tracheostomy tip or high-pressure balloon cuff, rarely into the innominate artery which lies anteriorly.

Further information

Commercial video of Cook/Ciaglia Blue Rhino insertion. ℘ https://www.cookmedical.com/products/cc_ptis_webds/

McGrath BA et al. Multidisciplinary guidelines for the management of tracheostomy and laryngectomy airway emergencies. *Anaesthesia* 2012;**67**: 1025–1041.

Royal College of Anaesthetists recommendations on tracheostomy displacement. ℘ http://www.rcoa.ac.uk/document-store/nap4-section-3-appendices (Appendix 2, p. 205).

Young D et al. Effect of early versus late tracheostomy placement on survival in patients receiving mechanical ventilation: the TracMan randomized trial. *JAMA* 2013;**309**: 2121–2129.

Grant CA et al. Tracheo-innominate artery fistula after percutaneous tracheostomy: three case reports and a clinical review. *Br J Anaesth* 2006;**96**: 127–131.

Appendices

A1 Blood gases and acid–base balance *921*

A2 BMI calculator *935*

A3 CT anatomy of the thorax *937*

A4 CT patterns of lung disease *945*

A5 Drugs used for bronchoscopy and sedation *957*

A6 Lung function and cardiopulmonary exercise testing *963*

A7 Plain radiograph *979*

A8 Radiological investigations and radiation exposure *983*

A9 Useful websites *987*

Blood gases and acid–base balance

Interpretation of ABGs 1 922
Interpretation of ABGs 2 924
Use of A–a gradient diagram: examples 926
Acid–base balance 928
Conversion between arterial O_2 saturation and O_2 tension
  (Hb dissociation curve) 932

Interpretation of ABGs 1

Normal ranges

Breathing air: PaO_2 >12 kPa (>10 in normal elderly), $PaCO_2$ 4.6–5.9 kPa.

How to take

- **ABGs** Best taken from radial, rather than brachial, artery due to dual radial/ulnar supply to hand. Use a heparinized syringe; analyse immediately or within 30 min if kept on ice.

  Always record date, time, and the % inspired O_2.
- **Arterialized capillary sample** An underused technique. Uses small glass pre-heparinized tube to draw up blood from a lancet puncture on the **bottom end** of the ear lobe. Blood gas machine must take microsamples (most do). $PaCO_2$ levels are accurate enough for clinical practice, but good arterialization, with rubefacients (Algipan/Deep Heat) or heat and vigorous rubbing, are required for an accurate PaO_2; the latter is less important, as oxygenation can be assessed by oximetry. Can easily be performed by nursing staff to monitor response to NIV and O_2 therapy.

The three main things blood gases tell you about gas exchange
- How is the patient ventilating their alveoli? This is derived from the $PaCO_2$. $PaCO_2$ ≥6 kPa ≈ underventilating, $PaCO_2$ ≤4.5 kPa ≈ overventilating
- Is the PaO_2 high enough to adequately oxygenate tissues and prevent anaerobic metabolism? PaO_2 >6 kPa (SaO_2 ≈ 80%) is probably adequate; PaO_2 >7 kPa (SaO_2 >87%) is definitely adequate
- Is there evidence of ventilation-perfusion (V/Q) mismatch? Evidence of low V/Q units is derived from the calculated A–a O_2 gradient.

The two main things blood gases tell you about acid–base balance
(see section Acid–base balance)
- What is the respiratory component to an abnormal pH? This is derived from the $PaCO_2$
- What is the metabolic component to an abnormal pH? This is derived from the standard base excess/deficit.

The A–a gradient calculator graph sets out the graphical representation of gas exchange

(see Fig. A1.1)
- Point ① = pO_2 and pCO_2 (virtually zero) of **inspired air** (atmospheric pressure ≈ 100 kPa; air is 21% O_2, and air is slightly 'diluted' by water vapour pressure (7 kPa) following humidification by upper airways). 21% of 100–7 = 20 kPa. (Point ② = pO_2 and pCO_2 when breathing 24% O_2 via a Ventimask, and point ③ = pO_2 and pCO_2 when breathing 28% O_2 via a Ventimask.)
- Point ④ = theoretical pO_2/pCO_2 of **alveolar gas** when breathing air, if all the O_2 removed and replaced by CO_2 (equivalent to extreme hypoventilation and impossible!), when the respiratory quotient (RQ = CO_2 produced/O_2 consumed) is 0.8 (usual value)

- The line between ① and ④, with a gradient of 0.8, describes all possible combinations of alveolar gas, towards ① if ventilating more and towards ④ if ventilating less, called the *alveolar air line*
- Point ⑤ = area in which PaO_2 and $PaCO_2$ of *arterial blood* sit normally. If lungs are perfect gas exchangers, then blood leaving the lungs and entering systemic arterial circulation (⑤) should be perfectly equilibrated with the alveolar gas (A).

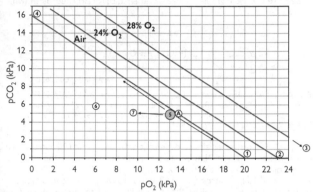

Fig. A1.1 pCO_2 vs pO_2: alveolar air lines and A–a gradient calculator.

- However, the *mixed venous point* = ⑥ (or the *pulmonary arterial* blood) is well to the left of the alveolar air line. This is because capillary PO_2 falls more kPa than the PCO_2 rises during gas exchange in the tissues (CO_2 solubility curve is steeper than PaO_2–SaO_2 solubility, or dissociation, curve)
- Thus, if the lungs fail to oxygenate returning mixed venous/pulmonary arterial blood properly (e.g. area of consolidation, or low V/Q due to asthma/chronic obstructive pulmonary disease (COPD)), then it is as if mixed venous blood has bypassed the lung and 'leaked' into the arterial blood, which therefore drags the eventual arterial PaO_2/$PaCO_2$ point to the left of the alveolar air line, e.g. point ⑦.

Interpretation of ABGs 2

- The horizontal distance between the actual arterial point and the 'ideal' alveolar air line (e.g. ⑤ minus ⑦, 3.5 kPa) is called the **alveolar to arterial (A–a) gradient** and is a measure of how efficiently mixed venous blood is equilibrated with alveolar gas, i.e. it is a measure of V/Q mismatch, right-to-left shunts, and very severe lung fibrosis (through reduced diffusion across the alveolar capillary membrane). As well as being read off the graph, it can be mathematically calculated, as shown in Fig. A1.2.

$$\text{Arterial } PO_2 \quad \text{Arterial } PCO_2$$

$$A - a \text{ gradient} = PIO_2 - \left(PaO_2 + \frac{PaCO_2}{0.8} \right)$$

Inspired PO_2 Respiratory quotient

Fig. A1.2 Calculation of inspired PO_2 breathing air, 24 or 28% O_2. **Air**, 21% of $(100 - 7) \approx 20$ kPa (where 100 kPa is atmospheric pressure, and 7 kPa is water vapour pressure due to the inspired air being humidified); **24%**, 24% of $(100 - 7) \approx$ 23 kPa; **28%**, 28% of $(100 - 7) \approx 26$ kPa.

In Fig. A1.1, the alveolar air line depends on the % inspired O_2, and the two extra lines for 24% and 28% O_2 are shown. In the calculation, the PIO_2 has to be adjusted accordingly (see Fig. A1.2).

In normal lungs, matching of V/Q is not totally perfect due to relative underperfusion of the apices and overperfusion of the bases (gravity effects on pulmonary arterial blood flow, not fully compensated for by hypoxic vasoconstriction of pulmonary arterioles). These imperfections in V/Q and direct drainage of some of the cardiac muscle venous blood into the left ventricular (LV) cavity, and hence systemic arterial circulation, lead to a small A–a gradient, 1–2 kPa in the young and middle-aged and 2–3 kPa in the elderly. Figures in excess of these values are abnormal and indicate areas of low V/Q or increased shunt.

Use of A–a gradient diagram: examples

Case 1

Consider point W in the pO_2–pCO_2 graph (see Fig. A1.3), the blood gases on air of a young non-smoker complaining of chest pain 7 days post-operatively. The PaO_2 of 13 is normal. Does this reassure you or does it provide supporting evidence for a PE? Ask the following questions:
- How much is the patient ventilating? $PaCO_2 \approx 2$; therefore ≤ 4.5 kPa and indicates hyperventilation
- Is the patient adequately oxygenated? $PaO_2 > 7$ kPa; therefore OK
- Is there an abnormal A–a gradient? Read off graph, horizontal line between W and alveolar line, or calculate:

$$20 - [13 + (2/0.8)] \approx 4.5 \text{ kPa}$$

>2 kPa, hence yes; therefore, the V/Q matching is not normal.

This provides supporting evidence for a PE but could just as well be due to consolidation from pneumonia, for example.
- *Remember*: PaO_2 cannot be used to assess V/Q matching in the lung without an associated $PaCO_2$ to tell you 'what the PaO_2 ought to be'.

Case 2

Consider point X on the pO_2–pCO_2 graph (see Fig. A1.3). These are the gases on air from a young man following an overdose of methadone.
- How much is the patient ventilating? $PaCO_2 \approx 11$; therefore ≥ 6 kPa and indicates hypoventilation
- Is the patient adequately oxygenated? PaO_2 only 6 kPa; therefore, it is not enough and he needs extra O_2
- Has the patient got an elevated A–a gradient?

$$20 - [6 + (11/0.8)] \approx 0.8 \text{ kPa}$$

<2 kPa, hence no; therefore, there is nothing wrong with the lungs, despite the abnormal gases; this represents pure hypoventilation.

After a messy stomach washout, he is sent to the ward and 24 h later is febrile. Gases on **24%** O_2 are point Y on the graph; thus, both $PaCO_2$ and PaO_2 are better.
- How much is the patient ventilating? $PaCO_2$ just ≥ 6 kPa; therefore, he is still hypoventilating a bit
- Is the patient adequately oxygenated? $PaO_2 > 7$ kPa; therefore, he is adequately oxygenated
- Has the patient got an A–a gradient?

$$23 - [11 + (6.5/0.8)] \approx 4.2 \text{ kPa}$$

(remember, the PIO_2 is 23 kPa, because he is on **24%** O_2.)

>2 kPa, hence yes; therefore, he may have developed an aspiration pneumonia.

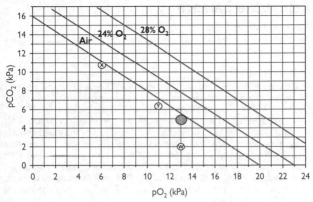

Fig. A1.3 Examples of using A–a gradient.

Three things blood gases tell you about gas exchange
- How much is the patient ventilating their alveoli?—$PaCO_2$
- Is the PaO_2 high enough to adequately oxygenate tissues and thus prevent anaerobic metabolism?
- Is there any evidence of a V/Q mismatch, assessed from the A–a gradient for O_2?

Acid–base balance

Normal ranges

pH 7.37–7.43 (H^+ 37–43 nmol/L), $PaCO_2$ 4.7–5.9 kPa, base excess ± 3 mmol/L.

Interpretation

Acid–base relationships are best plotted as a $PaCO_2$ vs pH graph, because these are the two 1° measurements made by a blood gas machine (everything else to do with acid–base balance is calculated). This is shown in Fig. A1.4.

Normal acid–base is the area labelled N, the pH between 7.37 and 7.43, the $PaCO_2$ around 5 kPa. As ventilation is decreased or increased ($PaCO_2$ going up or down, respectively), the pH will change, the amount depending on the buffering capacity of the blood (CO_2 is an acid gas, combining with water to give $[H^+]$ and $[HCO_3^-]$ ions). Without buffering, the pH would fall disastrously following small rises in $PaCO_2$. This buffering capacity depends mainly on Hb and other proteins, producing the normal buffer line running through N on the graph.

Therefore, **acute hypoventilation and hyperventilation** will move the patient up and down this line, in the direction *b* or *c*, respectively. If the **hypoventilation** at point *b* becomes **chronic** (e.g. as it may in COPD), then the kidney retains bicarbonate (by excreting $[H^+]$) to try and correct the pH towards normal, and the patient moves onto a new $[HCO_3^-]$ buffer line displaced to the right, e.g. the one labelled +10 meq/L (35 meq/L). The degree of displacement represents the **metabolic component to the acid–base status** and, in this case, because the $[HCO_3^-]$ has risen, will be higher than the normal figure of about 25 meq/L. When the raised figure is quoted relative to the normal 25 meq/L (by subtracting 25), this is called the **base excess**. Thus, buffer lines to the right of the normal buffer line represent a metabolic alkalosis or base excess.

These figures are calculated, assuming a normal or 'standard' $PaCO_2$, called the 'standard bicarbonate' (SBC on the blood gas machine printout) or 'standard base excess' (usually BE). The other similar figures on some printouts (usually HCO_3^- and TCO_2) are calculated at the patient's actual $PaCO_2$ and are not much use.

Chronic hyperventilation (e.g. at altitude due to the hypoxia) produces the opposite, a resorption of $[H^+]$ by the kidney, and the buffer line shifts to the left, giving a negative value for the 'base excess', a **base deficit**. Thus, a metabolic acidosis compensates for a respiratory alkalosis. Note that these corrections rarely bring the pH back to normal, as there needs to be an error signal to keep the correction process going.

A **metabolic acidosis** (such as in ketoacidosis) will also move the line to the left (*a*), producing a base deficit (or negative base excess), followed by hyperventilation to try and correct it (i.e. a respiratory alkalosis to correct a metabolic acidosis). This pure ventilatory stimulation in the absence of abnormal lungs often produces deep breathing, with little increase in rate, and is called **Kussmaul's breathing**. Thus, lines to the left of the normal buffer line represent a metabolic acidosis or base deficit.

Important point A metabolic acidosis, e.g. due to anaerobic metabolism (and hence lactic acid production), can reverse the compensatory metabolic alkalosis 2° to chronic hypercapnia, e.g. during a COPD exacerbation with severe hypoxia, thus removing the 'evidence' for previous chronic CO_2 retention.

Finally, a **metabolic alkalosis**, e.g. during hypokalaemia (when the kidney is forced to use [H⁺], instead of [K⁺], to swap for the sodium that needs resorbing from the tubular fluid), moves the buffer line to the right (*d*) but with only limited hypoventilation available to compensate, due to the inevitable ventilatory stimulation the attendant hypoxaemia produces.

Thus, the mixture of respiratory and metabolic contributions to a patient's acid–base disturbance can be established by plotting the PaCO₂ and pH on the graph.

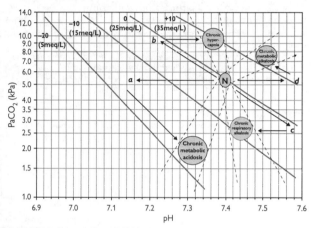

Fig. A1.4 Acid–base balance: PaCO2–pH.

Lines running top left to bottom right are the iso-bicarbonate lines labelled as absolute [HCO₃⁻] (in brackets) or as a base excess/deficit (relative to a [HCO₃⁻] of 25meq/L), hence can be – (metabolic acidosis) or + (metabolic alkalosis).

Anion gap

The anion gap [(Na⁺ + K⁺) – (Cl⁻ + HCO₃⁻)] shows the amount of other anions, apart from [Cl⁻] and [HCO₃⁻], that exists and helps differentiate the cause of any metabolic acidosis. Depending on methods of measurement, the normal value is between 8 and 16 mmol/L (or meq/L) and mainly due to albumin. High anion gap indicates loss of [HCO₃⁻] without a subsequent increase in [Cl⁻]. Electroneutrality is maintained by increase in anions such as ketones, lactate, [PO₄⁻], and [SO₄⁻]. Because these anions are not part of the anion gap calculation, the result is a high anion gap.

An acidosis with a normal anion gap will be a simple HCO₃⁻/Cl⁻ exchange such as might occur, e.g. in:
• Renal tubular acidosis
• Acetazolamide therapy
• [HCO₃⁻] loss from profuse diarrhoea.

An anion gap is likely to be present, e.g. when the metabolic acidosis is due to:

- Diabetes, starvation, or alcohol-induced ketoacidosis (ketones are acids)
- Renal failure (although can be in the normal range, too)
- Lactic acidosis
- Salicylate poisoning
- Methanol poisoning
- Ethylene glycol (antifreeze) poisoning.

Three things arterial samples tell you about acid–base balance
- Is there a ventilatory/respiratory component from an abnormally high or low $PaCO_2$?
- Is there a metabolic component evidenced by a shift of the buffer line to the left or right, numerically the base excess (or deficit)?
- If there is a metabolic acidosis, is there an increased anion gap?

Further information
Williams AJ. Assessing and interpreting arterial blood gases and acid-base balance. *BMJ* 1998;**317**: 1213.

Conversion between arterial O₂ saturation and O₂ tension (Hb dissociation curve)

See Fig. A1.5 and Table A1.1.

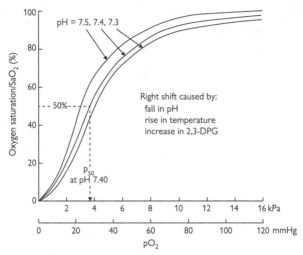

Fig. A1.5 Hb dissociation curve.

A *fall in pH* (more acidotic) or a rise in **body temperature** will move the dissociation curve to the **right**. This has the effect of making the **PaO2 higher for any given SaO2**, e.g. at pH 7.20, a measured saturation (e.g. by oximetry) of 90% is equivalent to a higher PaO₂ of 9.7 kPa (73 mmHg) than the usual 7.7 kPa (58 mmHg); a rise in body temperature to 41°C will do the same, and the effects of pH and temperature are additive.

Conversely, for a given PaO₂, pyrexia and acidosis will **lower the SaO2** and thus O₂ carriage to the tissues. A PaO₂ of 7.7 kPa (58 mmHg) will normally give an SaO₂ of 90%, but, if the temperature rises to 41°C and pH falls to 7.20, then the SaO₂ falls to 70%.

Increasing 2,3-DPG levels shift the curve to the right, but levels fluctuate unpredictably and any changes are small.

Changes in body temperature are often the reason why measured pulse oximetry saturations apparently 'do not agree' with the measured blood gases (pH is taken into account in the **theoretical** calculation of SaO₂ by blood gas analysers, but the patient's correct body temperature is rarely entered and thus is not taken into account). This is particularly important in hypothermia when the curve is left-shifted, leading to impaired O₂ unloading. Furthermore, an apparently adequate oximetry reading can mask a low PaO₂, which will further lessen O₂ availability to the tissues (although somewhat mitigated by the reduced metabolic rate of hypothermic tissues).

Table A1.1 Conversion chart*

% saturation	kPa	mmHg
98	15.0	112
97	12.2	92
96	10.8	81
95	9.9	74
94	9.3	70
93	8.8	66
92	8.4	63
91	8.1	60
90	7.7	58
88	7.3	55
86	6.8	51
84	6.5	49
82	6.2	47
80	5.9	45
75	5.4	40
70	1.9	37
65	4.5	34
60	4.2	31
55	3.8	29
50	3.5	27

* Assumes a normal position of the Hb dissociation curve; kPa and mmHg conversion factor: $7.5 \times$ kPa $\approx$ mmHg.

Appendix 2

BMI calculator

For BMI calculator, see Fig. A2.1.

BMI = weight in kilograms, divided by height in metres squared.

For example, for a 70 kg man who is 1.8 m tall:

$$BMI = 70/(1.8 \times 1.8) = 21.6$$

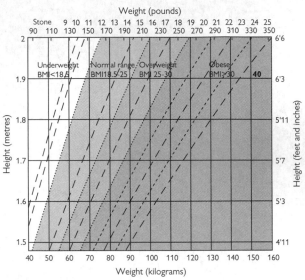

Fig. A2.1 BMI calculator.

CT anatomy of the thorax

Level of C7 *938*
Level of T2 *939*
Level of T4 *940*
Level of T6 *941*
Level of T7 *942*
Level of T9 *943*

These are **not** standard images set for mediastinal or lung viewing but have been adjusted to aid anatomical labelling (see Fig. A3.1 to Fig. A3.6).

NB: Contrast was used to highlight the vessels.

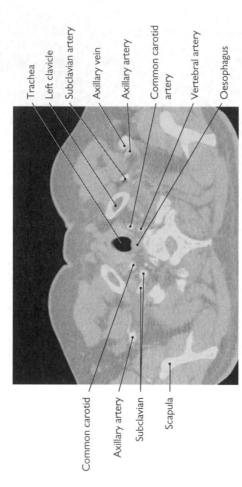

Fig. A3.1 CT anatomy of the thorax: level of C7.

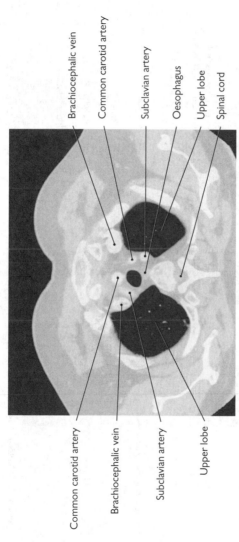

Fig. A3.2 CT anatomy of the thorax: level of T2.

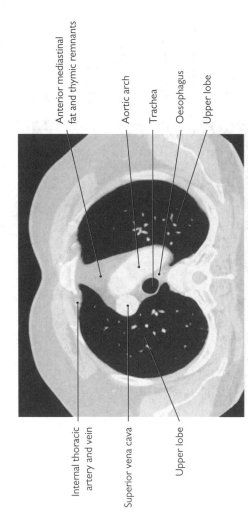

Anterior mediastinal
fat and thymic remnants

Aortic arch

Trachea

Oesophagus

Upper lobe

Internal thoracic
artery and vein

Superior vena cava

Upper lobe

Fig. A3.3 CT anatomy of the thorax: level of T4.

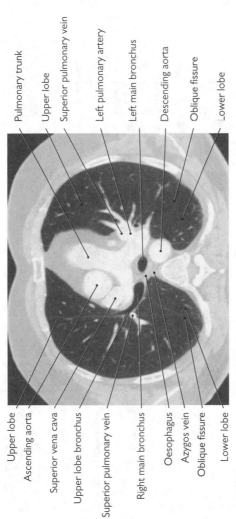

Pulmonary trunk
Upper lobe
Superior pulmonary vein
Left pulmonary artery
Left main bronchus
Descending aorta
Oblique fissure
Lower lobe

Upper lobe
Ascending aorta
Superior vena cava
Upper lobe bronchus
Superior pulmonary vein
Right main bronchus
Oesophagus
Azygos vein
Oblique fissure
Lower lobe

Fig. A3.4 CT anatomy of the thorax: level of T6.

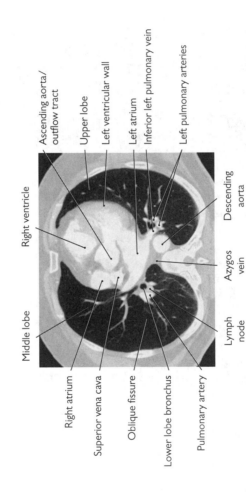

Fig. A3.5 CT anatomy of the thorax: level of T7.

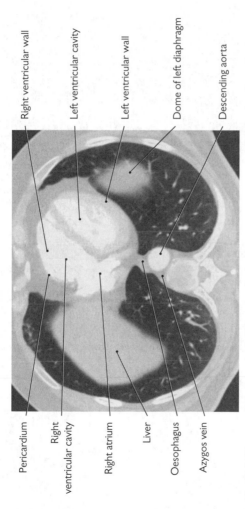

Right ventricular wall

Left ventricular cavity

Left ventricular wall

Dome of left diaphragm

Descending aorta

Pericardium

Right ventricular cavity

Right atrium

Liver

Oesophagus

Azygos vein

Fig. A3.6 CT anatomy of the thorax: level of T9.

CT patterns of lung disease

Airspace consolidation 946
Air trapping 947
Cystic airspaces 948
Fissural, bronchovascular, and subpleural nodularity 949
Ground-glass shadowing 950
Honeycomb lung 951
Mosaic attenuation pattern 952
Nodularity 953
Poorly defined centrilobular nodules 954
Reticular (or linear) pattern 955
Tree in bud 956

Airspace consolidation

Process	Causes
Fluid/secretion accumulation in alveoli	Pneumonia, pulmonary oedema, or haemorrhage, acute respiratory distress syndrome (ARDS), cryptogenic organizing pneumonia (COP), eosinophilic pneumonia, drugs, lung adenocarcinoma, lymphoma

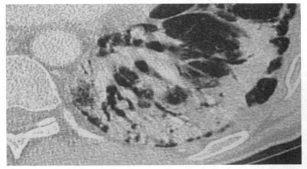

Fig. A4.1 Cryptogenic organizing pneumonia (COP). Air bronchograms clearly present.

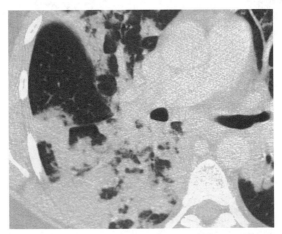

Fig. A4.2 Extensive airspace consolidation due to eosinophilic pneumonia.

Air trapping

Process	Causes
Partial small airway obstruction	Asthma, obliterative bronchiolitis, chronic obstructive pulmonary disease (COPD)

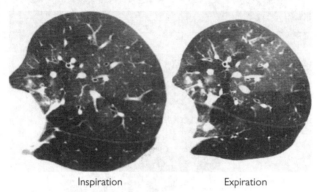

Inspiration   Expiration

Fig. A4.3 Air trapping.

Subject prone. There is a mosaic pattern, with geographical regions of varying density. On expiration, the denser area becomes more dense, indicating that portion of the lung has deflated; other parts of the lung remain lucent, indicating that air is trapped behind narrowed airways.

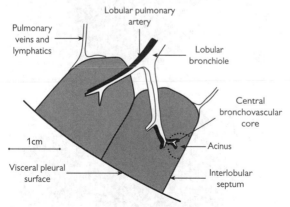

Fig. A4.4 Structure of two 2° pulmonary lobules abutting the pleural surface.

The 2° pulmonary lobule is the smallest anatomical area visible on CT. Tree-in-bud appearance will be in the acinus around the central bronchovascular core. Reticular patterns will be centred on the interlobular septae and/or draining lymphatics. Mosaic patterns and air trapping will tend to follow outlines of the lobule or sets of lobules.

Cystic airspaces

Process	Causes
Clearly defined air-containing space with definable wall	Lymphangioleiomyomatosis (LAM), Langerhans cell histiocytosis (LCH), end-stage usual interstitial pneumonia (UIP), Pneumocystis pneumonia (PCP), lymphoid interstitial pneumonia (LIP), septic emboli

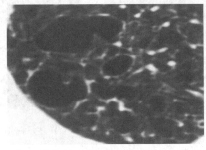

Fig. A4.5 Langerhans cell histiocytosis (LCH).
Walls are thin, but more pronounced, irregular, and widely spread than emphysematous holes.

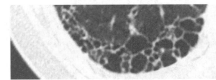

Fig. A4.6 Peripheral cysts (honeycombing) of usual interstitial pneumonia (UIP).
Characteristic subpleural distribution.

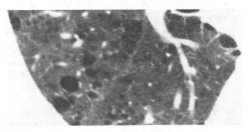

Fig. A4.7 Holes in the lungs due to emphysema.
No real 'walls'. Centrilobular vessels are often visible within the holes, which are not seen in true cysts.

Fissural, bronchovascular, and subpleural nodularity

Process	Causes
Nodules seen along the pulmonary fissures, along the bronchovascular bundles, and subpleurally	Sarcoidosis. Also described in Kaposi's sarcoma

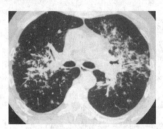

Fig. A4.8 Perihilar and bronchovascular distribution of nodularity in sarcoidosis.

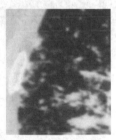

Fig. A4.9 Subpleural nodules in sarcoidosis.

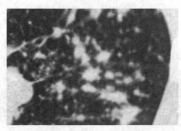

Fig. A4.10 Irregular/nodular thickening of fissures and bronchovascular bundles in sarcoidosis.

Ground-glass shadowing

Process	Causes
Grey appearance to lung interstitium; air in bronchus looks blacker	Parenchymal inflammatory conditions such as sarcoidosis, idiopathic interstitial pneumonias (IIPs), hypersensitivity pneumonitis (HP), pulmonary oedema or haemorrhage, PCP, alveolar proteinosis, drug/radiation injury

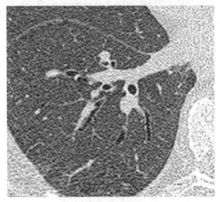

Fig. A4.11 Subtle diffuse ground-glass shadowing in subacute hypersensitivity pneumonitis (HP).

Note the 'black bronchus sign' where air in the bronchus looks blacker than the lung parenchyma (which is of increased density).

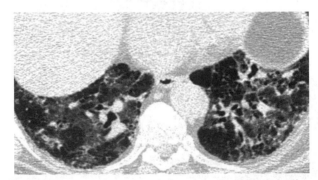

Fig. A4.12 More marked ground-glass shadowing in a patient with known usual interstitial pneumonia (UIP) pattern of interstitial lung disease (ILD) who has developed an acute exacerbation of idiopathic pulmonary fibrosis (IPF).

There is also very early honeycombing and traction bronchial dilatation (bronchiectasis).

Honeycomb lung

Process	Causes
End-stage fibrotic lung	Usual interstitial pneumonia (UIP), asbestosis

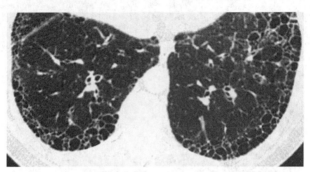

Fig. A4.13 Honeycombing in usual interstitial pneumonia (UIP). Usually mainly peripheral.

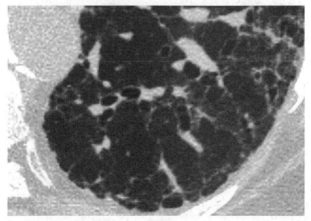

Fig. A4.14 More subtle honeycombing at the lung periphery with other features of usual interstitial pneumonia (UIP).

Traction bronchial dilatation due to surrounding lung fibrosis and a reticular pattern beginning to outline the 2° pulmonary lobule.

Mosaic attenuation pattern

Process	Causes
Well-defined areas of normal lung abutting abnormal lung, giving a mosaic pattern. If the pattern is accentuated in expiration, this indicates small airways disease	Small airways disease, such as asthma, bronchiectasis, bronchiolitis, and HP. Vascular disease, such as pulmonary embolus (PE), pulmonary hypertension (PHT). Causes of ground glass attenuation can cause a mosaic pattern when patchy

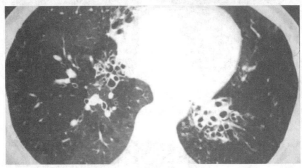

Fig. A4.15 Bronchiectasis with small airways disease that is causing the mosaic pattern.

In addition, there are markedly bronchiectatic airways in the left lower lobe, with considerable airway crowding due to distal lung collapse.

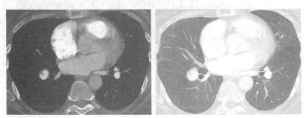

Fig. A4.16 Computed tomography (CT) demonstrating chronic pulmonary emboli (PEs) and consequent mosaic attenuation.

Whiter lung represents normally-perfused lung, while black areas represent hypoperfusion.

Nodularity

Process	Causes
Small discrete dots 1–10 mm, may be in airspaces or interstitium	Metastases, sarcoidosis, pneumoconiosis, hypersensitivity pneumonitis (HP), miliary tuberculosis (TB), fungal infection, idiopathic pulmonary haemorrhage, alveolar microlithiasis, varicella pneumonitis

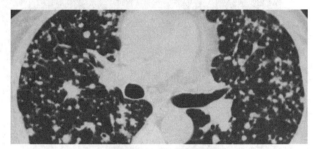

Fig. A4.17 Multiple dense nodules of varying size due to metastases.

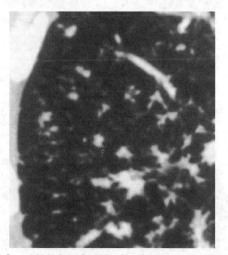

Fig. A4.18 Sarcoid. Multiple small nodules throughout lung but usually associated with other features of sarcoid such as fissural nodularity and bilateral hilar node enlargement.

Poorly defined centrilobular nodules

Process	Causes
Peribronchiolar inflammation in the absence of intraluminal secretion	HP, respiratory bronchiolitis-associated interstitial lung disease (RB-ILD)

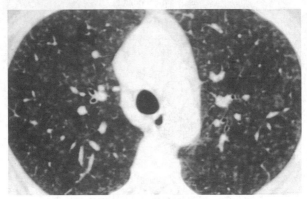

Fig. A4.19 Soft centrilobular nodularity due to hypersensitivity pneumonitis (HP) (previously called extrinsic allergic alveolitis, EAA).

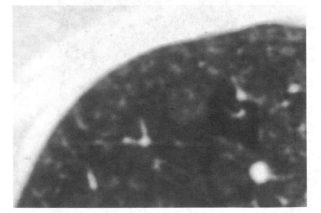

Fig. A4.20 Another example of HP, enlarged to show position of soft nodules in the centre of the 2° pulmonary lobules.

Reticular (or linear) pattern

Process	Causes
Linear fine lines, indicating thickened interlobular septa. Subpleural reticulation	Interstitial lung disease (ILD) (e.g. usual interstitial pneumonia (UIP), asbestosis), pulmonary oedema, drug-induced fibrosis, pulmonary haemorrhage, lymphangitis

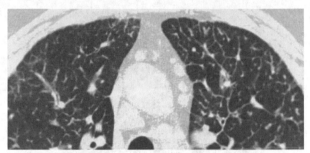

Fig. A4.21 Lymphangitis carcinomatosis. Infiltrated lymphatics widen and thicken the interlobular septa.

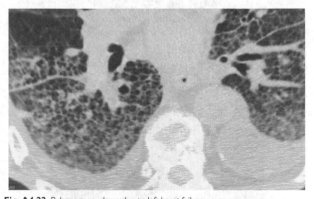

Fig. A4.22 Pulmonary oedema due to left heart failure.

Fluid-distended lymphatics outlining the 2° pulmonary lobules. Worse in dependent areas. Fluid in the fissures, bilateral pleural effusions, and some airspace filling with pulmonary oedema.

Tree in bud

Process	Causes
Mucus/pus/secretions filling bronchioles and causing dilatation	Small airways disease, particularly infection, including mycobacteria, *Haemophilus influenzae*, diffuse pan-bronchiolitis, cystic fibrosis (CF), yellow nail syndrome, 1° pulmonary lymphoma

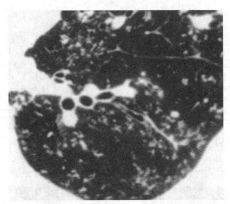

Fig. A4.23 Extensive tree-in-bud appearance in the left lower lobe from opportunistic mycobacterial disease.

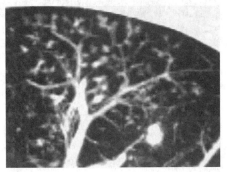

Fig. A4.24 Tree-in-bud appearance, enhanced by a post-processing technique called 'maximum intensity projection'.

Effectively, this squashes denser structures from several thin cuts into one, allowing branching structures to be viewed in their entirety.

Drugs used for bronchoscopy and sedation

Table A5.1 Commonly used drugs for sedation and bronchoscopy (continued on p. 959).

Drug	Dose	Pharmacology	Side effects
Midazolam	Slow IV injection—maximum rate 2 mg/min Initial dose: 2–2.5 mg (0.5–1 mg in the frail or elderly) given 5–10 min before procedure Supplemental doses, if required: 1mg (0.5–1 mg in frail or elderly), at 2–10 min intervals Usual maximum total dose: 3.5–7 mg (3.5 mg in frail or elderly) for standard bronchoscopic procedures. May be higher in longer procedures	Onset within 2 min, with maximum effect at 5–10 min (may be longer in frail or elderly or those with chronic illnesses) Duration of action variable, but typical range is 30–120 min Approximate half-life 1.5–2.5 h	Respiratory depression, apnoea, bronchospasm, laryngospasm, hypotension, heart rate alterations, cardiac arrest Life-threatening side effects and prolonged sedation are more likely in the elderly and those with impaired respiratory or cardiovascular status, hepatic impairment, renal impairment, myasthenia gravis, and with rapid IV injection
Fentanyl	Slow IV injection—usually over 1–3 min Initial dose: 25 micrograms Supplemental doses, if required: 25 micrograms Usual maximum total dose: 50 micrograms	Onset almost immediate, with maximum effect at 5 min Duration of action variable, but typical range is 30–60 min Approximate half-life 2–7 h	Nausea, vomiting, and other GI upset, myoclonic movements, respiratory depression, apnoea, bronchospasm, laryngospasm, hypo/hypertension, arrhythmia, cardiac arrest Caution in elderly patients and those with impaired respiratory or cardiovascular status, hepatic impairment, and myasthenia gravis

Alfentanil	Slow IV injection—usually over 30 s Initial dose: 250 micrograms Supplemental doses, if required: 250 micrograms Usual maximum total dose: 500 micrograms	Onset almost immediate onset and maximum effect Duration of action variable, but usually shorter than fentanyl Approximate half-life 1–2 h	See Fentanyl
Lidocaine (during bronchoscopy)	*Intranasal* Lidocaine 2% gel: 6 mL (120 mg) *Oropharynx* Lidocaine 10% spray: three actuations (30 mg) *Vocal cords, tracheobronchial tree* Lidocaine 1% solution: 2 mL boluses applied topically, as required Use minimum dose to achieve effective cough suppression and patient comfort. Subjective symptoms of lidocaine toxicity are common when ≥9.6 mg/kg is used; much lower doses are usually sufficient	Onset 3–5 min. Common mistake not to wait long enough for maximal effect, leading to unnecessary extra doses Duration of action variable, but typical range is 60–90 min Approximate half-life 1.5–2 h	CNS effects (confusion, blurred vision, dizziness, drowsiness, light-headedness, myoclonus, nausea, nystagmus, paraesthesiae, restlessness, tremulousness, coma, convulsions, respiratory failure) CVS effects (hypotension, bradycardia, arrhythmia, cardiac arrest) Methaemoglobinaemia (rare) Caution in those with hepatic and cardiac dysfunction, and with significant renal impairment
Adrenaline (during bronchoscopy)	Topical Adrenaline 1:10,000: 2–10 mL		Hypertension, tachycardia, arrhythmia, tremor

Adapted from British Thoracic Society guideline for diagnostic flexible bronchoscopy in adults. *Thorax* 2013;68:i1–i44, with permission from BMJ

Table A5.2 Antagonists available for sedative drugs

Drug	Dose	Pharmacology	Side effects
Flumazenil	To reverse midazolam Initial dose: 200 micrograms IV over 15 s Supplemental doses: 100 micrograms every 60 s if inadequate response Typical cumulative dose range: 300–600 micrograms Maximum total dose: 1 mg Note—when combined midazolam-opioid sedation used and reversal required, use flumazenil first (unless large dose of opioid given)	Onset 1min Duration of action 1–4 h Approximate half-life 40–80 min Duration of action may be shorter than midazolam → care to ensure sedation does not recur	Nausea, vomiting, anxiety, agitation, dizziness, hypertension, tachycardia May lower seizure threshold May cause withdrawal in chronic benzodiazepine users
Naloxone	To reverse opioids Initial dose: 100–200 micrograms IV Supplemental dose: 100 micrograms every 2 min, if inadequate response	Onset 2–3 min Duration of action 45 min to 4 h Approximate half-life 1–1.5 h Duration of action may be shorter than opioid → care to ensure sedation does not recur	Nausea, vomiting, dizziness, headache, tachycardia, hypo/hypertension May cause withdrawal in chronic opioid users

Adapted from BTS guideline for diagnostic flexible bronchoscopy in adults with permission.

Further information

Du Rand IA et al. British Thoracic Society guideline for diagnostic flexible bronchoscopy in adults. Thorax 2013;**68**: i1–i44.

Lung function and cardiopulmonary exercise testing

Flow–volume loop 1 *964*
Flow–volume loop 2 *966*
Spirometry and peak flow *968*
Lung volumes *970*
Gas transfer *972*
Respiratory muscle function *973*
Predicted values and peak flow reference ranges *974*
Cardiopulmonary exercise testing (CPET) *976*

Flow–volume loop 1

A good start to understanding lung function tests is the forced flow–volume loop (see Fig. A6.1). This plots inspiratory and expiratory flow against lung volume during a maximal expiratory and maximal inspiratory manoeuvre.

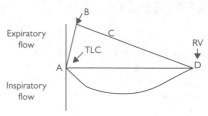

Fig. A6.1 Flow–volume loop.

At the beginning of **expiration** from a full breath in, the expiratory muscles are at their strongest, the lungs at their largest, and hence the airways are at their most open (A). Because the lungs are at their largest, the radial attachments to the airways, effectively the alveolar/capillary membranes and their connective tissue, are pulling the hardest and supporting the airways against **dynamic compression** during the exhalation manoeuvre.

This means that the highest flow rates are possible at the beginning of the blow, hence the sudden rise to a **PEFR** in the first 100 ms or so of the forced breath out (B). This is the **peak flow** and is essentially what a peak flow meter measures (see Fig A6.5).

As the lung empties and the lung volume drops, the dilatory pull on the airways from the radial attachments of the surrounding lung tissue reduces (C). Hence, the airways narrow and become less supported and are less able to resist dynamic compression. This means that the maximal airflow obtainable, regardless of effort, falls too.

Eventually, the expiratory muscles come to the end of their 'travel' and cannot squeeze the chest anymore. Also, increasingly with age, the small airways may actually close off, preventing any more emptying (D). The volume at which this begins to happen is called the **closing volume**.

As maximal **inspiration** starts, although the inspiratory muscles are at their strongest, the airways are at their smallest. Thus, flow rates start low and increase as the airways open up. However, as the lung expands, the inspiratory muscles are approaching the end of their 'travel' and are weakening; this means the flow rates fall again, hence the different rounded appearance of the inspiratory limb of the flow–volume curve.

Thus, normally, the inspiratory and expiratory flow rates depend on lung volume and are termed 'volume-dependent'. If there is a **fixed upper airway narrowing**, such as from a solid hard tumour partially blocking the trachea, then the size of the airway at this point may become so narrow that it now limits maximal flows. However, its diameter will **vary very little** with lung volumes, and hence flow will become 'volume-independent'. Fig. A6.2 shows this.

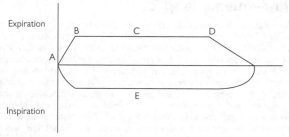

Fig. A6.2 Volume-independent flow.

At (A), the rise in flow will initially be normal, but, at some point, the maximum flow imposed by the upper airway narrowing will cut in (B). From that point onwards, the flow rate will be fixed at this maximum (C) until, at much lower lung volumes, the lower recoil and narrowing of the small airways again determine the maximum flow (D). The flow–volume curve has been severely 'clipped', with a square-ish appearance. The same clipped appearance will be present on the inspiratory limb (E), giving rise to the 'square box' appearance.

Sometimes, such upper airways restriction may be **variable**, rather than **fixed**, and only obstruct during inspiration (e.g. paralysed and collapsing vocal cords), due to the obstructing elements being sucked in and then blown open again on expiration.

Thus, a square inspiratory limb, but normal expiratory limb, provides evidence of a mobile **extrathoracic *upper airways obstruction.***

Conversely, a mobile intrathoracic upper airway obstruction (e.g. soft fleshy tumour at the carina or retrosternal thyroid) may obstruct more during expiration (when the expiratory effort is compressing the lung), compared with inspiration when the chest is being expanded.

Thus, a square expiratory limb, but normal inspiratory limb, is evidence of a **variable intrathoracic *upper airways obstruction.***

Sometimes, ratios of maximal inspiratory to maximal expiratory flows are used to characterize the intra- or extrathoracic airway obstruction.

Flow–volume loop 2

The other, more common, causes of airway obstruction are due to narrowing of the lower airways (asthma, chronic obstructive pulmonary disease (COPD)). In these conditions, the airway calibre (and thus flow rates) still remains dependent on lung volume. Hence, the flow rates decrease, as the lung volume decreases, but particularly decrease at low lung volumes. This is because resistance to flow is proportional to the airway radius raised to the power of 4 (r^4) and therefore most significant when airways are already small. Hence, increasing airflow obstruction produces expiratory flow–volume curves like those in Fig. A6.3. This greater effect of small airways narrowing at low lung volumes has led some to report flow rates at, for example, 25% expired lung volume or averaged between 25% and 75% of the total expired lung volume.

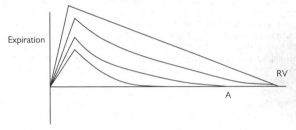

Fig. A6.3 Expiratory flow–volume curves—lower airways obstruction.

Airways can be so small that, during expiration, they begin closing off earlier than normal (the **closing volume**); hence, a full breath out is not possible, producing air trapping and a raised residual volume (RV) (A). Sensitive tests of small airways narrowing have to concentrate on flows at low lung volumes, and peak flow measurements are relatively insensitive.
• Note, however, that peak flow measurements are the most sensitive to **upper airway narrowing** and a good way to follow changes in upper airway narrowing during, for example, radiotherapy for a central airway obstructing lung cancer.

Spirometry and peak flow

- The ordinary spirometer (mechanical or electronic) records **volume against time**, rather than **flow against volume**
- The two essential measures are **FEV1** and **vital capacity (VC)**.

The VC is the maximum amount of air that can be blown out completely. This will be **reduced** if the lungs are **stiff** (preventing a full breath in), the **inspiratory muscles are weak** (preventing a full breath in), or the **airways are narrowed** such that the small airways collapse during expiration (preventing a full breath out).

The FEV_1 is the amount (forced expiratory volume) that can be blown out in 1 s. Because the value is taken over a second, a much longer period of flow is being captured during the breath out than the PEFR, but, despite this, the measurement is still being made when the airways are larger. It is less dependent on effort and generally more robust. The ratio of the two figures (FEV_1/VC) tells us about the degree of airflow obstruction.

A ratio of FEV_1/VC of less than about 70% indicates airflow **obstruction**. This ratio is very useful because it is hardly affected by sex, height, ethnic origin, and the lower limit of normal only slightly reduces with age. The individual measures of FEV_1 and VC **do** need corrections for the above factors and are usually quoted as either % predicted or with the lower/upper limits of normal. The range of normality is considerable, and it may not be clear if results are simply at the bottom end of normal or considerably reduced from the patient's normally much higher figures. Serial measurements indicating continuing deterioration may be the first clue. Only if the FEV_1/VC ratio is **normal**, can the VC be confidently used to infer whether there is a reduced total lung volume such as from interstitial lung disease (ILD). A low VC with normal FEV_1/VC ratio is called a **restrictive** pattern. A **low** FEV_1/VC ratio is called an **obstructive** pattern, and a reduced VC **cannot** then be confidently used to infer that the total lung volume is also reduced and indeed may even be increased because of air trapping. A small print fact is that the FEV_1/VC ratio may actually be raised in ILD, as the airways are better supported by the fibrosed radial attachments, which reduces dynamic compression, thus increasing expiratory flow, compared to that expected for the lung volume.

The **slope** of the volume–time plot from a spirometer is effectively the **flow** at any particular point; because flow is dropping during expiration, the slope progressively flattens off. However, if there is any fixed upper airways obstruction (as previously discussed), the expiratory flow rate will be constant for a while, and hence the spirometer line will be straighter than usual. An interesting index to detect possible upper airway obstruction the **Empey index** has been described:

Empey Index = $[FEV_1 \text{ (mL)} / PEFR \text{ (L/min)}]$

Because PEFR is clipped first by the presence of upper airflow obstruction, relative to the FEV_1, the above index gets larger with such a problem. A figure over 10 is suggestive of upper airflow obstruction, but it is only a pointer, and there will be false positives and negatives.

Although one-off measures of lung function can be made, more interesting information comes from serial measurements, e.g. in asthma, PEFR will fluctuate with characteristic morning 'dips'.

Spirometry—how to do it

Follow local guidance in choosing an appropriate location and personal protective equipment as lung-function manoeuvres are aerosol generating. A standardized approach to spirometry is important (see Table A6.1). Say to the patient, 'This is a test of how big your lungs are and how fast you can empty them. What I would like you to do is take an enormous breath in, the biggest you can manage, then seal your lips around the tube, and blow as hard and as fast and as long as you possibly can'. Then demonstrate the manoeuvre yourself with a spare tube (not necessarily connected to the spirometer) so that they can then mimic it. While they are blowing, say 'excellent, well done, keep blowing, come on, come on, come on, keep blowing'.

Table A6.1 Spirometry guidance

Certification, registration and calibration	The ATRP now offer training and certification in spirometry and hold a register of trained individuals and aim for full implementation by March 2021. The joint ATS/ERS statements stipulate requirements for standardization and calibration for lung-function departments to follow.
Standing or sitting?	Seated position is recommended. Normal values are based on a seated position. The high intrathoracic pressure generated may cause the patient to pass out. Therefore, sitting down is safer
Nose clip?	Prevents escape through the nose which would give falsely low figures but is uncomfortable. Is not required for forced expiration but slower expiratory measurements and maximal inspiratory flow requires clips.
Best of three blows?	Required to demonstrate that maximal blow has been consistently achieved, by seeing two identical tracings with the 2 best blows have both FEV_1 and FVC values within 150 ml of each other. Spirometry devices may automatically tell you if repeatability criteria have/have not been met. If not met further blows are required.
When to stop spirometry	Healthy individuals will have normally blown out fully by about 5 s but those with significant airflow obstruction will have longer forced expiratory times. Electronic spirometers will often stop once criteria for the end of expiration have been met, one of which is expiration for 15 s.
Contraindications	Relative contraindications include but are not limited to acute myocardial infarction, unstable PE, unstable arrhythmia, pneumothorax, recent thoracic/brain/sinus/ eye surgery, late-term pregnancy, haemoptysis, and TB (see ATS/ERS position statement in further reading)
Medications to avoid	SABA (4–6 h), SAMA (12 h), LABA e.g. formoterol, salmeterol (24 h), ultra-LABA e.g. indacaterol, vilanterol, olodaterol (36 h), LAMA (36–48 h)

Lung volumes

Lung volumes are essentially determined by a balance of the compliance of the lungs, the compliance of the chest wall and the contraction of the respiratory muscles. Static lung volumes measure mid-lung volumes or functional residual capacity (FRC) which is either determined by either inert gas dilution or body plethysmography. The total lung capacity (TLC) and residual volume (RV) are then derived spirometric values from FRC. The TLC is the volume of the lung at maximum inspiration and the RV is the volume at maximum expiration. See Fig. A6.4 and Table A6.2.

Inert gas dilution

Often used to measure gas transfer. An inert tracer such as helium is included in the inhaled gas mixture that is diluted by the air already in the lung; by comparing inspired helium concentration with expired, TLC can be calculated by gas dilution principles. In the presence of lower airways obstruction, the helium may not 'reach' all parts of the lung during the 10 s breath hold, and the volume calculated from this dilution will therefore be lower than the real TLC. An alternative technique is multiple breath nitrogen washout where inhaled 100% oxygen is used to displace the nitrogen resident in the lungs from prior breathing of room air. Estimations of lung volume are consistent with both gas dilution techniques in healthy individuals.

Body plethysmography

Requires the patient to sit in an airtight cabinet and breathe through a shuttered mouthpiece connected to the outside world. The subject breaths normally and the mouthpiece is shuttered close at the end of normal expiration. The subject then makes an inspiratory effort against a closed mouthpiece. This leads to decreased intrathoracic pressure and the lungs expand pushing the chest wall out. This in turn compresses the gas in the closed box. The pressure changes in the box and at the mouthpiece (which equates to the change in alveolar pressure) can then be used to calculate the unknown volume of the lung or FRC. Note that this volume will include any bullae or pneumothorax, and the difference between the plethysmographic lung volume and the helium dilution volume will reflect the bullae/pneumothorax volumes, as well as areas not reached by the helium due to increased airways resistance. Body plethysmography can also be used to calculate airways resistance.

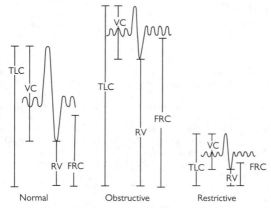

Fig. A6.4 Lung volumes in normal, obstructive, and restrictive lung conditions. TLC, total lung capacity (not always increased when obstructive pattern); VC, vital capacity; RV, residual volume; FRC, functional residual capacity; FEV$_1$, forced expiratory volume in 1 s.

Table A6.2 Lung volume patterns

Derivative	Obstructive	Restrictive
FEV$_1$ (% predicted)	↓↓	↓
VC (% predicted)	↓ or →	↓
FEV$_1$/VC ratio	↓	→ or ↑ (increased recoil)
TLC (% predicted)	↑ or →	↓
RV (% predicted)	↑	↓
FRC (% predicted)	↑	↓
RV/TLC ratio	↑ (gas trapping)	→ or ↓

Further information

Gibson GJ. *Clinical Tests of Respiratory Function*, 3rd edn. Hodder Arnold, 2008.

Gas transfer

Usually done in the lung function laboratory, and it essentially measures the amount of **gas-exchanging surface area** available. Commonly a gas mixture containing a 'diffusing' tracer (usually carbon monoxide (CO)) and a 'mixing' tracer (for example helium) is inhaled using a single-breath technique. Following maximal inspiration of the gas mix subjects hold their breath for 10 s, and then exhale. The amount of CO that has disappeared (by crossing the alveolar capillary membrane and being taken up by red cells) is calculated. A correction for the Hb concentration is required, as the amount of CO transferred will fall as the available Hb is reduced. The **total amount of CO transferred is the TLCO** (total lung, TL). When divided by the total lung volume during the breath-hold, it is called the **kCO, gas transfer per unit lung volume (TLC)**. The total lung volume 'reached' by the CO is the amount breathed in **plus** the amount of air already in the lung at the start of the breath in.

- The TLCO and kCO are **reduced** in emphysema when alveoli have been destroyed
- The TLCO and kCO are **reduced** in ILD where the alveolar capillary membrane may be thick enough to reduce CO passage
- The kCO may also be **raised** (and TLCO normal) when lungs are poorly expanded by, say, weak respiratory muscles, because the lung is 'more concentrated' and transfers CO **better** when quoted per unit volume
- The kCO may also be **raised** for a few days when there has been profuse lung haemorrhage, as can occur in, e.g. systemic lupus erythematosus (SLE), Wegener's, and Goodpasture's. This is because the free red cells lining the alveoli take up CO directly and 'falsely' elevate the figure. As the Hb is broken down, the kCO returns to normal, unless there is another bleed. This helps to distinguish re-bleeding from other causes of lung infiltrates such as infection.

This test requires more cooperation than simple spirometry, as well as a minimum inspired volume, and therefore cannot always be obtained.

Respiratory muscle function

Respiratory muscle function

Respiratory failure and small VCs may be due to compromised respiratory muscles. It is therefore useful to be able to assess inspiratory and expiratory muscle power. There may be global weakness or specific inspiratory weakness, usually due to diaphragm paralysis. In the clinic, the simplest test is a *lying and standing VC*. If the diaphragm is paralysed, then, on lying down, the abdominal contents will push up the diaphragm and limit inspiration. On standing, the abdominal contents drop and aid inspiration. It is worth noting that obesity can also cause a fall in supine VC due to compromising muscle function without the presence of muscle weakness (abdominal obesity compresses and reduces thoracic volumes in the supine position).

- A fall in VC of <10% on lying down is probably normal
- A fall of 10–20% is suspicious of diaphragm paralysis
- A fall of >20% is abnormal and suggests significant, usually bilateral, diaphragm paralysis.

In the laboratory, there are various ways to test respiratory muscle function. The patient can blow against a **pressure meter** after a maximum inspiration and inspire against the meter after a full expiration. This is, of course, highly effort-dependent. A manoeuvre, such as a *sniff*, is very stereotypic, and patients can reproduce this. Measuring the inspiratory pressure produced at the nose during this manoeuvre is a rough and ready way of screening for inspiratory muscle weakness. More accurate assessments of inspiratory muscle function, particularly the diaphragm, can be obtained using two semi-inflated balloons, introduced via the mouth and oesophagus, placed above and below the diaphragm, and connected to pressure transducers. The *transdiaphragmatic pressures* during maximal inspiratory efforts, sniffing, and breathing to TLC all provide reproducible measures of diaphragm function but depend on good cooperation and effort by the patient. Activating the phrenic nerve directly with a superficial electrical stimulator, or by using high-intensity magnetic stimulation over the nerve roots of C3–C5, while measuring transdiaphragmatic pressures, provides a non-effort-dependent way to test diaphragm function. While these maximal inspiratory and sniff pressures fall with diaphragm muscle weakness, COPD can also reduce these measures due to flattening of the diaphragm compromising muscle function. As with supine VC measurements, strictly speaking these are measurements of respiratory muscle compromise and not weakness.

Predicted values and peak flow reference ranges

The major determinants of lung volume are height, sex and age. Smaller differences are found in ethnic variations—generally due to differences in thorax-to-leg ratios. Historically, predicted values have been biased to a Caucasian, male working age group. Recent studies have attempted to rectify gaps in knowledge.

For the purposes of predictive values, the diversity of a population is reflected in the distribution around the mean value. The divergence from the mid-point is referred to as the Residual Standard Deviation (RSD). 90 % of the sample population should therefore fall within ±1.645 RSD. This allows calculation of the upper/lower limit (normal range) as well as the more familiar % predicted values. Whilst there is a move to using the lower limit of normal to define abnormality many treatment guidelines (e.g. the GOLD COPD guidelines and NICE anti-fibrotics in idiopathic pulmonary fibrosis (IPF)) still utilize % predicted cut-offs.

See Fig. A6.5.

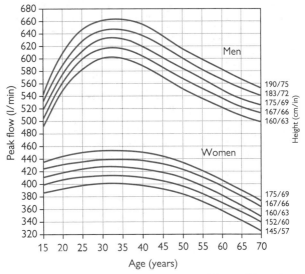

Fig. A6.5 Normal values for peak flow, based on original Gregg and Nunn values (*BMJ* 1973) but corrected for new EU scale peak flow meters. Normal range extends about ± 15% or roughly 100 L/min in men and 50 L/min in women.

Note: old Wright peak flow meters over-read in the middle of the scale (e.g. reading about 400 when actual value was 350 L/min) and were replaced from October 2004 by a corrected scale.

Further reading

Graham *et al*. Standardization of Spirometry 2019 Update. An Official American Thoracic Society and European Respiratory Society Technical Statement AJRCCM 2019;200: e70–e88

🔗 http://artp.org.uk
🔗 https://vitalograph.co.uk/resources/gli-normal-values

Cardiopulmonary exercise testing (CPET)

General points
- An exercise test, with additional measurement of ventilatory gases
- Useful for assessing:
  - Cardiorespiratory fitness
  - Relative contribution of cardiovascular (CV) and respiratory (RS) disease to exercise limitation
  - Disease severity assessment and prognostication
  - Risk stratification pre-lung resection, lung and cardiac transplantation, cardiac medical device therapy, other surgical evaluations
  - Response to an intervention.

Undertaking CPET
- Baseline spirometry and maximum voluntary ventilation (MVV)
- Measurements include serial electrocardiograms (ECGs), SpO_2, blood pressure (BP), heart rate (HR), expired concentrations of O_2 and CO_2, tidal volume, and breathing frequency (via face mask or mouthpiece with nose clips). Can include arterial blood gases (ABGs) on a bike or capillary blood gases (CBGs) with a bike or treadmill.
- Calculation of V_E (minute ventilation), VO_2 (O_2 consumption), VCO_2 (CO_2 production) at rest and throughout exercise
- Ventilatory threshold represents a point where several ventilatory parameters show a threshold-like behaviour, related to the onset of anaerobic respiration and lactic acidosis. Many ways of estimating; look for the inflection point on plots of VCO_2 vs VO_2 or V_E vs VCO_2
- ABGs (via an arterial line) are occasionally taken
- Usually performed on a cycle ergometer (alternatively, a treadmill)
- Cycle is initially unloaded, and then work is ramped (based on usual activity level; pre-test FEV_1 and MVV results can also be helpful)
- Doctor and physiologist monitor patient during test and ensure mask/mouthpiece closely fitting. Patient encouragement during testing enhances performance and can make results more meaningful
- Test usually stopped due to exhaustion (e.g. tired legs or too dyspnoeic). Stop immediately with significant arrhythmias, ST depression ≥2 mm, heart block, significantly falling BP, ischaemic-sounding chest pain, severe symptomatic hypoxaemia, or near syncope
- Unloaded pedalling at end of test.

Interpreting variables
- See Table A6.3.

Patterns in unexplained exertional dyspnoea
- Decreased VO_2 peak/max—defines degree of impairment, independent of mechanism
- V_E/VCO_2 slope increase and $P_{ET}CO_2$ decrease— could be due to hyperventilation but consider causes of exercise-related pulmonary hypertension (PHT)
- SpO_2 fall—suggests V/Q mismatching
- FEV_1/PEF decreases, V_E/MVV increases—suggests respiratory cause
- Lack of ventilatory threshold—suggests cause related to ventilation.
- Fall in FEV_1 can occur 30 min or longer post-exercise in exercise induced bronchospasm

Table A6.3 Interpreting CPET variables

Variable	Interpretation	Normal values
Peak VO_2 (mL/kg/min) (or VO_2 max)	Maximum O_2 utilization Global prognostic marker/severity assessment. Influenced by CV, RS, and muscular function	Influenced by age and sex (15–80 mL/kg/min) Reported as % predicted
VO_2 at ventilatory threshold (VT) (mL/kg/min)	Associated with anaerobic threshold. Limit of workload sustainable for prolonged periods	~ 50–65% peak VO_2 Influenced by training and genetic predisposition
Peak respiratory exchange ratio (RER)	RER = VCO_2/VO_2 ratio ↑work → ↑VO_2 but ↑↑VCO_2 → ↑RER Marker of effort during exercise	Good effort suggested by RER ≥1.1
V_E/VCO_2 slope (V_E on y-axis; VCO_2 on x-axis)	Determined by V/Q matching Marker of disease severity	<30 normal. Particularly high in PHT
V_E/VO_2 at peak exercise	Ventilatory cost of O_2 uptake at peak exercise	≤40 normal
End-tidal CO_2 partial pressure ($P_{ET}CO_2$)	Determined by V/Q matching and cardiac function Marker of disease severity	Rest: 4.8–5.6 kPa At VT: ↑ 0.4–1.1 kPa Above VT: ↓ due to increased ventilatory response to metabolic acidosis
V_E/MVV V_E measured at peak exercise, MVV at rest	Helps determine if dyspnoea is related to a pulmonary cause	≤0.8 normal >0.8 suggests pulmonary limitation
O_2 pulse (mL O_2/beat)	O_2 pulse = VO_2/HR Surrogate for stoke volume response to exercise Helpful for assessing possible myocardial ischaemia	Normally rises during exercise, reduced rise in chronic heart failure
Change in VO_2/change in workload ($\Delta VO_2/\Delta W$)	Helpful for assessing possible myocardial ischaemia	Normally linear rise of VO_2 with work Average 10 mL/min/W
FEV_1 and PEF (L/min)	Compare pre- and post-exercise Changes suggest respiratory cause of dyspnoea (not asthma-specific)	<15% reduction with exercise
Heart rate recovery (HRR)	Compares max HR with HR after 1 min recovery. Related to parasympathetic activation	Normally HRR >12 beats lower at 1 min. If <12, suggests cardiac cause

(Continued)

Table A6.3 (*Contd.*)

Exercise BP	CV response to exercise	Usual to have modest increase in SBP with exercise. DBP usually static or decreases due to vasodilatation
SpO_2	Useful for assessing for respiratory causes of exertional dyspnoea	Should not fall >5%. Greater fall in RS disease and PHT

Further information

Guazzi M et al. Clinical recommendations for cardiopulmonary exercise testing data assessment in specific patient populations. *Eur Heart J* 2012;**33**: 2917–2927.

Plain radiograph

Posterior-to-anterior view (see Fig. A7.1) 980
Left lateral view (see Fig. A7.2) 981
Lobar collapses (see Fig. A7.3) 982

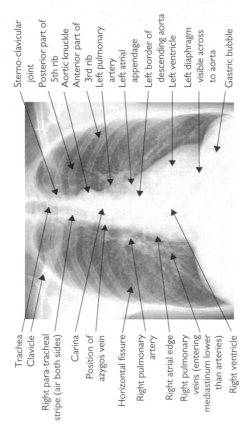

Trachea
Clavicle
Right para-tracheal stripe (air both sides)
Carina
Position of azygos vein
Horizontal fissure
Right pulmonary artery
Right atrial edge
Right pulmonary veins (entering mediastinum lower than arteries)
Right ventricle

Sterno-clavicular joint
Posterior part of 5th rib
Aortic knuckle
Anterior part of 3rd rib
Left pulmonary artery
Left atrial appendage
Left border of descending aorta
Left ventricle
Left diaphragm visible across to aorta
Gastric bubble

Fig. A7.1 Normal PA chest radiograph.

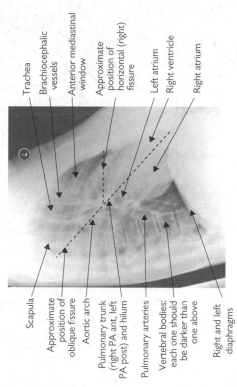

Trachea

Brachiocephalic vessels

Anterior mediastinal window

Approximate position of horizontal (right) fissure

Left atrium

Right ventricle

Right atrium

Scapula

Approximate position of oblique fissure

Aortic arch

Pulmonary trunk (right PA ant, left PA post) and hilum

Pulmonary arteries

Vertebral bodies: each one should be darker than one above

Right and left diaphragms

Fig. A7.2 Normal left lateral chest radiograph.

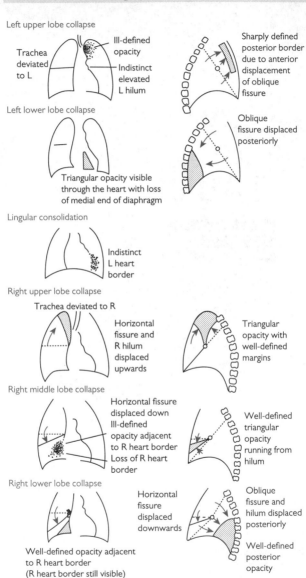

Left upper lobe collapse

Trachea deviated to L

Ill-defined opacity

Indistinct elevated L hilum

Sharply defined posterior border due to anterior displacement of oblique fissure

Left lower lobe collapse

Triangular opacity visible through the heart with loss of medial end of diaphragm

Oblique fissure displaced posteriorly

Lingular consolidation

Indistinct L heart border

Right upper lobe collapse

Trachea deviated to R

Horizontal fissure and R hilum displaced upwards

Triangular opacity with well-defined margins

Right middle lobe collapse

Horizontal fissure displaced down
Ill-defined opacity adjacent to R heart border
Loss of R heart border

Well-defined triangular opacity running from hilum

Right lower lobe collapse

Horizontal fissure displaced downwards

Oblique fissure and hilum displaced posteriorly

Well-defined posterior opacity

Well-defined opacity adjacent to R heart border (R heart border still visible)

Fig. A7.3 Lobar collapse.

Radiological investigations and radiation exposure

Table A8.1 Common radiological investigations used in respiratory practice (continued on ➡ p. 985)

Investigation	Plain CXR (AMBER), one view	Staging chest and abdo CT	HRCT	CTPA	Low-dose CT	V/Q scan ^{99m}TcMAA and ^{133}Xe	PET scan	MRI	Head CT
Indication	Best technique for plain chest radiography	For example, for staging lung cancer, usually with IV contrast to identify vascularity of structures	For diffuse lung disease, giving good resolution at level of 2° pulmonary lobule	For PE and visualization of pulmonary vasculature	Used in lung cancer screening and lung nodule follow-up	For identifying perfusion defects without accompanying ventilation defects, as in PE	For detection of malignant deposits and increasingly for areas of inflammation	Better detection of malignant tissue invasion	For example, for brain metastases
Technique	Multiple beam equalization improves contrast by varying beam intensity, depending on tissue density	Commonly, multidetector CT, which acquires thin (0.625 mm) slices and can reconstruct images in the axial, coronal and sagittal planes. 200–400 mA beam intensity	For older patients, multidetector CT, which acquires thin (0.625 mm) slices and can reconstruct images in multiple planes. For younger patients, 1.25 mm at 10 mm intervals, i.e. only about 10% of the lung scanned	Multidetector CT, which acquires thin (0.625 mm) slices and can reconstruct images in multiple planes	Multidetector CT, which acquires thin (0.625 mm) slices and can reconstruct images in multiple planes. 50 mA beam intensity	IV radiolabelled albumin macroaggregates that lodge in the pulmonary arterioles to image vasculature, and inhaled xenon gas to image ventilated areas.	Radiolabelled glucose (^{18}F-FDG)—uptake proportional to metabolic activity		Multidetector CT, which acquires thin (0.625 mm) slices and can reconstruct images in multiple planes

Radiation dose mSv or mGy (× 100 for mrad)	0.04	Variable, ~1-2 mSv with modern CT scanners but can be as high as 4 mSv Larger doses of contrast medium scatter more radiation into nearby tissues	1	1-2 mSv with modern CT scanners	Variable, <0.5–1 mSv	Variable, up to 1 mSv	7	0	1-2
Radiation dose (time equivalent to background radiation in the UK)	5 days	8 months	4 months	8 months	4 months	4 months	2.3y	0	8 months
Radiation dose (equivalent to numbers of CXRs)	1	50	25	50	25	25	175	0	50
Limitations	Poorer resolution, so 2° pulmonary lobule not visualized	Early cancers may be missed if performed as widely spaced thin sections	Same as ordinary CT	Lower beam intensity produces lower resolution	No structural information or the ability to make alternative diagnoses	Usually combined with CT, so add on up to another 6 mSv	Lower resolution		

Different departments/countries will use different protocols, e.g. some will always do a standard CT as well as an HRCT in case a malignant nodule is missed.

Radiation dose estimates are fraught with many assumptions, and there is significant uncertainty in some areas.

1 mSv is the dose of absorbed radiation produced by exposure to 1 mGy of radiation.

1 mSv ≈ 100 mrad absorbed dose (mSv includes quality factor (type of radiation and nature of tissue), but, for X-rays and most tissues, mSv and mGy are numerically identical (for alpha emitters, 1 mGy causes 20 mSv)).

Background radiation ~3 mSv/y (mainly from radiation in the home and varies across the country); transatlantic flight ≈ extra 0.03 mSv.

Useful websites

Thoracic societies and charities

American College of Chest Physicians. http://www.chestnet.org
American Thoracic Society. http://www.thoracic.org
British Lung Foundation. http://www.lunguk.org
British Society for Allergy and Clinical Immunology. http://www.bsaci.org
British Thoracic Society. http://www.brit-thoracic.org.uk
Canadian Thoracic Society. http://cts-sct.ca
European Respiratory Society. http://www.ersnet.org
Society of Thoracic Surgeons. http://www.sts.org
Thoracic Society of Australia and New Zealand. http://www.thoracic.org.au

Thoracic journals

American Journal of Respiratory and Critical Care Medicine ('Blue journal').
http://www.atsjournals.org
BMJ Open Respiratory Research. http://bmjopenrespres.bmj.com
Chest. http://www.chestjournal.org
European Respiratory Journal. http://erj.ersjournals.com
Lancet Respiratory Medicine. http://www.thelancet.com/journals/lanres/
home
Respirology. http://onlinelibrary.wiley.com/journal/14401843
Thorax. http://thorax.bmj.com

General journals

British Medical Journal. http://www.bmj.com
Journal of the American Medical Association. http://jamanetwork.com
The Lancet. http://www.thelancet.com
National Library of Medicine (Pub Med). http://www.ncbi.nlm.nih.gov/
pubmed
New England Journal of Medicine. http://www.nejm.org

Clinical and educational resources

Drugs that cause respiratory disease. http://www.pneumotox.com
Fitness to drive. Driver and Vehicle Licensing Agency. http://www.gov.uk/
health-conditions-and-driving
Radiopaedia. Useful 'wiki' style radiology website. http://radiopaedia.org
Respiratory training in the UK. Details and curriculum on Joint Royal
College of Physicians Training Board's website. http://www.jrcptb.org.uk/
specialties/respiratory-medicine
Respiratory Specialty Certificate Exam. Details and sample questions
on Royal College of Physicians' website http://www.mrcpuk.org/
mrcpuk-examinations/specialty-certificate-examinations/specialties/
respiratory-medicine

Index

Note: Tables, figures, and boxes are indicated by an italic *t*, *f*, and *b* following the paragraph number.

A

abbreviated mental test
    score 521*b*
Abram's pleural needle
    biopsy 872–3
abscess
    lung 544–5, 546–7
    peripheral cold 589
Access to Work Grant 737
ACE inhibitor cough 19
acetaldehyde 274
Achromobacter
    xylosoxidans 245
acid–base balance 928–30
actinomycosis 550–1
acute bronchitis 711
acute chest syndrome 674–5
acute interstitial
    pneumonia 332–3
acute mountain sickness
    300, 301
acute pharyngitis 710
acute pleuritic chest pain 9
acute respiratory assessment
    service 207
acute respiratory distress
    syndrome 115–22
    clinical features 117
    complications 121
    definition and
        epidemiology 116
    diagnosis 118
    future developments 122
    management 120, 121*f*
    pathophysiology 116–17
    prognosis 121
acute rhinitis 708
acute rhinosinusitis 709
acute upper airway
    obstruction 704
adaptive
    servo-ventilation 700–1
adenocarcinoma 338
adenovirus 640
adiaspiromycosis 583
adrenaline
    anaphylaxis 707*b*
    bronchoscopy 835, 958*t*
    central airway
        obstruction 842
    haemoptysis 47*b*, 252
advance decisions 729

advance statements 729
air embolism 486
air trapping 947
air travel 298–9
airway
    acute upper airway
        obstruction 704
    central airway
        obstruction 842–3
    endotracheal
        intubation 830–1
    initial assessment 23
    intubation 830–1
    laryngeal mask 829
    management 827–31
    nasopharyngeal 828
    obstruction 142,
        704, 842–3
    oropharyngeal 828
    simple adjuncts 828
    supraglottic airway
        devices 829
aldehydes 274
alfentanil 888, 958*t*
ALK1 454
allergic bronchopulmonary
    aspergillosis 253,
        292, 562–3
    bronchiectasis 560
    seropositive only 560
allergic rhinitis 18, 168
altitude sickness 300–1
alveolar haemorrhage
    see diffuse alveolar
        haemorrhage
alveolar
    lipoproteinosis 508–9
alveolar microlithiasis 490
ambrisentan 461
ambulatory oxygen 794
aminophylline 150*b*, 207
amiodarone 264
ammonia 274
amniotic fluid embolism 486
amoebic pulmonary
    disease 625
amylase, pleural fluid 60
amyloidosis 492–6
    classification 492*b*
    laryngeal 494
    mediastinal and hilar 494
    parenchymal amyloid 494
    pleural effusion 494

    tracheobronchial
        amyloid 494
anaphylaxis 706–7
ANCA 715*b*, 716–17
angiomyolipoma 502
anion gap 929–30
ankylosing spondylitis 225
anthrax 552–3
antibiotic therapy
    community-acquired
        pneumonia
        526–7, 530
    COPD 206
    cystic fibrosis 242–3,
        243*b*, 248
    desensitization 248
    lung abscess 547
    non-HIV immuno
        compromised 81
    parapneumonic effusion
        and empyema 416
    ventilator-associated
        pneumonia 539
    see also macrolides
anti-GBM disease
    (Goodpasture's) 721
anti-MDA5 antibodies 220
antimicrobials 88
antineutrophil cytoplasmic
    antibodies see ANCA
anti-synthetase
    syndrome 220
anti-TNF α-therapy
    264, 610–11
α1-antitrypsin
    deficiency 210–11
argon–plasma
    coagulation 848
asbestos 123–39
    asbestosis 128–9
    asbestos-related lung
        disease 124–5, 138–9
    benign asbestos-related
        pleural disease 126–7
    diffuse pleural
        thickening 127
    domestic exposure 124
    mechanisms of
        exposure 124
    mesothelioma 130–2
    occupation exposure 124
    pleural effusion 423
    rounded atelectasis 127

aspergilloma 566
Aspergillus 560, 568
  and bronchiectasis 181
  post-lung transplant 767
aspiration pneumonia 540
  antibiotic treatment 530*t*
  bacterial infection 542–3
  chemical pneumonia 542
  clinical features 542–3
  idiopathic inflammatory
      myopathies 221
  mechanical obstruction 543
  risk factors 540
  systemic sclerosis 223
asthma 16, 141–68
  action plan 155
  acute severe 148–51
  aetiology 143
  allergen avoidance 158
  and allergic
      bronchopulmonary
      aspergillosis 292
  and allergic rhinitis (hay
      fever) 168
  aspirin-induced 145*b*
  breastfeeding 163
  breathing techniques 158
  childhood 396
  chronic cough 16
  clinical features 144
  cystic fibrosis 253
  deaths 148
  diagnosis 144, 145*b*, 160
  differential diagnosis 147*b*
  difficult/refractory 160–1
  discussing with ITU 151*b*
  diving 302, 303*b*
  epidemiology 142
  examination 144
  hospital treatment of acute
      asthma 150*b*
  investigations 146–7
  management 152–5
  monitoring morbidity 155*b*
  non-pharmacological
      management 158
  occupational asthma 164–5
  oral allergy syndrome 145*b*
  outpatient reviews 152*b*
  pathophysiology 142
  pharmacological
      management 152–5
  pregnancy 162–3
  risk factors 148
  severe asthma with fungal
      sensitization 561
  smoking cessation 158
  steroid-resistant 161
  treatment 156–7
  vocal cord dysfunction 167
atelectasis

rounded 127
  shrinking pleuritis with 127
systemic lupus
      erythematosus 218
atrial septostomy 464–5
Attendance Allowance 736
atypical, opportunistic,
      and environmental
      mycobacteria 618–19
autofluorescence
      bronchoscopy 846
autonomic nervous system
      tumours 386
azathioprine 264, 742
azithromycin see macrolides

B

bacterial infections 648–9
barotrauma 302
base deficit 928–9
base excess 928–9
BCGosis 616
BCG vaccination 613–14
Behçet's syndrome 226
bends 302
benefits system 733–7
benralizumab 154
benzodiazepines 888
berylliosis 432–3
beryllium lymphocyte
      proliferation test 433
bi-level positive airway
      pressure 772
blastomycosis 580–1
bleomycin 262*b*, 265, 878
Blesovsky syndrome 127
blunt dissection drains 852
BMPR2 454
Bochdalek hernia 398
BODE index 194*t*
body mass index 102, 180–1,
      194*t*, 254
bone morphogenetic protein
      receptor type II 454
bosentan 461
brachytherapy 849
brain metastases 807
breakthrough pain 802–3
breastfeeding
  asthma 163
  tuberculosis 602
breathing, initial
      assessment 23
breathlessness 3–6
  causes 5*b*, 6
  clinical assessment 4
  distinguishing cardiac and
      respiratory causes 6
  investigations 5
  lung cancer 805*b*

non-malignant respiratory
      disease 808
  palliative care 804
  physiological mechanisms 4
  post-operative 63–8
  pregnancy 69–72
Brett's syndrome 399
bronchial angiogram 46
bronchial artery
      embolization 46
bronchial biopsies 840
bronchial brushings 840
bronchial laser
      resection 848
bronchial provocation
      testing 868
bronchial thermoplasty 156
bronchial washings 840
bronchiectasis 169–81
  aetiology 170, 171*t*
  antimicrobial
      chemotherapy 176
  and *Aspergillus* 181
  clinical features and
      diagnosis 174–5
  complications 181
  definition 170
  epidemiology 170
  exacerbations 176–7
  investigations 174–5
  lung transplantation 760–1
  macrolide antibiotics 178
  management 176–81
  pathophysiology 170
  rheumatoid arthritis 217
  severity index 178
  systemic sclerosis 223
bronchiolitis 183–7
  acute 187
  causes 185*b*
  clinical features 184
  constrictive 184, 185*b*
  definition 184
  diffuse
      pan-bronchiolitis 186–7
  epidemiology 184
  investigations 186
  management 186
  pathophysiology 184
  proliferative 184, 185*b*
  small airways disease
      and obliterative
      bronchiolitis 217
bronchiolitis obliterans
      syndrome 765, 768
bronchioloalveolar/
      bronchoalveolar cell
      carcinoma 338
bronchoalveolar lavage
      97, 840
  bronchoscopy with 82, 97

diffuse lung disease 39
bronchopulmonary
  dysplasia 394–5
bronchoscopy 833–49
  with BAL 82, 97
  bleeding and 835
  central airway
    obstruction 842–3
  contraindications 834
  diagnostic 844–6
  indications 834
  lung cancer 344
  navigation 845
  patient preparation 836
  procedure 836–7
  rigid 846
  risks 834
  sampling techniques 840
  therapeutic 848–9
bullectomy 208
bupropion 822
Burkholderia cepacia
  complex 244
Burkholderia
  pseudomallei 555
busulfan 265–6

C

cadmium fumes 276
caisson disease 302
Candida infection
  oral 708
  pneumonia 575
candidiasis 708
capacity 728–9, 729b
Caplan's syndrome 217, 429
carbon monoxide
  poisoning 278–9
cardiac sarcoidosis 667
cardiogenic pulmonary
  oedema 71b, 774
cardiopulmonary exercise
  testing 815b
Carer's Allowance 736
Castleman's disease 390
catamenial
  pneumothorax 447
central airway
  obstruction 842–3
central sleep apnoea 694–5
  causes and clinical
    features 696–9
  definition and
    epidemiology 694
  future developments 701
  investigations 700–1
  management 700–1
  sleep study 700
cepacia syndrome 244
CFTR modulators 251

CFTR-related disease 239
chemical pleurodesis
  443, 878–9
chemical pneumonitis 542
chest drains 440–1, 851–9
  clamping 856
  complications 853
  contraindications 852
  indications 852
  indwelling pleural
    catheters 858–9
  insertion technique 854–5
  management 856
  removal 856
  types 852
chest pain 8
  acute pleuritic 9
  chronic 10
chest wall deformity,
  and neuromuscular
    weakness 782–3
chest wall limitation 223
chest wall restrictive
  diseases 697
Cheyne-Stokes breathing
  associated with
    altitude 699
  associated with heart
    failure 698
chickenpox 643
children see paediatric lung
  disorders
Chlamydophila
  pneumoniae 529
Chlamydophila psittaci 529
chlorambucil 266
chlorine 274
chloroquine 649–50
chronic asthma 152–5
chronic chest pain 10
chronic cough
  aetiology and clinical
    assessment 12–13
  causes 15
  examination 13
  idiopathic 19
  investigations 13
  treatment 14
chronic lung allograft
  dysfunction 768–9
chronic lung disease of
  prematurity 394–5
chronic necrotizing
  aspergillosis 566–7
chronic obstructive
  pulmonary disease
  (COPD) 189–211
  acute respiratory
    assessment
    service 207
  aetiology 190

antibiotics 206
α1-antitrypsin
  deficiency 210–11
BODE index 194t
bronchodilators 206
bronchoscopic lung
  volume reduction
  surgery 208
bullectomy 208
clinical features 191
CXR 192
DECAF score 203–4, 204t
definition 190
diagnosis 193–4
diet 197
education 196
ethical
  considerations 730–1
exacerbations
  202–7, 203b
history 191
inhaled therapy 198
intubation/intensive
  care 207
investigations 192–4
lung transplantation
  208, 760
lung volume reduction
  surgery 208, 209
management 203b, 206–7
modified MRC dyspnoea
  scale 193b
mucolytics 199b
non-invasive ventilation
  199, 207, 774, 784
non-pharmacological
  management 196–7
outpatient clinic 197b
oxygen therapy 199, 206
palliative care/respiratory
  sedation 200
pathology 190–1
prognostic scores 203–4
psychosocial support 197
pulmonary function
  tests 192
pulmonary
  hypertension 458
pulmonary
  rehabilitation 196–7
rehabilitation and
  nutrition 207
self-management plan 197
signs 191
smoking cessation 196
surgical/bronchoscopic
  treatment 208–9
treatment 206–7, 209
vaccination 199
chronic pulmonary
  aspergillosis 566–7

chronic rejection
phenomenon 185b
chronic respiratory
failure, non-invasive
ventilation 782–4
chronic rhinosinusitis 18
chronic thromboembolic
pulmonary
hypertension 459
Churg–Strauss
syndrome 722–3
chylothorax 60
cidofovir 515
coal workers
chest disease in 427
pneumoconiosis 428–9
cocaine 274
coccidioidomycosis 582
coeliac disease 254–5
colon cancer 254–5
community-acquired
pneumonia 518–19
abbreviated mental test
score 521b
adjunctive treatment 524
aetiology 518
antibiotics 526–7, 530
cardiovascular risk 532
clinical features 519
combination treatment
including a
macrolide 527
CXR 532
definition 518
diagnosis 519
discharge from
hospital 532
epidemiology 518
examination 519
follow-up 532
ICU admission 525
investigations 522–3
management 524–5
monitoring 525
non-invasive
ventilation 775
pathogens 528–9
prognostic factors 520
risk factors 518
severity assessment 520–1
specific pathogens 528–9
supportive treatment 524
treatment failure
531, 531b
vaccination 533
viral causes 528
computed tomographic
pulmonary angiogram
46, 72, 452–3, 476–7
computed tomography (CT)
82, 93, 437, 646

see also high-resolution
computed
tomography
congenital
abnormalities 398–9
congenital lobar
emphysema 398
connective tissue
disease 213–28
ankylosing spondylitis 225
autoantibodies 228
Behçet's syndrome 226
differential
diagnoses 214–15
idiopathic inflammatory
myopathies 220–1
investigations 215b
rheumatoid
arthritis 216–17
Sjögren's syndrome 224
systemic lupus
erythematosus 218–
19
systemic sclerosis 222–3
Constant Attendance
Allowance 737
constrictive
bronchiolitis 184
continuous positive airway
pressure 647–8, 773
coronavirus disease
(COVID-19) 645–50
clinical features 645
clinical trials 649–50
complications 648–9
differential
diagnosis 646–7
imaging 646
laboratory features 645–6
management 647–8
outcome 649
risk factors 645
severity assessment 647
cor pulmonale 231–5
corticosteroids 433, 649–50,
742–3, 878
Corynebacterium
diphtheriae 710
cough
ACE inhibitor 19
chronic see chronic cough
lung cancer 806
non-malignant respiratory
disease 809
post respiratory tract
infections 19
cough hypersensitivity
syndrome 12–13
cough syncope 12
COVID-19 645–50
Coxiella burnetii 529

CREST syndrome 222–3
cricoarytenoid arthritis 217
cricothyroidotomy
861–3, 863b
critical illness with
respiratory
disease 21–5
Crohn's disease 310
cryotherapy/
cryoextraction 848
cryptococcosis 574
cryptogenic fibrosing
alveolitis see idiopathic
pulmonary fibrosis
cryptogenic haemoptysis 47
cryptogenic organizing
pneumonia 330–1
CURB65 520–1
cyclophosphamide
266, 744–5
cystic airspaces 948
cystic change 37
cystic fibrosis 170, 237–59
acute kidney injury 257
antibiotics 242–3, 243b,
244–5, 248
asthma 253
CFTR modulators 251
CFTR-related disease
239, 239t
chronic rhinosinusitis 257
definition 238
diabetes 256
diagnosis 239
distal intestinal obstructive
syndrome 254–5
electrolyte
abnormalities 257
exacerbations 246–7
fertility 256–7
future developments 259
gastrointestinal
disease 254–5
genetics 238–9
lung transplantation
258, 760–1
macrolides 250
microbiology 240
mucoactive agents 250
multidisciplinary
care 238
non-invasive
ventilation 783
non-tuberculous
mycobacteria 245
nutritional
management 254
palliative care 258
pathophysiology 238
physiotherapy 250
pneumothorax 447

Pseudomonas aeruginosa
    infection 242–3
psychosocial support 258
pulmonary
    complications 252–3
pulmonary
    interventions 250–1
respiratory support 251
screening 239
steroids 251
stress incontinence 257
vaccination 258
cysts 390
    enteric or
        bronchogenic 390
    pleuropericardial 390
    thymic 389
cytokine release
    syndrome 648–9
cytokines 157
cytomegalovirus
    pneumonia 638–9
    post-lung
        transplantation 767

D

daytime sleepiness 101*b*
D-dimers 474–5
deep vein thrombosis 72,
    474–5, 4/4*t*
    see also pulmonary
        thromboembolic
        disease
dermatomyositis 220–1
desquamative interstitial
    pneumonia 335
diabetes
    cystic fibrosis 256
    TB 605
diaphragm
    hernia 398
    thoracic ultrasound 904
diet
    asthma 158
    COPD 197
    cystic fibrosis 254
    lymphangio
        leiomyomatosis 504
diffuse alveolar
    haemorrhage
    27–30, 219
diffuse cutaneous systemic
    sclerosis 222–3
diffuse lung disease 31–41
    acute respiratory
        failure 40–1
    anatomy 32
    blood tests 38
    bronchoalveolar lavage 39
    cardiac investigations 38
    causes 32, 33*t*
    CXR 35
    examination 35
    history 34–5
    HRCT 35, 36–7
    imaging 35, 37
    investigations 38–9
    lung biopsy 39
    pulmonary function
        tests 38
    Sjögren's syndrome 224
    sputum 38
    systemic lupus
        erythematosus 218
    urine tests 38
diffuse
    pan-bronchiolitis 186–7
diffuse parenchymal
    disease 32
diffuse pleural
    thickening 127
dirofilariasis 626
disability assessment 23
disability premiums 737
Disabled Facilities Grant 737
Disabled Students'
    Allowance 737
disseminated BCG infection
    (BCGosis) 616
diuretics 88
diving 302–4, 303*b*
dornase alfa 180–1
driving, sleep apnoea
    100–1, 690–1
drug-induced lung
    disease 261–81
    clinical presentations 262
    examples of specific
        drugs 264–8
    lupus 219*b*
    pulmonary eosinophilia 293
    see also toxin-induced lung
        disease
dupilumab 154
dysfunctional
    breathing 283–7
    clinical features 284
    definition 284
    diagnosis 285
    management 286
    Nijmegen hyperventilation
        score 287
    pathophysiology 284
    prognosis 286
dyspnoea *see* breathlessness

E

Echinococcus granulosus 624
*Echinococcus
    multilocularis* 624
e-cigarettes 823
economy class
    syndrome 471
electrocautery 848
electronic cigarettes 823
embolectomy 481
emphysema
    congenital lobal 398
    COPD 190–1
    subcutaneous (surgical)
        437, 447
Employment and Support
    Allowance 736
empyema 412–18
endemic mycoses 576
    adiaspiromycosis 583
    blastomycosis 580–1
    coccidioidmycosis 582
    histoplasmosis 578–9
    paracoccidioid
        omycosis 583
    penicilliosis
        (Talaromycosis) 583
endobronchial ultrasound
    590–1, 844–6
endoglin 454
endothelin receptor
    antagonists 461
endotracheal
    intubation 830 1
engraftment syndrome 84–5
Entamoeba histolytica 625
eosinophilic bronchitis 16
eosinophilic granulomatosis
    with polyangiitis
    (Churg–Strauss
    syndrome) 295, 722–3
eosinophilic lung
    disease 289–95
epiglottitis, acute
    (supraglottitis) 708
epoprostenol 460–1
Epworth Sleepiness Scale
    103*f*, 682
erionite 130
erythema nodosum 666
ethambutol 596–7
ethical
    considerations 727–32
excessive dynamic airways
    collapse 712
expiratory positive airways
    pressure 772
extensively drug-resistant
    TB 607
extreme environments
    297–304
exudative pleural effusion
    see pleural effusion,
    exudative
ex vivo lung perfusion 765

F

fat embolism 487
fentanyl 958t
financial entitlements 733–7
flumazenil 958t
flying 298–9
folded lung 127
formaldehyde 274
Francisella tularensis 554
fungal respiratory
    infections 559–83

G

gastrointestinal disease
    305–10, 669
gastro-oesophageal reflux
    disease 16–17, 254–5
Gefapixant 19
germ cell tumours 389
giant cell arteritis 724
gold 266
granulomatosis with
    polyangiitis
    (Wegener's) 716–19
Group A *Streptococcus* 710

H

haematopoietic stem cell
    transplant 86
Haemophilus influenzae 244
haemoptysis 43–7, 567
    causes 44–5
    cryptogenic 47
    cystic fibrosis 252
    diagnostic approach 44
    examination 44
    history 44
    investigations 46–7
    management 46, 47b
    massive 47b, 252
hantavirus pulmonary
    syndrome 644
hay fever 18, 168
heart–lung
    transplantation 764
heparin 479, 648
hepatic hydrothorax 306
hepatopulmonary
    syndrome 306–7
hereditary haemorrhagic
    telangiectasia 497
hernia, diaphragmatic 398
high altitude cerebral
    oedema 300–1
high altitude pulmonary
    oedema 300, 301
high-resolution computed
    tomography
    amyloidosis 495

diffuse lung disease 32,
    35, 36–7
    pneumoconiosis 429
    see also computed
        tomography (CT)
Histoplasma capsulatum 578
histoplasmosis 578–9
HIV-related respiratory
    disease 91–7
    causes 96
    clinical assessment 92–3
    investigations 92, 97
    pneumothorax 447
    TB 605, 608–9
    treatment 97
Hodgkin's lymphoma 390
hospital-acquired
    pneumonia
    clinical features 534–5
    management 536–7
    risk factors 534b
human metapneumovirus 641
hydrocarbons/mineral
    oils 275
hypercalcaemia 364,
    364b, 666
hypereosinophilic
    syndrome 295
hypersensitivity
    pneumonitis 311–16
    acute 314
    causes 312, 312t
    chronic 314
    clinical features 314
    definition 312
    diagnosis 314–15
    differential diagnosis 315
    epidemiology 312
    investigations 314–15
    management 316
    pathophysiology 313
    prognosis 316
hyperventilation syndrome
    284, 287
hypnosis 823
hypoventilation, sleep
    apnoea and 677–02
hypoxia
    challenge test 298, 299b
    COVID-19 647–8
    flying 298
    high altitude 300–1
    non-malignant respiratory
        disease 808

I

icterohaemorrhagic fever 556
idiopathic chronic cough 19
idiopathic inflammatory
    myopathies
    220–1, 221b

idiopathic interstitial
    pneumonias 317–36
idiopathic pulmonary
    fibrosis 318
    acute exacerbations 327b
    causes 320
    clinical features 320
    clinical trials 324
    definition 320
    diagnosis 321
    differential diagnosis 322
    epidemiology 320
    future developments 326
    histology 321
    investigations 321
    lung transplantation 760
    management 324–5
    pathophysiology 320
    prognosis 326
    see also pulmonary fibrosis
idiopathic pulmonary
    hemosiderosis 498–9
    aetiology 498
    clinical features 498
    clinic appointments 499
    examination 499
    investigations 499
    management 499
    pathophysiology 498
    prognosis 499
iloprost 460–1
immune reconstitution
    inflammatory
    syndrome *see* IRIS
immunocompromised
    patients
    antibiotic treatment 81
    assessment 80–1
    bronchoscopy with
        BAL 82
    causes of pulmonary
        disease 84–5
    CT 82
    differential diagnosis 86–7
    HIV 91–7
    infection 84
    investigations 81, 82
    lung biopsy 82
    multiple disease
        processes 85
    non-HIV 79–89
    non-invasive
        ventilation 775
    pleural effusion 80b
    treatment 88–9
    see also HIV-related
        respiratory disease
immunosuppressive
    drugs 739–46
    patient advice 740b, 740
    tests before and during
        treatments 740t

immunotherapy
asthma 158
drug and toxin-induced
lung disease 280–1
live attenuated BCG 616
PD-1 and PD-L1 354b
subcutaneous allergen 706
income support 737
inducible laryngeal
obstruction 712
Industrial Injuries
Disablement
Benefit 737
indwelling pleural
catheters 858–9
infections see respiratory
infections
inflammatory bowel
disease 310
influenza 632–3
avian 632–3
clinical and laboratory
features 634
diagnosis 635
differential diagnosis 634
imaging 634
infection control 636
management 636–7
outcome 637
severity assessment 636
treatment 636–7
vaccination 199, 533, 637
inhalational lung
injury 274–6
inhalers 748–54, 752t
inspiratory positive airways
pressure 772
intensive care unit 755–7
interferon alfa 515
interstitial lung disease
32, 220
intubation 830–1
invasive aspergillosis 564–5
IRIS 93, 94b, 572

K

ketamine 889
Kussmaul's breathing 928–9

L

Lady Windermere
syndrome 618
Langerhans cell
histiocytosis 500–1
laryngeal and tracheal
disorders 712
laryngitis 711
lasting power of
attorney 728

Legionella
pneumophila 528–9
Lemierre's
syndrome 544b
leptospirosis 556–7, 557b
leukotriene receptor
antagonists 162
lidocaine 958t
liver disease 255, 604
Löffler's syndrome 292
lopinavir 649–50
low molecular weight
heparin 479, 648
lung abscess
antibiotics 547
clinical features 544–5
complications 547
differential diagnosis 546b
drainage 547
management 546–7
prognosis 547
surgery 547
lung biopsy 344, 346b
diffuse lung disease 39
immunocompromised
patients 82
open 39
percutaneous
image-guided 39
lung cancer 337–79
adenocarcinoma
338, 339b
anxiety and
depression 806
brain metastases 807
breathlessness 805b
bronchoscopy 344
chemotherapy 358
clinical features 340–1
cough 806
CT/US-guided biopsy 344
diagnostic
procedures 344–5
epidemiology 338
epithelial lung
tumours 339b
ethical considerations 732
hypercalcaemia 364
investigations 342–3
liquid biopsies 359
mediastinoscopy 345
mediastinotomy 345
multidisciplinary team 343
non-small cell lung cancer
338, 350–2, 354–5
palliative care 802–4
pleural effusion 806
poor appetite 807
pulmonary carcinoid
tumours 368–70
pulmonary nodules 372

radiofrequency ablation/
microwave
ablation 359
radiologically guided lung
biopsy 346b
radiotherapy 356, 358
recurrent laryngeal nerve
palsy 807
screening 378–9
small cell lung cancer
338–9, 358
spinal cord
compression 366–7
squamous cell
carcinoma 338
staging 348–9, 348t, 349b
superior vena caval
obstruction 360–3
surgery 345, 350–2, 358
symptoms and signs 340–1
syndrome of inappropriate
secretion of
antidiuretic
hormone 365
targeted molecular
therapy 359
thoracoscopy 345
transbronchial needle
aspiration 344
treatment 358
types 338–9
lung transplantation 759–69
acute cellular rejection 766
airway complications 766
assessment process 763
bilateral sequential 764
chronic lung allograft
dysfunction 768–9
complications
766–7, 768–9
contraindications 762
follow-up 764
future developments 765
heart–lung 764
indications 760–1
infection 767
investigations 763
living lobar 764
malignancy 769
management of patients
on waiting list 763
outcomes 765
patient selection 760–1
primary graft
dysfunction 766
recurrence of primary
disease 769
routine surgery after 764
single lung 764
surgical approaches 764
timing of referral 761

lung transplantation (Contd.)
underlying conditions 760
urgent and super-urgent
lung allocation
schemes 761
lupus pneumonitis 218
lymphangio
leiomyomatosis 502–5
clinical features 502
definition and
aetiology 502
diagnosis 504
examination 503
investigations 503
management 504
organs affected 502–3
pathology 502
prognosis 505
lymphangitis
carcinomatosis 341
lymphoid interstitial
pneumonia 336
lymphoma
Hodgkin's 390
Sjögren's syndrome 224

M

macitentan 461
MacLeod's syndrome 399
macrolides 250
bronchiectasis 178
chronic asthma 156
cystic fibrosis 250
see also antibiotic therapy
malignant pleural
effusion 404–10
causes 404
clinical features 404
differential diagnosis 404
epidemiology 404
indwelling pleural catheter
insertion 409
intercostal chest drainage
and pleurodesis 408
investigations 404–5
LENT score 405–6, 406t
management 408–10
prognosis 405–6
therapeutic pleural
aspiration 408
trapped lung or failed
pleurodesis 409–10
treatment 408–10
Mantoux skin test 591b
measles 640
mediastinal
abnormalities 381–91
anatomy 384
anterior (prevascular)
384, 385
cysts 390

enlarged lymph nodes 390
inflammation 391
lymphoma 390
Masaoka–Koga thymoma
staging system 387b
mediastinal
emphysema 391
neural tumours 386
paravertebral (posterior)
384, 385
thymoma 386
thyroid 389
vascular 391
visceral (middle) 384, 385
mediastinal lymph node
stations 845f
mediastinoscopy 345
mediastinotomy 345
melioidosis 555
mepolizumab 154
MERS-coronavirus 654
mesothelioma 130–2
anxiety and
depression 806
brain metastases 807
clinical course 135
cough 806
future
developments 135–6
lung cancer 806
palliative care 802–4
peritoneal 135
pleural effusion 806
poor appetite 807
staging 132, 132t, 133b
treatment 134–5
metal fumes 274
methaemoglobin 278
methotrexate 266–7, 744
methyl isocyanate 275
microscopic polyangiitis 720
microvascular embolic
disease 648–9
midazolam 958t
Middle East respiratory
syndrome (MERS) 654
Modified Observer's
Assessment of
Alertness/ Sedation
(MOAAS) scale 887t
monoclonal antibody
therapy 154, 162
Morgagni hernia 398
MRSA 244
mucoactive agents 250
mucolytics 199
mycobacterial respiratory
infections 585–621
Mycobacterium abscessus
245, 621
Mycobacterium avium
complex 245, 620

Mycobacterium chelonae 621
Mycobacterium fortuitum 621
Mycobacterium gordonae 620
Mycobacterium kansasii 620
Mycobacterium
malmoense 620
Mycobacterium xenopi 620
Mycoplasma pneumoniae 529

N

naloxone 958t
National Early Warning
Score (NEWS2) 757
nebulizers 747–54
necrobacillosis 544b
negative pressure
ventilators 773
neuromuscular weakness,
non-invasive ventilation
775, 782–3
nicotine replacement
therapy 196, 819–20
Nijmegen hyperventilation
score 287, 287t
nitrofurantoin 267
nitrogen dioxide 275
Nocardia 548
nocardiosis 548–9
nocturnal
hypoventilation 694–5
nodules see pulmonary
nodules
non-cardiogenic pulmonary
oedema 71b
non-invasive
ventilation 771–86
abbreviations 772
acute respiratory
failure 778–9
chronic respiratory
failure 782–4
community-acquired
pneumonia 775
continuous positive airway
pressure 773
contraindications 776
COPD 784
cystic fibrosis 783
end-of-life weaning 786
high-flow nasal
oxygen 773
immunocompromised
patients 775
indications 774–5
negative pressure
ventilators 773
positive pressure
ventilators 772
sleep apnoea 783
terminology 772–3
troubleshooting 780t

non-malignant respiratory
    disease 808–9
  anxiety and
      depression 808
  cough 809
  dyspnoea 808
  hypoxia 808
  palliative care 808–9
non-small cell lung cancer
    338, 350–2
  adjuvant therapy 355
  radiotherapy 356
  surgery 350–2
  systemic anti-cancer
      therapy 354–5
non-specific
    bronchoprovocation
    testing 868
non-specific interstitial
    pneumonia 328–9
  causes/associations 328
  clinical features 328
  definition 328
  diagnosis 329
  epidemiology 328
  histology 329
  investigations 328–9
  management 329
  prognosis 329
non-tuberculous
    mycobacteria 618–21
  clinical features 618
  diagnosis 619
  investigations 618
  management 619
  risk factors 618
  species 620–1

O

obesity 702
obesity hypoventilation 774
obstructive lung disease 760
obstructive sleep apnoea
    100, 102, 678–80
  advice to patients 690–1
  alternative
      diagnoses 688–9
  clinical features 682
  CPAP 688–9
  decompensated 774
  definition 678, 684–6
  epidemiology 678
  examination and
      investigations 682
  future developments 692
  management 686–7
  obesity-related respiratory
      problems 702
  pathophysiology 678
  problems 688

screening tool 77b
sleepiness 682
sleep studies 684–7
occupational asthma 164–5
  causes 165t
  diagnosis 164–5
  management 166
  risk factors 164
occupation exposure
  asbestos 124
  asthma 164–5, 166
omalizumab 154
opioids
  conversion 803b
  sedation 888
oral allergy syndrome 145b
oral anti-inflammatory
    drugs 157
oral methylxanthines 198
organizing pneumonia 220,
    223, 224
organophosphate
    poisoning 270–1
osteoporosis, steroids
    and 742
oxygen therapy 787–97
  alert card 791
  ambulatory 794
  COPD 199, 206
  drug-induced lung
      disease 267
  emergency
      therapy 788–91
  flying 299b
  high-flow nasal oxygen 773
  home therapy
      792–4, 796–7
  long-term 792–3
  pneumothorax 441
  short burst 794
ozone 275

P

paediatric lung disorders
    393–400
  chronic lung disease of
      prematurity 394–5
  congenital
      abnormalities 398–9
  transition to adult
      services 400
  virus associated
      wheeze 396
palliative care 799–809
  COPD 200
  dyspnoea 804
  general points 800
  lung cancer and
      mesothelioma
      802–4, 806–7

non-malignant respiratory
    disease 808–9
  opioids 803b
  pain 802–3
pancreatitis 254–5, 310
paracoccidioidomycosis 583
paradoxical reaction see IRIS
paragonimiasis 627
paraneoplastic
    syndromes 340–1
parapneumonic
    effusion 412–13
  bacteriology 414
  chest tube drainage 416
  clinical features 412f, 413
  definition 412, 412f
  differential diagnosis 413
  difficulties in
      management 417
  intrapleural
      fibrinolytics 416
  investigations 414
  management 416–17
  nutritional support 416–17
  outcome 418
  risk factors 413
  surgery 417
  thromboprophylaxis 417
paraquat poisoning 270
parasitic respiratory
    infections 623–7
pectus carinatum 399
pectus excavatum 399
penicillamine 267
penicillins
    (Talaromycosis) 583
peripheral cold
    abscess 589
Personal Independence
    Payment 736
phosgene 275
phosphodiesterase-4
    inhibitors 199
phosphodiesterase-5
    inhibitors 460
photodynamic therapy 848
pleural biopsy
  Abram's pleural needle
      biopsy 872–3
  techniques 869–73
pleural disease 218
pleural effusion
    49–61, 401–23
  amyloidosis 494
  asbestos exposure 423
  clinical assessment 50–1
  clinical features 402
  coronary artery bypass
      graft 423
  CT 402
  CXR 402

pleural effusion (Contd.)
  diagnostic algorithm 52f
  exudative 51, 56–7
  haemothorax 422
  imaging 402–3
  investigations 51
  lung cancer 806
  malignant 404–6
  mesothelioma 806
  MRI 403
  non-HIV immuno
    compromised 80b
  PE 422
  PET/CT 403
  pleural thickening 423
  rheumatoid arthritis
    216, 422
  thoracentesis 50
  thoracic ultrasound 903
  transudative 51, 54
  tuberculous pleural
    effusion 420–1
  ultrasound 402
pleural fluid analysis 58
  amylase 60
  cholesterol 60
  differential cell count 59t
  fluid characteristics 58t
  glucose 60
  pH 60
  triglyceride 60
pleural infection 905
pleural thickening 903
pleuritis
  ankylosing spondylitis 225
  rheumatoid arthritis 216
  shrinking pleuritis with
    atelectasis 127
pleurodesis 875–9
pneumococcal
  pneumonia 528
pneumococcal
  vaccination 533
pneumoconioses 425–33
  berylliosis 432–3
  coal miners 427
  mineral dusts 426–7, 426t
  silicosis 430–1
pneumocystis
  pneumonia 570–1
  antimicrobial
    treatment 572
  causes 570
  clinical features 570
  definition 570
  investigations 570–1
  outcome 572–3
  treatment 572–3
pneumonia
  acute eosinophilic 294
  acute interstitial 332–3
  chronic eosinophilic 294

desquamative
    interstitial 335
  hospital-acquired 534–7
  idiopathic interstitial
    pneumonias 317–36
  lymphoid interstitial 336
  non-specific
    interstitial 328–9
  organizing 217, 326, 330–1
  pneumococcal 528
  varicella 643
  ventilator-associated 538–9
  viral 630
  see also aspiration
    pneumonia;
    community-acquired
    pneumonia;
    pneumocystis
    pneumonia;
    ventilator-associated
    pneumonia
pneumothorax 435–48
  aspiration 440, 881–3
  catamenial 447
  causes and
    pathophysiology 436
  chemical pleurodesis 443
  chest drainage 440–1
  clinical features 437
  cystic fibrosis 252, 447
  definition 436
  discharge from
    hospital 441
  epidemiology 436
  flying 299
  HIV 447
  iatrogenic 446
  investigations 437
  management
    440–1, 442–3
  outpatient follow-up 442
  oxygen therapy 441
  persistent air leak 441
  pregnancy 447
  prognosis 438
  re-expansion pulmonary
    oedema 448
  subcutaneous (surgical)
    emphysema 447
  surgical management 442
  tension 446b, 446
  thoracic ultrasound 902
  traumatic 447
  treatment algorithm 444–5
polyarteritis nodosa 724
porto-pulmonary
    hypertension 308–9
positive end expiratory
    pressure 772
positive pressure
    ventilators 773
post-nasal drip 18

post-operative
    breathlessness 63–8
post-polio syndrome 696
pregnancy
  asthma 162–3
  breathlessness 69–72
  cystic fibrosis 256–7
  pneumothorax 447
  pulmonary arteriovenous
    malformations 514
  TB 602
  thromboembolic
    disease 484
preoperative
    assessment 73–6
primary ciliary
    dyskinesia 506–7
programmed death ligand
    1 354b
programmed death
    protein-1 354b
progressive massive
    fibrosis 428–9
progressive neurological
    disease 732
proliferative
    bronchiolitis 184
propofol 889
prostanoids 460–1
pseudochylothorax 60
Pseudomonas aeruginosa
    177, 242–3
psittacosis 529
pulmonary alveolar
    proteinosis
  clinical features 509
  diagnosis 510
  epidemiology 508
  histology 508
  pathophysiology 508
  prognosis 511
  treatment 510
pulmonary arterial
    aneurysms 226
pulmonary arterial
    hypertension 308–9,
    453b, 761
pulmonary arteriovenous
    malformations 512–14
  aetiology 512
  clinical features 513
  complications 514
  diagnosis 512
  management 514
  pregnancy 514
  shunt
    quantification 512–13
pulmonary ascariasis 625
pulmonary carcinoid
    tumours 368–70
pulmonary embolism
  acute 474–5

examination of
    patient 472–3
haemodynamic
    effects 469
management of acute
    massive/high
    risk 481b
response teams 482
systemic lupus
    erythematosus 218
Wells's score 475t
see also pulmonary
    thromboembolic
    disease
pulmonary embolism
    massive 481b
pulmonary fibrosis
ankylosing spondylitis 225
rheumatoid arthritis 216
systemic sclerosis 222–3
see also idiopathic
    pulmonary fibrosis
pulmonary function
    tests 192
pulmonary hydatid
    disease 624
pulmonary hypertension
    220, 232–3, 449–65
chronic
    thromboembolic 459
clinical classification 451b
cystic fibrosis 256–7
definition 450
due to left heart
    disease 458
due to lung diseases and/or
    hypoxia 458
end-of-life care 465
future developments 465
investigations 452–3
management
    460–2, 464–5
National Pulmonary
    Hypertension
    Service 453
pathophysiology 450
presenting features 450–1
prognosis 465
pulmonary arterial
    hypertension 454–6
surgical treatments 464–5
systemic lupus
    erythematosus 218
systemic sclerosis 223
with unclear and/or
    multifactorial
    mechanisms 459
pulmonary nodules
benign 376
causes 372t
definition 372

with extrathoracic
    malignancy 377
malignant 376
management 373–4
rheumatoid arthritis 216
pulmonary oedema
acute cardiogenic 774
diving 303–4
pulmonary
    rehabilitation 811–14
aims 812
candidates 813
future developments 814
outcome assessment
    measures 814
pre-rehabilitation
    assessment 814
programme 814
shuttle walk test 815b
pulmonary sequestration/
    sequestrated
    segment 398
pulmonary thromboembolic
    disease 467–87
acute pulmonary
    embolism 472, 474–5
aetiology 470–1
air embolism 486
amniotic fluid
    embolism 486
anticoagulation 479–80
causes 486–7
chronic thromboembolic
    disease 472
clinical features 472–3
definition 468
diagnosis 474–5
'economy class
    syndrome' 471
embolectomy 481
epidemiology 468
estrogen-containing
    oral contraceptive
    pills 485
examination 472–3
fat embolism 487
follow up 482
HRT 485
inferior vena cava filter
    placement 482
inherited
    thrombophilia 471
investigations 476–7
pathophysiology 468
pregnancy 484
response teams 482
risk of malignancy 471
risk stratification 478
septic, hydatid, and
    tumour emboli 487
severity index 478, 478t

thrombolysis 480–1
treatment 478–82
see also deep vein
    thrombosis
pulmonary vasculitis see
    vasculitis

Q

Q fever 529

R

radiation-induced
chronic eosinophilic
    pneumonia 272
organizing pneumonia 272
pulmonary disease 272
radiation pneumonitis 272
Ramsay scale 887t
rare lung diseases 489–515
recurrent respiratory
    papillomatosis 515, 807
reduced earning
    allowance 737
re-expansion pulmonary
    oedema 448
remdesivir 648
reslizumab 154
respiratory bronchiolitis-
    associated interstitial
    lung disease 334
respiratory failure 105–11
apparent rapid onset 108
causes 106–8
clinical presentation 108
definition 106
examination 110
history 110
management 111
neuromuscular
    weakness 775
pathophysiology 106–8
pulmonary function
    tests 110
slow onset 108
respiratory infections
bacterial 517–57
fungal 559–83
mycobacterial 585–621
parasitic 623–7
viral 629–54
respiratory sedation 200
respiratory support 251
respiratory syncytial
    virus 642
restrictive allograft
    syndrome 769
Revised National Early
    Warning Score
    (NEWS2) 757

rheumatoid arthritis 216–17
bronchiectasis 217
Caplan's syndrome 217
cricoarytenoid
arthritis 217
organizing pneumonia 217
pleural effusion 216
pleuritis 216
pulmonary fibrosis 216
pulmonary nodules 216
Sjögren's syndrome 217
small airways disease
and obliterative
bronchiolitis 217
vasculitis 217
rhinitis 18
allergic 18
non-allergic 18
post-nasal drip 18
vasomotor 18
rhinosinusitis 709
riociguat 460
ritonavir 649–50
rituximab 745
rounded atelectasis 127

S

sarcoidosis 655–69
aetiology 656
chest disease
658–9, 660–1
definition 656
differential diagnosis
657b, 659b
drug treatment 662–4
epidemiology 656
extrathoracic disease
666–7, 668–9
immunopathology 656–7
immunosuppressive
treatment 663b
lung transplantation 664
management 662b, 662–4
prognosis 664
thoracic 658b
SARS-coronavirus
(SARS-CoV) 651–3
schistosomiasis 626
sclerosants 878
sedation 885–90
administration 886
drugs 888–9
Modified Observer's
Assessment of
Alertness/Sedation
(MOAAS) scale 887t
Ramsay scale 887t
safe sedation 885–90
specific circumstances 890
selexipag 461

severe acute respiratory
syndrome
coronavirus 2
(SARS-CoV-2) 645–50
severe acute respiratory
syndrome
(SARS) 651–3
case definition 651
clinical features 652
epidemiology 651
hospital admission 653
incubation period 652
investigations 652
laboratory case
definition 651
pathophysiology 651
prognosis 653
treatment 652
shingles 643
shrinking lung syndrome 218
shuttle walk test 815b
sickle cell disease 671–5
acute chest
syndrome 674–5
background 672
pulmonary
complications 672
silicosis 430–1
management 431
pathophysiology 430
types 430–1
silicotuberculosis 430–1
simple pulmonary
eosinophilia 292
sinusitis 18–19
Sjögren's syndrome
217, 224
skin prick tests 866
sleep and breathing
problems 99–104
see also central sleep
apnoea; obstructive
sleep apnoea
small airways disease
and obliterative
bronchiolitis 217
small cell lung cancer 338–9
chemotherapy 358
radiotherapy 358
surgery 358
treatment 358
smoke 275
smoking cessation 817–23
aims of
interventions 818–19
nicotine replacement
therapy 819–20
non-nicotine replacement
therapy 822–3
solid organ
transplantation 86–7

spinal cord
compression 366–7
spontaneous pneumo
mediastinum 221
squamous cell
carcinoma 338
Staphylococcus aureus
244, 529
statutory sick pay 736
Stenotrophomonas
maltophilia 245
steroids
chronic asthma 157
cystic fibrosis 251
inhaled 157
oral 199
osteoporosis 742
pneumocystis
pneumonia 572
pulmonary disease 88
systemic 206
steroid-sparing drugs 156
Streptococcus
pneumoniae 528
stress incontinence 257
strongyloidiasis 625
subacute invasive pulmonary
aspergillosis 566–7
subcutaneous (surgical)
emphysema 437, 447
sulfasalazine 268
sulphur dioxide 276
superior vena caval
obstruction
360–3, 362b
supraglottic airway
devices 829
SWORD scheme 427
Swyer–James
syndrome 399
syndrome of inappropriate
secretion of
antidiuretic hormone
365b
systemic lupus
erythematosus
acute lupus
pneumonitis 218
atelectasis 218
classification 219b
connective tissue
disease 218–19
diffuse ILD 218
drug-induced lupus 219b
pleural disease 218
systemic sclerosis
connective tissue
disease 222–3
diffuse cutaneous 222–3
environmentally
induced 222–3

limited cutaneous 222–3
overlap syndromes 222–3
pulmonary fibrosis 222–3
sine scleroderma 222–3

T

Takayasu's arteritis 724
Talaromyces marneffei 583
talc 268
terbutaline 156
thoracentesis 891–4
  diagnostic 893
  pleural effusion 50
  therapeutic 894
thoracic ultrasound 895 06
  abnormal lung 904
  aerated lung 902f, 902
  appearances 902–3, 904–6
  cautions 906
  diagnostic and therapeutic
    utility 896, 896t
  diaphragm 904
  guided intervention 905
  malignancy 905
  performing the
    examination 900–1
  pleural effusion 903
  pleural infection 905
  pleural thickening 903
  pneumothorax 902
  training 897
  see also ultrasound
thoracoscopy 907–11
  contraindications 909
  indications 909
  lung cancer 345
  post-thoracoscopy
    care 911
  preparation of patient and
    consent 910
  procedure 910
  risks associated
    with 909
  technique 910–11
thymic carcinoid 389
thymic cysts 389
thymoma 388b
thyroid 389
tonsillitis 710
toxin-induced lung
  disease 213–28
  organophosphate
    poisoning 270–1
  paraquat poisoning 270
  see also drug-induced lung
    disease
toxocariasis 626
tracheal disorders, laryngeal
  and 712
tracheitis 711

tracheobronchial stent
  insertion 849
tracheobronchitis 8, 711
tracheobronchomalacia 712
tracheomalacia 398
tracheostomy 913–18
  complications 918
  decannulation 915
  indications 914
  percutaneous vs surgical 914
  temporary 914
  tube options 916
transbronchial lung
  biopsy 840
transbronchial needle
  aspiration 344, 844
transport assistance 737
transudative pleural
  effusions see pleural
  effusion: transudative
treprostinil 460–1
tropical pulmonary
  eosinophilia 293, 627
tuberculosis 430–1, 586–7
  adverse drug
    reactions 598–9
  anti-TB drugs 596–7, 597t
  anti-TNF-α
    treatment 610–11
  BCG vaccination 613–14
  cattle TB 614
  chemotherapy 595,
    604–5, 607t
  in coal miners 427
  directly observed
    treatment 592
  disseminated BCG
    infection 616
  drug resistance
    598–9, 599t
  drug-sensitive 594–5
  drug treatment 592
  epidemiology 586
  extensively drug-resistant
    TB 607
  extrapulmonary disease 589
  flying 299
  follow-up 601
  future developments 617
  inpatient admission 600–1
  investigations 590–1
  latent infection 608–9
  liver function tests 604b
  management 592–3, 594–5
  Mantoux skin test 591b
  multidrug-resistant
    601, 606–7
  pathophysiology 586–7
  pericardial 589
  pregnancy 602
  pulmonary disease 588

risk factors 586–7
screening and contact
  tracing 612–14
treatment failure/disease
  relapse 600–1
tuberculous pleural
  effusion 420–1
tularaemia 554

U

ulcerative colitis 310
ultrasound
  guided intervention 905
  physics of 898–9
  see also thoracic ultrasound
upper airway and tracheal
  disease 703–12
  acute upper airway
    obstruction 704
  anaphylaxis 706–7
  laryngeal and tracheal
    disorders 712
  see also upper respiratory
    tract infections
upper airway cough
  syndrome 18
upper respiratory tract
  infections 630,
    708–9, 710–11
  acute bronchitis,
    tracheitis, and trache
    obronchitis 711
  acute epiglottitis
    (supraglottitis) 708
  acute pharyngitis and
    tonsillitis 710
  acute rhinitis 708
  candidiasis 708
  laryngitis 711
  rhinosinusitis 709
urinothorax 60

V

vaping 268
varenicline 822
vasculitis 713–24
  anti-GBM disease
    (Goodpasture's) 721
  classification 714–15
  eosinophilic
    granulomatosis
    with polyangiitis
    (Churg–Strauss
    syndrome) 722–3
  granulomatosis with
    polyangiitis
    (Wegener's) 716–17
  idiopathic inflammatory
    myopathies 221

vasculitis (Contd.)
microscopic polyangiitis 720
rare pulmonary
vasculitides 724
rheumatoid arthritis 217
small-vessel 714–15, 715t
venous thromboembolism
470t, 648–9
ventilator-associated
pneumonia 538–9
antibiotics 539
definition 538
diagnosis 538

differential
diagnosis 538b
investigations 538–9
risk factors 539b
ventilatory failure 221
Vincent's angina 710
viral pneumonia 630
viral respiratory
infectins 629–54
virus associated
wheeze 396
vocal cord
dysfunction 167

W

walking speed test 815b
Wegener's
granulomatosis with
polyangiitis 716–19
Weil's disease 556
welding fumes 276
Working Tax Credit 737

Z

zinc fumes 276